3 3073 00363311 0

DATE DUE

MAR 1 3 1996	
JUL 6 1998	

GAYLORD   PRINTED IN U.S.A.

PEDIATRIC ONCOLOGY AND HEMATOLOGY
Perspectives on care

PEDIATRIC ONCOLOGY AND HEMATOLOGY

Perspectives on care

Edited by

Marilyn J. Hockenberry, RN, MSN, PNP

Pediatric Hematology-Oncology, Nurse Practitioner,
Duke University Medical Center,
Clinical Associate,
Graduate School of Nursing,
Duke University,
Durham, North Carolina

Deborah K. Coody, RN, MSN, CPNP

Pediatric Endocrinology Nurse Practitioner,
University of Texas Health Science Center, Houston, Texas;
Formerly Pediatric Oncology Nurse Practitioner,
University of Texas, M.D. Anderson Hospital and Tumor Institute,
Houston, Texas

with 140 *illustrations*

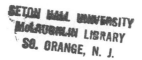
SETON HALL UNIVERSITY
McLAUGHLIN LIBRARY
SO. ORANGE, N. J.

THE C. V. MOSBY COMPANY

ST. LOUIS · TORONTO · PRINCETON   1986

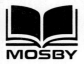

MOSBY

A TRADITION OF PUBLISHING EXCELLENCE

Editor: Barbara Ellen Norwitz
Developmental editor: Sally Adkisson
Editing supervisor: Peggy Fagen
Project editor: Barbara Merritt
Manuscript editor: Melissa Neves
Book design: Joanne Kluba (Top Graphics)
Cover design: Susan E. Lane
Production: Florence Fansher

RC
281
C4
P435
1986

Copyright © 1986 by The C.V. Mosby Company

All rights reserved. No part of this publication may be reproduced, stored in a retrieval system, or transmitted, in any form or by any means, electronic, mechanical, photocopying, recording, or otherwise, without prior written permission from the publisher.

Printed in the United States of America

The C.V. Mosby Company
11830 Westline Industrial Drive, St. Louis, Missouri 63146

Library of Congress Cataloging in Publication Data

Main entry under title:

Pediatric oncology and hematology.

   Includes bibliographies and index.
   1. Tumors in children—Nursing. 2. Blood—
Diseases—Nursing. 3. Pediatric hematology.
4. Pediatric nursing. I. Hockenberry, Marilyn J.
II. Coody, Deborah K. [DNLM: 1. Hematologic Diseases—
in infancy & childhood. 2. Hematologic Diseases—
nursing. 3. Neoplasms—in infancy & childhood.
4. Neoplasms—nursing. WY 156 P371]
RC281.C4P435 1986   618.92'992   85-21368
ISBN 0-8016-2253-0

GW/VH/VH 9 8 7 6 5 4 3 2 1   02/A/287

Contributors

DAVID BECTON, MD

Assistant Professor of Pediatrics, Division of Hematology-Oncology, Arkansas Children's Hospital, Little Rock, Arkansas

HALLIE A. BOREN, RN, MSN, CPNP

Pediatric Oncology Nurse Practitioner, University of Texas, M.D. Anderson Hospital and Tumor Institute, Houston, Texas

ROSALIND BRYANT, RN, MSN

Pediatric Hematology-Oncology Nurse Clinician, Duke University Medical Center, Durham, North Carolina

HOPE ANNE CASTORIA, RN, BSN

Nurse Clinician, Pediatric Hematology-Oncology, Mt. Sinai Medical Center, New York, New York

DEBORAH K. COODY, RN, MSN, CPNP

Pediatric Nurse Practitioner, Division of Pediatric Endocrinology, University of Texas Medical School, Houston, Texas

PATRICIA H. COTANCH, RN, PhD

Associate Professor of Nursing, Assistant Professor of Psychiatry, Duke University Medical Center, Durham, North Carolina

JOANN ELAND, RN, MA, PhD

Assistant Professor of Nursing, University of Iowa, Iowa City, Iowa

JOHN M. FALLETTA, MD

Professor of Pediatrics, Chief, Division Hematology-Oncology, Duke University Medical Center, Durham, North Carolina

JEAN H. FERGUSSON, RN, MSN, CRNP

Director, Pediatric Nurse Practitioner Project—Oncology, Children's Hospital of Philadelphia; Assistant Adjunct Professor, Widener School of Nursing, Chester, Pennsylvania

MARTHA BLECHAR GIBBONS, RN, MS, CPNP

Doctoral Student, Human Development, University of Maryland, College Park, Maryland

ALEXANDER M. GORDON, BA, MEd

Director, Play Therapy, Duke University Medical Center, Durham, North Carolina

ALEXANDER GREEN, MD

Member, Hematology-Oncology, St. Jude Children's Research Hospital, Memphis, Tennessee

EDWARD C. HALPERIN, MD

Assistant Professor, Division of Radiation Oncology, Department of Radiology, Duke University Medical Center, Durham, North Carolina

MICHAEL HARRIS, MD

Chief, Department of Pediatric Hematology-Oncology, Mt. Sinai Medical Center, New York, New York

F. ANN HAYES, MD

Member, Hematology-Oncology, St. Jude Children's Research Hospital, Memphis, Tennessee

SUZANNE B. HERMAN, RN, MSN, PNP

Clinical Instructor, School of Nursing, University of North Carolina, Chapel Hill, North Carolina

MARILYN J. HOCKENBERRY, RN, MSN, PNP

Pediatric Hematology-Oncology Nurse Practitioner, Duke University Medical Center, Clinical Associate, Graduate School of Nursing, Duke University, Durham, North Carolina

WILLIAM KEITH HOOTS, MD

Assistant Professor of Pediatrics, M.D. Anderson Hospital and Tumor Institute; Assistant Professor of Pediatrics and Internal Medicine, University of Texas Medical School; Medical Director, Gulf States Hemophilia Diagnostic and Treatment Center, Houston, Texas

SAMUEL L. KATZ, MD

Professor and Chairman, Department of Pediatrics, Duke University Medical Center, Durham, North Carolina

JOLEEN KELLEHER, RN, MSN

Director of Nursing, Fred Hutchinson Cancer Research Center, Seattle, Washington

THOMAS R. KINNEY, MD

Associate Professor of Pediatrics, Division of Pediatric Hematology-Oncology, Duke University Medical Center, Durham, North Carolina

JOHN KOEPKE, MD

Professor of Pathology, Associate Medical Director of Hospital Labs, Duke University Medical Center, Durham, North Carolina

CAMPBELL W. McMILLAN, MD

Professor of Pediatrics, School of Medicine, University of North Carolina, Chapel Hill, North Carolina

NANCY FERGUSON NOYES, RN, BSN

Former Pediatric Oncology Nurse Clinician, West Virginia University Medical Center, Morgantown, West Virginia

BECKY PACK, RN, MSN, PNP

Pediatric Oncology Nurse Practitioner, University of Texas, M.D. Anderson Hospital and Tumor Institute, Houston, Texas

CHARLES PRATT, MD

Member, Hematology-Oncology, St. Jude Children's Research Hospital, Memphis, Tennessee

PAT STANFILL, RN, MSN

Director of Nursing, St. Jude Children's Research Hospital, Memphis, Tennessee

MARGARET P. SULLIVAN, MD

Pediatrician and Professor of Pediatrics, Department of Pediatrics, University of Texas, M.D. Anderson Hospital and Tumor Institute, Houston, Texas

JAN VAN EYS, PhD, MD

Mosbacher Professor of Pediatrics, Head, Division of Pediatrics, University of Texas, M.D. Anderson Hospital and Tumor Institute; Professor of Pediatrics, University of Texas Medical School, Houston, Texas

RALPH VOGEL, RN, CPNP

Pediatric Oncology Nurse Practitioner, Solid Tumor Division, St. Jude Children's Research Hospital, Memphis, Tennessee

MARTHA S. WARREN, RN, BSN

Nurse Clinician, Comprehensive Hemophilia Diagnostic Treatment Center, University of North Carolina, Chapel Hill, North Carolina

MARY J. WASKERWITZ, RN, BSN, CRNP

Department of Pediatric Hematology-Oncology, University of Michigan, Ann Arbor, Michigan

To

Matthew, Les, Aimee, Todd,

**and all the children like them,
who have touched our lives and
made us the better for it**

M. J. H.
D. K. C.

Preface

Major advances in the treatment of children with malignancies and blood diseases have occurred in the past three decades. Many of the malignancies once viewed as universally fatal now can be perceived as chronic illnesses that often are curable. Children with certain inherited blood dyscrasias similarly are now living longer, more productive lives. Associated with the changing prognosis of children with malignancies and blood disorders have been significant changes in the role of the nurse providing care for these children. Today nurses administer primary care, which may encompass physical assessment, performance of diagnostic procedures, and the administration of therapeutic agents. These specialized and expanded roles make it imperative for nurses to acquire a foundation of knowledge regarding the specific disease entities.

The purpose of this book is to provide nurses with a comprehensive approach to diagnosis and management of hematologic and oncologic disorders in children. We have emphasized clinical features, pathophysiology, and current therapies for these disorders and the psychosocial sequelae of the disease and its treatment. We hope not only to provide a knowledge base for the beginning practitioner but also to broaden the perspectives for the experienced nurse. Although the text has been designed for nurses, it should also provide a reference source for other professionals including physician's assistants, social workers, psychologists, play therapists, and dieticians.

The organization of the book reflects an attempt to provide a comprehensive review of both pediatric oncology and hematology. The first section is devoted to childhood malignancies. Each chapter discusses the etiology, clinical features, diagnostic studies, prognostic factors, current therapy, and pertinent nursing considerations. Each chapter also contains representative case studies and nursing protocols for the specific diseases.

The second section of the book discusses hematologic disorders of childhood. Although this section is organized in the same manner as the childhood malignancies, the hematologic section is unique. It is the first comprehensive presentation of pediatric hematology in a nursing textbook.

Section three of the book provides a conceptual basis for treatment, reviewing the principles of chemotherapy, radiation therapy, and bone marrow transplantation. This section also describes the principles of supportive care, which include management of infection, pain, and nutrition in children with cancer. The use of blood products is also discussed from both a hematologic and an oncologic perspective.

The last section of the book presents an overview of the psychosocial aspects of care of the child with cancer. Issues regarding perceptions of cancer and its impact on the family are discussed. Methods to increase coping strategies and assist the child in returning to school are presented. Late effects of cancer are reviewed, stressing their impact on the child's future. Finally, dealing with the child who may die is addressed, emphasizing its effect on all who have been involved.

We are grateful to our contributors for sharing their expertise in this book. We would like to acknowledge the Nursing In-service Education Division of St. Jude Children's Research Hospital for the use of their nursing care protocols. A special thanks goes to Nancy Henn, medical illustrator at Duke University. We appreciate the constant effort of the editorial staff at The C.V. Mosby Company, especially Sally Adkisson. We are most indebted to Martha Timmons, without whom this book would have been impossible. Her constant support and dedication to this book has made the idea become reality.

Marilyn J. Hockenberry
Deborah K. Coody

Contents

PEDIATRIC ONCOLOGY
AND HEMATOLOGY
Perspectives on care

PART I

CHILDHOOD MALIGNANCIES

CHAPTER 1

Introduction to childhood cancer

MARILYN J. HOCKENBERRY, DEBORAH K. COODY, and JOHN M. FALLETTA

There is a new sense of awareness in the 1980s regarding childhood cancer. This change has come with the increasing success of treatment for cancer. There are approximately 6000 new cases occurring in children under 15 years of age in the United States each year.[1] Over one half of these children will be cured of their disease. Although cancer is still a life-threatening illness, improved survival has altered the approach to the child with cancer.

Those involved in the comprehensive care of children with cancer must be knowledgeable about all aspects of the illness and its treatment. This chapter is intended to provide an overview of pediatric oncology and to assist in forming a knowledge base for the professional working in this area. Subsequent chapters of this section will discuss the major childhood malignancies in detail. These chapters will review typical clinical presentations of specific childhood cancers, their incidence and etiology, therapeutic management, and prognostic details.

INCIDENCE

Cancer is the most frequent cause of death from disease in children under 15 years of age.[1] Only accidents kill more children than do cancers (Table 1-1). The incidence of childhood cancer, or the number of children newly diagnosed with a cancer per number at risk in the population within a given time period, is more difficult to determine than the mortality, since cancer is not a required reportable disease throughout the United States. Data on the U.S. incidence of cancer in children are available from two major sources: the National Cancer Sur-

veys of the Biometry Branch of the National Cancer Institute and the Surveillance, Epidemiology and End-Results Program (SEER) of the National Cancer Institute. Although these two sources are not exactly comparable, they do give estimates of the occurrence of new cancers in children under the age of 15 in the United States. Based on a 10% sample of the population, SEER is an ongoing system that provides the annual data on diagnosis, treatment, and survival of cancer patients.

Race

The most frequent tumor types for both white and black children in the United States are leukemias, brain tumors, and lymphomas, accounting for about 62% of all cancers in children[1] (Table 1-2). Leukemias and lymphomas constitute 34% and 39% of the cancers in white and black children, respectively. Solid tumors comprise 66% and 61%, respectively, of cancers in the two racial groups. Most tumors have similar frequencies among the white and black children in the United States, with the exception of leukemia, which occurs more frequently in whites, and melanoma and Ewing's sarcoma, which occur very rarely in blacks (Table 1-3).

Childhood cancer rates vary markedly among different countries. The lowest rate of childhood cancer is reported from Bombay, India (6.5/100,000), whereas the highest incidence is seen in Israel (18/100,000 Jewish population) and Nigeria (17.4/100,000).[2] Of all childhood cancers, Wilms' tumor has the most constant worldwide incidence, whereas the incidence of leukemia varies greatly

Table 1-1. Leading causes of death among children aged 1 to 14, both sexes (United States, 1980)

Rank	Cause of death	Number of deaths	Percent of deaths	Death rate per 100,000 population ages 1-14
1.	Accidents	8,537	45.2	17.7
2.	Cancer	2,070	11.0	4.3
3.	Congenital anomalies	1,587	8.4	3.2
4.	Homicide	734	3.9	1.5
5.	Heart diseases	668	3.5	1.4
6.	Pneumonia and influenza	461	2.4	0.9
7.	Meningitis	274	1.5	0.5
8.	Cystic fibrosis	240	1.3	0.5
9.	Cerebral palsy	227	1.2	0.5
10.	Cerebrovascular diseases	154	0.8	0.4
11.	Meningococcal infections	144	0.8	0.3
12.	Anemias	142	0.8	0.3
13.	Suicide	142	0.8	0.3
14.	Benign neoplasms	142	0.8	0.3
15.	Chronic obstructive lung disease	132	0.7	0.3
	All others	3,222	16.9	6.6
	All causes	18,876	100.0	39.0

From American Cancer Society: Cancer Statistics, 1985, CA **35**(1):34, 1985.

Table 1-2. Cancer incidence by site for children under 15, SEER program

Rank	Site	Number of deaths	Percent of total	Rate per 1,000,000 children
1.	Leukemia	664	30.2	33.6
2.	Central nervous system	409	18.6	20.7
3.	Lymphomas	298	13.6	15.1
4.	Sympathetic nervous system	170	7.7	8.6
5.	Soft tissue	141	6.5	7.1
6.	Kidney	135	6.1	6.8
7.	Bone	101	4.6	5.1
8.	Retinoblastoma	58	2.6	3.0
9.	Liver	26	1.2	1.3
	All others	195	8.9	9.9
	All sites	2,197	100.0	111.1

From American Cancer Society: Cancer Statistics, 1985, CA **35**(1):34, 1985.

Table 1-3. Relative frequency of major categories of malignant neoplasms in U.S. children under 15 years of age

Histologic category	Percent of total	
	White	Black
Leukemia	30.9	24.3
Central nervous system	18.3	21.6
Lymphoma	13.8	11.3
Sympathetic nervous system	7.8	7.2
Soft tissue	6.2	8.6
Kidney	5.8	9.0
Bone	4.7	3.6
Retinoblastoma	2.5	4.1
Gonadal and germ cell	2.0	3.6
Liver	1.3	—
Teratoma	0.4	0.5
Miscellaneous	6.3	6.4

Based on SEER Program Data, National Cancer Institute. From Sutow, W.W., Fernbach, D.J., and Vietti, T.J.: Clinical pediatric oncology, ed. 3, St. Louis, 1984, The C.V. Mosby Co.

Table 1-4. Comparison of incidence of major forms of childhood cancer between sexes

Site	Male/female ratio by 5-year age groups		
	Up to 4 years	5-9 years	10-14 years
All sites	1.31	1.40	1.03
Leukemias	1.49	1.21	1.38
Central nervous system	1.16	1.33	0.89
Lymphomas	1.62	3.89	1.32
Sympathetic nervous system	1.48	0.63	0.33
Soft tissues	1.68	1.31	1.18
Kidney	0.77	0.90	0.11
Bone	1.18	1.20	1.60
Eye	0.93	—	—
Other sites	1.41	1.06	0.52

Based on SEER Program Data, National Cancer Institute. From Sutow, W. W., Fernbach, D. J., and Vietti, T. J.: Clinical pediatric oncology, ed. 3, St. Louis, 1984, The C.V. Mosby Co.

among countries. Liver cancer occurs more frequently in the Far East; retinoblastoma, in India; neuroblastoma, in Western Europe; and pineal tumors, in Japan.

Age

Incidence and mortality from specific tumor types reported in children vary with age. Forty-one percent of all childhood cancers occur between birth and 4 years of age.[3] Cancer incidence in newborns less than 29 days old is 36.5/1 million and in infants less than 1 year of age is 183.4/1 million.[4] The tumor frequency order in infants younger than 1 year of age is different from that for children of older age. Neuroblastoma is the most common malignancy, followed by leukemia, kidney tumors, sarcomas, retinoblastomas, and tumors of the central nervous system. Leukemia ranks first in mortality because of greater survival rates among neuroblastoma patients. Hodgkin's disease, bone tumors, and acute myelocytic leukemia exhibit a peak incidence after 10 years of age.

Sex

In general, males are affected slightly more often than females in a ratio of approximately 1.2:1 (Table 1-4). Acute lymphocytic leukemia (ALL), lymphomas, and central nervous system tumors, especially medulloblastoma, account for the higher incidence in males. There are no significant differences between rates of cancers in male and female newborns.

MAJOR MALIGNANCIES
Leukemia

Leukemia is the most common neoplasm in U.S. white children, accounting for 30% of all childhood neoplasms and affecting 1/20,000 to 25,000/year.[5] ALL is the most frequently occurring childhood leukemia in U.S. white children but is much less common in black children. Males are affected slightly more than females. Nonlymphocytic leukemias do not have a peak incidence in childhood but have a relatively constant incidence by age, sex, and race in the United States.

Brain tumors

Brain tumors are the second most common group of childhood neoplasms in the United States.[5] The overall incidence is the same for both black and white children and for males and females. However, there is a male preponderance of about 3:2 for medulloblastoma and intracranial germ cell tumors. Brain tumors occur most frequently between the ages of 5 and 10 years, yet age-specific incidence rates vary depending on histologic types.

Neuroblastoma

Neuroblastoma is the third most common malignancy of childhood, accounting for 11% of malignant tumors seen in the first 14 years of life.[6,7] It represents 20% to 50% of all neonatal malignancies and up to 14% of the malignancies in older children.[7] Neuroblastoma occurs at a rate of 1 in every 10,000 live births.

Hodgkin's disease

Hodgkin's disease is the most common lymphoma in U.S. white children, affecting 1 in 175,000 children per year.[5] The incidence of Hodgkin's disease is low before the age of 5 years. Before the age of 10 years, males are affected more than females. However, during adolescence the sexes are affected in almost equal numbers.[8,9] Hodgkin's disease has a bimodal age incidence curve that varies with geography and socioeconomic condition. The overall incidence of Hodgkin's disease is increased in developed countries and in high socioeconomic groups, although its occurrence in individuals less than 15 years of age is relatively low. In underdeveloped countries and in low socioeconomic groups, the overall incidence is lower, but there is an earlier onset, with a peak age before 15 years.

Non-Hodgkin's lymphoma

Non-Hodgkin's lymphomas account for approximately 6% of malignant neoplasms in U.S. white children, yet in some African countries, non-Hodgkin's lymphomas may account for the majority of tumors. They occur at an annual rate of about 7 per 1 million children and adolescents. The peak incidence is between the age of 7 and 11. There is a 3:1 male to female predominance.

Wilms' tumor

Wilms' tumor is an embryonal tumor occurring in 1 per 200,000 to 250,000 children per year. It accounts for about 10% of all malignant tumors in children, with approximately 500 new cases in the United States annually.[10] The tumor has a peak incidence before 5 years of age, with 30% occurring in children less than 1 year of age and 70% occurring before the age of 4. Wilms' tumor rarely occurs in children past the age of 7. The distribution of cases is roughly equal in all countries. There is no sexual predominance, but familial cases have been reported.

Bone tumors

Bone tumors account for approximately 5% of malignant neoplasms in U.S. children under the age of 15 years.[3] Osteogenic sarcoma is the most common bone tumor in the pediatric age group, occurring most often during the adolescent growth spurt. Ewing's sarcoma is the second most common bone tumor in children, appearing between 5 to 15 years of age.

Soft tissue tumors

Soft tissue tumors account for 6.5% of malignancies in U.S. children. Rhabdomyosarcoma is the most common pediatric soft tissue sarcoma. The peak ages of incidence of rhabdomyosarcoma are in early childhood and late adolescence.[11] The incidence varies little with race.

Retinoblastoma

Retinoblastoma is an embryonal tumor occurring in approximately 1 in 20,000 to 30,000 live births in U.S. blacks and whites.[12] It accounts for 1% to 3% of all childhood malignancies. The incidence is increased in the Bantu of South Africa.[13] This tumor has a peak incidence before 5 years, and males and females are affected equally.

ETIOLOGY

The causes of childhood cancer are unknown. Genetic and environmental influences are difficult to evaluate. Specific genetic predisposition to some cancers exists in children but are not common. Environmental influences occurring in childhood may actually lead to cancer in the adult. Specific environmental relationships to the onset of cancer are shown in Tables 1-5 and 1-6.

Ionizing radiation

Since initiation of more stringent protective measures in the use of radiologic procedures, carcinogenic effects of x-ray exposure in childhood or in utero have been greatly reduced. Numerous studies establishing effects of radiation in children have addressed this issue. These studies include survivors of the atomic bomb in Hiroshima and other nuclear explosions and patients given high-dose radiation for malignancies.[14] ALL, myelogenous leukemia, and thyroid cancer have occurred following exposure to ionizing radiation.[15] Although the radiation exposure may occur during childhood, most malignancies do not appear until later in life. Leukemia in victims of the atomic bombs was seen as early as 3 to 10 years after the occurrence.[14] Most tumors in children, however, cannot be clearly attributed to radiation exposure because of the long latent period for most radiogenic cancers, which extends the clinical onset of malignancy well beyond the pediatric age.

Ultraviolet radiation

Excessive exposure to sunlight may predispose a child to basal cell carcinoma later in life.[15] However, skin cancers during childhood are rarely observed.

Asbestos

The latent period for exposure to asbestos is too long to be defined yet as a cause of childhood cancer. Its association with adult lung cancer, however, has been established. Major concern continues regarding the number of classrooms with asbestos walls and ceilings. Determination of the magnitude of the deleterious effects of this exposure in children remains to be made.

Drugs during intrauterine life

In 1971 it was established that diethylstilbestrol (DES), given to pregnant women to prevent spontaneous abortion, predisposes to clear cell adenocarcinoma of the vagina occurring years later in their daughters.[15] This study further established that

Table 1-5. Factors associated with childhood cancer—intrauterine exposure

Agent	Tumor type
Ionizing radiation	
Obstetric x-rays	All childhood cancers
	Negative findings, same data
Atomic bomb	No effect
Drugs	
Synthetic nonsteroidal estrogens (diethylstilbestrol)	Clear cell carcinoma of the vagina, cervix
Dilantin: fetal hydantoin syndrome	Neuroblastoma, ganglioneuroblastoma (5)*, mesenchymoma (1), Wilms' tumor (1), neuroectodermal tumor (1)
Alcohol: fetal alcohol syndrome	Adrenocortical carcinoma (1), neuroblastoma (2), ganglioneuroblastoma (1), hepatoblastoma (1), teratoma (1)
"Pregnancy drugs" (sedative and others, not hormones)	All childhood cancers

From Sutow, W.W., and Fernbach, D.J., and Vietti, T.J.: Clinical pediatric oncology, ed. 3, St. Louis, 1984, The C.V. Mosby Co.
*Number of reported cases is given in parentheses.

Table 1-6. Environmental factors associated with childhood cancers—postnatal exposure

Agent	Tumor type	Mode of exposure
Ionizing radiation		
Therapeutic radiation	Many tumor types including leukemia, thyroid, skin, brain, bone, soft tissue	Therapeutic radiation
Atomic bomb	Leukemia, thyroid, many adult tumors	Whole body
Nuclear fallout, Marshallese	Thyroid cancer	Ingestion of radionuclides
Nuclear fallout, Utah	Acute leukemia	Ingestion of radionuclides
	Negative study, same data	
Drugs		
Alkylating agents	Acute nonlymphocytic leukemia	Treatment for cancer, autoimmune disease, or organ transplantation
Cyclophosphamide	Bladder cancer	Treatment for cancer, autoimmune disease, or organ transplantation
Immunosuppressant drugs	Non-Hodgkin's lymphoma	Treatment for autoimmune disease or organ transplantation
Anabolic androgenic steroids	Liver tumors	Treatment for aplastic anemia
Phenytoin (Dilantin)	Lymphoma	Treatment for seizure disorders
Barbiturates	Brain tumors	In utero exposure and early infancy
	No effect	Treatment for seizure disorder

From Sutow W.W., Fernbach D.J. and Vietti, T.J.: Clinical pediatric oncology, ed. 3, St. Louis, 1984, The C.V. Mosby Co.

Table 1-7. Constitutional chromosome disorders associated with childhood cancer

Chromosomal abnormality	Childhood tumor
Down's syndrome	Leukemia, testicular, retinoblastoma*
Turner's syndrome	Neurogenic tumors, postestrogen endometrial, leukemia, gonadal
Klinefelter's syndrome	Nonlymphocytic leukemia, germ cell tumors (gonadal and mediastinal)
Other sex aneuploidy (XXYY, XXXY, XXX including XXY)	Retinoblastoma*
XY gonadal dysgenesis	Gonadoblastoma, dysgerminoma
Trisomy 13	Teratoma, leukemia, neurogenic
Trisomy 18	Neurogenic, Wilms'
XYY, XYY mosaic	Osteosarcoma (1)†, medulloblastoma (1), CML (2), ALL (1)

From Sutow, W.W., Fernbach, D.J., and Vietti, T.J.: Clinical pediatric oncology, ed. 3, St. Louis, 1984, The C.V. Mosby Co.
*Often trisomy 21 is associated with sex chromosome aneuploidy.
†Number of cases reported given in parentheses.

any carcinogen crossing the placenta may be carcinogenic to the offspring. As yet, there is no direct evidence to establish the effect exposure to other chemical carcinogens in utero has on the occurrence of malignancies later in life. Chemicals such as benzene, styrene, plastics, and food additives have been identified in cord blood. However, these and other chemicals remain as questionable causes that may predispose an individual to cancer.[15]

Drugs during childhood

There is an increased frequency of cancer related to exposure to radioisotopes and prolonged immunosuppressive therapy after transplantation.[14] Lymphoma and hepatobiliary tumors have been seen in children after renal transplantation. Androgenic steroids used in the treatment for Fanconi's aplastic anemia have been associated with hepatocellular carcinoma. Chemotherapy for other types of tumors have been shown to predispose leukemia and solid tumors (see Chapter 31 on late effects).

Viruses

The Epstein-Barr virus (EBV) has been linked to the African Burkitt's lymphoma and with X-linked lymphoproliferative disorders. Nasopharyngeal carcinoma has also been associated with EBV.

Genetics

Certain hereditary diseases predispose a child to cancer. Four general categories of abnormalities have been associated with a predisposition for the development of cancer[16]: (1) ataxia-telangiectasia and xeroderma pigmentosum in which defective repair of DNA occurs[17]; (2) immunodeficiency disorders causing increased risk for development of lymphomas; (3) renal dysplasia, which is associated with Wilms' tumor; and (4) chromosomal abnormalities such as Down's syndrome. Specific types of chromosomal disorders associated with childhood cancer are shown in Table 1-7.

Retinoblastoma is the only cancer with enough survivors over several generations to serve clearly as a genetic model for childhood cancers.[18] It is now established that a number of cases may be hereditary and attributable to an autosomal dominant mutation with high penetrance.[19] Retinoblastoma has also been associated with the chromosomal deletion 13q14. These findings have been found in children with heritable retinoblastoma or with nonheritable retinoblastoma. The presence of the chromosomal delection 13q14 supports the belief that the same genetic events occur in both types of retinoblastoma and may be inherited defects or acquired.[15]

Wilms' tumor also appears to present as a hereditary and nonhereditary form of cancer. However, only 1% to 2% of these children have reported relatives also having Wilms' tumor. The hereditary type of Wilms' tumor is thought to be autosomal dominant and is associated with an earlier than average age of diagnosis.[20] It is frequently a bilateral or multifocal tumor.

Neuroblastoma also appears to present in a hereditary and nonhereditary pattern.[21] As in Wilms' tumor, siblings and cousins are most frequently affected. This type of cancer may be associated with a germinal mutation in about 22% of cases.[15]

HISTORY OF MANAGEMENT

Curing cancer was the goal set by those providing care to children with cancer 30 years ago. At that time the major emphasis in childhood cancer had been in defining specific types of malignancies.[22] Surgical removal of a neoplasm was the only treatment modality established, and cure was rare. The first successful use of a medicine for the treatment of cancer occurred in 1948, with Farber's introduction of aminopterin for the therapy of ALL.[23] This landmark in the treatment of childhood cancer was followed by a number of major events leading to the increasing cure rates in recent years. These events include the following:

1. Development of cytotoxic agents such as 6-mercaptopurine and methotrexate based on the principle of antimetabolite processes[24]

2. Identification of a specific therapy for a specific disease (e.g., actinomycin D for Wilms' tumor; vincristine and prednisone for ALL)[25]
3. Recognition of the most effective manner in which to use chemotherapeutic agents in combination with localized therapy, including radiation therapy and surgery, now called multimodal therapy[26]
4. Development of specific drugs most effectively used in ALL for induction, maintenance, and treatment of occult disease[27]
5. Initiation of more effective supportive care (blood products and antibiotics) used with the development of more aggressive therapeutic regimens[18]
6. Development of centers designed to perform research and provide comprehensive care for children with cancer
7. Cooperation among treatment institutions to pool patients to provide more information for the development of effective therapeutic programs
8. Recognition of the psychologic effects childhood cancer has on the entire family

Pediatric oncology is now a model for the cure of cancer, since most treatment successes in cancer have been with children.[22] Childhood ALL has been the single most important model in the development of new principles for cancer cure. Most of the early work in chemotherapeutic agents was in childhood ALL.[22] In the mid-1950s prednisone, methotrexate, and 6-mercaptopurine were used to induce remissions; however, these children had only brief remissions and did not survive. Increasing the length of complete remission then became one of the major goals of chemotherapy.

Various chemotherapeutic agents were tried in combinations. By the early 1960s combination chemotherapy regimens were being used in childhood ALL, with the length of remission being extended. Nearly all of these children, however, soon relapsed. The absolute need for maintenance therapy was established by 1965. As maintenance programs began to prevent disease recurrence, an increased incidence of extramedullary disease began to be apparent. In response to this new threat, central nervous system prophylaxis was initiated. After 1965 the therapeutic approach to childhood ALL had developed into a systematic approach using combination therapy to induce complete remissions, central nervous system prophylaxis to prevent overt central nervous system disease, and maintenance therapy to prevent disease recurrence. The prognosis changed in 30 years from a uniformly fatal disease to a disease curable in as many as 60% of children. Fig. 1-1 represents the change in prognosis for ALL over the past two decades. The success of these strategies has paved the way for the development of effective therapeutic regimens used in other cancers.

New findings that further define prognostic groups for leukemia have been established. Immunologic characterization of ALL cells has permitted investigators to distinguish those children at high risk risk for relapse from those with a better prognosis.

Wilms' tumor has also been successfully treated using multimodal and adjuvant therapy, establishing the concept of such treatment for many types of solid tumors. Use of radiation therapy and chemotherapy following surgery for Wilms' tumor began in the 1960s and helped define the importance of adjuvant therapy, which is therapy administered in the absence of measurable disease, aimed at eradicating microscopic residual disease. The National Wilms' Tumor Study was established during this time and helped lead to an improved 2-year survival rate from 20% three decades ago to over 80% within the last 10 years. The National Wilms' Tumor Study now places emphasis on evaluating and reducing side effects of treatment. The most recent study is quantifying disturbances in growth and development, functional impairments, genetic damage, interference with sexual function, and oncogenesis.[15] Current therapy is now aimed at obtaining cure with fewer late effects.

Many of the principles found to be important in improving the treatment for patients with Wilms' tumor have been applied to other malignancies, with the result of improved survival rates. Solid

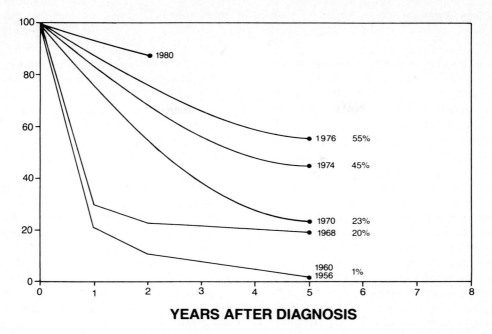

YEARS AFTER DIAGNOSIS

Fig. 1-1. Progress over the last two decades in treatment and survival rate of ALL. (From Sutow, W.W., Fernbach, D.J., and Vietti, T.J.: Clinical pediatric oncology, ed. 3, St. Louis, 1984, The C.V. Mosby Co.)

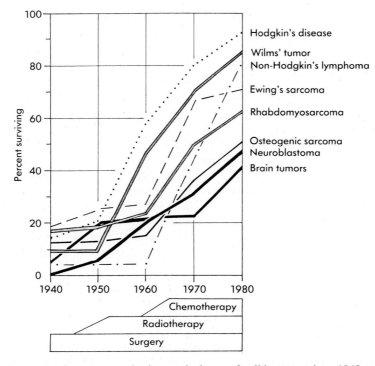

Fig. 1-2. Progressive improvement in the survival rate of solid tumors since 1940s. (From Burchenal, J.H., and Oettgen, H.F., editors: Cancer achievements, challenges and prospects for the 1980's, New York, 1981, Grune & Stratton, Inc., by permission.)

tumors are now better classified histologically, with favorable and unfavorable patterns being recognized. As yet, however, better treatment for those high risk groups has not been clearly established, but the group that must receive more innovative therapy has been identified. Fig. 1-2 shows the progressive improvement in survival of children with solid tumors over the past 40 years. Table 1-8 demonstrates projected survival rates of all childhood cancers.

A plateau appears now to have been reached in the improvement of therapy for most childhood cancers. Most recent advances are descriptive rather than therapeutic. Efforts continue to better understand the kinetics of cancer cells. Research in the biochemistry and immunology of the tumor cell is becoming more active.

Genetics research is now making a major contribution to the identification of specific subtypes of cancers and their possible causes. The discovery of specific genes, labeled oncogenes, has led to a better understanding of a genetic code for these cancer genes. Over two dozen of these oncogenes have been detected.[28] The mechanism by which oncogenes participate in the development of cancer is carefully being unraveled.

SUMMARY

Numerous events have led to increased survival for children with cancer. These have included the organization of comprehensive oncology teams, successful clinical research trials, improved supportive care measures, and the identification of significant prognostic variables within disease categories.[29] Changes in management and treatment modalities have improved the outcome for many children. Prolonged survival in childhood cancer has created new dilemmas, which now must be pursued. Establishment of innovative treatment modalities for children with poor prognosis must be evaluated. Therapy designed to decrease the late effects and to reduce the acute toxicities of treatment are major issues. Studies into the possible causes of childhood cancer are now a major initiative because progress is being made in research in biochemistry, genetics, and immunology. Psychosocial issues caused by cancer as a chronic illness are now essential areas of research.

Table 1-8. Survival in childhood cancers—current projections

	Predicted 3-year survival rates (%)	Putative biologic cure rates (%)
Acute lymphoid leukemia	60	40-50
Myeloid leukemia	25	
Hodgkin's disease	90	70-80
Non-Hodgkin's lymphoma	50	
Neuroblastoma	25	30
Wilms' tumor	75	70-80
Retinoblastoma	90	
Brain tumors	45*	40†
Osteosarcoma	40	40
Ewing's sarcoma	50	40
Rhabdomyosarcoma	50	40
Other malignant neoplasms	50	
All types	50	

From Sutow, W.W., Fernbach, D.J., and Vietti, T.J.: Clinical pediatric oncology, ed. 3, St. Louis, 1984, The C.V. Mosby Co.
*Including nonmalignant brain tumors.
†Medulloblastoma.

REFERENCES

1. American Cancer Society: Vital statistics of the United States: 1980, CA **35**(1):34, 1985.
2. Waterhouse, J., and others, editors: Cancer incidence in five continents, vol. 3, Lyons, France, 1976, International Agency for Research on Cancer.
3. Young, J., and others: Cancer incidence, survival and mortality for children under 15 years of age, New York, 1978, ACS Professional Educational Publication.
4. Bader, J., and Miller, R.: U.S. cancer incidence and mortality in the first year of life, Am. J. Dis. Child. **133**:157, 1979.
5. Young, J., and Miller, R: Incidence of malignant tumors in U.S. children, J. Pediatr. **86**:254, 1975.
6. Carter, S., and Glastein, E: Neuroblastoma. In Carter, S.: Principles of cancer treatment, New York, 1982, McGraw-Hill, Inc.
7. Hayes, F., and Green, A.: Neuroblastoma. In Kelley, V.C.: Practice of pediatrics, vol. 5, Philadelphia, 1984, Harper & Row, Publishers, Inc.

8. Jenkin, R., and others: Hodgkin's disease in children: a retrospective analysis 1958-73, Cancer **35:**979, 1975.

9. Tan, C., and others: The changing management of childhood Hodgkin's disease, Cancer **35:**808, 1975.

10. Aren, B.: Wilms' tumor: a clinical study of 81 children, Cancer **33:**637, 1974.

11. Li F., and Fraumeni, J., Jr.: Rhabdomyosarcoma in children: epidemiologic study and identification of a familial cancer syndrome, J. Natl. Cancer Inst. **43:**1365, 1969.

12. Devesa, S.: The incidence of retinoblastoma, Am. J. Ophthalmol. **80:**263, 1975.

13. Freedman, J., and Goldberg, L: Incidence of retinoblastoma in the Bantu of South Africa, Br. J. Ophthalmol. **60:**655, 1976.

14. Levine, A.S.: Cancer in the young, New York, 1982, Masson Publishing USA, Inc.

15. Sutow, W.W., Fernbach, D.J., and Vietti, T.J.: Clinical pediatric oncology, ed. 3, St. Louis, 1984, The C.V. Mosby Co.

16. Marks, P.A.: Genetically determined susceptibility to cancer, Blood **58**(3):415, 1981.

17. Mauer, A.M., Simone, J.V., and Pratt, C.B.: Current progress in the treatment of the child with cancer, J. Pediatr. **91**(4):523, 1977.

18. Wollner, N., and others: Non-Hodgkin's lymphoma in children, Med. Pediatr. Oncol. **1:**235, 1975.

19. Vogel, F.: Genetics of retinoblastoma, Hum. Genet. **52:**1, 1979.

20. Breslow, N.E., and Beckwith J.B.: Epidemiological features of Wilms' tumor: results of the National Wilms' Tumor Study, J. Natl. Cancer Inst. **68:**429, 1982.

21. Knudson, A.J., and Strong, L.C.: Mutation and cancer: neuroblastoma and pheochromocytoma, Am. J. Hum. Genet. **24:**514, 1972.

22. Roberts, L.: Cancer today, origins, prevention and treatment, Washington, D.C., 1984, National Academy Press.

23. Van Eys, J., and Sullivan, M.P.: Status of the curability of childhood cancers, New York, 1980, Raven Press.

24. Elion, G.B., Burgi, E., and Hitchings, G.H.: Studies on condensed pyrimidine systems, the synthesis of some 6-substituted purines, J. Am. Chem. Soc. **74:**411, 1952.

25. Farber, S., and others: Clinical studies of actinomycin-D with special reference to Wilms' tumor in children, Ann, N.Y. Acad. Sci. **39:**421, 1960.

26. Wolf, J.A., and others: Single versus multiple dose dactinomycin therapy of Wilms' tumor, N. Engl. J. Med. **279:**290, 1968.

27. Pinkel, D., and others: Nine years' experience with "total therapy" of childhood acute lymphocytic leukemia, Pediatrics **50:**246, 1972.

28. Knudson, A.G.: Hereditary cancer, oncogenes, and anti-oncogenes, Cancer Res. **45:**1437, 1985.

29. Waskerwitz, M.J., and Ruccione, K.: An overview of cancer in children in the 1980's, Nurs. Clin. North Am. **20**(1):5, 1985.

CHAPTER 2

Childhood leukemias

HOPE ANNE CASTORIA and MICHAEL HARRIS

This chapter will discuss the major forms of leukemia in children. Improvements in the understanding and treatment of these diseases will be stressed. These include a better understanding of the process of hematopoiesis and a more precise classification of cell types. Clinical observations have led to an improved understanding of the pathophysiologic process in the dissemination of leukemia, resulting in recognition of the importance for early treatment of central nervous system (CNS) and testicular involvement. Advances in chemotherapy and the results of many cooperative study group drug trials have greatly improved the effectiveness of this specific form of therapy. An understanding and improvement of general supportive care in these patients may have contributed to the success of the newer chemotherapeutic protocols. Finally, the role of the nurse in the management of children with leukemia will be discussed.

THE LEUKEMIAS
Etiology and incidence

There were approximately 6000 new cases of cancer in children in 1984. Acute lymphocytic leukemia (ALL) accounted for about 1800 of these cases, an incidence rate of 3.5/100,000/year for leukemia in children under 15 years of age.[1]

As in all types of malignancy, the exact cause of leukemia is unknown. However, several factors associated with an increased risk of disease may have etiologic significance. Among these are infection, radiation, chemical and drug exposure, and genetic factors.

Many studies have shown a relationship between viral infection and the cause of leukemia in animals. Until recently there has been little evidence for such an association in humans. However, infection with the human T cell leukemia virus (HTLV) has been shown to be strongly associated with the occurrence of T cell leukemia in Japanese adults.[2] Clusters of cases of leukemia have also been cited as evidence for an infectious origin, although prospective studies have failed to find any significance for these outbreaks, attributing them to a chance phenomenon.[3,4]

Ionizing radiation is leukemogenic. This is substantiated by the high incidence of leukemia in radiologists exposed to high doses of gamma radiation.[5] Children treated with radiation for a large thymus and patients with ankylosing spondylitis treated with radiation have also been found to have an increased risk of leukemia.[6,7] Follow-up of atomic bomb survivors revealed that the closer an individual was to the epicenter of the explosion, the greater was the risk of leukemia.[8]

Exposure to benzene has been implicated as an etiologic factor in adults.[9] Chemotherapy of Hodgkin's disease and Wilms' tumor has been followed by the emergence of acute leukemia.[10,11] In the case of Hodgkin's disease, chlorambucil seems to be the leukemogenic agent.[12]

The increased incidence of leukemia in various syndromes with chromosomal abnormalities is evidence for a genetic susceptibility to this disease. Down's syndrome, Fanconi's syndrome, Bloom's syndrome, and other diseases characterized by chromosome fragility are associated with an increased risk of leukemia. Family studies have revealed that the risk of leukemia for siblings of an affected child is four times greater than that in the general population.[13] The group with the greatest risk of developing leukemia is an identical twin of a child with leukemia, in whom the risk is 20% to 25%.[14] The risk is greatest when the unaffected child is less than 1 year of age and decreases to the risk for other siblings after 7 years of age. Of particular interest are the recent findings of an association of susceptibility to Hodgkin's disease and chronic lymphocytic leukemia with human leukocyte antigen (HLA) genes of the major histocompatibility complex.[15,16] Individuals expressing human immune-related (Ia) gene HLA-DR5 have a threefold greater risk of developing Hodgkin's disease than a matched control population.[15]

Classifications. Leukemias are classified in several ways. Acute leukemia is distinguished by the predominantly blast cells, as opposed to more mature cells found in the chronic leukemias. A second method of classification is the differentiation between lymphocytic and myelogenous or nonlymphocytic types of acute and chronic leukemia. Finally, different subtypes of the acute leukemias are now recognized. Several techniques are applied to make these distinctions, including cellular morphology, cytochemistry, and immunologic markers. Classification of leukemia grew out of the belief that the course of disease varied according to the several criteria mentioned. This has been borne out in a number of studies.[17,18] Clinical features, response to therapy, and prognosis may now be accurately predicted depending on the cell type involved. In addition, results of studies from various institutions regarding any of these factors can now be reliably compared.

Morphology. The standard classification scheme for morphologic differentiation of leukemic subtypes is that described by the French-American-British working group (FAB).[19] Several criteria are used to distinguish between ALL and acute non-lymphocytic leukemia (ANLL) and between each of the subtypes of these diseases, including cell size; nuclear/cytoplasmic ratio; number of nucleoli;

and presence or absence of cytoplasmic vacuoles, granulocytes, and Auer rods. A summary of the distinguishing features between ALL and AML is shown in Table 2-1. Further subdivision of ALL into three subgroups, L1, L2, and L3, and of ANLL into six subgroups, M1 through M6, is also described. In ALL L1 and L2 subtypes are commonly associated with non-T non-B and T cell forms of this disease. B cell ALL is associated with an L3 morphology similar to that in Burkitt's lymphoma.

Cytochemistry. The reaction of leukemic cells with various cytochemical stains provides a second means of distinguishing lymphocytic from nonlymphocytic leukemia. To some degree they are also helpful in determining the subtypes of the disease. In general, lymphocytic cells are positive with periodic acid–Schiff (PAS) stain and negative with Sudan black stain and with stains for myeloperoxidase and various esterases. The reverse is true of the myelogenous leukemias. Positivity with an acid phosphatase stain is most characteristic of T cell acute lymphocytic leukemia. These features are summarized for the lymphocytic and nonlymphocytic leukemias in Table 2-1. An immunofluorescent stain for the enzyme terminal deoxynucleotidyl transferase (TdT), not a true cytochemical test, is also helpful. The enzyme is absent in cells from patients with nonlymphocytic and B cell leukemia but is positive in T cell and non-T non-B cell ALL.

Immunology. Using current knowledge of the functional subsets of lymphocytes, ALL can be subdivided into several subgroups, including T cell, B cell, pre-B cell, and non-T non-B (common or null) cell leukemia. Various cell markers are used to distinguish between these subgroups. The common ALL antigen is found in patients with the pre-B and non-T non-B cell types of ALL. Although not present on normal lymphocytes, it is not specific for leukemia.[20] Ia antigens are cell membrane proteins encoded by the major histocompatibility complex responsible for graft rejection. These antigens are found on non-T non-B, B, and pre-B leukemic blasts and some of the ANLL subgroups. B cell leukemia is characterized by the presence on the cell surface of immuno-

Table 2-1. Morphologic characteristics of acute lymphoblastic leukemia (ALL) and acute myeloblastic leukemia (AML)*

Feature	ALL	AML
Nuclear chromatin	Clumped	Spongy
Nuclear/cytoplasmic ratio	High	Low
Nucleoli	O-2	2-5
Auer rods	Absent	Present
Granules	Absent	Present
Cytoplasm	Blue	Blue-gray
Cytochemistry		
Nonenzymatic methods		
PAS	Positive	Negative
Sudan black	Negative	Positive
Enzymatic methods		
Myeloperoxidase	Negative	Positive
Esterases:		
α-Napthyl acetate	Negative	Positive (AMML, AMol)
Naphthol ASD chloroacetate	Negative	Positive (AML, AMML)

From Lanzkowsky, P: Pediatric hematology oncology, New York 1980, McGraw-Hill, Inc.
*The AML group includes acute myelocytic leukemia (AML), acute myelomonocytic leukemia (AMML), acute monocytic leukemia (AMoL), and erythroleukemia. This group is commonly referred to as *acute nonlymphocytic leukemia.*

globulin molecules. Pre-B cells lack surface immunoglobulin, but using a fluorescent stain on fixed cells, they can be shown to contain the heavy chain of IgM in their cytoplasm. T cells are characterized by their ability to form rosettes with sheep erythrocytes or by the presence of T cell specific membrane antigens recognized by several antisera or monoclonal antibodies. Normal T cells may also be divided into helper and suppressor subgroups based on their separate reaction with additional monoclonal antibodies, and T cell leukemias are now being evaluated with these markers.[21] The diagnosis of a particular immunologic type of ALL is associated with a predictable clinical course, response to therapy, and prognosis, described in subsequent sections. The use of cell surface markers in the analysis of the nonlymphocytic leukemias is in its infancy and has not as yet improved on the classification using morphologic and cytochemical criteria.

Clinical features

Almost all the clinical signs and symptoms of ALL are a result of either replacement of normal bone marrow components or infiltrates of extramedullary sites by leukemic cells. The clinical features of ALL described here are much the same in all the acute lymphocytic leukemias in children. Particular variations in the clinical presentation of the various subgroups of ALL will be described in the following sections.

The onset of disease may be insidious or acute, but most patients seek medical help within 2 to 6 weeks after the onset of symptoms. Early in the disease the patient's signs and symptoms may be relatively mild. Occasionally the disease may have been clinically evident for months. especially in a child who demonstrates symptoms of bone and joint pain. Those children with the briefest clinical history often have the most rapidly growing leukemic cell populations. A review of the presenting complaints in 724 children evaluated by members of the Southwest Oncology Group is shown in Table 2-2.[1]

Replacement of normal bone marrow by leukemic cells results in anemia, neutropenia, and thrombocytopenia. Anemia causes fatigue, weakness, pallor, and lethargy. Bleeding as a result of

Table 2-2. Presenting clinical and laboratory findings in 724 children with acute lymphoblastic leukemia

Clinical features	Percent	Laboratory findings	Percent
Age (yr)		Hepatosplenomegaly	
<1.5	6	None	32
1.5-3	18	Moderate	55
3-10	54	Marked	13
>10	22	WBC ($\times 10^9$/liter)	
Sex (male)	57	<10	53
Race		10-49	30
White	89	≥50	17
Nonwhite	11	Hemoglobin (gm/dl)	
Fever	61	<7	43
Hemorrhage	48	7-11	45
Bone pain	23	≥11	12
Lymphadenopathy		Platelets ($\times 10^9$/liter)	
None	50	<20	28
Moderate	43	20-99	47
Marked (>3 cm)	7	≥100	25
Splenomegaly		Blasts in bone marrow (%)	
None	38	25-64	25
Moderate	49	65-94	50
Marked	14	≥95	25
Immunological markers		Mediastinal mass	7
Null	80	Central nervous system disease	4
T	18		
B	2		
Lymphoblast morphology			
L_1	84		
L_2	15		
L_3	1		
Immunoglobulins			
Normal	82		
Depressed (1 or more classes)	18		

From Miller, D.R.: Acute lymphoblastic leukemia, Pediatr. Clin. North Am. **27**(2):270, 1980.

thrombocytopenia is common and includes cutaneous bruises or purpura, petechiae, epistaxis, melena, and gingival bleeding. More serious gastrointestinal and intracranial hemorrhage may occur with platelet counts of less than 20,000/mm³. Fever is a very common presenting complaint and in many cases results from the leukemia itself. However, since neutropenia is present in a majority of patients at the time of diagnosis, the patient is immunocompromised and at risk for an opportunistic infection.

Leukemic cells may infiltrate almost any organ of the body and thus cause a number of different symptoms. It is this feature that has led to leukemia being called the "great imitator."

Enlargement of the liver and spleen is seen in about two thirds of the patients and is associated with a feeling of abdominal fullness and anorexia with subsequent weight loss. Lymphadenopathy is present in half of the children at the time of diagnosis. Clinical evidence of CNS involvement is present in less than 10% of cases at diagnosis and may be associated with increased intracranial pressure, resulting in headache, vomiting, and visual disturbances. CNS disease and testicular leukemia are more common during relapse of leukemia following prolonged remission and are described in separate sections.

Bone and joint pain may be the initial complaint in 25% to 30% of patients. Pain is caused by leukemic infiltration of bone or joints or expansion of the marrow. Tenderness to palpation is evident over involved bones. The presence of a limp and associated joint pains often lead to a misdiagnosis of juvenile rheumatoid arthritis, and acute leukemia must be included in the differential diagnosis of this disease.

Enlargement of the kidneys because of leukemic infiltration may occur but is usually asymptomatic. Priapism is seen usually in association with a high white blood cell (WBC) count. This may result from either sludging of leukocyte-rich blood in the penile vasculature or leukemic involvement of sacral nerve roots.[22] Infiltration of the gastrointestinal tract can result in vague abdominal pain but is usually asymptomatic except in very advanced disease. Skin involvement, usually seen only in congenital leukemia, consists of nodular purpuric lesions of the face and trunk.

Diagnostic evaluation

Anemia and thrombocytopenia are present in approximately 90% of the patients at the time of diagnosis. WBC counts can range from $100/mm^3$ to 1 million $cells/mm^3$, but in two thirds the count is less than 20,000 to $25,000/mm^3$.[1]

Blast cells may or may not be seen in a peripheral blood smear. The diagnosis, however, requires that a bone marrow examination be performed. The marrow is usually hypercellular and contains 60% to 100% blast cells in contrast to the normal number of less than 5% (see Fig. 2-1). In ALL these blasts usually have a morphology termed L1 or L2 (see the section in this chapter on classification). In contrast to the granulocytic blasts of ANLL, they are strongly positive with PAS stain, contain the enzyme TdT, and may be positive with one or more immunologic markers of lymphocytes. Unlike the blasts seen in acute myelocytic leukemia (AML), they do not contain cytoplasmic granules or Auer rods and are negative for stains with peroxidase

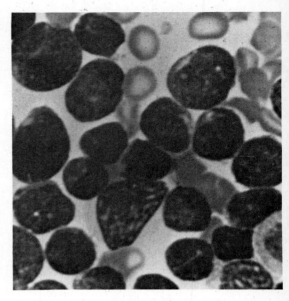

Fig. 2-1. Blasts present in bone marrow film.

and esterase. Normal marrow components such as megakaryocytes and erythroid and granulocyte precursors are reduced or absent.

A lumbar puncture should be performed to examine the CNS for leukemic involvement. Cerebrospinal fluid (CSF) pressure, protein, and glucose levels should be measured and a cytocentrifuge sample of CSF examined for the presence of leukemic blasts.

A chest x-ray examination may reveal a mediastinal mass, commonly seen in the T cell type of ALL. Pulmonary infiltrates may signify pneumonia or the uncommon finding of leukemic infiltrates. An intravenous pyelogram or ultrasonography may show renal enlargement. A skeletal survey should be performed in children with bone and joint pain. Changes are most often seen in the long bones and include generalized rarefaction of the bone, transverse radiolucent lines (leukemic lines), and pathologic features.[23]

A variety of biochemical abnormalities may occur but are not specific for leukemia. Most result in some way from release of chemical substances from dying leukemic cells. Hyperuricemia as a result of release of uric acid by leukemic cells is common and often becomes worse following chemotherapy. It may result in symptoms of anorexia, nausea, vomiting, and lethargy and can cause renal damage. Elevated serum levels of serum glutamic oxaloacetic transaminase (SGOT) and lactic dehydrogenase (LDH) also reflect release of these enzymes from leukemic cells. Tetany may be caused by hypocalcemia and hyperphosphatemia, a result of leukemic cell turnover with the release of organic phosphates.

A variety of chromosomal abnormalities is seen in ALL. The report of the Third International Workshop on Leukemia in 1980 showed that 66% of 330 patients with ALL had abnormal chromosomes.[24] These included structural abnormalities, such as the translocation of 8q− to 14q+ seen most commonly with L3 marrow morphology, and an abnormal number of chromosomes (hypodiploidy or hyperdiploidy), seen in 75% and 39% of patients with null cell or T cell ALL, respectively. A hypodiploid karyotype is associated with a poorer prognosis.[25]

ACUTE LYMPHOCYTIC LEUKEMIA
Subclassification

Non-T non-B cell leukemia. Non-T non-B cell leukemia accounts for approximately 66.9% of cases of ALL in children, making it the most common form of this disease.[26] Fortunately, it is also the most responsive to chemotherapy and carries the best prognosis of all types of ALL. Clinical features of this disease are similar to those in other forms of ALL. The leukemic blasts lack both B and T cell markers. They are also negative for surface membrane immunoglobulin, sheep erythrocyte receptors, and T cell specific antigens. They do express, however, the common ALL and Ia antigen. This cell type appears to represent an early stage in the development of lymphocytes, before acquisition of mature T and B cell antigens. Treatment involves the usual phases of induction, CNS prophylaxis, and maintenance. Approximately

45% of children with this type of ALL can be expected to achieve long-term cure.[27]

T cell leukemia. T cell leukemia makes up approximately 14.2% of cases of ALL in children.[27] The cell of origin is a lymphocyte that has developed within the thymus (thymus dependent). These cells are distinguished by their ability to spontaneously form heat-stable rosettes with sheep erythrocytes (E rosette positive). The cell membrane receptor for sheep erythrocytes and other T cell specific membrane antigens may also be identified by various xenoantisera and monoclonal antibodies. Surface membrane immunoglobulins and common acute lymphoblastic leukemia (cALL) antigen are not present in these cells. Cytochemically, the cells are acid phosphatase positive in 75% of patients, which helps distinguish them from other types of ALL. Like most lymphoblasts, however, they are negative for peroxidase and naphthol chloracetate esterase. The cytologic FAB classification of the blast cells in this disease is usually that of an L1 or L2 morphology.

Clinically, T cell leukemia presents with many of the same signs and symptoms of other forms of ALL. However, infiltration of the CNS, liver, spleen, lymph nodes, and mediastinum is more common. A mediastinal mass may be found in up to 75% of children with T cell ALL and when present suggests the T cell origin of the leukemia (Fig. 2-2). T cell leukemia is four times more common in males than females and is especially prevalent in older children and adolescents.[26] It must be differentiated from T cell lymphoblastic lymphoma, which also may present with a mediastinal mass.

The prognosis of patients with T cell leukemia is significantly worse than that of patients with common ALL, in part because of a greater tumor burden at diagnosis, as mentioned previously.[28] Both the rate of induction and duration of remission are worse in these patients. The incidence of early CNS and testicular relapse is significantly greater compared to that for non-T non-B cell leukemia.[29] Treatment failure, defined as failure to achieve remission or development of relapse, is 13% for null

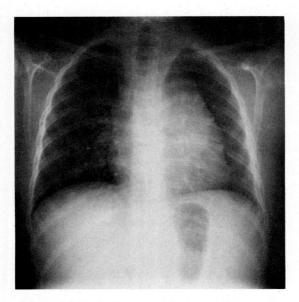

Fig. 2-2. Mediastinal mass in child with T cell leukemia.

cell leukemia compared to 33% for patients with the T cell phenotype.[30]

B cell leukemia. B cell leukemia is the rarest form of ALL, comprising 0.6% of cases of ALL in children.[26] It is slightly more common in adults. This disease probably represents an extension to the peripheral blood and bone marrow of B cell lymphomas of the Burkitt's or diffuse, poorly differentiated, lymphocytic type.[31] Extension to the blood is a feature of these diseases seen primarily in children. The blast cells contain surface membrane immunoglobulin like normal mature B cells, but are negative for the sheep erythrocyte receptor found on T cells, TdT, PAS, acid phosphatase, and alpha naphthyl esterase. Lymphadenopathy is uncommon, and mediastinal masses are rare; but the CNS is frequently involved. B cell leukemia is the most refractory to treatment of all types of ALL. It usually runs a rapidly fatal course, with most children not surviving more than 1 year.

Pre-B cell leukemia. Pre-B cell leukemia is the most recently recognized phenotype of acute lymphoblastic leukemia, first described by Vogler and others in 1978, and accounts for 18.3% of ALL in children.[26,32] Similar to non-T non-B cell leukemia, pre-B leukemia blasts lack detectable B and T cell markers like sheep erythrocyte receptors and surface immunoglobulin. They also have in common the expression of Ia and cALL antigen on their surface. However, the blasts in pre-B leukemia contain heavy chains of IgM demonstrable by immunofluorescent techniques on fixed cells. These blast cells represent an early stage in the development of B cells, at which the cells cannot manufacture complete immunoglobulin molecules, and therefore cannot express immunoglobulin on their surface. This subgroup of ALL probably accounts for 25% of leukemias previously designated common ALL antigen (cALLa) positive non-T non-B cell leukemia.[32]

Pre-B cell leukemia has a similar clinical presentation to that of non-T non-B leukemia. However, a recent study by Crist and others[33] described several interesting features. A significantly higher incidence of pre-B leukemia has been noted in black children. Presently the remission induction rate is similar, but children with pre-B cell leukemia have a greater frequency of relapse while on maintenance therapy. The average duration of remission in pre-B cell leukemia is therefore shorter than that for non-T non-B leukemia. Relapse in pre-B cell leukemia is also more frequently complicated by involvement of the CNS. Prognosis for pre-B leukemia must therefore be considered poorer than for the more common non-T non-B cell leukemia.

CNS leukemia

CNS leukemia is an infiltrate of the meninges by leukemic lymphoblasts. Factors associated with a high rate of CNS involvement include age less than 12 months, T-cell or B-cell type ALL, and a high WBC count at diagnosis.[34-36] CNS involvement is present at the time of diagnosis in approximately 8% of new patients.[36,37]

The pathogenesis of the meningeal proliferations of leukemic cells is not certain. It has been suggested that these lesions originate from blood-borne seeding of leukemic cells from the bone marrow before treatment is initiated or during relapse.[37]

The child with CNS leukemia is usually asymptomatic. The disease is discovered following the initial lumbar puncture or during one of the routine follow-up CSF studies. When they occur, symptoms are caused by an increase in intracranial pressure. Most common among these are vomiting, headache, lethargy, and papilledema. Any of these signs or symptoms should alert the practitioner to the possibility of CNS involvement. Involvement of the oculomotor nerves resulting in visual disturbances such as diplopia is occasionally seen.

When the lumbar puncture is performed, the opening pressure may sometimes reveal an increased intracranial pressure. Cytocentrifugation of the spinal fluid is performed, and a WBC count with greater than 10 lymphoblasts per cubic millimeter is considered indicative of CNS involvement. The spinal fluid may also show a decreased glucose or increased protein concentration. Monoclonal antibodies and special staining are sometimes used to differentiate normal lymphocytes from lymphoblasts.

As mentioned above, patients with ALL may or may not have clinically evident CNS involvement at the time of diagnosis. Provided with a sanctuary by the blood-brain barrier, these leukemic cells may actually escape the effects of antileukemic drugs and become the source of a CNS relapse of disease. This is thought to be a result of poor penetration of the CNS by chemotherapeutic agents and slower proliferation of leukemic cells with the spinal fluid. Entry of leukemic cells into the CNS probably occurs either by direct infiltration around small meningeal vessels or during petechial bleeding. Prophylactic treatment of the CNS following induction therapy reduces the chances of this complication.

In the past two decades it has become possible to prevent the occurrence of CNS relapse in over 90% of patients using either cranial irradiation (1800 to 2400 rad) and intrathecal methotrexate (6 to 15 mg/m^2/injection) or intrathecal methotrexate alone immediately following remission induction.[38] This form of therapy has replaced the use of higher-dose craniospinal radiation alone. Presently the use of triple intrathecal medications including methotrexate, hydrocortisone, and cytosine arabinoside is being practiced at many institutions.[39] A relapse of meningeal leukemia, when it occurs, is usually microscopic and not clinical, but the prognosis is poor. In one recent report, however, five of ten patients treated with intrathecal methotrexate, craniospinal irradiation, systemic reinduction therapy, and continuation therapy with additional intrathecal methotrexate remained in second remission for 13 to 37 months following a CNS relapse.[40]

Although cranial radiotherapy and intrathecal methotrexate have been very efficacious in preventing relapse and relieving the symptoms of meningeal leukemia, they are not without adverse side effects. Short-term toxic reactions to repeated doses of intrathecal methotrexate include nausea and vomiting, headache, fever, dizziness, weakness, and leg pain. In addition, there are several long-term complications associated with CNS prophylaxis. The most disturbing of these is the increased incidence of learning disabilities, particularly in children less than 5 years of age at the time of diagnosis. A 35% incidence of learning disabilities has been described in this age group.[41] This long-term complication occurs more frequently in children who develop the postradiation "somnolence syndrome" 4 to 6 weeks after CNS prophylaxis. This syndrome consists of lethargy, nausea, vomiting, low-grade fever, irritability, and weight loss without infection or other causes. Also disturbing is a report of second malignancies occurring within the area of the radiotherapy field.[42] Thus, although the use of craniospinal irradiation and intrathecal methotrexate has been very successful in preventing CNS relapse of ALL, research must continue to reevaluate alternative treatment modalities, so as to lower the late morbidity associated with this form of therapy (see Chapter 31).

Gonadal leukemia

With increasing long-term survival of children with ALL, testicular relapse has become more common. The incidence of confirmed testicular relapse varies from less than 5% in some studies to

40% in others.[43,44] The reason for these differences is important and may be a result of the presenting characteristics of the disease.

Testicular relapse can occur while a patient is on chemotherapy but is more common after discontinuation of chemotherapy. Rarely, testicular disease is present at the time of diagnosis. Patients with high WBC counts tend to have testicular relapse earlier in the course of their disease than those who have normal or low WBC counts at diagnosis.[45] Painless enlargement of one or both testes and scrotal discoloration or an increased firmness should alert the clinician to a possible testicular relapse. Therefore it is very important that the testes are inspected and palpated during each physical examination. Confirmation of testicular disease is made by histologic examination of the testes either following orchidectomy, needle aspiration, or wedge biopsy.

The pathophysiology of testicular leukemia is uncertain. It has been suggested that a blood-gonad barrier similar to the blood-CSF barrier exists, shielding leukemic cells in the gonads from the effects of chemotherapy.[46] However, no anatomic structure similar to the glial cell–blood barrier of the CNS is present in the testicles. Another possibility that has been suggested is the resistance to chemotherapy of cells in a relatively cold environment.[47] Alternatively, blasts may be present in the testicles early in the course of disease but for some reason remain dormant, thus avoiding the effects of drugs that act only on dividing cells.[45]

The treatment of testicular leukemia includes radiation to the testes. If biopsy confirms involvement of only one testis, radiation may be given to that side alone, but this method is controversial because of the possibility of false-negative biopsies. Usually, 2000 rad in 100- to 200-rad doses are given to both testes. Radiation renders the male patient sterile, but Leydig's cell function and testosterone level may remain normal so that sexual development is unaffected.[48]

Most patients with testicular relapse, if treated only with local radiation, will subsequently develop a hematologic and/or CNS relapse. The best results have been obtained when local radiation has been combined with vigorous reinduction chemotherapy and CNS prophylaxis. Nevertheless, the length of remission and prognosis for those who develop overt testicular disease while on chemotherapy is poor. However, in those whose testicular relapse occurs more than 1 year following cessation of therapy, or in those who have asymptomatic testicular infiltration detected by a remission biopsy, such aggressive treatment may lead to long-lasting remissions.[49]

Two practices with regard to testicular relapse of leukemia deserve special mention. One is routine biopsy of the testicles before cessation of therapy. This has the potential of early diagnosis of residual disease. The second, prophylactic radiation of the testes following attainment of remission, has been shown to decrease the frequency of subsequent testicular relapse. However, neither practice has succeeded in lowering the rate of bone marrow relapse.[50] One reason may be the occasional occurrence of false-negative testicular biopsies. Biopsy specimens represent a very small portion of the testicle, and a scanty leukemic infiltrate may not be included in the biopsy sample. Failure of prophylactic testicular radiation may be caused by the inability of this approach to prevent reseeding of the bone marrow, or testicular involvement may be merely a marker of residual disease in other sites as well. In addition, this therapy would render all patients sterile while only a minority have testicular involvement.

Involvement of the ovaries has been found at autopsy in 11% to 50% of cases.[51,52] Antemortem diagnosis of extramedullary involvement of the ovaries has been rare until recently. Seven cases have been described of girls with leukemic infiltration of the ovaries at the primary site of extramedullary relapse.[53-55] All were in bone marrow remission at the time their ovarian disease was detected. Difficulty in the detection of ovarian involvement may be one reason for the infrequent antemortem diagnosis of ovarian leukemia.

Treatment

Elimination of disease and long-term survival are goals of therapy in ALL that are now possible in many cases. Current treatment regimens require progress through several phases including remission induction, consolidation, CNS prophylaxis, and maintenance. Following successful completion of these phases, the patient may be removed from therapy and continue to remain in long-term remission. It is well established that in all phases of treatment, multiple-drug therapy is superior to the use of single agents.[56] It has also been determined that the type of therapy used in any phase has an effect on the success of particular treatment regimens in subsequent phases of therapy. Many studies have been performed examining the multiple permutations of different drug regimens at different phases of therapy. This is especially pertinent today when treatment is tailored to risk category at presentation and immunologic phenotype of ALL. These findings have increased the survival role of high-risk and T cell leukemia patients over the last few years. Finally, general supportive care, as in newly diagnosed disease, remains of vital importance in preventing serious consequences from the toxic effects of treatment and the disease itself.

General measures. Inhibition of normal hematopoiesis by leukemic bone marrow infiltration results in the anemia, thrombocytopenia, and neutropenia present at diagnosis. Transfusion with packed red blood cells should be used to correct symptomatic anemia. Likewise, patients with clinical bleeding or, at some institutions, those with platelet counts less than 20,000/mm^3 should receive transfusions of platelets. A dose of 0.2 unit/kg usually results in an increase of the platelet count of 80,000 to 100,000/mm^3.

Although fever may be a consequence of the disease itself, any febrile patient with an absolute neutrophil count (calculated as the sum of segmented neutrophil and band forms) of less than 500/mm^3 should be suspected of being septic, and broad-spectrum multiple-antibiotic therapy should be started immediately. Patients with leukemia are immunosuppressed and are therefore at risk for graft versus host disease following transfusion of immunocompetent cells. Therefore at some institutions all blood products are irradiated with a dose of 1800 rad before transfusion to inactivate any immunocompetent cells.

Pulmonary infection with *Pneumocystis carinii* was once a major complication during remission. This is now prevented by the prophylactic administration of trimethoprim-sulfamethoxazole. Disseminated varicella-zoster continues to be a problem during therapy, particularly in patients receiving multiple-drug regimens. This may be treated prophylactically with zoster immune globulin (ZIG) or therapeutically with acyclovir.

Biochemical problems arising from the lysis of leukemic cells, such as hyperuricemia and hypercalcemia associated with hyperphosphatemia, may become even worse following the initiation of cytotoxic chemotherapy. Hyperuricemia can result in kidney damage that prevents the use of optimum doses of chemotherapeutic drugs. Hydration, urinary alkalinization, and allopurinol are successful in preventing significant clinical effects of elevated serum uric acid. Amphojel is also effective in lowering phosphate levels and restoring homeostasis.

Induction and consolidation. The goal of induction therapy is to rapidly eliminate as many leukemic cells as possible, thereby allowing restoration of normal hematopoiesis. Rapid induction reduces the likelihood of drug resistance developing during treatment and the chance of serious infection or hemorrhage. Successful therapy is associated with a reduction of leukemic cells in the bone marrow to less than 5% of the total number of cells.

Although remission can be obtained with single agents, combinations of drugs have been shown to result in a higher rate and duration of remission. Prednisone combined with vincristine has been the most successful such combination, resulting in remission in 90% of patients treated with this regimen.[57] Several studies have examined the use of additional agents, particularly asparaginase.[58] Although an improvement in the remission rate of several percent can be achieved using asparaginase in addition to prednisone and vincristine, this difference is not always significant. Importantly though, the duration of remission with this three-drug regimen is longer than that following prednisone and vincristine alone, an example of one phase of therapy influencing another.[59] Daunorubicin has also been used successfully as a third drug.[60] Addition of a fourth drug has not been found superior to the three-drug combinations described and was more toxic.[61]

Other treatment strategies include aggressive drug combinations during or immediately following induction, called consolidation, to further reduce leukemic cell load. Preliminary results of a study using this strategy are promising, with a 99% rate of remission in both standard and high-risk patients.[62]

From 5% to 10% of patients will not achieve a remission with one of the induction protocols just mentioned. Prognosis for these patients is poor. However, it has been possible to obtain remission in these cases using drugs other than the standard induction agents. Cytosine arabinoside, cyclophosphamide, and VM-26 have been used successfully in various combinations.[63,64]

Treatment of the CNS during or immediately following induction has become mandatory in the therapy of ALL. As discussed in the section on CNS leukemia, this area may be protected from the effects of systemic chemotherapy and serve as a source of occult disease. Thus cranial irradiation with intrathecal methotrexate or use of intrathecal therapy consisting of methotrexate, hydrocortisone, and cytosine arabinoside following induction has become part of the standard therapy of ALL and is able to prevent CNS relapse in 90% of patients.[65] In standard-risk or low-risk patients, intrathecal methotrexate alone during induction and throughout maintenance therapy or high-dose systemic methotrexate plus intrathecal methotrexate early in remission is sufficient.[66,67] The long-term side effects of CNS radiation and chemotherapy are discussed in the section on CNS leukemia.

Maintenance therapy. Although few leukemic cells are detectable once remission is obtained, it is important to remember that a large number of leukemic cells are still present. Clinical remission can occur when the total body load of leukemic cells is reduced from 10^{12} to 10^{10} cells.[68] If these remaining cells are not removed, relapse is inevitable. Thus continued therapy is necessary to achieve long-term remissions or cures.

The most successful combination in this phase of therapy has been oral or parenteral methotrexate plus 6-mercaptopurine. Up to 50% of standard-risk patients can be expected to remain in long-term remission with this protocol.[69] Variations of this regimen have included the intermittent rather than continuous use of chemotherapy during remission and periodic reinforcement with induction agents, including prednisone, vincristine, and asparaginase or daunorubicin. However, no significant differences in the rate of relapse have been found among these various maintenance strategies.[70,71]

Chemotherapy cannot be continued indefinitely because of toxicity and the possible emergence of drug-resistant clones of leukemic cells. No reliable method exists, however, to determine if any residual disease is present. Current practice is to continue maintenance therapy for 2½ to 3 years. Before treatment is discontinued, patients should have a complete physical examination and bone marrow and CSF examinations. These should be repeated at 2- to 3-month intervals during the first year after therapy and less frequently or not at all in later years. Results of several studies show a relapse rate of approximately 20% following cessation of therapy.[72] Most relapses occur within the first year, and the rate declines in subsequent years. After 4 to 6 years after therapy, relapse rarely occurs. The risk of relapsing after therapy cannot be predicted by clinical features that may have been present at diagnosis.[73]

Relapse. With first and subsequent relapses, the chances of survival become less and less, probably because of the emergence of increasingly drug-resistant subpopulations of leukemic cells. Patients who relapse after therapy is discontinued respond better to treatment than those who relapse during maintenance therapy. Of the latter group 70% to 80% can achieve a second remission using various three-or four-drug regimens, including prednisone, vincristine, daunorubicin, and asparaginase.[74] Intensive early consolidation using VM-26 and cytosine arabinoside may prolong the disease-free interval.[75] Although the majority of children enter second remission, the long-term survival is rare after such an event. Bone marrow transplantation from an HLA-identical sibling donor has proved to be an effective form of therapy, with long-term cure rates of approximately 33%.[76,77] Transplants between HLA-nonidentical individuals uses a relatively new technology in which the possibility of a graft versus host reaction is reduced by the removal of immunocompetent cells from the donor marrow[78] (see Chapter 22). However, the major cause of failure of this approach continues to be relapse of leukemia.

A higher rate and duration of remission can be obtained in patients who relapse after cessation of therapy. Treatment of the CNS and systemic chemotherapy have been found to lengthen the duration of remission. However, an overwhelming majority of these patients will also suffer a subsequent relapse.

Prognosis

Approximately 50% of children with ALL can now be expected to achieve a long-term cure (Fig. 2-3 and Table 2-3). The marked improvement in overall survival for childhood leukemia is a result of newer chemotherapeutic agents and refined protocols for the administration of these drugs. As discussed in the section on classification, morphologic and other features of the leukemic blast are associated with a somewhat predictable clinical course. Other prognostic variables have also been described, some of which have great predictive

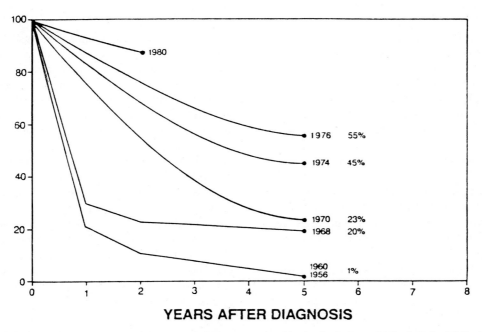

Fig. 2-3. Survival curve for ALL. (From Sutow, W.W., Fernbach, D.J., and Vietti, T.J.: Clinical pediatric oncology, ed. 3, St. Louis, 1984, The C.V. Mosby Co.)

Table 2-3. Prognostic factors in acute lymphoblastic leukemia of childhood

Factor	Favorable	Unfavorable
Demographic		
Age	3-7 yrs	<2, >10 yrs
Race	White	Black
Sex	Female	Male
Leukemic burden		
Initial white blood cell count	$<10 \times 10^9$/liter	$>50 \times 10^9$/liter
Adenopathy	Absent	Present
Central nervous system disease at diagnosis	Absent	Present
Hemoglobin	<7 gm per dl	>10 gm per dl
Platelet count	$>100 \times 10^9$/liter	$<100 \times 10^9$/liter
Mediastinal mass	Absent	Present
Morphology and histochemistry		
Lymphoblasts	L_1	L_2 or L_3
Periodic acid–Schiff stain	Positive	Negative
Ph^1 chromosome	Absent	Present
Immunologic factors		
Immunoglobulins	Normal IgG,A,M	Decreased IgG,A,M
Surface markers	"null cell" ALL	T- or B-cell All
Response to induction therapy	M_1 marrow (<5% blasts) on day 14	M_3 marrow (>25% blasts) on day 14

From Miller, D.R.:Acute lymphocytic leukemia, Pediatr. Clin. North Am. **27**(2):271, 1980.

value. Together these factors are important to the clinician for four reasons. First, the ability to assign a patient to a low-, standard-, or high-risk group allows the clinician to modify the therapy appropriately. Thus, although aggressive therapy may be called for in high-risk patients, less toxic treatment may suffice for low-risk patients. Second, assignment to an immunologic phenotype (e.g., B cell, T cell) also dictates the use of a specific therapeutic regimen. Third, clinical trials of new drugs or treatment strategies depend on the ability to describe the study and control groups in terms of prognostic subgroups. For example, if a group of predominantly high-risk patients were chosen to receive a new drug, comparison with a lower-risk group not receiving the drug would seriously impair the validity of the results. Finally, it is important for the clinician to be able to accurately discuss his or her expectations for the patient's outcome with the family.

The most important prognostic indicator is the WBC count at diagnosis. Patients with a WBC less than 10,000/mm³ have the best prognosis, whereas those with a WBC over 50,000/mm³ are a poor-risk group.[79] Age is the second most important prognostic variable. Children between the ages of 2 to 10 years may be expected to have a better outcome than those less than 1 and greater than 10 years of age.[17] The Children's Cancer Study Group has described several other factors associated with a poor prognosis, including L2 or L3 FAB morphology, male sex, low platelet count, hemoglobin greater than 10 g/dl, presence of a mediastinal mass, and depressed immunoglobulin levels.[18]

The T, B, and pre-B cell subgroups of ALL are associated with a poorer prognosis than the more common non-T non-B cell type of ALL. However, high-risk clinical features associated with a particular subgroup, such as a high WBC count associated with a mediastinal mass frequently seen in T cell ALL, may be responsible for these differences. The number of cases is too small at this time to allow the separate evaluation of immunologic and clinical variables in predicting the outcome.

Recent studies have identified two other prognostic variables. Presence of a left shift in the peripheral blood at diagnosis, defined as 1% or more of metamyelocytes, myelocytes, or promyelocytes, was associated with a 92-month duration of remission in 74% of such patients, compared with only 42% in those without a left shift.[80] It was suggested that a left shift represented a smaller degree of myelosuppression following a reduced tumor cell load, compared with patients in whom it was absent. Alternatively, the presence of 10% or more hand mirror cells, lymphoblasts with a distinctive morphology similar to that of a hand mirror, was associated with a shorter survival, compared with patients with less than 10% hand mirror cells.[81] In both these studies the contribution of other prognostic variables was taken into account before these conclusions were made.

Once a patient has been in complete remission for a certain period of time, some of the prognostic factors have been found to lose their predictive value.[73] After 18 months of complete remission, for example, the rate of survival is no longer associated with the WBC count at the time of diagnosis. Weaker prognostic variables lose their predictive value even earlier. Thus age at diagnosis and sex are no longer predictive of eventual outcome following 15 months of complete remission. Interestingly, sex of the individual again becomes a significant prognostic factor after 24 months of remission, with females again having an advantage. This may be a result of late testicular relapse in males or other endocrine functions not yet defined.

NONLYMPHOID LEUKEMIAS
Acute nonlymphocytic leukemia

ANLL is a term that includes several morphologic variants of malignancy of a multipotent hemopoietic stem cell. These include acute myeloid leukemia (AML), promyelocytic leukemia (APL), myelomonocytic leukemia (AMMoL), monocytic leukemia (AMoL), and erythroleukemia (AEL, Di

Guglielmo's syndrome). Together they account for about 20% of all acute leukemias in children. AML is the most common acute leukemia in children less than 1 year of age. The incidence of disease appears unrelated to sex or race.[82] As a group, these diseases have many clinical similarities to ALL, but they are not as responsive to treatment.

Etiology. Several factors predisposing to ANLL have been identified. A number of congenital conditions characterized by chromosomal abnormalities, such as Down's syndrome and Turner's syndrome and some congenital immunodeficiency diseases like Wiskott-Aldrich syndrome and ataxia-telangiectasia, are associated with an increased risk of ANLL.[74] Persons exposed to high doses of ionizing radiation, such as occurred as Hiroshima, are also predisposed to ANLL.[6] Of particular concern to pediatric oncology clinicians is the increased risk of ANLL in patients in long-term remission of Hodgkin's disease following therapy with radiation and alkylating agents.[83]

Of recent interest is the finding of specific chromosomal abnormalities associated with a particular type of ANLL. For instance, a translocation between chromosome 15 and 17 is frequently seen in APL.[84] These abnormalities are found only in the malignant cells and not in normal cells of blood or other tissues. Perhaps relevant in this regard are the recent observations concerning chromosome translocations in the B cell neoplasm Burkitt's lymphoma.[85] Translocation between chromosomes 8 and 14 in this disease involves a portion of the c-myc oncogene, which under certain conditions can transform normal cells into malignant cells in vitro.

Classification. The standard scheme for classifying the various types of ANLL is that described by FAB.[19] This scheme classifies the cell types based on several morphologic features that include the number of nucleoli, size, and abundance of granules and the presence or absence of Auer rods (tubular cytoplasmic structures derived from primary granules). Further delineation is provided by the reaction of the involved cells with several cytochemical stains, including peroxidase, naphthol AS-D chloracetate esterase, and acid phosphatase (see Table 2-1). Assignment to one of the M1 to M6 subclasses and either AML, AMML, AMoL, or AEL depends on a combination of these features. The aim of classification is to enable valid comparisons between different individuals and institutions regarding the incidence, clinical course, and response to therapy of the several subtypes of ANLL.

Clinical features. Clinical manifestations of ANLL, like ALL, are mostly a result of leukemic cell infiltration of the marrow that replaces normal marrow components. The resulting anemia leads to pallor, fatigue, and weakness. Anorexia and weight loss are also common. Neutropenia predisposes the patient to infection and fever. Thrombocytopenia is also frequent and results in petechiae, easy bruisability, nose bleeds, and bleeding of the gums. More severe bleeding is associated with the acute promyelocytic type of ANLL. These patients may have severe disseminated intravascular coagulation (DIC) caused by procoagulants released from leukemic granulocytes, and pulmonary or intracranial hemorrhages can result in death.

Collections of leukemic blasts can form localized masses in soft tissues, skin, gonads, bones, and sinuses and are called granulocytic sarcomas. Occasionally, these masses contain a large amount of the enzyme myeloperoxidase, which gives them a greenish color. They are then termed chloromas. A characteristic of AMoL is infiltration of the gingiva, lungs, meninges, and gastrointestinal tract. Hepatosplenomegaly and lymphadenopathy are seen in less than half of patients at the time of diagnosis. Bone and joint pain are common.

Laboratory features. Laboratory findings include anemia, neutropenia, and thrombocytopenia in over 90% of the patients. WBC counts are usually less than 50,000/mm³, but high counts are not uncommon in the monocytic type of ANLL. Blast cells are seen in the blood and bone marrow and range from less than 20% up to 100% of the cells. APL and AMMoL/AMoL are associated with a larger percentage of cells of promyelocytic and monocytic morphology, respectively. Blasts of

ANLL can be distinguished with almost 100% certainty from blasts of ALL by the finding of cytoplasmic Auer rods or peroxidase activity. In APL plasma fibrinogen levels may be decreased and prothrombin (PT) and partial thromboblastin time (PTT) prolonged because of the coagulation defects just mentioned. As in other leukemias, serum LDH and uric acid levels may be elevated. Serum muramidase, an enzyme found in normal granulocytes and monocytes, is normal to elevated in AML but is usually high in AMMoL and AMoL.

Induction of remission in patients with ANLL is much more difficult than in patients with ALL. The drug combinations used are not specific for leukemic cells but also destroy normal bone marrow precursor cells, thus resulting in marrow aplasia and pancytopenia. General supportive measures include transfusions of platelets and packed red blood cells in those patients with thrombocytopenia and anemia, respectively. Blood products may be irradiated before therapy to prevent graft versus host disease. However, packed red cells should be given with caution to patients with WBC counts greater than 200,000/mm³ in whom hyperviscosity may result in intravascular thrombosis and hemorrhage in the CNS. These patients require leukophoresis, low-dose cranial irradiation, or chemotherapy to reduce the total leukocyte count. Plasma fibrinogen levels with PT and PTT should be evaluated and heparin therapy begun in those patients with evidence of DIC, particularly in the promyelocytic type of ANLL. Fever should warn of infection and, when associated with an absolute neutrophil count of less than 500 to 1000/mm³, should be treated with broad-spectrum antibiotic therapy using a combination of drugs. Hyperuricemia should be treated with hydration, alkalinization of the urine, and allopurinol.

Treatment. Advances in chemotherapy have significantly improved the outlook for patients with AML. Multiple-drug therapy has replaced the use of single agents, since the effects of different drugs may be additive, and resistance to a particular drug by a subpopulation of cells can be avoided. The goal of therapy is to eliminate the leukemic population of cells from the blood and bone marrow so that the remaining normal cells can regenerate. Therapy is thus invariably associated with severe marrow aplasia and pancytopenia, requiring transfusions of the various blood components and intense supportive care for infection. From 10% to 30% of patients may die from infection or hemorrhagic complications as a result of therapy.[82] The reason for this difference in the initial outcome from ALL may be that AML is a disease of the early precursors of the bone marrow whereas ALL is a disease of lymphocytes that are not primarily involved in hematopoiesis. Thus the treatment of AML is directed at the stem cells of the bone marrow, leading to severe aplasia and a longer recovery to normal.

The most successful combinations of chemotherapeutic agents in remission induction have included one of the anthracycline antibiotics daunorubicin or doxorubicin (Adriamycin) with the pyrimidine antimetabolite cytosine arabinoside (ara-C). Other drugs used in combination with one or both of these include 6-thioguanine, cyclophosphamide, prednisone, and vincristine. Additional courses of chemotherapy, early or late in remission (called consolidation), are an attempt to further reduce the leukemic cell load and prolong remission. Remission can now be obtained in 60% to 85% of children with ANLL.[86]

Maintenance therapy has not been proved as valuable in prolonging remission in all study groups. Several studies have shown an improvement in the length of remission, whereas others have found no benefit from maintenance therapy.[87,88] Likewise, the usefulness of immunotherapy during remission is uncertain. A recent controlled study of the comparison of immunotherapy with chemotherapy during remission of AML in 508 adult patients showed a significantly longer duration of remission and median survival time in patients given chemotherapy.

One recent study reported a relapse rate of 75% for patients with ANLL in remission.[89] However, a study from the German Cooperative Study Group reported a relapse rate of 40% after 3 years in 199

children who were treated with an intensive regimen of induction, consolidation, and maintenance chemotherapy in addition to cranial irradiation.[90] CNS relapse has become an increasing problem in children with ANLL now that longer remissions are possible. Approximately one fifth of patients may experience a CNS relapse.[89] A recent study, however, suggests that prophylaxis using cranial irradiation and intrathecal methotrexate can improve this figure.[90] Reinduction of remission is more difficult to obtain than in the de novo disease, perhaps because of selection of a particularly drug-resistant subpopulation of cells. However, using ara-C and daunorubicin, 25% to 50% of patients can achieve a second remission.[82] Reinduction with high-dose ara-C and m-AMSA was shown by Hines and others[91] to be successful in obtaining remission in 28 of 40 patients (70%) with ANLL in relapse. Other drugs used for this purpose include VP-16-213, 6-thioguanine, and 5-azacytidine.

A recent therapeutic modality is the transplantation of allogeneic bone marrow into patients with ANLL in remission. This form of treatment is particularly successful in children during first remission and when an HLA-identical sibling is available.[92] Ablation of the bone marrow using intensive chemotherapy and radiation followed by bone marrow transplantation has resulted in complete remission for a period of 2 years in 70% to 80% of children with ANLL in first remission. It remains to be determined whether this form of therapy will prove superior to the use of chemotherapy alone.

Prognosis. The median survival of patients with ANLL has increased from 3 months before the induction of chemotherapy to longer than 1 year, and 55% of patients will remain in remission for at least 24 months.[89] Prognosis is unrelated to the morphologic type of ANLL. Patients with ANLL usually have longer remission if they survive the initial phase of disease and induction when DIC and bleeding become a problem. Infection, extramedullary disease, and high total leukocyte counts tend to be associated with poorer outcome.

Chronic myelogenous leukemia

Chronic myelogenous leukemia (CML) is uncommon in children, accounting for less than 5% of all childhood leukemias.[91] Two distinct types of CMLs are recognized. The adult form of CML is seen most commonly in children 10 to 12 years of age or older and is clinically similar to the disease in adults. The juvenile form of CML is distinct from the adult form with respect to clinical presentation and prognosis and is seen mainly in infants and children less than 2 years of age (Table 2-4).

Adult form. The adult form of CML develops insidiously and may occasionally be discovered in an asymptomatic patient when splenomegaly or hematologic abnormalities are found during a routine physical examination. Usually, however, the patient is admitted with malaise, pallor, weight loss, and fatigue as a result of anemia and frequently an increased metabolic rate. Bone pain caused by replacement of the normal marrow components by an overgrowth of leukemic cells may occur. The lower half of the sternum is a characteristic site, and tenderness is often found there. Splenomegaly is the most common physical finding and may be accompanied by hepatomegaly. The spleen may enlarge to fill half the abdomen, resulting in increased abdominal girth. By compressing the stomach, splenomegaly results in a feeling of gastric fullness and anorexia. Enlargement of the lymph

Table 2-4. Differences between adult and juvenile forms of chronic granulocytic leukemia*

	Adult	Juvenile
Age of onset	Usually more than 2 years	Usually less than 2 years
Physician findings		
Facial rash	Absent	Present
Lymphadenopathy	Occasional	Frequent, with tendency to suppuration
Splenomegaly	Marked	Variable
Hemorrhagic manifestations	Absent	Frequent
Hematologic findings*		
White blood cell count at onset	Usually $>100 \times 10^9$/liter	Usually $<100 \times 10^9$/liter
Monocytosis of peripheral blood and bone marrow	Absent	Usually present[26]
Eosinophilia and basophilia	Common	Uncommon
Thrombocytopenia	Uncommon at onset	Frequent at onset
Red blood cell abnormalities		
Ineffective erythropoiesis	Absent	Present
I antigen on red blood cell	Normal	Reduced
Fetal hemoglobin level	Normal	15%-50%
Normoblasts in peripheral blood	Unusual	Frequent
Other laboratory findings		
Chromosome studies	Ph[1] chromosome positive	Ph[1] chromosome negative
Urinary and serum muramidase levels	Slightly elevated	Markedly elevated
Immunologic abnormalities	None	Strikingly high immunoglobulin levels, high incidence of antinuclear antibodies (52%) and anti-IgG antibodies (43%)
Nature of colonies produced in vitro from peripheral blood	Predominantly granulocytic	Almost exclusively monocytic
Response to busulfan	Uniformly good	Poor
Median survival	2½ to 3 years	Less than 9 months

From Baehner, R.L.: Hematologic malignancies: leukemia and lymphoma. In Miller, D.R., and others: Smith's blood disorders of infancy and childhood, St. Louis, 1978, The C.V. Mosby Co.
*Both forms have low alkaline phosphatase levels in blood neutrophils.

nodes is rare in the chronic phase of the disease.

Laboratory findings include a marked leukocytosis with WBC counts usually greater than 50,000/mm³. A differential count reveals that these cells represent all stages of development of the granulocyte (myeloid) series, from the most immature myeloblasts to normal, mature polymorphonuclear leukocytes. Rarely, an increase in the basophilic and eosinophilic granulocyte count may be observed and is generally regarded as a poor prognostic sign. Platelet counts may be normal or elevated, and a mild anemia is usually present.

Bone marrow examinations reveal a hypercellular marrow overpopulated with granulocytes in all stages of development. The granulocyte/erythroid ratio is 10:1 to 50:1 rather than the usual 2:1 to 5:1. If peripheral blood eosinophil, basophil, or platelet counts are elevated, these cells and their precursors are also increased in the bone marrow.

Because of rapid cell turnover, levels of uric acid in blood and urine may be elevated even before treatment. Granulocyte destruction may also lead to highly elevated levels of vitamin B₁₂ because of their release of transcobalamin I, the serum carrier of vitamin B₁₂. Leukocyte alkaline phosphatase (LAP), an enzyme found in granulocytes, is very low in CML and may help to distinguish it from other disorders in which there is a marked leukocytosis, such as infection or polycythemia vera.

The most characteristic finding in CML, however, is the Philadelphia chromosome (Fig. 2-4).

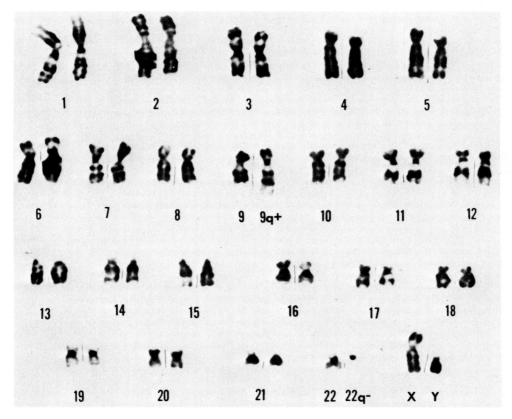

Fig. 2-4. Philadelphia chromosome in CML exemplifying deletion of long arm of chromosome 22, which has translocated to chromosome 9.

This is the result of a deletion in the long arm of chromosome 22, which becomes translocated to another chromosome, usually chromosome 9. This anomaly is found in 80% to 90% of all patients with CML. Patients without the Philadelphia chromosome have a very different clinical course and a poorer response to therapy, and it has even been suggested that it be considered a separate disease.[93] Presence of the Philadelphia chromosome appears to be an acquired trait, since only the affected member of a pair of identical twins, in which one developed CML, had the abnormal chromosome.[94] The abnormality is seen in 90% to 100% of all dividing cells in the granulocyte series, suggesting that the leukemia derives from the malignant transformation of a single clone.

Course and treatment. CML usually progresses through three distinct phases. The preclinical stage, which may last months to years, is characterized only by subtle hematologic abnormalities, such as slight leukocytosis with a left shift and decreased LAP activity. Patients at this stage are asymptomatic but may be discovered on routine examination. In the chronic phase, typical signs and symptoms of CML have developed. With therapy the patients average a remission of 1 to 4 years, after which they inevitably undergo a transition to an acute phase of disease called the blast crisis. This phase is very refractory to treatment with a median survival of less than 12 months.

The prognosis of CML has not changed appreciably in over 80 years. This stems partially from the ease with which remission is obtained and the general well-being of patients in the chronic phase of disease if it is well controlled. However, almost all patients eventually undergo a blast crisis and no therapy has proved effective in either treating this phase or preventing its occurrence. The median survival of 40 to 50 months from diagnosis was once very favorable in comparison to that of ALL and AML. However, advances in the treatment of these diseases with no corresponding advancement in therapy of CML has now reversed the situation.

Irradiation of the spleen was the standard treatment of CML for many years. It is very effective in rapidly reducing splenomegaly, lowering the leukocyte count, and alleviating symptoms. It is currently used only when rapid reduction in splenic size is essential.

Today, chemotherapy is the mainstay of treatment, and busulfan (Myleran) has been the most useful drug. A study of 102 randomized patients showed busulfan therapy to be better than irradiation in controlling signs and symptoms of disease and in the lack of adverse side effects.[95] Median survival of the group treated with busulfan was 1 year longer than that treated with irradiation. The goal of therapy is to control the abnormal granulocyte proliferation. Busulfan is an alkylating agent that acts at the level of precursor cells in the marrow. For this reason, its effects are not seen until 10 to 14 days after treatment is begun, and WBC counts may continue to drop for 2 to 3 weeks after treatment is stopped. Once a WBC of 10,000 to 20,000/mm^3 is achieved, therapy should be discontinued, since bone marrow depression, especially thrombocytopenia, may occur. Other adverse effects of busulfan are pulmonary fibrosis, which is rare, and increased skin pigmentation. Hydration and treatment with allopurinol before chemotherapy is important to prevent the effects of hyperuricemia following destruction of the granulocyte pool.

Other chemotherapeutic agents, such as dibromomannitol, 6-mercaptopurine, and hydroxyurea, are also successful at inducing and maintaining remission of the chronic phase of CML and may have some advantages in select patients. However, none of these drugs has proved superior to busulfan in terms of preventing blast crisis or median survival time.[96]

Splenectomy has also been used in the treatment of CML. Its use in patients with hypersplenism or refractory splenomegaly may result in clinical and hematologic improvement. However, a high operative mortality in patients with rapidly progressive disease mitigates against splenectomy.[97] Elective splenectomy has been suggested as a means of preventing or delaying the onset of blast crisis, since it is felt that the spleen may be the site where this metamorphosis occurs. A recent study, however, showed that in a group of 189 patients randomized to splenectomy or no splenectomy, median survival was the same in the two groups as a whole or in several subgroups based on clinical presentation.[98]

It is important to note that even following reduction of the WBC count to normal levels with busulfan, the majority of bone marrow cells remain Philadelphia chromosome positive. Thus the patient is not in a true remission but functions with a malignant population of granulocytes. This suggests that elimination of all cells containing the Philadelphia chromosome may result in a cure. Various drugs have been used in this regard, including busulfan, 6-thioguanine, ara-C, and vincristine. However, reduction in the number of Philadelphia chromosome positive cells is still often incomplete and difficult to maintain, and patients are subject to hemorrhage and infection following bone marrow hypoplasia. An alternative approach is the combination of aggressive chemotherapy and total body irradiation followed by bone marrow transplantation. Four patients who underwent transplantation were found to be completely free of Philadelphia chromosome positive cells for up to 31 months after transplantation.[99]

Acute phase. Virtually 100% of CML patients who do not succumb to intercurrent illness or the adverse effects of treatment will eventually enter blast crisis. Early manifestations are malaise, fatigue, weight loss, recurrence of splenomegaly, and the appearance of lymphadenopathy. This is accompanied by slowly decreasing red blood cell and platelet counts and neutropenia. Eventually, overt involvement of the blood and bone marrow with leukemic blasts is evident. Varying degrees of myelofibrosis and extension of the tumor to the skin, lymph nodes, CNS, and other sites may be present. In 70% of the patients the blasts have a myeloid morphology and resemble AML. However, remission is much more difficult to maintain compared

with patients with AML, and the median survival time is only several months. In 20% to 30% of patients the blasts have a lymphoblastic morphology, contain the enzyme TdT, and are positive for the common ALL antigen, thus resembling ALL. Although these patients are more responsive to therapy with vincristine and prednisone, this remission usually only lasts for 8 to 10 months.

Juvenile CML. Juvenile CML is a rare disease, with less than 100 cases reported. Signs and symptoms include lymphadenopathy, hemorrhage as a result of thrombocytopenia, variable splenomegaly, and an erythematous facial rash. The blood and bone marrow show an increase in myeloid cells consisting of granulocytes and monocytes. The peripheral WBC is usually less than 100,000/mm³. A mild anemia is usually present and is associated with various red blood cell abnormalities, including an increase in the amount of fetal hemoglobin. A polyclonal elevation of immunoglobulin levels is found in about half the cases. The Philadelphia chromosome is not seen in patients with juvenile CML. The disease follows a relentless course and is extremely resistant to conventional forms of treatment. A recent study of 38 children with juvenile CML revealed a median survival time of 16 months.[100] Especially poor prognosis was associated with age greater than 2 years, hepatomegaly, bleeding and thrombocytopenia, and high numbers of blasts in the peripheral blood.

CASE STUDY

C.P. is a 5-year-old boy who initially had a 2-week history of headache, low-grade fever, and multiple bruises without obvious trauma. A complete blood count done at the local pediatrician's office revealed a WBC count of 11,000/mm³ with 40% blast cells in the differential, a hemoglobin of 8 g/dl, and a platelet count of 15,000/mm³.

The patient was transferred to a major medical center. C.P. was accompanied by both parents and was alert and playful. Physical examination revealed shoddy cervical lymphadenopathy, with the spleen 2 cm and a liver 3 cm below the left and right costal margins, respectively. Ecchymoses were found on all four extremities.

The complete blood count now revealed a WBC count of 10,500/mm³ with 55% blasts, 40% lymphocytes, 9% neutrophils, and 1% eosinophils. The hemoglobin was 8.2 g/dl, and the platelets were 17,500/mm³. On the same day a lumbar puncture and a bone marrow examination were performed. The bone marrow was hypercellular with 85% blasts of LI, FAB morphology. Sudan black and myeloperoxidase stains were negative, whereas the PAS was positive. Immunoglobulin guides revealed cells to be positive for common ALL and Ia antigen and negative for surface membrane immunoglobulin and T cell–specific antigen. The lumbar puncture did not reveal any blast cells or an increase in the number of normal cells, and the protein and glucose were in normal limits. A chest x-ray examination and intravenous pyelogram with negative for evidence of leukemia. The patient's blood chemistries were normal except for an elevated LDH. C.P. was diagnosed with non-T, non-B acute lymphoblastic leukemia. Treatment was initiated with vincristine 2 mg/m² and prednisone 60 mg/m².

NURSING CONSIDERATIONS

The nurse is the member of the health team who is with the child and the family most frequently and is in the best position to evaluate their changing needs. From initial diagnosis through discontinuation of therapy, which may or may not include the dying process, the nurse is the coordinator of all aspects of the patient's care. To meet this challenge the nurse must first understand the pathogenesis of leukemia. The nurse should be present with the child, family, and physician when prognosis and treatment plan are discussed so that the nurse may review all or part of this information as needed and identify any misconceptions. A care plan should be developed that includes daily teaching during the initial hospitalization, as well as with each subsequent visit. With a better understanding of leukemia and its side effects, the patient will be better able to cope and adjust to the impact of cancer in his or her life-style. The nurse should also involve other members of the health team, including the social worker, child life specialist, clergy, or nutritionist as needed.

The most common side effects of leukemia and its treatment are those that affect the hematopoietic system: neutropenia, thrombocytopenia, and anemia. The side effects are caused by either tumor cells in the bone marrow as in initial diagnosis or relapse or myelosuppression following intensive chemotherapy.

Neutropenia, a decrease in granulocytes, will put the child at a greater risk for infection. Close observation for signs of infection by assessing the child's mouth, skin puncture sites, and rectum should be performed. Good mouth and skin care should be encouraged. Only oral or axillary temperature should be taken. A fever over 101° F or 38.3° C requires that a sepsis workup be implemented and the administration of broad-spectrum antibiotics be started (see Chapter 24 on infections). Cultures of the blood, urine, nasopharynx, and other questionable sites should be obtained along with a chest x-ray film. Controversy around granulocyte transfusions varies with each institution and is further discussed in Chapter 24.

Bleeding resulting from thrombocytopenia may occur either spontaneously or after trauma. Pressure should be applied for at least 10 minutes after venipuncture, bone marrow aspiration, intravenous line discontinuation, or any other time the skin is punctured. Soft sponge toothettes along with good mouth care should be used to cleanse the mouth and teeth. Urine, stool, emesis, and sputum should be examined for blood. If epistaxis occurs, the child should be in an upright position and pressure applied to the bridge of the nose for 10 minutes. The nose may be packed with gel foam with epinephrine if the bleeding continues despite pressure. Platelets should be administered for active bleeding during thrombocytopenia. Any increase in petechiae or hematomas should be reported immediately.

Weakness, fatigue, pallor, shortness of breath, headache, tachycardia, tachypnea, or orthostatic hypotension can be signs of anemia. Depending on the severity, anemia is treated with a blood transfusion. Thorough observation of these signs and symptoms and prompt reporting will enable the child to be treated in accordance with the criteria of each institution. Usually after the transfusion, the patient looks and feels better.

The child will continue to need support throughout and beyond the treatment period. Chapter 27, "Impact of Cancer," discusses issues at specific developmental stages that must be addressed with each child. It also looks at issues such as the adolescent's difficulty in dealing with the loss of hair and weight gain versus the young child's fear of leukemia being punishment for something done wrong. The family and child require continued support after the child's therapy has been discontinued. Chapter 28, "Crisis Points in Cancer," addresses the issues concerning discontinuing therapy, along with relapse and end stage disease.

Great strides have been made in improving the outlook for a child with leukemia. Newer chemotherapeutic regimens have lead to significant decreases in the mortality of this disease. Improvement in the general supportive care of children with leukemia, including blood and platelet transfusions, aggressive control of infection, and the use of improved venous access devices, have led to better general well-being of the patient during chemotherapy. The increasing use of home care has also improved the quality of life for these patients during therapy.

Advances in several areas will continue to improve the outlook for a child with leukemia. Newer and more specific chemotherapy will continue to be evaluated. Advances in DNA technology and molecular biology are beginning to improve our understanding of the etiologic origins of these diseases. Genetic engineering may become a viable form of treatment for leukemia and other diseases in the near future. Advances in immunology have also contributed to improvements in the diagnosis and management of leukemia. Monoclonal antibodies have become an important tool in the classification of the disease and may in the future be an effective leukemia-specific agent in the treatment of this disease. Improvements in allogeneic and syngeneic bone marrow transplants will also improve the outlook for some children with leukemia. Professionals involved in the care of the child with leukemia have a much more optimistic attitude than was possible two decades ago.

NURSING CARE PROTOCOL FOR THE CHILD WITH NEWLY DIAGNOSED LEUKEMIA

Nursing diagnoses (problems/needs)	Goals/objectives (patient/family will:)	Interventions (nurse will:)
1. Knowledge deficit (related to the diagnosis of leukemia)	Understand treatment management and major precautions for the child with leukemia	Discuss disease process and its treatment in detail with pediatric oncology team Daily review questions regarding the child's progress Reemphasize information the oncologist has given family Discuss precautions necessary for the child

Continued.

Nursing diagnoses (problems/needs)	Goals/objectives (patient/family will:)	Interventions (nurse will:)
2. Knowledge deficit (need for information related to chemotherapy)	Be able to state names of drugs, amounts to be taken at home, and broad purpose Identify expected side effects (early) and proper methods for follow-up Have side effects within expected limits and control; demonstrate absence of complications	Evaluate level of understanding and teach accordingly; document teaching and evaluation Teach, evaluate, and document side effects related to chemotherapy (see Chapter 20); emphasize needs for precautionary measures when counts are low (e.g., stay away from crowds, call for fever over 101° F; do not manipulate the rectum)
	Have minimum late side effects; compliance with follow-up care to allow for prompt recognition and treatment of late side effects	(See Chapter 20 for further nursing implications) Teach importance of return visits for follow-up; observe carefully for possible late effects Stress good general and dental hygiene
3. Anxiety (emotional distress related to diagnosis, testing, possible hospitalization, treatment, and side effects)	Have decreased anxiety Express feelings regarding diagnosis	Encourage verbalization of fears and concerns Contact other health professionals as necessary Encourage family to explore support groups and other resources available
4. Injury: potential for (infection)	Detect signs and symptoms of infection Minimize risks and complications of infections	Assess daily: mouth for ulcerations and redness; skin punctures for edema, redness; anal region for fissures or breakdown; auscultate lungs Check temperature every 4 hr and record; report immediately: temperature greater than 38.3° C, changes in depth and rate of respiration, dysuria, cloudy or foul smelling urine

Nursing diagnoses (problems/needs)	Goals/objectives (patient/family will:)	Interventions (nurse will:)
		Assist in sepsis workup if fever occurs: blood cultures, throat cultures, urine culture, chest x-ray (CXR) Initiate antibiotics per physician order and continue with strict adherence to schedule (initiating antibiotics on neutropenic patient with suspicion of sepsis should be considered an emergency procedure; initial doses should be administered immediately) Administer acetaminophen (Tylenol) for fever as ordered; initiate tepid sponging if does not respond within 30 min or if temperature is greater than 40° C (104° F)
5. Injury: potential for (bleeding)	Detect signs of active bleeding Maintain precautions to prevent bleeding	Do not perform intramuscular injections Put pressure at each puncture site for at least 5 to 10 min Use toothettes to clean mouth and teeth Check urine, emesis, and stools for blood every shift Record new areas of petechiae and ecchymosis If epistaxis occurs, set child up and hold bridge of nose for 10 min; nose may need to be packed with gel foam soaked in epinephrine If platelets are ordered, assess vital signs and patient closely for reaction Take precautions against head injury

Continued.

NURSING CARE PROTOCOL FOR THE CHILD WITH NEWLY
DIAGNOSED LEUKEMIA—cont'd

Nursing diagnoses (problems/needs)	Goals/objectives (patient/family will:)	Interventions (nurse will:)
6. Injury: potential for (kidney damage following rapid destruction of leukemic cells)	Prevent metabolic imbalance	Ensure adequate hydration with ordered IV fluids (1½ × maintenance) Administer allopurinol on schedule (Lysis of leukemia cells causes increased uric acid which can cause kidney impairment) Maintain strict intake and output (I & O) Obtain daily weights. Daily review: lytes, blood urea nitrogen, creatinine, and uric acid Force PO fluids
7. Coping (ineffective, individual)	Prevent developmental delays	Discuss with family importance of continuing usual discipline; endeavor to keep child on usual routines for nap, arousal, bedtime, and meals as much as possible Encourage daily school for children of age Make daily trips to playroom Provide stimulus at bedside: favorite toys, mobiles if appropriate age, books, picture
8. Knowledge deficit (related discharge and subsequent management at home)	Adequate management of the child at home	Review considerations for home care emphasizing major areas of concern: fever, bleeding, and change in behavior
	Prevention of complications caused by lack of knowledge	Review medications to be given at home

NURSING CARE PROTOCOL FOR THE CHILD WITH NEWLY
DIAGNOSED LEUKEMIA—cont'd

Nursing diagnoses (problems/needs)	Goals/objectives (patient/family will:)	Interventions (nurse will:)
9. Coping, ineffective family: compromised	Develop adequate coping mechanisms	Explain all procedures in detail; allow for verbalization of fears and frustrations
	Display basic understanding of leukemia	Use play therapy to allow patient to express fears 1. Read *You and Leukemia* with child 2. Perform procedures on doll with child 3. Make a doctor's kit 4. Take daily walk with child Support parents Make use of social worker's services daily If possible, do not allow venipunctures at the younger child's bedside

REFERENCES

1. Miller, D.R.: Acute lymphoblastic leukemia, Pediatr. Clin. North Am. **27**:269, 1980.
2. Cory, S.: Oncogenes and B-lymphocyte neoplasia, Immunology Today **4**:1, 1983.
3. Heath, C.W., Jr., and Hasterlik, R.J.: Leukemia among children in a suburban community, Am. J. Med. **34**:796, 1963.
4. Clemmesen, J.: On the epidemiology of leukemia. In Clenton, F.J., Crowther, D., and Malpas, J.S., editors: Advances in acute leukemia, New York, 1974, American Elsevier Publishing Co., Inc.
5. Brill, A.B., Tomonaga, M., and Heyssel, R.M.: Leukemia in man following exposure to ionizing radiation, Ann. Intern. Med. **56**:590, 1962.
6. Murray, R., Heckel, P., and Hepelmann, L.H.: Leukemia in children exposed to ionizing radiation, N. Engl. J. Med. **261**:585, 1959.
7. Court, Brown, W.M., and Doll, R.: Mortality from cancer and other causes after radiotherapy for ankylosing spondylitis, Br. Med. J. **2**:1327, 1965.
8. Bizzozero, O.J., Jr., Johnson, K.G., and Ciocco, A.: Radiation-related leukemia in Hiroshima and Nagasaki 1946-64. I. Distribution, incidence and appearance time, N. Engl. J. Med. **274**:1095, 1966.
9. Vigliani, E., and Sarta, G.: Benzene and leukemia, N. Engl. J. Med. **271**:872, 1964.
10. Cadman, E.C., Capizzi, R.L., and Bertino, J.R.: Acute nonlymphocytic leukemia: a delayed complication of Hodgkin's disease therapy, Cancer **40**:1280, 1977.
11. Schwartz, A.D., Lee, H., and Baum, E.S.: Leukemia in children with Wilms' tumor, J. Pediatr. **87**:374, 1975.
12. Cameron, S.: Chlorambucil and leukemia, N. Engl. J. Med. **296**:1065, 1977.
13. Nora, A.H., Nora, J.J., and Fernbach, D.J.: Hereditary predisposition to leukemia. In Proceedings of the International Congress of the Twelfth International Society of Hematology, New York, 1968.
14. Miller, R.W.: Persons with exceptionally high risk of leukemia, Cancer Res. **27**:2420, 1967.
15. LoGalbo, P.R., and others: Association of certain Ia allodeterminants with susceptibility to Hodgkin's disease, Ann. Clin. Res. **31**:478A, 1983.

16. Nunez-Roldan, A., and others: Association of certain Ia allotypes with the occurrence of chronic lymphocytic leukemia: recognition by a monoclonal anti-Ia reagent of a susceptibility determinant not in the DR series, J. Exp. Med. **156**(6):1872, 1983.

17. George, S.L., and others: Factors influencing survival in pediatric acute leukemia: the SWCCSG experience 1958-1970, Cancer **32**:1542, 1973.

18. Miller, D.R., and others: Prognostic factors and therapy in acute lymphoblastic leukemia of childhood: CCG -141, Cancer **51**:1041, 1983.

19. Bennett, J.M., and others: Proposals for the classification of acute leukemias: French-American-British (FAB) Cooperative Group, Br. J. Haematol. **33**:451, 1976.

20. Metzgar, R.S., and others: Distribution of common acute lymphoblastic leukemia: antigens in non-hematopoietic tissues, J. Exp. Med. **154**:1249, 1981.

21. Reinberz, E.L., and others: Discrete stages of human intrathymic differentiation: analysis of normal thymocytes and leukemic lymphoblasts of T lineage, Proc. Natl. Acad. Sci. **77**:1958, 1980.

22. Baehner, R.L.: Hematologic malignancies: leukemia and lymphoma. In Miller, D.R., and others, editors: Smith's blood diseases of infancy and childhood, ed. 5, St. Louis, 1984, The C.V. Mosby Co.

23. Thomas, L.B., and others: The skeletal lesions of acute leukemia, Cancer **14**:608, 1961.

24. Third International Workshop: July 21-25, 1980, Cancer Genet. Cytogenet. **4**:95-142, 1981.

25. Sandberg, A.A.: The chromosomes in human cancer and leukemia, New York, 1980, Elsevier North-Holland, Inc.

26. Freeman, A.I.: Childhood acute lymphocytic leukemia progress and prospects, Wayne, N.J., 1983, Lederle Laboratories.

27. Sallan, S.E., and others: Cell surface antigens: prognostic implications in childhood acute lymphoblastic leukemia, Blood **55**:395, 1980.

28. Simone, J.V.: Outlook for acute lymphocytic leukemia in children in 1982, Ann. Rev. Med. **32**:207, 1981.

29. Pullen, D.J., and others: ALinC 13 classification protocol for acute lymphoblastic leukemia, characterization of immunologic phenotypes and correlation with treatment results: a Pediatric Oncology Group study. Presented at St. Jude's Children's Research Hospital International Symposium on Leukemia Cell Biology and Therapy (5/19 to 22/82). Murphy, S., and Gilbert, J., editors: Elsevier, North Holland, Excerpta Medica Publishers, New York (in press).

30. Pullen, D.J., and others: Southwest Oncology Group experience with immunologic phenotyping in acute lymphocytic leukemia of childhood, Cancer Res. **41**:4802, 1981.

31. Henderson, E.S.: Clinical diagnosis. In Gunz, F.W., and Henderson, E.S., editors: Leukemia, New York, 1983, Grune & Stratton, Inc.

32. Vogler, L.B., and others: Pre-B cell leukemia: a new phenotype of childhood lymphoblastic leukemia, N. Engl. J. Med. **298**:872, 1978.

33. Crist, W., and others: Pre-B cell leukemia responds poorly to treatment: a Pediatric Oncology Group study, Blood **63**:407, 1984.

34. Cangir, A., George, S., and Sullivan, M.: Unfavorable prognosis of acute leukemia in infancy, Cancer **36**:1973, 1975.

35. Pullen, D.J., and others: Modified LSA$_2$-L$_2$ treatment on 53 children with E-rosette-positive T-cell leukemia: results and prognostic factors (a Pediatric Oncology Group Study), Blood **60**:1159, 1982.

36. George, S.L., and others: Factors influencing survival in pediatric acute leukemia: the SWCCSG experience 1958-1970, Cancer **32**:1542, 1973.

37. Gaddy, D.S., and Wood, A.: Cancer in children: the leukemias. In Fochtman, D., and Foley, G.V., editors: Nursing care of the child with cancer, Boston, 1982, Little, Brown & Co.

38. Freeman, A.I., and others: Comparison of intermediate-dose methotrexate with cranial irradiation for the post-induction treatment of acute lymphocytic leukemia in children, N. Engl. J. Med. **308**:477-484, 1983.

39. Sullivan, M.P.: Equivalence of intrathecal chemotherapy and radiotherapy as central nervous system prophylaxis in children with acute lymphocytic leukemia: a Pediatric Oncology Group study, Blood **60**:948, 1982.

40. Wells, R.J., Weetman, R.M., and Bachner, R.L.: The impact of isolated central nervous system relapse following initial complete remission in childhood acute lymphocytic leukemia, J. Pediatr. **97**:429, 1980.

41. Inati, A., and others: Efficacy and morbidity of central nervous system "prophylaxis" in childhood acute lymphoblastic leukemia: eight years' experience with cranial irradiation and intrathecal methotrexate, Blood **61**:297, 1983.

42. Nesbit, M., and others: Evaluation of long-term survivors of childhood acute lymphoblastic leukemia (ALL), Proc. Am. Assoc. Cancer Res. **23**:107, 1982.

43. Nesbit, M.E., and others: Testicular relapse in childhood acute lymphoblastic leukemia: association with pretreatment patient characteristics and treatment: a report for Children's Cancer Group, Cancer **45**:2009, 1980.

44. Land, V.J., and others: Long-term survival in childhood acute leukemia, late relapses, Med. Pediatr. **7**:9, 1979.

45. Wong, K., and others: Clinical and occult testicular leukemia in long-term survivors of acute lymphoblastic leukemia, J. Pediatr. **96**:569, 1980.

46. Kuo, T.I., Tschang, T.P., and Chu, J.Y.: Testicular relapse in childhood acute lymphocytic leukemia during bone marrow remission, Cancer **38**:2604, 1976.

47. Van Eys, J., and Sullivan, M.P.: Testicular leukaemia and temperature, Lancet **2**:256, 1976.

48. Blatt, J., Poplack, D.G., and Sherins, R.J.: Testicular function in boys after chemotherapy for acute lymphoblastic leukemia, N. Engl. J. Med. **304:**1121, 1981.

49. Bowman, W.P., and others: Isolated testicular relapse in acute lymphoblastic leukemia of childhood: categories and influence on survival, J. Clin. Oncol. **2:**924, 1984.

50. Kaj, H., and Rankin, A.: Testicular irradiation in leukemia, Lancet **2:**1115, 1981.

51. Sullivan, M.P., and Hrgovck, M.: Extramedullary leukemia. In Sutow, W.W., Vietti, T.J., and Fernbach, D.J., editors: Clinical pediatric oncology, ed. 2, 1977, St. Louis, The C.V. Mosby Co.

52. Himelstein-Braw, R., Peters, H., and Farber, M.: Morphological study of the ovaries of leukemic children, Br. J. Cancer **38:**82, 1978.

53. Cecalupo, A.J., Lawrence, S.F., and Sullivan, M.P.: Pelvic and ovarian extramedullary leukemic relapse in young girls, Cancer **50:**587, 1982.

54. Chu, J.Y., and others: Ovarian tumor as manifestation of relapse in acute lymphoblastic leukemia, Cancer **48:**377, 1981.

55. Zarrouk, S.O., and others: Leukemic involvement of the ovaries in childhood lymphocytic leukemia, J. Pediatr. **100:**422, 1982.

56. Frei, E., III, and others: The effectiveness of combinations of antileukemic agents inducing and maintaining remission in children with acute leukemia, Blood **26:**642, 1965.

57. Selawry, O.S., and Frei, E., III: Prolongation of remission in acute lymphocytic leukemia, Br. J. Haematol. **32:**465, 1976.

58. Ortega, J.A., and others: L-asparaginase, vincristine and prednisone for induction of first remission in acute lymphocytic leukemia, Cancer Res. **57:**535, 1977.

59. Jones, B., and others: Optimal use of L-asparaginase (NSC-109229) in acute lymphocytic leukemia, Med. Pediatr. Oncol. **3:**387, 1977.

60. Haghbin, M.: Chemotherapy of acute lymphoblastic leukemia in children, Am. J. Hematol. **1:**201, 1976.

61. Aur, R., and others: Multiple combination therapy for childhood acute lymphocytic leukemia, N. Engl. J. Med. **291:**1230, 1974.

62. Henzi, G., and others: Treatment strategy for different risk groups in childhood acute lymphoblastic leukemia: a report from the BFM study group. In Neth, R., and others, editors: Haematology and blood transfusion: modern trends in human leukemia IV, vol. 26, Berlin, 1981, Springer-Verlag.

63. Lay, H.N., Ekest, H., and Colebatch, J.H.: Combination chemotherapy in children with ALL who failed to respond to standard remission induction therapy, Cancer **36:**1220, 1975.

64. Rivera, G., and others: Combined VM-26 and cytosine arabinoside in treatment of refractory childhood lymphocytic leukemia, Cancer **45:**1284, 1980.

65. Komp, D.M., and others: CNS prophylaxis in acute lymphoblastic leukemia: comparison of two methods: a Southwest Oncology Group study, Cancer **50:**1031, 1982.

66. Freeman, A.I., and others: Comparison of intermediate dose methotrexate (IDM) with cranial radiation (CRT) in acute lymphocytic leukemia (ALL), Proc. A.S.C.D. **1:**130, 1982.

67. Haghbon, M., and others: Intensive chemotherapy in children with acute lymphoblastic leukemia (L-2 Protocol), Cancer **33:**1491, 1974.

68. Henderson, G.S.: Acute lymphocytic leukemia. In Gunz, F.W., and Henderson, E.S., editors: Leukemia, New York, 1983, Grune & Stratton, Inc.

69. Aur, R.J.A., and others: Childhood acute lymphocytic leukemia: study VIII, Cancer **42:**2123, 1978.

70. Aur, R.J.A., and others: Comparison of two methods of preventing central nervous system leukemia, Blood **42**(3):349, 1973.

71. Goff, J.R., Anderson, H.R., and Cooper, P.F.: Distractibility and memory deficits in long-term survivors of acute lymphocytic leukemia, Dev. Behav. Pediatr. **1**(4):158, 1980.

72. George, S.L., and others: A reappraisal of the results of stopping therapy in childhood leukemia, N. Engl. J. Med. **300:**269, 1979.

73. Sather, H., and others: Disappearance of the predictive value of prognostic variables in childhood acute lymphoblastic leukemia: a report from Children's Cancer Study Group, Cancer **48:**370, 1981.

74. Stimone, J.V., and Rivera, G.: Management of acute leukemia. In Sutow, W.W., Vietti, T.J., and Fernbach, D.J., editors: Clinical pediatric oncology, ed. 3, St. Louis, 1984, The C.V. Mosby Co.

75. Rivera, G., and others: Prolonged second marrow remission in children with lymphocytic leukemia (ALL) treated with VM-26 and cytosine arabinoside (ARA-C), Proc AACR/ASCO **22:**481, 1981.

76. Johnson, F.L., and others: A comparison of marrow transplantation with chemotherapy for children with acute lymphoblastic leukemia in second or subsequent remission, N. Engl. J. Med. **305:**846, 1981.

77. Johnson, F.L., and Thomas, E.D.: Treatment of relapsed acute lymphoblastic leukemia in childhood (letter), N. Engl. J. Med. **310:**263, 1984.

78. Reisner, Y., and others: Transplantation for acute leukemia with HLA-A & B non-identical parental marrow cells fractionated with soybean agglutinin and sheep red blood cells, Lancet **2:**327, 1981.

79. Smithson, W.A., Gilchrist, G.S., and Burgett, E.D., Jr.: Childhood acute lymphocytic leukemia, Cancer **30:**158, 1980.

80. Shen, B.J., and others: Left shift in the peripheral blood count and diagnosis in acute lymphocytic leukemia is significantly correlated with duration of complete remission, Blood **63:**216, 1984.

81. Miller, D.R., and others: Unfavorable prognostic significance of hand mirror cells in childhood acute lymphoblastic leukemia: a report from the Children's Cancer Study Group, Am. J. Dis. Child. **137**:346, 1983.

82. Dampier, C., and Chilcote, R.R.: Acute non-lymphocytic leukemia, Pediatr. Ann. **12**:293, 1983.

83. Coleman, C.N., and others: Hematologic neoplasia in patients treated for Hodgkin's disease, N. Engl. J. Med. **297**:1249, 1977.

84. Kancko, Y., and others: Chromosome pattern in childhood acute non-lymphocytic leukemia (ALL), Blood **60**:389, 1982.

85. Gallo, R.C., and Reitz, M.S., Jr.: Human retrovirus and adult T-cell leukemia-lymphoma, J. Natl. Cancer Inst. **69**:1209, 1982.

86. Pizzo, P.A., Henderson, E.S., and Leventhal, B.G.: Acute myelogenous leukemia in children: a preliminary report of combination chemotherapy, J. Pediatr. **88**:125, 1976.

87. Ellison, R.R., and others: Arabinosyl cytosine: a useful agent in the treatment of acute leukemia in adults, Blood **32**:507, 1968.

88. Preisler, H.D., and others: Treatment of acute nonlymphocytic leukemia: use of anthracycline-cytosine arabinoside induction therapy and a comparison of two maintenance regimens, Blood **53**:455, 1979.

89. Lampkin, B.C., and others: Current status of the biology and treatment of acute non-lymphocytic leukemia in children (report from the ANLL Strategy Group of the Children's Cancer Study Group), Blood **61**:215, 1983.

90. Creutzig, V., and others: Improved treatment results in childhood acute myelogenous leukemia: a report of the German Cooperative Study AML-BFM-78, Blood **65**:298, 1985.

91. Hines, J.D., and others: High-dose cytosine arabinoside and m-AMSA is effective therapy in relapsed acute nonlymphocytic leukemia, J. Clin. Oncol. **2**:545, 1984.

92. Thomas. E.D., and others: Marrow transplanation for acute non-lymphoblastic leukemia in first remission, N. Engl. J. Med. **301**:597, 1979.

93. Barfinkel, L.S., and Bennett, D.E.: Extramedullary myeloblastic transformation in chronic myelocytic leukemia simulation a coexistent malignant lymphoma, Am. J. Pathol. **51**:638, 1969.

94. Bauke, J.: Chronic myelocytic leukemia, Cancer **24**:643, 1969.

95. Medical Research Council: Chronic granulocytic leukemia: comparison of radiotherapy and busulphan therapy, Br. Med. J. **1**:201, 1968.

96. Kaung, D.T., and others: Comparison of busulfan and cyclophosphamide in the treatment of chronic myelogenous leukemia, Cancer **27**:608, 1971.

97. Wolf, D.J., Silver, R.T., and Coleman, M.: Splenectomy in chronic myeloid leukemia, Ann. Intern. Med. **89**:684, 1978.

98. Italian Cooperative Study Group on chronic myeloid leukemia: results of a prospective randomized trial of early splenectomy in chronic myeloid leukemia, Cancer **54**:333, 1984.

99. Fefer, A., and others: Disappearance of Ph-positive cells in four patients with chronic granulocytic leukemia after chemotherapy, irradiation and marrow transplantation from an identical twin, N. Engl. J. Med. **300**:333, 1979.

100. Castro-Malaspina, H., and others: Subacute and chronic myelomonocytic leukemia in children (juvenile CML), Cancer **54**:675, 1984.

CHAPTER 3

Non-Hodgkin's lymphoma

PAT STANFILL and JOHN M. FALLETTA

DEFINITION

The non-Hodgkin's lymphomas (NHL) are solid tumors of the hematopoietic system whose cells of origin represent the malignant counterpart of subclasses of normal lymphocytes.[1] In children the disease tends to disseminate early and is commonly widespread at diagnosis. Because of this dissemination, lymphomas in children must be considered as systemic diseases. Histologically, the lymph node is diffusely involved with malignant lymphoblasts of either T or B cell origin.[1,2]

There are four common types of non-Hodgkin's lymphoma occurring among children and adolescents (Table 3-1 and Fig. 3-1). Lymphoblastic lymphoma is the most common and in its thymic presentation is generally a proliferation of malignant T cells. In its nonthymic presentation it resembles acute lymphoblastic leukemia in its possible range phenotypes.

Undifferentiated lymphoma of the Burkitt's type (BL) is a B cell malignancy characterized by rapid onset of primarily extranodal disease. It is endemic to parts of tropical Africa and New Guinea and occurs sporadically elsewhere in the world. An association between BL and the Epstein-Barr virus has been reported in 95% of the African cases and approximately 15% to 25% of American cases. BL has played an important role in the study of oncogene expression because of the varying immune phenotypes displayed and their characteristic chromosomal translocations. This is the fastest proliferating human tumor, with a cell cycle of 28 hours. Burkitt's lymphoma predominantly affects the abdominal and/or pelvic viscera, retroperitoneal soft tissue, jaw, gonads, and the central nervous system.

Non-Burkitt's type (NB) undifferentiated lymphomas appear to differ from Burkitt's lymphoma only morphologically. BL demonstrates uniform cells with basophilic nucleoli, whereas non-Burkitt's lymphoma cells are more pleomorphic and usually have single eosinophilic nucleoli. Clinical features are almost indistinguishable in these two types of non-Hodgkin's lymphoma.

Large cell lymphomas generally affect older children and adolescents and represent a more heterogeneous group than the first three histologic types. The sites affected by large cell lymphomas vary and may include mediastinal, nodal, and skin tissue or the gastrointestinal tract.

INCIDENCE

Non-Hodgkin's lymphoma is the third most frequent category of malignancies in children and occurs at an annual rate of about 71 million children and adolescents.[3,4] The peak incidence is between the ages of 7 and 11, with 9 years of age as the median.[3] The frequency of occurrence increases with age, especially after the age of 2. There is a 3:1 male to female predominance.

ETIOLOGY

There is no known cause for NHL although several theories link the disease to an impaired immune system. Since NHL is a malignancy of the immune system, and immunodeficient patients have a high risk of developing NHL, lymphoma may arise as a result of excessive antigenic stimulation of an

Table 3-1. Comparison of morphologic, cytochemical, and immunologic features of childhood non-Hodgkin's lymphoma

	Lymphoblastic	Burkitt's	Non-Burkitt's	Large cell
Cytology	L_1* or L_2	L_3	L_3	Variable
Periodic acid–Schiff (PAS) stain	Occasionally positive	Negative	Negative	Ocassionally positive
Methyl green pyronine stain	Weak or focal positive	Strongly positive	Strongly positive	Variable, usually positive
Terminal deoxynucleotidyl transferase	Positive	Negative	Negative	Negative
Immunologic markers	T, pre-B or non-T non-B	B	Usually B; may be non-T non-B, rarely T	Usually B; may be non-T non-B, occasionally T, rarely histiocytic

*French-American-British classification of acute lymphocytic leukemia (ALL).

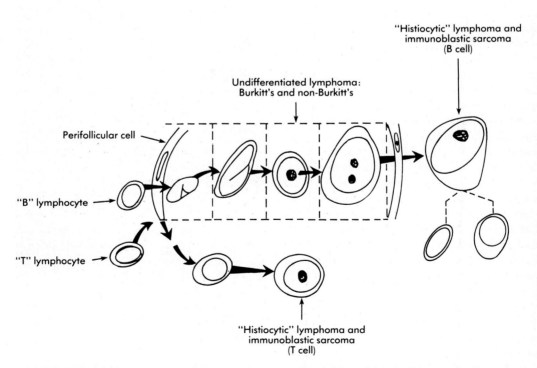

Fig. 3-1. Cytologic types of non-Hodgkin's lymphoma in children. (Courtesy J.J. Butler, MD, and M.P. Sullivan, MD.)

immune system lacking appropriate regulatory controls. Genetic considerations also exist, given that chromosomal anomalies are evident, particularly in Burkitt's lymphomas. Also the marked male predominance of NHL plus the X-linked lymphoproliferative syndrome reports suggest X-linked recessive predisposition.[5] A possible viral cause for some types of NHL is also of intense current interest. In most African children with Burkitt's lymphoma the genome for Epstein-Barr virus is incorporated into the DNA, whereas similar associations are uncommon in American Burkitt's lymphoma.[5]

CLINICAL PRESENTATION

The clinical presentation of non-Hodgkin's lymphoma depends on the site and extent of tumor.[1] Common sites in order of their occurrence are the abdomen, mediastinum, head and neck (Fig. 3-2), and peripheral nodes (Table 3-2). The predominant site of clinically detectable disease is usually extranodal.

An intra-abdominal presentation occurs in about 35% of NHL patients and usually involves the gastrointestinal tract. In favorable cases the tumor is small, involving the intestinal wall, and is detected rapidly when intussusception occurs. Painful attacks of cramping abdominal pain often accompanied by vomiting occur, and complete obstruction of the intestine may follow. Intussusception in children after the age of 2 usually points to a structural defect or a mass. Non-Hodgkin's lymphoma is second only to Meckel's diverticulum as the causative factor. When NHL is more widespread in the abdomen, the presentation involves more diffuse abdominal pain, abdominal distention, and intestinal symptoms. Often children are diagnosed as having appendicitis, and then tumor is found at the time of surgery.

Constipation, an increase in the size of the abdomen caused by ascites, and a decrease in the general health of the child may be presenting symptoms of abdominal NHL. Obstructive jaundice is rare but may occur. As the intra-abdominal tumor grows, widespread dissemination can occur, with bone marrow invasion, pleural effusion, enlarged testes, and peripheral lymphadenopathy.

Children with American Burkitt's lymphoma generally have extensive abdominal disease with or without central nervous system or bone marrow involvement. The pleura, kidneys, and pericardium are often involved. The tumor is rapidly growing, and rarely do symptoms persist longer than 6 to 8 weeks before diagnosis.

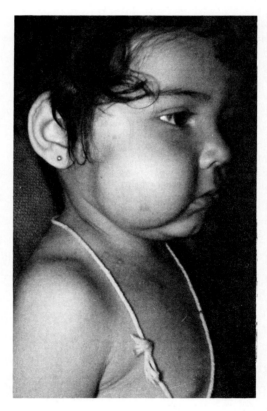

Fig. 3-2. Large soft tissue mass in right cheek, American Burkitt's tumor. (Courtesy Medical Communications, University of Texas, M.D. Anderson Hospital and Tumor Institute.)

Table 3-2. Correlation of primary site of presentation with histologic type*

Lymphoma	Mediastinum	Abdomen	Lymph nodes	Other
Lymphoblastic	63 (81)	8 (6)	27 (37)	38 (30)
Burkitt's	0 (—)	46 (36)	9 (12)	31 (25)
Non-Burkitt's	4 (5)	52 (41)	17 (23)	31 (25)
Large Cell	9 (11)	15 (12)	19 (25)	23 (18)
Other	2 (3)	7 (5)	3 (4)	3 (2)
TOTAL	78 (100)	128 (100)	75 (100)	126 (100)

Modified from data presented in Schweisguth, O.: Solid tumors in children, New York, 1982, John Wiley & Sons.
*Percentages in parentheses.

Mediastinal primary disease occurs in 25% of all cases of non-Hodgkin's lymphoma and generally is a result of lymphoblastic lymphoma (see Table 3-2). The diagnosis of mediastinal NHL is sometimes delayed because the symptoms mimic acute bronchitis. The child experiences a frequent cough and may have transient fever and have increasing respiratory distress. Full jugular veins, facial edema, and significant dyspnea caused by tracheal-bronchial compression follow, focusing attention on the upper thorax as the site of disease. Percussion demonstrates anterior and posterior dullness that leads the examiner to suspect pleural effusion. Cervical and supraclavicular adenopathy may be evident. Thoracentesis, radiation therapy, or other immediate interventions to relieve respiratory distress are indicated to prevent respiratory failure. Other primary sites of lymphomas include the nasopharynx and the peripheral lymph nodes in addition to variable sites grouped as extralymphatic in nature.

DIAGNOSTIC EVALUATION AND STAGING

The diagnosis of non-Hodgkin's lymphoma requires histologic and/or cytologic evidence for the presence of malignant lymphoblasts. Assessment to determine the extent of disease follows. The diagnostic evaluation should include a careful physical examination and detailed history, complete blood count, chest x-ray examination, hepatic and renal function studies, skeletal and skull survey or bone scan, biopsy of accessible clinically abnormal tissue, bone marrow aspiration with biopsy, and lumbar puncture (Table 3-3).[6] These studies are adequate to identify the site and extent of disease and serve as pretreatment baseline values. Additional studies are indicated depending on the site of the disease and whether the disease is determined to be local or disseminated. The clinical differentiation between non-Hodgkin's lymphoma and acute lymphoblastic leukemia (ALL) is sometimes difficult, because NHL may be so widely disseminated at diagnosis. An acceptable method to distinguish NHL from ALL involves the percentage of lymphoblasts in the bone marrow. Bone marrow aspiration in lymphoma demonstrates from zero to 25% lymphoblasts, whereas 25% lymphoblasts or more are seen in acute leukemia.[3]

Intravenous pyelography, contrast studies of the gastrointestinal tract, lymphangiography, ultrasonography, and computerized axial tomography may be appropriate. An exploratory laparotomy to determine extent of disease is unnecessary. The initial workup may be delayed if a life-threatening situation such as intestinal obstruction or respiratory distress is evident on arrival at the treatment center. In this instance prompt therapeutic intervention is essential, and the detailed diagnostic studies are of secondary concern.

The diagnosis of NHL can sometimes be confirmed by the detection of pathologic lymphoblasts in aspirates of bone marrow, ascitic fluid, or pleural fluid. Mediastinal disease is usually accompanied

Table 3-3. Studies used in the diagnosis and staging for non-Hodgkin's lymphoma

Studies	Findings
History and physical examination	Measure all lymph nodes and involved organs to determine extent of disease.
Complete blood count with differential and platelet count	Abnormal count may be a result of bone marrow infiltration.
Serum chemistry: electrolytes, uric acid, creatinine, calcium, phosphorus, bilirubin, alkaline phosphatase, albumin, immunoglobulin quantitation.	Serum chemistry abnormalities occur frequently after rapid cell turnover; increased uric acid, decreased calcium and increased phosphorus are common findings; on implementation of treatment, rapid tumor lysis may occur increasing these abnormalities.
Bone marrow aspirate	May demonstrate bone marrow infiltration.
Cerebral spinal fluid examination	Necessary to determine central nervous system involvement.
Urinalysis	Allows for assessment of kidney function.
Chest x-ray examination	Mediastinal mass may be present.
Abdominal ultrasound on computerized tomographic (CT) scan	May indicate abdominal mass, enlarged lymph nodes, or enlarged organs such as spleen or kidneys.
Bone scan	May be necessary to determine boney involvement.
Other tests recommended dependent on site of presentation	
Coagulation profile	
Intravenous pyelogram	
Liver-spleen scan	
Barium studies of the small and/or large bowel	

Table 3-4. A staging system for childhood non-Hodgkin's lymphoma

Stage I
   A single tumor (extranodal) or single anatomic area (nodal), with the exclusion of mediastinum or abdomen.
Stage II
   A single tumor (extranodal) with regional node involvement.
   Two or more nodal areas on the same side of the diaphragm.
   Two single (extranodal) tumors with or without regional node involvement on the same side of the diaphragm.
   A primary gastrointestinal tract tumor, usually in the ileocecal area, with or without involvement of associated mesenteric nodes only.*
Stage III
   Two single tumors (extranodal) on opposite sides of the diaphragm.
   Two or more nodal areas above and below the diaphragm.
   All the primary intra-thoracic tumors (mediastinal, pleural, thymic).
   All extensive primary intra-abdominal disease.*
   All paraspinal or epidural tumors, regardless of other tumor site(s).
Stage IV
   Any of the above with initial CNS and/or bone marrow involvement.†

From Murphy, S.B., and Donaldson, S.S.: Pediatric lymphoma. In Carter: Principles of cancer treatment, New York, 1982, McGraw-Hill, Inc. With permission.

*A distinction is made between apparently localized GI tract lymphoma versus more extensive intra-abdominal disease because of their quite different pattern of survival after appropriate therapy. Stage II disease typically is limited to a segment of the gut plus or minus the associated mesenteric nodes only, and the primary tumor can be completely removed grossly by segmental excision. Stage III disease typically exhibits spread to para-aortic and retroperitoneal areas by implants and plaques in mesentery or peritoneum, or by direct infiltration of structures adjacent to the primary tumor. Ascites may be present, and complete resection of all gross tumor is not possible.

†If marrow involvement is present initially, the number of abnormal cells must be 25% or less in an otherwise normal marrow aspirate with a normal peripheral blood picture.

Table 3-5. Clinical staging of Burkitt's lymphoma

Stage	Extent of tumor
A	Single extra-abdominal site
B	Multiple extra-abdominal sites
C	Intra-abdominal tumor with involvement of one or more extra-abdominal sites
D	Stage C but greater than 90% of tumor surgically resected

Reprinted by permission of The New England Journal of Medicine. Ziegler, J.L.: N. Engl. J. Med. **305**(13):735, 1981.

by peripheral lymph node enlargement, and the pathologic disease can be confirmed by peripheral lymph node biopsy. However, if no peripheral disease is detectable, involved mediastinal tissue must be obtained for histology, either by mediastinoscopy or thoracotomy.

A variety of NHL staging systems are currently in use, but the one most helpful in children is the system developed by Murphy and Wollner (Table 3-4).[6,7] Burkitt's lymphoma is generally staged according to Ziegler's classification (Table 3-5).[8] Since stage of disease helps define proper therapy in non-Hodgkin's lymphoma, careful attention to the diagnostic workup and accuracy in staging are necessary.

TREATMENT AND MANAGEMENT

An aggressive, multimodal approach using surgical intervention, multiple agent chemotherapy, and involved field radiation is the treatment of choice for NHL. With the knowledge gained through the determination of prognostic factors and the recognition of non-Hodgkin's lymphoma as a systemic disease, each patient's therapy can be individualized. Rapid tumor reduction, selective use of radiation therapy, and central nervous system prophylaxis are all principles of NHL treatment.

Surgical intervention has recently gained a more active role in the management of non-Hodgkin's lymphoma. Lymph node biopsy or biopsy of a mass

as a diagnostic measure, surgical intervention to manage side effects of disease such as obstruction of the intestine, or complete tumor removal without creating functional impairment are examples of the role the surgeon assumes in current therapy. Some surgeons suggest that more aggressive attempts to remove tumor bulk in Burkitt's lymphoma may improve treatment results.

The role of the radiation therapist in the treatment of NHL is controversial at present.[3] The value of radiation therapy in localized disease is under study by the Pediatric Oncology Group. Approaches to therapy include radiation to local disease and total nodal irradiation including the abdomen.

The combined use of several antineoplastic agents with radiation therapy was developed in the early 1970s and is responsible for an improved future for children with non-Hodgkin's lymphoma. A variety of multiagent regimens have been used to treat NHL. Wollner and others[9] reported positive results in a series of 86 children using cyclophosphamide, prednisone, vincristine, daunomycin, and intrathecal methotrexate as induction therapy, with maintenance or oral thioguanine, cyclophosphamide, BCNU, ara-C, vincristine, and oral and intrathecal methotrexate. Toxicity posed a serious problem, and subsequent therapies by others attempted to obtain similar survival rates with less toxicity. Miser reported a 70% disease-free survival rate with a modified approach to therapy based on Wollner's LSA_2L_2 protocol, as did the Pediatric Oncology Group whose reported survival rate was 64%.[10,11]

Chemotherapy regimens in current use for the treatment of NHL vary, but most incorporate high doses of cyclophosphamide and moderate to high doses of methotrexate, adriamycin, vincristine, and prednisone. A complete response is usually noted within 4 to 6 weeks. Maintenance therapy for patients with limited disease (Stage I to II) combines a comparatively simple two- or three-drug combination, often with pulses of more intensive drug cycles.[7] For patients with advanced (Stage III to IV) disease, therapy must be intensive to maintain remission and improve the likelihood of cure. Burkitt's lymphoma generally responds well to chemotherapy, specifically cyclophosphamide, but frequently the tumor reappears in a short period of time.[5]

Central nervous system prophylaxis is recommended for all patients with advanced NHL, including patients with head or neck primaries, mediastinal primaries, and unresectable abdominal disease. Intermittent intrathecal methotrexate with or without cytosine arabinoside is used in an attempt to prevent the usually fatal outcome of central nervous system relapse.

PROGNOSTIC FACTORS

A greater than 60% disease-free survival rate is reported in all non-Hodgkin's lymphoma patients when a multimodal approach is employed.[7] Survival rates before 1970 were less than 20% when localized radiation with or without chemotherapy was the treatment employed. Children with localized disease can expect cure rates approaching 100%.[12]

The use of multiple-drug regimens, first reported in the early 1970s, has significantly contributed to the dramatic advances in cure rates.[8,9] Wollner and others[9] analyzed two groups of patients with regard to primary site, histology, and staging and concluded that the most important prognostic factor was early and aggressive therapy.

There are several other factors considered to be prognostically significant in childhood non-Hodgkin's lymphoma. These include tumor site, origin as lymphatic or extralymphatic, stage, histology, and surface marker status. Extralymphatic tumors arising in the head and neck or peripheral nodes have a more favorable prognosis than lymphatic tumors of the mediastinum or abdomen.[13] The prognosis of children with intra-abdominal tumors is dependent on tumor bulk and resectability.

Stage at diagnosis has been demonstrated to be prognostically significant.[9,14,15] Stage II patients (see Table 3-3) are curable with survival rates approaching 100% when multiagent chemotherapy and radiation are combined.[9] Stage III and IV disease is much less responsive, with 2-year survival rates of approximately 50%.[9]

CASE STUDY

A 10-year-old white male was in good health until he developed anterior chest pain. He was seen by his local physician, who obtained a chest roentgenogram, which was read as normal. Two days later the child developed numbness of the lower lip and then right jaw pain which persisted for about 2 hours. Two weeks later he developed left wrist and forearm pain, followed 1 week later by return of his jaw pain, and his gums began to swell. He had night sweats, a low-grade fever, and a 5-pound weight loss. His teeth started to loosen. An oral surgeon biopsied the right mandibular gingiva, revealing Burkitt's lymphoma.

On physical examination gingival hypertrophy was noted bilaterally, and a 2 by 2 cm purple mass was noted in the second molar area of the palate. The abdominal girth was 55.5 cm at the umbilicus and 59 cm below the xiphoid, well above normal. The abdomen was distended, with prominent veins in the skin. The liver descended 6.5 cm below the right costal margin in the midclavicular line. Cervical lymph node enlargement was noted.

Laboratory values included a white blood cell count of 9700/mm³, hemoglobin of 12.2 g/dl, and a differential count of 78% neutrophils, 17% lymphocytes, and 5% monocytes. Arterial blood gases on room air were pH 7.41, Pco_2, 45.2 mmHg, Po_2 55.5 mm Hg. A chest film demonstrated a left pleural effusion. The bone marrow aspirate revealed 10% tumor cells.

Additional roentgenograms of the sinus and facial bones showed bilateral mandibular bone destruction, bilateral maxillary clouding, and a mass in the right maxillary sinus. The bone scan was normal. An intravenous pyelogram showed delayed and poor function on the right. The left kidney was normal.

A diagnosis was made of non-Hodgkin's lymphoma, Burkitt's type, Stage IV with involvement of the gingiva, maxilla, jaw, cervical lymph nodes, liver, spleen, and bone marrow. In addition, other diagnoses included bilateral alveolar disease of unknown cause, cellulitis of the right thumb with septic shock and *Candida* colonization of throat, sputum, and urine.

The child died 9 months from diagnosis after a stormy course of treatment. Autopsy revealed malignant lymphoma, Burkitt's type, of both jaws with leukemic conversion and involvement of the lymph nodes, bone, chest wall, liver, spleen, pancreas, diaphragm, kidneys, left adrenal gland, and omentum.

NURSING CONSIDERATIONS

The toxicity of therapy employed to treat non-Hodgkin's lymphoma mandates an intensive supportive care regimen. Presenting complaints of respiratory distress or abdominal pain must be immediately assessed and nursing strategies determined while medical or surgical intervention is occurring. A complete assessment of the respiratory status of the child with auscultation, percussion, and observation of general appearance is essential. Evidence of increasing respiratory distress as demonstrated by nasal flaring or chest wall retractions, shortness of breath, pallor, or cyanosis must be reported to the attending physician. An assessment of the abdomen should include presence or absence of bowel sounds, measurement of abdominal girth, elimination patterns, and questions about pain.

The initiation of therapy creates the potential for complications from tumor lysis, with uric acid nephropathy, hypocalcemia, hyperphosphatemia, and renal failure.[5] This syndrome must be avoided by careful attention to the patient's fluid and electrolyte management, the restriction of uric acid formation by allopurinol therapy, and a controlled lysis of tumor by careful introduction of antineoplastic agents. The site of the tumor may also cause compression of vital organs. During induction therapy, infection (either suspected or documented) must be aggressively managed. Frequent transfusions with blood products may be necessary. Maintenance of adequate nutrition, especially in children with a large abdominal mass, is a priority.

The psychosocial support necessary for the child with non-Hodgkin's lymphoma is similar to that for patients with other catastrophic diseases. Support for the child and family during the diagnosis and treatment of the disease is an aspect of the emotional care required to help the child fully recover from the malignancy. The child and family's knowledge of the disease and its treatment will reduce some of their anxiety, and they will be better participants in the recovery process.

Non-Hodgkin's lymphoma requires a multidisciplinary approach to care. If used thoughtfully, this approach increases the probability that the child with NHL will recover fully, both medically and psychologically.

NURSING CARE PROTOCOL FOR THE CHILD WITH NON-HODGKIN'S LYMPHOMA

Nursing diagnoses (problems/needs)	Goals/objectives (patient/family will:)	Interventions (nurse will:)
1. Knowledge deficit (related to diagnostic work-up)	Verbalize purpose of and methods for testing	Assist with and teach regarding workup procedures (physical examination, laboratory work, urine testing, chest x-ray examination, CT scans, skeletal survey and other scans, bone marrow aspirate, lumbar puncture; possible panorex, skull x-ray films, and abdominal CT scan; biopsy)

NURSING CARE PROTOCOL FOR THE CHILD WITH
NON-HODGKIN'S LYMPHOMA—cont'd

Nursing diagnoses (problems/needs)	Goals/objectives (patient/family will:)	Interventions (nurse will:)
2. Anxiety (emotional upset related to diagnosis, testing)	Have decreased level of anxiety	Teach (workup, disease, protocol, definitions of remission and relapse)
	Share feelings with support people	Assist with referrals to other services (chaplain, social work, psychology)
		Use active listening and offer support
		Use therapeutic play
3. Injury: Potential for (kidney damage following rapid destruction of lymphoma cells)	Exhibit metabolic balance	Ensure adequate hydration with ordered IV fluids ($1\frac{1}{2}$ × maintenance)
		Administer allopurinol on schedule. (Lysis of lymphoma cells causes increased uric acid, which can cause kidney impairment)
		Maintain strict I & O
		Weigh patient daily
4. Knowledge deficit (related to therapy)	Be able to state names of drugs, amounts to be taken at home, and broad purpose	Evaluate level of understanding and teach accordingly; document teaching and evaluation
	Identify expected side effects (early) and proper methods of follow-up	Teach, evaluate, and document side effects related to chemotherapy (Chapter 20)
	Have (early) side effects within expected limits and control; demonstrate absence of complications resulting from side effects	Emphasize need for precautionary measures when counts are low because of chemotherapy
		Stress good general and dental hygiene
		Reinforce need for prompt notification of physician for exposure to varicella or herpes zoster in patients who have not had varicella
	Have minimum late side effects; comply with follow-up care to allow for prompt recognition and treatment of late side effects	Teach importance of return visits for follow-up; observe carefully for possible late effects (growth retardation; sterility; secondary malignancies; pulmonary, renal, and hepatic complications)

Continued.

NURSING CARE PROTOCOL FOR THE CHILD WITH
NON-HODGKIN'S LYMPHOMA—cont'd

Nursing diagnoses (problems/needs)	Goals/objectives (patient/family will:)	Interventions (nurse will:)
5. Knowledge deficit (related to radiation therapy)	Be able to state broad purpose of therapy; identify expected side effects and follow-up appropriately; recognize post radiation syndromes	Teach, evaluate, and document information related to radiation therapy
	Have side effects within expected limits and control; absence of complications resulting from side effects	Prevent side effects when possible; carry out nursing and physician orders; instruct patient and parents on specific side effects of drugs
	Have minimum late side effects; comply with follow-up.	Teach importance of follow-up; observe for late effects (dependent on site)
6. Injury: potential for (recurrence and/or metastasis or failure to achieve remission)	Identify signs and symptoms of relapse (return of mass, increased nodes) central nervous system symptoms	Evaluate and document presence of signs and symptoms of relapse; notify physician
	Verbalize understanding of individualized treatment	Teach, evaluate, document
	Develop adequate coping methods in dealing with recurrence or failure to achieve remission	Identify significant others for support
		Initiate nursing care specific to patient needs
		Refer to chaplain or social worker when appropriate
7. Coping: ineffective family: compromised	Be able to cope with adjustment needed and return to maximum functioning	Provide support and teaching; refer as needed; encourage return to school with participation in activities as possible

REFERENCES

1. Schweisguth, O.: Solid tumors in children, New York, 1982, John Wiley & Sons.
2. Wilson, J.F., and others: Studies on the pathology of non-Hodgkin's lymphoma of childhood cancer, Cancer 53(8):1695, 1984.
3. Arenson, E.: Management of childhood non-Hodgkin's lymphoma, Curr. Concepts Oncol. p. 17, Summer 1984.
4. Fernbach, D.J.: Natural history of acute leukemia. In Sutow, W.W., Fernbach, D.J., and Vietti, T.J., editors; Clinical pediatric oncology, St. Louis, 1984, The C.V. Mosby Co.
5. Simone, J.V., Cassady, J.R., and Filler, R.M.: Cancers of childhood. In DeVita, V.T., Hellman, S., and Rosenberg, S., editors: Cancer, principles and practice of oncology, Philadelphia, 1982, J.B. Lippincott Co.
6. Murphy, S.B., and Donaldson, S.S.: Pediatric lymphoma. In Carter, S.K.: Principles of cancer treatment, New York, 1982, McGraw-Hill, Inc.
7. Murphy, S.B., and Hustu, H.O.: A randomized trial of combined modality therapy of childhood non-Hodgkin's lymphoma, Cancer 45(4):630, 1980.
8. Aur, R.J.A., and others: Therapy of localized and regional lymphosarcoma of childhood, Cancer 27:1328, 1971.
9. Wollner, N., and others: Non-Hodgkin's lymphoma in children: a comparative study of two modalities of therapy, Cancer 37:123, 1976.
10. Moss, W.T., Brand, W.N., and Battifora, H.: Radiation oncology: rationale, technique, results, St. Louis, 1979, The C.V. Mosby Co.
11. Miser, J.S., and others: Seventy percent survival in childhood non-Hodgkin's lymphoma: report of 21 cases treated with a less toxic LSA-L regimen, Am. J. Pediatr. Hematol. Oncol. 2(4):317, 1980.
12. Sullivan, M.P., and others: Pediatric Oncology Group experience with modified LSA_2-L_2 therapy in 107 children with non-Hodgkin's lymphoma (Burkitt's excluded), Cancer (in press).
13. Murphy, S.B.: Classification, staging and end results of treatment of childhood non-Hodgkin's lymphomas: dissimilarities from lymphomas in adults, Semin. Oncol. 7(3):337, 1980.
14. Glatstein, E., and others: Non-Hodgkin's lymphomas. VI. Results of treatment in childhood, Cancer 34:204, 1974.
15. Murphy, S.B., Frizzera, G., and Evans, A.E.: A study of childhood non-Hodgkin's lymphoma, Cancer 36:2121, 1975.

CHAPTER 4

Hodgkin's disease

HALLIE A. BOREN and MARGARET P. SULLIVAN

Hodgkin's disease is a malignancy of the lymphoid system, differentiated from other lymphomatous neoplasms by its histology, cell lineage, clinical behavior, and response to treatment [1,2] Characteristically, Hodgkin's disease arises in a single lymph node or anatomic group of lymph nodes. The malignancy usually follows a predictable pattern of progression: painless regional nodal enlargement, extension to contiguous nodes, and, if left untreated, extension to other organs such as spleen, liver, lung, or bone marrow.

HISTORY

Malpigh, in 1661 using postmortem findings, is credited with the earliest gross description of Hodgkin's disease. In 1832 Thomas Hodgkin contributed the first clinical and pathologic description of the disease entity based on his evaluation of seven patients with lymph node and splenic enlargement. The diagnosis of Hodgkin's disease withstood re-evaluation in only three of Hodgkin's case studies, one of which was a 10-year-old-child.[3,4] Wilks in 1856 classified Hodgkin's disease as a constitutional disorder of the lymph nodes.[3] Subsequent researchers believed the disease to be neoplastic in nature. During the late nineteenth century, ideas changed, and Hodgkin's disease as an infectious process was given considerable consideration.[4] The controversy over the exact nature of the disease has continued until modern times. Hodgkin's disease has been classified by the International Classification of Causes of Death as a non-neoplastic disease of the blood (1930-1938), an infectious disease (1939-1948), and now as a malignant neoplasm of the lymph system (1949).[5]

INCIDENCE AND ETIOLOGY

According to the Third National Cancer Survey, the annual diagnostic rate for Hodgkin's disease in the United States is 5.8/1 million in white children and 6.1/1 million in black children.[6] The incidence of Hodgkin's disease is rare before the age of 5 years, but occurrences have been documented in very young children.[7-10] Before the age of 10 years, boys are more frequently the victims of Hodgkin's disease, with studies reporting the male-to-female ratio as 1.4:1, 2.3:1, and 3.8:1.[7,9,11] During the preteen and teenage years, the frequency of occurrence in girls escalates so that the sexes are affected in almost equal numbers by the adolescent years.[4,9,11] One series even found teenage girls outnumbered boys 2:1.[12]

Hodgkin's disease has an unusual bimodal age-incidence curve that varies with geographic location and socioeconomic condition. In developed countries and in high-socioeconomic groups, the overall incidence of Hodgkin's disease is increased, but its occurrence in individuals less than 15 years of age is low. For example, Hodgkin's disease virtually does not exist in Japan's pediatric population.[13] The Hodgkin's disease age-incidence curve of countries such as the United States, Canada, Germany, Denmark, and England peaks in the 20-30 age range, declines until about 45 years of age, and steadily increases thereafter.[13] In contrast, in underdeveloped and developing countries and in low-socioeconomic groups, the overall occurrence of Hodgkin's disease is decreased, but the incidence in the pediatric population comprises a considerable percentage of the total.[14,15] Additionally, in countries such as Lebanon, Egypt, South Africa,

India, and Jordan, the bimodal age-incidence curve peaks one decade earlier than in the populations of developed regions.[16-23] For instance, Gad-el-Mawla and others[17] found that in Egypt one third of those people with Hodgkin's disease were less than 18 years old and almost 50% of those were less than 10 years old. Also of interest is the high incidence rate found by Aghai, Brenner, and Ramot[18] in Arab and oriental Jewish children in Israel.

As the exact nature of Hodgkin's disease has been subject to uncertainty, so has the origin. MacMahon in 1966 relied on the bimodal age-incidence curve of Hodgkin's disease to formulate his hypothesis that Hodgkin's disease is really a heterogeneous entity: a malignant inflammatory disease of the young and malignant neoplasm of the old.[13] Since that time, numerous researchers have examined the epidemiology of Hodgkin's disease looking for clues to its cause. Some investigators liken Hodgkin's disease, its occurrence, and behavior to viruses such as paralytic poliomyelitis or infectious mononucleosis.[24,25] Based on these similarities and the age-incidence curve, speculation has been that Hodgkin's disease may develop as an unusual consequence of a common infectious agent with social class factors influencing the age at which infection occurs.[26] For example, childhood Hodgkin's disease occurs with more frequency in low-socioeconomic conditions in which little protection from infectious agents exists. Conversely, the risk is lowest among young adults who had social factors such as small family size, few playmates, single-family housing, and relatively high education. These variables are some that protect children from early infections.[27]

Attempts to demonstrate clustering and interpersonal transmission of Hodgkin's disease have been mostly unsuccessful.[28-30] Nevertheless, Greenberg, Gutterman, and Cole[28] did find some clustering of young adult and Catholic cases during their survey of the greater Boston area. Gutensohn and Cole[27] have found that Jews with a history of infectious mononucleosis are at high risk for Hodgkin's disease. Some investigations have suggested that a history of tonsillectomy,[31,32] appendectomy, amphet-

amine use,[33] and chemical exposure[32] is associated with increased risk of Hodgkin's disease, but other studies have not confirmed these findings.[24,32]

Razis, Diamond, and Craven,[34] in a review of a large series of Hodgkin's disease cases, discovered 1.5% of the subjects to have close relatives with Hodgkin's disease. In another series, siblings of persons with Hodgkin's disease were found to have a sevenfold increased risk of developing the disease.[35] Also of interest in this study was that siblings of the same sex had a disproportionately increased incidence compared with siblings of the opposite sex. A common environmental exposure may be suspected in such cases.[14]

Torres and others[36] found identical or haplo-identical human leukocyte antigen (HLA) types in siblings with Hodgkin's disease, which suggests host susceptibility associated with the major histocompatibility system.[14] The association of Hodgkin's disease with parental consanguinity in Israel[37] and the analysis a Newfoundland family with a large number of lymphoreticular malignancies suggest that an autosomal recessive genetic locus associated with susceptibility to Hodgkin's disease and/or general immunodeficiency exists.[38]

HISTOLOGY

Histologic descriptions of Hodgkin's disease date back to 1872 when Langhans described the presence of giant cells in the malignant lesions.[3] Succeeding pathologists advanced the histologic description of Hodgkin's disease to include multinucleated cells, increased fibrotic tissue, and the frequent presence of eosinophils. Eventually, these giant, multinucleated cells came to be known as Reed-Sternberg cells (based on the contributions of these two researchers to the histology of Hodgkin's disease)[3] and are diagnostic of Hodgkin's disease when associated with certain cellular and architectural type lesions.[1] However, these cells alone are not sufficient for the diagnosis of Hodgkin's disease, since they can be found in other disorders such as infectious mononucleosis, nodular histiocytic lymphoma, and graft versus host reactions.[1,39,40] Diagnostic Reed-Sternberg cells are

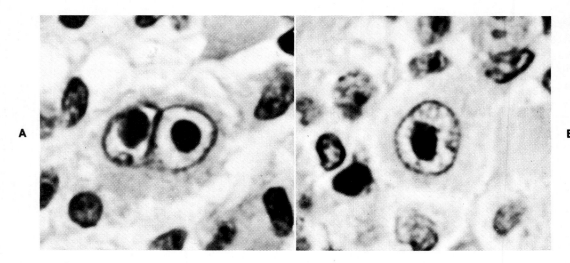

Fig. 4-1. A, Diagnostic Reed-Sternberg cell. **B,** Mononuclear form with large nucleolus. (From Sullivan M.P., Fuller, L.M., and Butler, J.J.: Hodgkin's disease. In Sutow, W.W., Fernbach, D.J., and Vietti, T.J.: Clinical pediatric oncology, ed 3, St. Louis, 1984, The C.V. Mosby Co.)

large and multinucleated, with each nucleus containing a nucleolus at least one fourth the size of the nucleus it occupies (Fig. 4-1). Mononuclear Reed-Sternberg cells, or immunoblasts, are also present in Hodgkin's disease and are considered by some to be the proliferative component in Hodgkin's disease while Reed- Sternberg cells represent the degenerative end stage component.[40] Again, immunoblasts are not diagnostic of Hodgkin's disease, since they are also found in reactive processes.[41] Immunologic and functional studies of these cells indicate that they are malignant monocytes and macrophages.[2,42]

The Rye modification of the Lukes and Butler histologic classification of Hodgkin's disease has been adopted worldwide.[43-45] The Rye classification divides Hodgkin's disease into four histologic classifications: lymphocytic predominance, nodular sclerosis, mixed cellularity, and lymphocytic depletion[44] (Table 4-1).

The histologic categories of Hodgkin's disease were thought to have prognostic implications, but with the advent of combination chemotherapy and high-energy radiotherapy, they have become less significant.[40] Of interest, however, is the intercon-

tinental and age distribution of childhood Hodgkin's disease by histologic classification. In the United States and other similarly developed countries, nodular sclerosing, a histology of supposedly good prognosis, is most common.[14,45] White, Siegel, and McCourt[46] found in their review of Hodgkin's disease in U.S. children under 7 years of age that mixed cellularity was the most common histologic type in children less than 4 years of age. In contrast, developing countries have a histologic predominance of mixed cellularity and lymphocyte depletion, categories that indicate a poorer prognosis.[14]

Strum and Rappaport[47] demonstrated with sequential biopsies of untreated Hodgkin's disease that the disease has a histologic progression. Studying sequential biopsy specimens, 0.1 to 17.3 years after the initial biopsy, they found that lymphocytic predominance may remain unchanged, evolve to mixed cellularity, or progress to lymphocytic depletion. The mixed cellularity type either remained the same or become lymphocytic depletion. Initial biopsy specimens that confirmed lymphocytic depletion were consistent with later specimens. Therefore the data do not suggest that a reversal

Table 4-1. Histologic subtypes of Hodgkin's disease according to the Rye classification

Rye: modified Lukes and Butler	Characteristics
Lymphocytic predominance	Predominantly small lymphocytes and reactive histiocytes
	Sparse Reed-Sternberg cells
	No necrosis
Nodular sclerosing	Collagen septa dividing lymphoid tissue into nodules
	Few Reed-Sternberg cells
	Numerous eosinophils
	Areas of necrosis
Mixed cellularity	All Hodgkin's disease cell types present
	Fewer lymphocytes and greater number of Reed-Sternberg cells
	Eosinophils and necrosis may be seen
Lymphocytic depletion	Decreased number of lymphocytes and other cells types
	Disorderly noncollagen connective tissue
	Rare bizarre-appearing Reed-Sternberg cells

Data compiled from Sullivan, M.P., Fuller, L.M., and Butler, J.J.: Hodgkin's disease. In Sutow, W.W., Fernbach, D.J., and Vietti, T.J., editors: Clinical pediatric oncology, ed. 3, St. Louis, 1984, The C.V. Mosby Co.; Lukes, R.J., and others: Cancer Res. **26:**1311, 1966; Moayeri, H., and Han, T.: Hodgkin's disease. In Tebbi, C.K., editor: Major topics in pediatric and adolescent oncology, Boston, 1982, G.K. Hall & Co.

of the progress exists. The nodular sclerosing histologic variety did not seem to follow this orderly progress. Thus the histologic progression appeared to be from the more cellular forms to the more acellular, sclerotic types.

Hodgkin's disease in the liver and bone marrow has important prognostic and therapeutic implications. Therefore special considerations are required for biopsy and histologic examination of these areas.[48] In the absence of a previously established diagnosis, the criteria are the same as the lymph nodes or tissue from any other site. Bone marrow specimens should be obtained by biopsy rather than aspiration as biopsy produces a superior specimen. Even with fibrotic infiltrations indicating disease presence, multiple bone marrow and liver biopsies may be required to find the diagnostic Reed-Sternberg cell. In instances when none is found, large mononuclear cells with large nucleoli may be considered diagnostic of Hodgkin's disease.[1]

IMMUNOLOGIC IMPAIRMENT

Hodgkin's disease is characterized by altered T lymphocyte function, clinically manifested as impaired cell-mediated immunity.[1,2,40,45] Delayed or anergic responses to allergens such as tuberculin (PPD), diphtherotoxoid, streptokinase-streptodornase, mumps, and *Trichophyton* and *Candida* species have been demonstrated.[1,49,50] Anergy to chemical antigens may also exist.[40] Additionally, the abnormal cellular immunity of Hodgkin's disease is reflected in the host's impaired ability to reject skin homografts.[51] Histologic studies of immunologic function in long-term disease-free survivors indicate cell-mediated immunity defects persist after cure,[51-53] although reactivity to skin test usually recovers as Hodgkin's disease activity subsides.[1,54]

The results of quantitative studies of T lymphocytes at diagnosis have been conflicting, with both normal values and T lymphopenia being reported.[55,56] Lauria and others[57] suggest that the significantly abnormal T lymphocyte subsets found in patients after therapy has been discontinued may be attributable to Hodgkin's disease alone or its treatment with chemotherapy or radiotherapy. As with quantiative studies of T lymphocytes, B lymphocyte numbers have been reported in conflicting studies as normal and significantly lower than normal at the time of diagnosis of Hodgkin's disease.[58,59] Nevertheless, antibody responses are active until extensive disease progression.[1] Han[60] suggests that in Hodgkin's disease the function of the peripheral blood B lymphocytes remains intact, and it is the activity of helper T lymphocytes that may be impaired. The number of B lymphocytes in patients treated for Hodgkin's disease and long-term survivors has been found to be increased.[61,62]

CLINICAL FEATURES

Hodgkin's disease, as reported in 60% to 90% of cases, typically presents as painless adenopathy in the lower cervical region.[40,63,64] Silent mediastinal disease is associated with about half of these cases.[1,65] Primary mediastinal involvement is rare, with an incidence of only about 4%.[40] Other nodal sites such as the axillary and inguinal groups are unusual presenting areas of adenopathy except in cases of generalized disease.[1]

Splenomegaly, an initial finding in 10% to 48% of cases, and hepatomegaly, initially found in 10% to 39% of cases, indicate advanced disease.[63,64] Childhood Hodgkin's disease presenting in an extranodal site is exceedingly rare.[1] In one large series that included 109 children, none presented in an extranodal site.[9] Other series have reported a low incidence of primary extranodal involvement. These sites are reported to include the lungs, pleura, kidneys, nervous system, and skin.[1,7,11]

Anorexia, malaise, and lassitude are common symptoms present at the time of diagnosis of Hodgkin's disease.[63] Other constitutional symptoms such as weight loss, fever, and night sweats were seen in 43% of the children in one series.[40] The fever has a usual pattern of intermittent elevations of 1° to 2° C (2° to 3° F) above normal. Seen less frequently are "picket fence" fevers in which sharp late afternoon or early evening fevers (40° C or 104° F) often are accompanied by chills. Pel-Ebstein fevers, recurrent and relapsing fever patterns, are unusual in children. Pruritus occurs on occasion in adolescents with large mediastinal and/or para-aortic disease.[1] At the time of diagnosis of Hodgkin's disease, the presence of an unexplained fever with temperatures above 38° C (100.4° F), weight loss of 10% of the normal body weight in 6 months, and drenching night sweats are thought to be of prognostic value. Pruritus is no longer

considered part of this prognostic complex of symptoms. When these symptoms are present, the case is classified as B; asymptomatic cases are classified as A. As the extent of disease progresses, so does the likelihood of systemic symptoms, reaching 75% and 100% in stage IV disease.[9,11]

DIAGNOSTIC WORKUP

The diagnosis of Hodgkin's disease is established by lymph node biopsy. Preferably, the largest available node is removed with its capsule intact. Needle biopsies and frozen-section diagnoses are contraindicated when Hodgkin's disease is suspected because such procedures do not allow pathologic examination of the node with architectural features undisturbed. When possible, biopsy of inguinal and submaxillary lymph nodes should be avoided, since changes following repeated chronic infections may mask a malignant process.[1]

History and physical examination

Once pathologic diagnosis of Hodgkin's disease has been established, the extent of disease involvement must be identified. Therapy will be determined based on age, sex, histology, and stage (extent of disease). Most patients could probably be cured of Hodgkin's disease with intensive chemotherapy and radiotherapy, but the severe early and late side effects of these modalities prohibit their excessive use. Essential to accurate clinical staging of Hodgkin's disease is a thorough history that explores the presence of constitutional symptoms (such as weight loss and fever) and a physical examination that carefully evaluates peripheral lymph node regions and the abdomen.

The importance of precise lymph node evaluation cannot be overstressed. Lymph node palpation entails rolling the balls of the fingers over the lymph node–bearing regions, first in a cephalad-caudad direction and then in a right-to-left direction. Nodes of the neck are best palpated by approaching patients from behind and examining one side at a time. The axilla should be examined with the patient in a sitting or recumbent position with the arm abducted and relaxed. The examiner uses his right hand to examine the patient's left axilla while his left hand steadies the patient's left shoulder and vice versa. To palpate epitrochlear nodes, the patient's elbow should be flexed about 90°. The right epitrochlear region is examined by grasping the patient's right wrist with the examiner's right hand, using the examiner's left hand to wrap around the patient's right elbow, and placing the fingers over the epitrochlear area. Inguinal nodes are found along the inguinal ligament in the horizontal plane, whereas femoral nodes are arranged vertically along the femoral canal below the inguinal ligament.[66]

The physical examination of the lymphatic system should include determination of lymph node size, location, consistency or character (matted, soft, freely movable, or fixed), tenderness, condition of overlying skin, involvement of other lymph nodes, and enlargement of abdominal organs.[66,67] Nodes less than 1 cm in size may be referred to as "shoddy." These nodes usually are normal. Firm to hard lymph nodes usually suggest a malignancy; whereas soft to fluctuant ones usually indicate infection.[67] The spleen is part of the lymphatic system and therefore should be carefully palpated for size and consistency.[68]

Before a final diagnosis of Hodgkin's disease, children are often presumed to have an adenitis related to infection and are treated with antibiotics. Other possibilities in the differential diagnosis of lymphadenopathy include cat-scratch disease, infectious mononucleosis, tuberculosis, toxoplasmosis, and coccidioidomycosis.[1]

Laboratory and radiographic evaluations

Additional clinical investigations of Hodgkin's disease include a battery of hematologic, biochemical, and radiographic evaluations. Anemia, although rare in Hodgkin's disease (less than 1%) and not specifically considered in the staging procedure, usually does indicate more than local disease (stage III or IV).[1,45] Two mechanisms have been identified in Hodgkin's disease that may singly or concurrently create anemia: hemolysis and/or impaired mobilization of iron stores.[1] The white blood cell count is usually normal, although occasionally patients will initially have marked leukocytosis or leukopenia. The cause is unknown, but presentation with one or the other of these white blood cell abnormalities is usually associated with an unfavorable course.[1] Absolute lymphocyte counts may be normal or slightly decreased, progressing to profound lymphocytopenia in advanced disease.[1,45] The erthyrocyte sedimentation rate is commonly elevated and usually correlates with disease activity and stage.[69] Bone marrow aspirations produce specimens that are unsatisfactory for demonstrating Hodgkin's disease. The fibrous and granulomatous nature of Hodgkin's disease prevents aspiration of bone marrow particles, and the bone marrow architecture is disrupted by the aspiration procedure. Although Silverman or Jamshidi needle biopsies of the posterior iliac crest produce satisfactory specimens, maximum diagnostic reliability is obtained from the bone marrow wedge of an open biopsy.[1,70]

Biochemical assays of liver function do not correlate well with hepatic involvement.[1] Elevated serum alkaline phosphatase levels in adults with Hodgkin's disease are primarily a result of elevated hepatic phosphatase levels.[3] This determination is not as helpful in children and adolescents, since levels may be physiologically elevated as a result of the bone isoenzyme. Additionally, osseous Hodgkin's disease is usually lytic, causing minimum abnormalities in the alkaline phosphatase levels.[40,71] Serum copper levels are frequently elevated in active Hodgkin's disease. Although no correlation has been demonstrated between actual serum copper level and extent of disease, the parameter is useful in monitoring disease activity and in detecting recurrence before it is otherwise demonstrable.[72,73]

Intrathoracic evaluation for Hodgkin's disease is an important component of the diagnostic workup because at least 50% of the patients will have mediastinal adenopathy and some of which will have pleural effusions. Tomography or computed tomography (CT) is helpful when there are questions of parenchymal or pleural disease.[1,45] Additionally, CT scans with contrast are useful in evaluating and delineating retrosternal mediastinal disease. Radiographs of patients with mediastinal

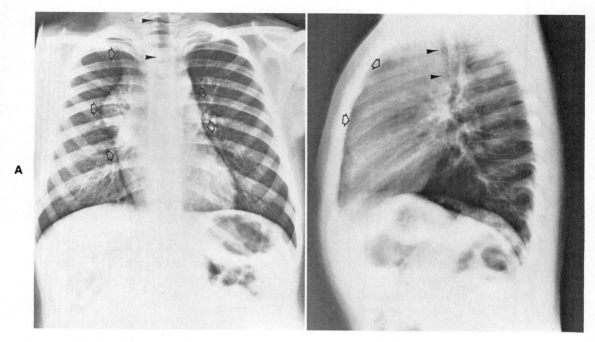

Fig. 4-2. Posteroanterior (**A**) and lateral (**B**) radiographs of 10-year-old male with Hodgkin's disease showing enlarged anterior mediastinal and paratracheal lymph nodes (open arrows) deviating tracheal air column (arrowheads) to left and posteriorly. (Courtesy F. Eftekhari, MD, University of Texas, M.D. Anderson Hospital and Tumor Institute.)

Hodgkin's disease typically demonstrate adenopathy in the anterosuperior mediastinum and in the paratracheal areas (Fig. 4-2). Nodes of the aortopulmonary space (ductus nodes) and those along the hilar structure (bronchiopulmonary nodes) are also commonly enlarged.[1]

Lymphangiography is a routine staging procedure in the evaluation of infradiaphragmatic Hodgkin's disease. It allows visualization of the iliac and para-aortic lymph nodes up to the level of the renal pedicles (Fig. 4-3) and has a diagnostic reliability of greater than 90% as confirmed by laparotomy.[68,74] CT scans with contrast of the abdomen and pelvis may detect enlarged nodes in the mesentery and elsewhere but cannot define nodal architecture. By lymphangiogram, changes in lymph node architecture such as a foamy, reticular appearance or filling defects can be detected before actual enlargement occurs.[11] Additionally, the opaque medium of lymphangiogram is retained in lymph nodes for 6 months or longer and can, with abdominal radiographs, serve as markers for disease regression, progression, or relapse. Since a lymphangiogram does not delineate celiac, porta hepatis, splenic pedicle, and mesenteric nodes (rarely involved), it is not useful in ruling out abdominal involvement. The primary contraindication for lymphangiography is massive mediastinal and pulmonary involvement because of the high risk of pulmonary oil embolism (manifested as fever and dyspnea). Other risks include allergic reaction to the contrast dyes and local infection at the site of cutdown.[5,11] Age is not a contraindication of lymphangiography, although general anesthesia is usually required for patients under the age of 10 years for obtaining the best results.[11]

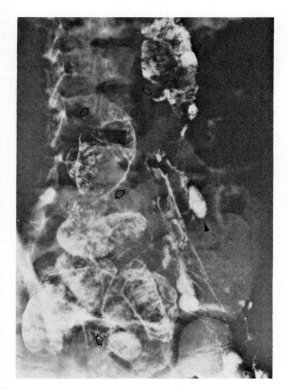

Fig. 4-3. Left posterior oblique view of bipedal lymphangiogram in 7-year-old girl with Hodgkin's disease demonstrating massive enlarged para-aortic, parailiac and inguinal nodes replaced by tumor (arrows). Note normal node (arrowhead). (Courtesy F. Eftekhari, MD, University of Texas, M.D. Anderson Hospital and Tumor Institute.)

Imaging studies commonly used in staging Hodgkin's disease are intravenous pyelograms (IVP), CT scans, ultrasonography, and nuclear scanning. IVPs, although not always helpful in defining disease, are important for accurate localization of the kidneys before abdominal radiotherapy. Neither CT scan nor ultrasound has the sensitivity of lymphangiography for disease detection; lymphangiography can detect local nodal involvement of only a few millimeters,[75] whereas nodes must be 1 cm or greater for CT detection and at least 2 to 3 cm for identification by ultrasound.[1,45] Nevertheless, ultrasound imaging can define neck and abdominal masses, determine spleen size and intrahepatic masses, monitor response to therapy, and detect early relapse. It also has a role in delineating bulky tumor margins for radiotherapy. Since ultrasound in noninvasive, does not involve radiation, and does not require contrast dyes, it is well tolerated by children.[1]

CT, as mentioned previously, is particularly useful in the evaluation of mediastinal and pulmonary Hodgkin's disease but has limited usefulness in delineating abdominal disease. CT scans of the abdomen do not have great diagnostic value in Hodgkin's disease because of the poor fat planes in the young that are necessary for adequately outlining organs and masses and the greater sensitivity of lymphangiogram.[1]

Gallium citrate (^{67}Ga), a tumor-seeking radionuclide that has shown great affinity for lymphomas, particularly Hodgkin's tissue, is used in many centers to determine extent of disease in the initial staging procedure. It also has been employed in designing radiotherapy portals, assessing response to therapy, and detecting new or recurrent disease. Nuclear scanning is especially useful in Hodgkin's disease patients sensitive to radiopaque dye or who have large mediastinal or pulmonary lesions that contraindicate a lymphangiogram.[1] ^{67}Ga imaging is more sensitive above the diaphragm (61% accuracy) than below (40% accuracy).[76] Nevertheless, this method has proved valuable in evaluating recurrent disease and demonstrating sites of involvement. Recurrent Hodgkin's disease has been identified with ^{67}Ga scanning 1 to 10 months before detection by physical examination or radiograph was possible.[77] Although liver and spleen scanning with technetium-99m sulfur colloid can effectively exclude liver involvement and accurately delineate spleen and location, the low probability of liver involvement at the time of diagnosis makes clinical usefulness of the study doubtful.[78]

PATHOLOGIC STAGING

As previously mentioned, precise determination of disease extent is vital to Hodgkin's disease treatment design and adequate therapy with a minimum of toxicities and sequelae. Hodgkin's disease is staged according to nodal regions as depicted in Fig. 4-4. Staging is usually assigned according to the classification proposed at the Ann Arbor Conference,[79] as depicted in Fig. 4-5.

Staging laparotomy with splenectomy is the most accurate means of determining abdominal involvement not detectable by clinical investigations.[80,81] With information available from laparotomy, therapy can be tailored to the extent of disease and needs of the individual child, minimizing iatrogenic complications most relevant to that age child (i.e., bone growth retardation).[82] The procedure was initially performed to clarify equivocal lymphangiogram findings and to seek occult disease of nodes beyond the scope of the lymphangiogram (celiac axis, mesenteric, and retrogastric nodes).[83-85] En bloc removal of the spleen along with precise histologic evaluation is essential for accurate pathologic staging; 30% to 40% of patients with clinically staged I or II Hodgkin's disease have unsuspected involvement of the spleen.[73] Furthermore, Green and others,[86] in an extensive review of the literature, found that the pathologic stage was different from the clinical stage in 29% of pediatric patients following staging laparotomy. And for those who had a change in stage, the pathologic stage was higher (i.e., from a stage II to a stage III) in 86% of the cases.[86] Thus staging laparotomy and splenectomy should be undertaken at the earliest opportunity following clinical studies on all patients over 5 years of age who do not have obvious stage IV disease at the time of diagnosis. Intubation and general anesthesia are contraindicated when a massive mediastinal disease is present. Therefore patients with such a presentation should receive mediastinal irradiation to shrink the bulky tumor before surgical staging.[87]

A midline incision extending from the xiphoid process to the midpelvis is the procedure most often used in the surgical staging of Hodgkin's disease patients.[85] After removal of the entire spleen and splenic hilar nodes, the splenic pedicle is marked with silver clips. Next, two needle biopsy specimens of each lobe of the liver are obtained, followed by wedge biopsy of the left liver lobe. Representative lymph nodes and those that appear ab-

normal are removed sequentially from the course of the common hepatic artery near the celiac artery, the common hepatic duct, the para-aortic and iliac lymph node-bearing regions, and the mesentery of the small bowel. The lymph node removal sites are marked with clips. While the patient remains on the table, obtaining a plain radiograph of the abdomen ensures that nodes shown by lymphography to be abnormal have been removed for histologic study. When present, the appendix is removed. In females who are potential candidates for abdominal radiation, the ovaries are moved to the midline or far laterally. A wedge bone marrow biopsy specimen is obtained from the iliac crest. (Bilateral iliac crest biopies are done at some centers.)[1]

Postoperatively, nasogastric suction is required in most cases for paralytic ileus, the result of splenectomy and bowel manipulation required for inspection and sampling of nodes. The tube is removed once peristalsis returns and flatus is passed. Early ambulation and frequent deep breathing with coughing exercises are essential in preventing pneumonia, an occurrence that could delay the beginning of chemotherapy. On the seventh postoperative day, sutures are usually removed, and chemotherapy may be initiated. Thrombocytosis, with platelet counts exceeding 1×10^6/ml, is not uncommon postoperatively.[1] Other acute complications following staging laparotomy in the pediatric population have included wound infection (0.6%), subphrenic abscess (0.1%), and hemobilia (0.1%).[81]

Encapsulated bacteria pose a lifelong threat of fulminating infection to children and adolescents having experienced splenectomy.[88-91] Hence, children under 5 years of age are not usually subjected to splenectomy so that their immature immune system may be preserved. One series that followed 200 splenectomized children observed that 10% developed septicemia and meningitis up to 20 years postsplenectomy and that 4.5% died of fulminating infections.[91] The causative organisms were *Streptococcus pneumoniae* (45% of the patients), streptococci (15% of the patients), and *Haemophilus influenzae* and *Neisseria meningitidis* (5% each). Cultures were sterile in 20% of the cases. Another series found that the only increase in infections in

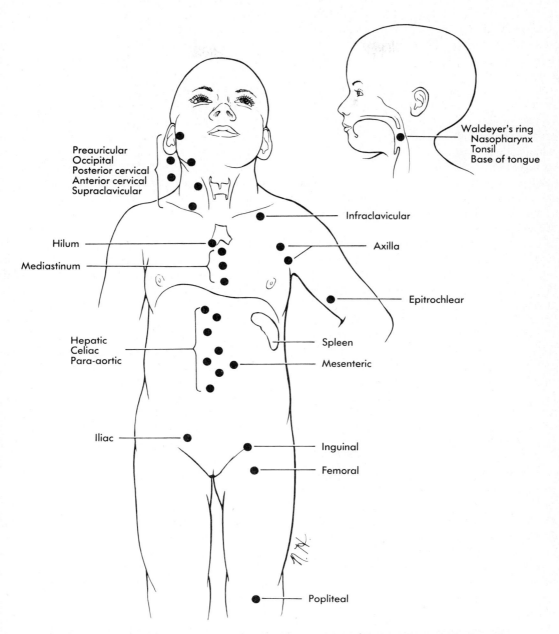

Fig. 4-4. Nodal regions for defining stage of Hodgkin's disease. (Adapted from Sullivan, M.P., Fuller, L.M., and Butler, J.J.: Hodgkin's disease. In Sutow, W.W., Fernbach, D.J., and Vietti, T.J.: Clinical pediatric oncology, ed 3, St. Louis, 1984, The C.V. Mosby Co.)

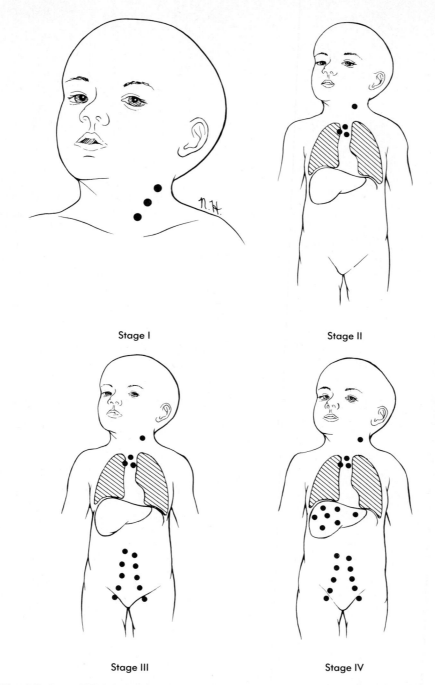

Stage I

Stage II

Stage III

Stage IV

Fig. 4-5. Stage I disease is limited to one lymphatic region. Stage II disease is limited to lymph nodes on one side of diaphragm. Stage III disease involves lymph nodes on both sides of diaphragm. Stage IV disease has disseminated diffusely to involve lung, liver, bone marrow, skin, and central nervous system. Each stage is further classified by ''A,'' asymptomatic and ''B,'' symptomatic (fevers, night sweats, weight loss of greater than 10% of body weight). (Adapted from Sullivan, M.P., Fuller, L.M., and Butler, J.J.: Hodgkin's disease. In Sutow, W.W., Fernbach, D.J., and Vietti, T.J.: Clinical pediatric oncology, ed 3, St. Louis, 1984, The C.V. Mosby Co.)

the recipients of splenectomy in children under 10 years of age was in the incidence of *S. pneumoniae* and *Haemophilus influenzae* bacteremia-meningitis.[92] In the Intergroup Hodgkin's Disease in Childhood study, 234 children and adolescents with stage I or II disease were followed postsplenectomy. Only four blood culture-proved cases of sepsis and three possible cases of sepsis without positive blood culture were reported 1 to 19 months after laparotomy. Two of the proved septic episodes occurred during chemotherapy for relapse, these causative organisms being *H. influenzae* and *S. pneumoniae*.[93] Others have noted that splenectomy does not enhance the risk of zoster and varicella infections.[94] Because of the severity of infections created by encapsulated bacteria, particularly *S. pneumoniae* in children and adolescents with Hodgkin's disease and splenectomy, attempts have been made to protect them by immunization with polyvalent pneumococcal polysaccharide vaccine.[95,96] The response to the vaccine is unpredictable if administered after the institution of therapy, but appears to be normal if administered before treatment. Conclusive data demonstrating that the vaccine actually decreases the incidence of bacteremia in splenectomized patients are lacking.[97] Therefore antibiotic prophylaxis, such as 250 mg of oral penicillin twice daily, is recommended for splenectomized children.[1] The Intergroup Hodgkin's Disease in Childhood study reported only one episode of sepsis *(H. influenzae)* in a patient complying with prophylactic recommendations.[93]

Late complications of splenectomy include the aforementioned infections and intestinal obstruction.[1,86] Intestinal obstructions occur in a small number of pediatric patients (3.9%)[94] and are seen more often in conjunction with abdominal radiotherapy.[1]

TREATMENT

In 1950 Peters[98] published survival data on radiologically treated Hodgkin's disease patients that indicated the disease was curable. Today, radiotherapy along with multiagent chemotherapy produces a 90% or better 4-year survival for stages I and II disease.[1] Differences in the details of therapy exist from institution to institution and specific chemotherapy regimens reflect the persuasion of the individual chemotherapist, but a general consensus exists for treatment plans. The intensity of treatment is dependent of disease presentation and stage (Table 4-2).

Chemotherapy

Childhood and adolescence, in which growth and maturation are still in progress, create special therapeutic concerns. Deviations from adult treatment regimens are necessary to assure freedom, insofar as possible, from late undesirable effects of therapy. In the very young, chemotherapy is used for disease control, and radiation therapy is delayed if possible until age 8 years to prevent severe retardation of bone growth and soft tissue development. Even in older children the objective of the chemotherapist and radiotherapist should be effective, minimum therapy.[1] Chemotherapy regimens employed to treat childhood Hodgkin's disease are as follows:

MAC (multiagent chemotherapy) (Memorial Hospital)[99]
  Doxorubicin, 20 mg/m^2/day × 3, days 1, 2, and 3
  Prednisone, 1 mg/kg/day, PO, for 3 weeks
  Procarbazine, 50 mg/day, PO, first 2 to 3 days then 100 mg/day for total of 3 weeks if tolerated
  Vincristine, 1 to 2 mg/m^2/week for 3 doses
  Cyclophosphamide, 40 mg/kg, IV, single dose as soon as hematologic status permits on completion of procarbazine
  Rest 2 week
  Repeat cycle every 3 months
A-COPP (M.D. Anderson Hospital)[100]
  Doxorubicin, 60 mg/m^2, IV, day 1
  Prednisone, 40 mg/m^2/day, PO, days 1 to 27 first and fourth cycles only; days 14 to 27 second, third, fifth, and sixth cycles
  Vincristine, 1.5 mg/m^2/week × 2, IV, days 14 and 20
  Cyclophosphamide, 300 mg/m^2/week × 2, IV, days 14 and 20
  Prednisone, 40 mg/m^2/day, days 14 to 27
  Procarbazine, 100 mg/m^2/day, PO, days 14 to 28
  Rest days 27 to 41
  Repeat cycle every 6 weeks

MOPP[101,102]

    Nitrogen mustard (HN_2), 6 mg/m^2, IV, days 1 and 8

    Vincristine, 1.4 mg/m^2, IV, days 1 and 8

    Prednisone, 40 mg/m^2/day, PO, days 1 to 14

    Procarbazine, 100 mg/m^2, PO, days 1 to 14

        Rest days 15 to 27

        Repeat cycle every 4 weeks

MOPP-lo Bleo (Southwest Oncology Group)[103]

    Nitrogen mustard (HN_2), 6 mg/m^2, IV, days 1 and 8

    Vincristine, 1.5 mg/m^2, PO, days 1 and 8

    Bleomycin, 2.0 mg/m^2, IV, days 1 and 14

    Procarbazine, 100 mg/m^2, PO, days 2 to 7 and 9 to 12

    Prednisone, 40 mg/m^2, PO, daily in 4 divided doses, days 2 to 7 and 9 to 12

        Rest days 13 to 27

        Repeat cycle every 4 weeks

CVPP (Cancer and Leukemia Group B[104])

    CCNU, 75 mg/m^2, PO, day 1

    Vinblastine, 4.0 mg/m^2, IV, days 1 and 8

    Procarbazine, 100 mg/m^2, PO, days 1 to 14

    Prednisone, 40 mg/m^2, PO, daily in 4 divided doses, days 1 to 14

        Rest days 15 to 27

        Repeat cycle every 4 weeks

ABVD (Bonadonna, Stanford modification)[105,106]

    Doxorubicin, 25 mg/m^2, IV, day 1

    Bleomycin, 10 mg/m^2, IV, day 1

    Vinblastine, 6 mg/m^2, IV, day 1

    Imidazole carboxamide (DTIC), 150 mg/m^2, IV, day 1

        Repeat cycle every 2 weeks

B-CAVe (Stanford)[107]

    Bleomycin, 2.5 mg/m^2, days 1, 28, and 35

    CCNU, 100 mg/m^2, IV, day 1

    Doxorubicin, 60 mg/m^2, IV, day 1

    Vinblastine, 5 mg/m^2, IV, day 1

        Repeat cycle every 6 weeks

ABDIC (M.D. Anderson Hospital)[108]

    Doxorubicin, 45 mg/m^2, IV, day 1

    Bleomycin, 5 mg/m^2, IV, days 1 and 5

    CCNU, 50 mg/m^2, PO, day 1

    Prednisone, 40 mg/m^2, PO, days 1 to 5

        Repeat cycle every 3 to 4 weeks

The number of chemotherapy cycles used with each of the regimens in this list is determined by multiple factors, including stage of disease, cumulative dose of agents with dose-limiting toxicities (e.g., doxorubicin), marrow tolerance of therapy, and long-range treatment plans.[1]

Before 1970 multiagent chemotherapy was gen-

Table 4-2. Treatments for Hodgkin's disease

Disease stage	Treatment
Favorable stage I disease (high cervical and inguinal)	Involved field radiotherapy
Stages I and II mediastinal presentations	
Small mediastinal "A" disease with negative hila	"Mantle" or neck and mediastinum radiotherapy
All other mediastinal disease	Mantle or neck and mediastinum radiotherapy followed by combination chemotherapy
	Para-aortic node irradiation only if adequacy of staging laparotomy is questionable
All other stages I and II presentations	Involved field radiotherapy
	Mantle radiotherapy possibly indicated in patients with supraclavicular nodes or for stage II disease
	Para-aortic node irradiation only if adequacy of staging laparotomy is questionable
Stage III	Combination chemotherapy-radiotherapy
Stage IV	Chemotherapy and optional radiotherapy for bulky disease

erally reserved for patients with stages III and IV of Hodgkin's disease, but more recently it has been used in combination with radiotherapy for all stages. The principle behind use of multiagent chemotherapy is that by combining several agents with differing toxicities, an additive or even synergetic antitumor effect will be achieved. The use of multiagent chemotherapeutic agents has been successful in markedly improving remission and survival times in stages III and IV.[1] Thus single-agent chemotherapy is given infrequently, only when patients become resistant to or intolerant of multiagent chemotherapy. Vinblastine is the most effective single-agent chemotherapy.[109]

Radiotherapy

Irradiation alone is curative for localized Hodgkin's disease, provided a high enough dose (3000 to 4000 rad) is delivered.[40] Kaplan reported, based on a review of the literature, that permanent local disease control can be achieved in 80% of cases using 3000 rad.[110] But again the long-term effects of heavy irradiation on developing bones and tissue make its use less than optimum. Additionally, such doses of radiation to the mediastinum are poorly tolerated by the heart and spinal cord. Excessive radiotherapy to the inguinal or femoral areas can create a blockage to lymphatic flow resulting in edema of the leg.[1]

Various radiotherapy fields have been used in treating Hodgkin's disease. Extended field refers to radiation portals that include the tumor-bearing site and the next echelon of lymph nodes.[40] Involved field radiation encompasses only the region of involvement: in stage I disease, treatment is limited to the involved area (Fig. 4-6); in stage II disease, adjacent fields are treated as one, whereas noncontiguous regions are treated as separate fields (Fig. 4-7). When all major lymph node chains above the diaphragm are in the radiation portal, it is referred to as a mantle field, and when all infradiaphragmatic nodes are covered, the field is commonly called an inverted "Y." The combination of these two portals constitutes total nodal irradiation. Adults tolerate extended field or total

nodal radiotherapy relatively well in terms of systemic effect and late complications; children and adolescents do not.[1]

In recent years a new approach to treatment of Hodgkin's disease has been to interpose involved field radiotherapy between courses of multiagent chemotherapy. Results indicate that such a design may be more effective and produce less growth disturbance than total nodal radiotherapy. Some centers have also successfully reduced the dose of irradiation when combined with chemotherapy.[40,111]

Surgical intervention

Surgical intervention in the treatment of Hodgkin's disease is confined primarily to biopsy procedures. Adequate operative treatment would require en bloc removal of involved nodal regions, resulting in disfigurement and interference with lymphatic drainage. Thus the sequelae of the surgical management of Hodgkin's disease exceeds that which radiotherapy may create and therefore exclude surgical intervention as a treatment.[1]

Relapse

Post-treatment disease surveillance should be most vigilant in the first 2 to 3 years after completing therapy because historically that is when the majority of relapses occur.[1] Less than 3% of patients relapse after more than 4 years after therapy,[40] making detection and management of the late effects of therapy the focus of long-term follow-up. Recurrence may be heralded by constitutional symptoms or biochemical abnormalities such as an elevated serum copper level or an increased sedimentation rate. When possible, a biopsy should be obtained to confirm recurrent disease. Staging studies are repeated as necessary to define extent of disease. Stage I and II patients with new disease in the radiotherapy field are treated with chemotherapy alone. Recurrent disease adjacent to or at the margin of radiotherapy portals may be treated with radiotherapy. Other manifestations of new disease should receive chemotherapy and radiotherapy. Relapsed or new stages III and

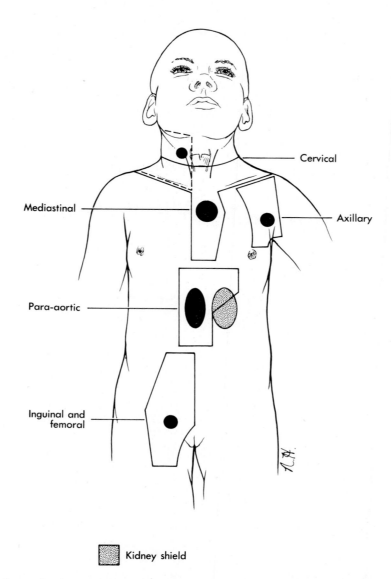

Cervical

Mediastinal

Axillary

Para-aortic

Inguinal and
femoral

Kidney shield

Fig. 4-6. Composite drawing for involved field radiotherapy for common anatomic nodal presentations of stage I Hodgkin's disease in either upper or lower torso. (Radiotherapy fields courtesy L. Fuller, MD, University of Texas, M.D. Anderson Hospital and Tumor Institute.)

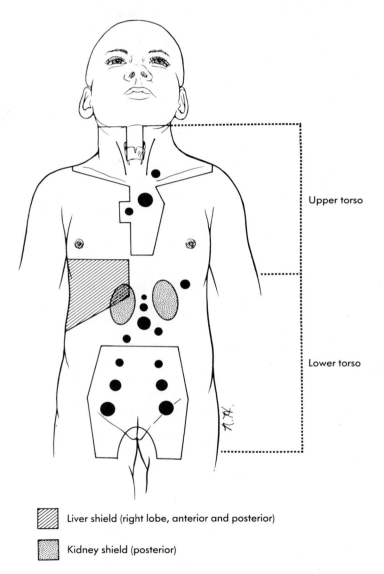

Upper torso

Lower torso

Liver shield (right lobe, anterior and posterior)

Kidney shield (posterior)

Fig. 4-7. Composite drawing for involved field radiotherapy for common anatomic nodal presentations of stage II Hodgkin's disease in either upper or lower torso. (Radiotherapy fields courtesy L. Fuller, MD, University of Texas, M.D. Anderson Hospital and Tumor Institute.)

IV disease present management problems that must be individualized.[1]

Diagnostic and therapeutic side effects

Diagnostic and therapeutic maneuvers involved in the management of children or adolescents with Hodgkin's disease can create a number of complications or side effects. These consequences of medical procedures may occur very early in treatment or not be apparent for many years. Potential side effects of lymphangiogram (i.e., oil emboli) and staging laparotomy with splenectomy (i.e., infection) have been previously reviewed. Most patients experience nausea and vomiting associated with chemotherapy and radiotherapy. The occurrence of complete or partial alopecia depends on the type of chemotherapy used and position of radiotherapy fields. Myelosuppression results from chemotherapy or irradiation. In adults up to 15% of the bone marrow volume is included in the mantle radiation field, whereas 50% of the bone marrow falls in the inverted "Y" portal.[40]

Children and adolescents who receive both chemotherapy and radiotherapy for Hodgkin's disease have a reported incidence of herpes zoster or varicella infections that ranges from 34% to 56%. The incidence among those who receive only radiotherapy is from 5.5% to 23.8%.[112,113] The frequency of infection in stage I disease is 13%, but in stages II, III, and IV the incidence is 35%, a phenomenon that may reflect the aggressiveness of therapy.[113] Splenectomy does not seem to influence the occurrence of this infection. Sullivan, Ramirez, and Bronell[112] found that in a series of 92 children with Hodgkin's disease, zoster episodes occurred during the third chemotherapy course following completion of radiotherapy. Eruptions of the virus occur primarily in the irradiated field.[112,113] Currently, two theories are proposed as to the frequent reactivation of latent herpes zoster virus during or following Hodgkin's disease treatment: local nerve root reaction to irradiation versus generalized immunosuppression.[112-114] Adenine arabinoside (ara-A) or acyclovir administered intravenously is used to shorten the clinical course and decrease the pain associated with zoster infections.[112-117]

Radiotherapy effects on the skin range from erythema and dry desquamation to moist desquamation and ulceration.[118] Exposure of irradiated skin to sunlight should be kept to a minimum. Chronic or late effects of irradiation of the skin include telangiectasia, hyperpigmentation, and even areas of hyperkeratosis[118] (see Chapter 21). Salivary glands in the path of the radiotherapy beam (cervical fields) undergo progressive glandular atrophy, fibrosis, and reduction in output beginning shortly after the initial exposure and intensifying thereafter.[119] By functioning as a deterrent to oral microflora and as a cleansing, mineralizing, and buffering agent, saliva protects teeth against caries.[120] When saliva output is impaired, rampant dental caries invariably ensue unless stringent measures are taken to protect the teeth.[119,120]

Early effects of radiotherapy on the thoracic organs may include pericarditis and radiation pneumonitis.[40,118] Late effects on these organs may manifest as pericardial fibrosis and pleural fibrosis.[121] With less frequency, myocardial fibrosis and myocardial insufficiency have been noted.[1]

Wilimas, Thompson, and Smith,[122] in a review of long-term survivors of childhood and adolescent Hodgkin's disease, found that growth retardation is the major long-term effect of radiotherapy. Growing cartilage is radiosensitive[118] and therefore growth disturbances are greatest when radiotherapy is administered during periods of accelerated growth. Children who receive extended field radiotherapy, especially those less than 6 years of age or between 12 to 13 years of age, primarily manifest growth retardation in decreased height.[122]

Significant hypoplasia of the breast may result when the breast buds of prepubertal girls are irradiated.[1,118]

Scatter radiation from inverted "Y" radiotherapy, even with testicles shielded, can be enough to create prolonged periods of either azoospermia or oligospermia, or even permanent sterility.[118] In females, ovarian function is afforded some protection when the ovaries are relocated to the midline or laterally at the time of staging laparotomy.[123] Menstruation may cease during treatment but resume some months later.[124] Children have been born to women who have had their ovaries relocated before inverted "**Y**" radiotherapy.[125]

The incidence of overt hypothyroidism occurring after therapeutic neck irradiation for childhood Hodgkin's disease is between 15.3%[107] and 57.1%.[126] Compensated hypothyroid states (normal T_4, elevated thyroid-stimulating hormone [TSH] levels) occur in 14.2%[108] to 48.5%[127] of cases. When radiation doses exceed 2600 rad, the incidence of elevated TSH levels significantly increases. Multiagent chemotherapy does not effect the incidence of hypothyroidism.[128] The exact role of the lymphangiogram in the development of thyroid dysfunction remains unclear; previous supposition had been that lymphangiogram was a predisposing factor in thyroid dysfunction, but more recent investigations suggest that it acts as a protective mechanism[129] or plays no role at all in the development of an abnormal thyroid.[128] The incidence of thyroid dysfunction increases over time after irradiation; therefore monitoring of thyroid function levels is important in long-term follow-up. One series has demonstrated spontaneous improvement in radiation-induced hypothyroidism in more than one third of their childhood Hodgkin's patients.[128]

The risk of developing a second cancer after experiencing a childhood malignancy is 17%.[130] Solid tumors associated with previous radiation for Hodgkin's disease include breast carcinoma, thyroid carcinoma, multiple basal cell carcinomas, and osteosarcoma.[1]

Late effects of chemotherapy are most evident in two areas, gonadal dysfunction and second malignancies. MOPP chemotherapy produces aspermia, the duration of which has not yet been fully determined.[124,131] Generally, less is known of the effects of chemotherapy on ovarian function. British investigations suggest that MOPP chemotherapy in women induces ovarian failure in 41% and irregular ovarian activity in 34%; 17% retain normal ovarian function.[132] The incidence of second malignancies among lymphoma patients receiving both intensive radiotherapy and chemotherapy has been much higher than expected; ratio of observed-to-expected second cancers is 29:1. At particular

risk are those patients receiving chemotherapy for relapse of Hodgkin's disease treated with intensive radiotherapy,[133,134] especially if the treatments are given within 12 months of each other.[135] In the adult population at least 177 cases of acute myelogenous leukemia have been documented following treatment for Hodgkin's disease.[136] Non-Hodgkin's lymphomas (4.4%) have also occurred as sequelae of treatment for Hodgkin's disease.[39] The incidence of leukemia and second malignant neoplasms is lower in children and adolescents with Hodgkin's disease but does occasionally occur.[1]

PROGNOSIS

The outlook for children and adolescents with Hodgkin's disease is very good. Patients with stage I Hodgkin's disease and some stage II disease (depending on presentation and specific histology) who are treated with definitive radiotherapy have experienced a 90% or better 4-year survival.[1] Patients with stage III disease managed with chemotherapy-radiotherapy regimens have an 80% or better survival at 4 years. And in stage IV disease 4-year survivals of 79% of the patients have been achieved.[1]

CASE STUDY

L.R., a 14-year-old Latin American female, was found to have palpable supraclavical lymph nodes on the left side during a routine school physical examination. No other adenopathy was noted. These nodes were again noted on follow-up 3 weeks later. Initially, the adenopathy had consisted of two nontender nodes. During the interval between examinations, there was progression to several, slightly tender nodes. The physical examination was otherwise normal; chest x-ray examination was normal; tine test negative; and white blood cell count was 9.4 with 68% neutrophils, 30% lymphs, 1% bands, and 1% basophils. There were no complaints of weight loss, fever, pruritis, night sweats, or change in activity level.

A lymph node biopsy of the left supraclavicular area was performed 1 month after the lymphadenopathy was first noted. The report was Hodgkin's disease, mixed cellularity. L.R. was referred to the pediatric department of a large cancer center.

Further diagnostic workup at the cancer center included a chest x-ray examination that now indicated mediastinal adenopathy, a lymphangiogram that was negative, an IVP that was normal, and blood work. Initial serum chemical survey was normal. Complete blood count was as follows: white blood cell count 12.3 (polys 60%, lymph 25%, monos 7%, eos 8%), platelets 409,000, hemoglobin 11.2 g/dl, and hematocrit 33.7%. Alkaline phosphatase isoenzyme (bone) was 111 miu/ml. Serum copper was 196 mcg/100 m with a sedimentation rate of 52 mm/hr. Staging laparotomy with splenectomy was negative for Hodgkin's disease. Thus clinical and pathologic investigations indicated L.R. had Hodgkin's disease stage II$_A$. Postoperatively, L.R. experienced a surgical wound abscess that necessitated her readmission to the hospital for intravenous antibiotics.

L.R. received a pneumococcal vaccination before splenectomy and postoperatively received prophylactic penicillin vk 250 mg PO b.i.d. Dental oncology evaluated L.R. before therapy and initiated prophylactic treatment for irradiation caries.

L.R.'s therapy consisted of two courses of CVPP, a rest period of 1 month, radiotherapy to the involved field (anterior and posterior mantle), another month's rest, and then four more courses of CVPP. All treatment was completed 9 months after diagnosis.

L.R. continues to do well 9 months after therapy. She is a cheerleader and plays on the school volleyball team.

NURSING CONSIDERATIONS

Successful management of Hodgkin's disease, in terms of disease control and freedom from harmful late effects of treatment, requires precise staging and careful monitoring for disease presence and development of treatment side effects. The nursing care of these children and adolescents is complex and demands a multitude of skills. In addition to providing comfort, taking vital signs, and administering chemotherapy, nursing expertise is required in supportive and educational interventions, physical assessment, surveillance for early and late sequelae of therapy, and coordination of the multiple diagnostic and treatment regimens in Hodgkin's treatment.

Much of the anxiety and emotional upset associated with the diagnosis of Hodgkin's disease can be lessened by educating the family as to what the disease is, what tests will be done to discover its distribution, and how it is treated. Many families and patients may be familiar with examinations, such as blood sampling or chest x-ray examina-

tions, but more sophisticated investigations, such as lymphangiograms, CT scans, and IVP's, may create considerable anxiety, especially in the young patients. Thorough explanations of the reason for the test, the testing procedure, and most importantly, how it will feel can decrease anxieties and enhance cooperation. Written material, in simple layman terms can augment and reinforce the information taught. Important to remember while teaching and throughout therapy is that families and patients are very anxious and often do not hear all that is said or misinterpret what is said.[137] Thus information may need to be repeated on several occasions or misinformation corrected. Again, written material can be a helpful resource.

Since Hodgkin's disease is frequently misdiagnosed (i.e., adentitis or cat-scratch fever), weeks or months may lapse between the time an enlarged lymph node is first noted and an accurate diagnosis is made. This delay in diagnosis and initiation of therapy can add to the family's anxiety. Not only does it introduce fear that the disease has had a chance to spread but that the family themselves are guilty of creating the delay. Nursing can help alleviate some of these stresses by allowing the family to voice their fears and providing reassurance that the delayed diagnosis was not the fault of the family.[138] Additional guilt or fears may stem from the family feeling they could have prevented their child from getting Hodgkin's disease had they taken better care of the child. Again, nursing can help quiet these feelings through listening, reassurance, and appropriate literature.

Since the diagnosis of Hodgkin's disease requires a lymph node biopsy, nursing care at that time focuses on explaining the procedure and teaching wound care postoperatively. Patients should be reminded to wear loose-fitting clothing over the surgical wound and wait until the sutures are removed before bathing the area. (These biopsies are usually done under local anesthesia but may require general anesthesia for younger children or uncooperative adolescents.)

Once diagnosis is established, the battery of x-ray examinations and blood work to follow must be scheduled and explained to the family. Chest x-ray examinations and blood sampling are usually not unfamiliar to the family or patient and require little nursing input. On the other hand, CT scans, lymphangiograms, and IVPs need careful explanations. Before these investigations, a history of allergy to iodine or contrast dyes should be obtained. If possible, the children (and even adolescents) should see the CAT scan machines before experiencing the examination; although not painful, the machinery can be very frightening. When IVPs are to be done, the family and the patient need to know that a laxative should be taken the night before and only liquids ingested the morning before the test.

Lymphangiograms can be performed with local anesthesia on adolescents, but younger children require general anesthesia. Families and patients should be warned that following this examination the patient's feet and urine may have a bluish discoloration. As each foot will have a small incision with stitches, patients need to be reminded to wear loose-fitting shoes and not immerse their feet in water until after the stitches have been removed. The incisions may be cleaned daily with alcohol. Symptoms of wound infection reviewed with the family can prevent a delay in initiation of therapy if such a procedural complication should occur. As previously mentioned, pulmonary oil embolism is a potential complication of lymphangiogram. Therefore patients must be observed postprocedure for dyspnea and fever. Warning families ahead of time that IVPs and lymphangiograms require follow-up films at 24 hours can save them the inconvenience of unexpected trips to the hospital.

The diagnostic workup of Hodgkin's disease is concluded by a staging laparotomy and splenectomy. Nursing considerations at this time include assuring that the patient receives a pneumococcal vaccine before surgery and intensive preoperative teaching. After surgery, nursing care that ensures frequent deep breathing, coughing, turning, and early ambulation is essential for a uncomplicated postoperative period. An uneventful recovery from surgery course allows chemotherapy to be initiated without delay at 10 days to 2 weeks after surgery.

As previously mentioned, saliva is important in the prevention of caries; when output is altered, as it is after salivary gland exposure to radiotherapy, care must be taken to prevent rampant caries. Thus nursing personnel should ensure that all Hodgkin's disease patients are referred to a dental oncologist for prophylactic care before irradiation treatment. Current recommendations are for daily brushing with a 0.4% stannous fluoride (SNF_2) gel. This application is to take place after the final oral hygiene procedure of the day and consists of placing about a ¾ inch of the SNF_2 gel on a toothbrush and carefully brushing the gel onto all tooth surfaces. After brushing, the patient swishes two to three times and expectorates without rinsing. Daily brushing with the SNF_2 gel is effective in control of postirradiation caries, but patients must comply for it to work.[139] Thus oral care of irradiated patients is also a focus of nursing care for children with Hodgkin's disease.

Since the incidence of herpes zoster infections is as high as 35% in children and adolescents with Hodgkin's disease,[99] nursing recognition of this malady is essential. Early recognition is important not only to protect those who have not had chickenpox, but prompt initiation of therapy can shorten the clinical course of the disease. Herpes zoster, or shingles, is thought to be caused by reactivation of latent varicella-zoster virus residing in sensory cells of the dorsal root ganglia, presumably present from a previous chickenpox infection.[124] The illness begins with pain and tenderness along the involved dermatome, usually having been in the irradiated field. Generalized malaise and fever are often also present. Within a few days, groups of red papules appear, distributed along one or two adjacent dermatomes. The individual lesions vesiculate, become pustular, dry up, and scab in the course of 5 to 10 days.[140] Ara-A given intravenously in a dosage of 15 mg/kg/24 hours over a 12-hour period for 5 days or acyclovir sodium 15 mg/kg/24 hours given IV in three divided doses every 8 hours over 1 hour seem to be effective in diminishing cutaneous spread and decreasing duration of pain.[114-117] Additionally, acyclovir ointments applied topically appear to increase lesion healing time, decreasing duration of viral shedding, and slightly decrease pain. Desquamation also seems to be diminished with the use of acyclovir topically. Important to keep in mind is that the neuralgia associated with varicella-zoster can be severe, requiring narcotics to relieve the pain.

The preceding overview of nursing considerations for the child or adolescent with Hodgkin's disease demonstrates the need for nursing expertise beyond traditional roles. As disease survival rates are maintained and improved, nursing attention must be focused on diminishing the sometimes devastating early and late effects of therapy. Additionally, nursing care tailored for the individual child or adolescent with Hodgkin's disease can facilitate the family's and patient's smooth and rapid return to home and their previous life patterns.

NURSING CARE PROTOCOL FOR THE CHILD WITH HODGKIN'S DISEASE

Nursing diagnoses (problem/needs)	Goals/objectives (patient/family will:)	Interventions (nurse will:)
1. Knowledge deficit (related to diagnostic workup)	Verbalize purpose of and methods for testing	Assist with and teach regarding workup procedures (P.E., lab work, CT scans, CXR, lymphangiogram, IVP) Encourage questions pertaining to workup Give any available teaching resources
2. Anxiety (emotional upset related to diagnosis, testing, possible hospitalization, treatment, and side effects)	Have decreased level of anxiety; share feeling with support people	Teach (workup, disease, protocol) Assist with referrals to other services (chaplain, social work, psychiatrist) Active listening, use of play, TLC, offer self
3. Knowledge deficit (need for initial surgery biopsy to establish definite diagnosis and staging laparotomy with splenectomy)	Verbalize general understanding of surgery Be able to state preoperative and postoperative routines	Assist with explanation of surgeries; explain need for staging laparotomy and splenectomy Teach preoperative and postoperative routines (NPO, IV, preoperative medicine, safety measures, turn, cough, deep breath, foley, NG, tour of recovery room preoperatively)
4. Injury: potential for (pneumococcal infection postsplenectomy)	Verbalize reason for pneumococcal vaccination Verbalize reason for daily prophylactic antibiotics; verbalize name and dose schedule of antibiotics	Teach reason for giving pneumococcal vaccination Teach reason for giving daily antibiotic prophylaxis and dose schedule

NURSING CARE PROTOCOL FOR THE CHILD WITH HODGKIN'S DISEASE—cont'd

Nursing diagnoses (problem/needs)	Goals/objectives (patient/family will:)	Interventions (nurse will:)
5. Injury: potential for (possible postoperative complications)	Have absence of postoperative complications	Implement preventive measures, identify complication, initiate prompt treatment of complication
Infection	Have clean, dry surgical incision that heals without any complications	Keep incision area dry and clean; observe for infection and report; teach how to care for wound and what to report; monitor laboratory work
Hemorrhage	Have minimum blood loss, stable vital signs	Monitor vital signs; note other signs and symptoms related to shock and pertinent lab work (Hgb, Hct); frequent dressing checks; observe for increase in drainage of fresh blood from any drainage tubes
Comfort, alterations in: Pain	Verbalize comfort: relaxed facial expression; progressive increase in mobility; decreasing request for pain medication	Comfort measures: positioning, touch, diversion, medication, emotional support
Mobility: impaired, physical	Have progressive increased participation in activities of daily living; chest clear, skin intact, bowel sounds present, tolerates PO intake, healing incision	Implement prevention measures, identify complications, initiate prompt treatment of complications
6. Knowledge deficit (needs related to chemotherapy)	Be able to state name of drug and broad purpose; be able to state how long therapy will be given Identify expected side effects (early) and proper methods of follow-up; have early side effects within expected limits and control absence of complications resulting from side effects	Evaluate level of understanding and teach accordingly; assist in having permits and consent forms signed Teach, evaluate, and document related to drugs; prophylaxis and treatment per nursing and physician orders related to individual protocol (see Chapter 20)
7. Knowledge deficit (related to radiation therapy)	Be able to state broad purpose of therapy; identify expected side effects and follow-up appropriately; Recognize postradiation syndromes	Teach, evaluate, and document (see Chapter 21)

Continued.

Nursing diagnoses (problem/needs)	Goals/objectives (patient/family will:)	Interventions (nurse will:)
	Have side effects within expected limits and control; absence of complications resulting from side effects	Prophylaxis and treatment per nursing and medical orders related to N & V, constipation, anorexia, stomatitis, skin breakdown, oral care
	Have minimum late side effects; compliance with follow-up	Teach importance of follow-up Observe for late effects: sterility, lung fibrosis in area radiated, the chance of fibrosis of the lining of the heart, low thyroid activity, caries and 1% risk of second tumors
8. Nutrition, alteration in: less than body requirements (following N & V, chemotherapy, radiation, disease)	Relief from N & V; weight stable; PO intake return to usual amount	Obtain order for antiemetics Arrange consultation with dietician Offer small, frequent appetizing meals Mouth care before all meals High-protein high-carbohydrate diet; well-balanced meals Monitor I & O carefully Eliminate unpleasant sights and smells Obtain order for topical mouthwash anesthetic Encourage fluids
9. Injury: potential for (reoccurrence and/or metastasis; potential for treatment failure)	Identify signs and symptoms of reoccurrence—enlarged lymph nodes; identify signs of treatment failure—progression of primary disease, lymph nodes do not regress	Teach, evaluate, document
	Verbalize understanding and individualized treatment	Teach, evaluate, and document according to individual treatment protocol
	Obtain remission or comfort during terminal phase	Nursing care specific to patient
10. Coping; ineffective family: compromised	Be able to cope with adjustments needed and return to maximum-grade functioning; maintain grade level in school	Provide emotional support and teaching; referral as needed; communicate with schools
	Maintain positive self-concept, return to activities of daily living and school	Follow-up as needed

REFERENCES

1. Sullivan, M.P., Fuller, L.M., and Butler, J.J.: Hodgkin's disease. In Sutow, W.W., Fernbach, D.J., and Vietti, T.J., editors: Clinical pediatric oncology, ed. 3, St. Louis, 1984, The C.V. Mosby Co.
2. Ford, R.J.: Immunobiology of Hodgkin's disease, The Cancer Bulletin **35:**204, 1983.
3. Hoster, H.A., and others: Hodgkin's disease. I. 1832-1947, Cancer Res. **8:**1, 1948.
4. Fraumeni, J.F., Jr., and Li, F.P.: Hodgkin's disease in childhood: an epidemiologic study, J. Natl. Cancer Inst. **42:**681, 1969.
5. Silverberg, E.: Leukemia and lymphomas: statistical and epidemiological information. American Cancer Society Professional Education Publication, 1977.
6. Young, J.L., and Miller, R.W.: Incidence of malignant tumors in U.S. children, J. Pediatr. **86:**254, 1975.
7. Teillet, F., and Schweisguth, O.: Hodgkin's disease in children: notes on diagnosis and prognosis based on experience with 72 cases in children, Clin. Pediatr. **8:**698, 1969.
8. Strum, S.B., and Rappaport, H.: Hodgkin's disease in the first decade of life, Pediatrics **46:**748, 1970.
9. Jenkin, R.D.T., and others: Hodgkin's disease in children: a retrospective analysis 1958-73, Cancer **35**(suppl.):979, 1975.
10. Bailey, R.J., Burgert, E.O., Jr., and Dahlin, D.C.: Malignant lymphoma in children, Pediatrics **28:**985, 1961.
11. Tan, C., and others: The changing management of childhood Hodgkin's disease, Cancer **35:**808, 1975.
12. Pierce, M.I.: Lymphosarcoma and Hodgkin's disease in children: proceedings of the National Cancer Conference, Sept. 13-15, 1960, Philadelphia, 1961, J.B. Lippincott Co.
13. MacMahon, B.: Epidemiology of Hodgkin's disease, Cancer Res. **26:**1189, 1966.
14. Strong, L.: Genetics, etiology, and epidemiology of childhood cancer. In Sutow, W.W., Fernbach, D.J., and Vietti, T.J., editors: Clinical pediatric oncology, ed. 3, St. Louis, 1984, The C.V. Mosby Co.
15. Chaves, E.: Hodgkin's disease in the first decade, Cancer **31:**925, 1973.
16. Azzam, S.A.: High incidence in Hodgkin's disease in children in Lebanon, Cancer Res. **26:**1202, 1966.
17. Gad-el-Mawla, N., and others: Pediatric Hodgkin's disease in Egypt, Cancer **52:**1129, 1983.
18. Aghai, E., Brenner, H., and Ramot, B.: Childhood Hodgkin's disease in Israel: a study of 17 cases, Cancer **36:**2138, 1975.
19. Solidoro, A., Guzman, C., and Chang, A.: Relative increased incidence of childhood Hodgkin's disease in Peru, Cancer Res. **26:**1204, 1966.
20. Doll, R., Payne, R., and Waterhouse, J.: Cancer incidence in five continents: a teaching report, New York, 1966, Springer-Verlag New York, Inc.
21. Jacobs, P., and others: Hodgkin's disease in children: a ten-year experience in South Africa, Cancer **53:**210, 1984.
22. Mani, A., Crowel, E.B., and Mathew, M: Epidemiologic features of Hodgkin's disease in Punjab, Indian J. Cancer **19:**183, 1982.
23. Tarawneh, M.S., and others: Hodgkin's disease in Jordanian children: a study of 26 cases, Clin. Oncol. **10:**21, 1984.
24. Gutensohn, N., and Cole, P.: Epidemiology of Hodgkin's disease in the young, Int. J. Cancer **19:**595, 1977.
25. Vianna, N.J., and Polan, A.K.: Immunity in Hodgkin's disease: importance of age at exposure, Ann. Intern. Med. **89:**550, 1978.
26. Gutensohn, N., and Shapiro, D.: Social class risk factors among children with Hodgkin's disease, Int. J. Cancer **30:**433, 1982.
27. Gutensohn, N., and Cole, P.: Childhood social environment and Hodgkin's disease, N. Engl. J. Med. **304:**135, 1981.
28. Greenberg, R., Gutterman, S., and Cole, P.: An evaluation of space-time clustering in Hodgkin's disease, J. Chron. Dis. **36:**257, 1983.
29. Grufferman, S., Cole, P., and Levitan, T.: Evidence against transmission of Hodgkin's disease in high schools, N. Engl. J. Med., **300:**1006, 1979.
30. Scherr, P.A., Gutensohn, N., and Cole, P.: School contact among persons with Hodgkin's disease, Am. J. Epidemiol. **120:**29, 1984.
31. Vianna, N.J., and others: Tonsillectomy and childhood Hodgkin's disease, Lancet **2:**338, 1980.
32. Hardell, L., and Bengtsson, N.O.: Epidemiological study of socioeconomic factors and clinical findings in Hodgkin's disease, and reanalysis of previous data regarding chemical exposure, Br. J. Cancer. **48:**217, 1983.
33. Henderson, B.E., and others: Risk factors for nodular sclerosis and other types of Hodgkin's disease, Cancer Res. **39:**4507, 1979.
34. Razis, D.V., Diamond, H.D., and Craver, L.F.: Familial Hodgkin's disease: its significance and implications, Ann. Intern. Med. **51:**933, 1959.
35. Grufferman, S., and others: Hodgkin's disease in siblings, N. Engl. J. Med. **296:**248, 1977.
36. Torres, A., and others: Simultaneous Hodgkin's disease in three siblings with identical HLA-genotype, Cancer **46:**838, 1980.
37. Abramson, J.H., and others: A case-control study of Hodgkin's disease in Israel, J. Natl. Cancer Inst. **61:**307, 1978.
38. Thompson, E.A.: Pedigree analysis of Hodgkin's disease in a Newfoundland genealogy, Ann. Hum. Genet. **45:**279, 1981.

39. Strum, S.B., Park, J.K., and Rappaport, H.: The observation of cells resembling Sternberg-Reed cells in conditions other than Hodgkin's disease, Cancer **26:**176, 1970.

40. Tan, C.T., and Chan, K.W.: Hodgkin's disease, Pediatr. Ann. **12:**306, 1983.

41. Butler, J.J.: Non-neoplastic lesions of lymph nodes of man to be differentiated from lymphomas, Natl. Cancer Inst. Monogr. **32:**233, 1969.

42. Kaplan, H.S., and Gartner, S.: "Sternberg-Reed" giant cells of Hodgkin's disease: cultivation in vitro, heterotians plantation, and characterization as neoplastic macrophages, Int. J. Cancer **19:**511, 1977.

43. Lukes, R.J., and Butler, J.J.: The pathology and nomenclature of Hodgkin's disease, Cancer Res. **26:**1063, 1966.

44. Lukes, R.J., and others: Report of the nomenclature committee, Cancer Res. **26:**1311, 1966.

45. Moayeri, H., and Han, T.: Hodgkin's disease. In Tebbi, C.K., editor: Major topics in pediatric and adolescent oncology, Boston, 1982, G.K. Hall & Co.

46. White, L., Siegel, S.E., and McCourt, B.A.: Patterns of Hodgkin's disease at diagnosis in young children, Am. J. Pediatr. Hematol. Oncol. **5:**251, 1983.

47. Strum, S.B., and Rappaport, H.: Consistency of histologic subtypes in Hodgkin's disease in simultaneous and sequential biopsy specimens, Natl. Cancer Inst. Monogr. **36:**253, 1973.

48. Rappaport, H., and others: Report to the committee on histological criteria contributing to staging of Hodgkin's disease, Cancer Res. **31:**1864, 1971.

49. Kelly, W.D., Good, R.A., and Varco, R.L.: Anergy and skin homograft survival in Hodgkin's disease, Surg. Gynecol. Obstet., **107:**565, 1958.

50. Aisenberg, A.C.: Studies on delayed hypersensitivity in Hodgkin's disease, J. Clin. Invest. **41:**1964, 1962.

51. Sokal, J.E., and Primikirios, N.: The delayed skin test response in Hodgkin's disease and lymphosarcoma: effect of disease activity, Cancer **14:**597, 1961.

52. Bjorkholm, M., Holm, G., and Mellstedt, H.: Immunologic profile of patients with cured Hodgkin's disease, Scand. J. Haematol. **18:**361, 1977.

53. Case, D.C., and others: Depressed *in vitro* lymphocyte responses to PHA in patients with Hodgkin's disease in continuous long remission, Blood, **49:**771, 1977.

54. Riiswiik, R.E., Sybesma, J.P., and Kater, L.: A prospective study of the changes in the immune status before, during, and after multiple-agent chemotherapy for Hodgkin's disease, Cancer **51:**637, 1983.

55. Anderson, E.: Depletation of thymus-dependent lymphocytes in Hodgkin's disease, Scand. J. Haematol. **12:**263, 1974.

56. Bobrove, A.M., and others: Quantitation of T- and B-lymphocytes and cellular immune function in Hodgkin's disease, Cancer **36:**169, 1975.

57. Lauria, F., and others: Increased proportion of suppressor/cytotoxic (OKT8 +) cells in patients with Hodgkin's disease in long-lasting remission, Cancer **52:**1385, 1983.

58. Han, T., and Minowada, J.: Impairment of cell-mediated immunity in untreated Hodgkin's disease: evaluation by skin test, lymphocyte stimulation test, and T-lymphocyte counts, N.Y. State J. Med. **78:**216, 1978.

59. Holm, G., and others: Lymphocyte abnormalities in untreated patients with Hodgkin's disease, Cancer **37:**751, 1976.

60. Han, T.: Role of suppressor cells in depression of T-lymphocyte proliferative response in untreated and treated Hodgkin's disease, Cancer **45:**2102, 1980.

61. Gergely, P., Szegedi, G., and Berenyi, E.G.: Lymphocyte surface immunoglobulins in Hodgkin's disease, N. Engl. J. Med. **289:**220, 1973.

62. Sutcliffe, S.B., and others: Intensive investigation in management of Hodgkin's disease, Br. Med. J. **2:**1343, 1976.

63. Evans, H.E., and Nyhan, W.L.: Hodgkin's disease in children, Bull. Johns Hopkins Hospital **114:**237, 1964.

64. Origenes, M.L., Jr., Need, D.J., and Hartman, J.R.: Treatment of the malignant lymphomas in children, Pediatr. Clin. North Am. **9:**769, 1962.

65. Kaplan, H.S.: Hodgkin's disease, Cambridge, Mass., 1972, Harvard University Press.

66. Carpentieri, V., Smith, L., Jr., and Daeschner, C.: Approach to a child with enlarged lymph nodes, Texas Med. **79:**58, 1983.

67. Keller, J.: Nodes, In Walker, K.H., Hall, W.D., and Hurst, J.W., editors: Clinical methods, ed. 2, Boston, 1980, Butterworth Publishers, Inc.

68. Jing, B.S., and McGraw, J.P.: Lymphangiography in diagnosis and management of malignant lymphomas, Cancer **19:**565, 1966.

69. Ray, G.R., Wolf, P.H., and Kaplan, H.S.: Valve of laboratory indicators in Hodgkin's disease: preliminary results, Natl. Cancer Inst. Monogr. **36:**315, 1973.

70. Webb, D.I., Ubogy, G., and Silver, R.T.: Importance of bone marrow biopsy in the clinical staging of Hodgkin's disease, Cancer **26:**313, 1970.

71. Aisenberg, A.C., and others: Serum alkaline phosphatase at the onset of Hodgkin's disease, Cancer **26:**318, 1970.

72. Hrgovcie, M., and others: Serum copper levels in lymphoma and leukemia: special reference to Hodgkin's disease, Cancer **21:**743, 1968.

73. Pagliardi, E., and Giangrandi, E.: Clinical significance of the blood copper in Hodgkin's disease, Acta Haematol. **24:**201, 1960.

74. Gamble, J.F., and others: Influence of staging celiotomy in localized presentations of Hodgkin's disease, Cancer **35:**817, 1975.

75. Kaplan, H.S.: Hodgkin's disease: unfolding concepts concerning its nature, management, and prognosis, Cancer **45:**2439, 1980.

76. Horn, M.L., Ray, R.C., and Kriss, J.P.: Gallium-67 citrate scanning in Hodgkin's disease and non-Hodgkin's lymphomas, Cancer **37**:250, 1976.

77. Handmaker, H., and O'Mara, R.E.: Gallium imaging in pediatrics, J. Nucl. Med. **18**:1057, 1977.

78. Harris, J.M., Tang, D.B., and Weltz, M.D.: Diagnostic tests and Hodgkin's disease: a standardized approach to their evaluation, Cancer **41**:2388, 1978.

79. Carbone, P.P., and others: Report of the committee on Hodgkin's disease staging classification, Cancer Res. **31**:1860, 1971.

80. Hays, D.M.: The staging of Hodgkin's disease in children reviewed, Cancer **35**(suppl.):973, 1975.

81. Paglia, M.A., and others: Surgical aspects and results of laparotomy and splenectomy in Hodgkin's disease AM. J. Roentgenol. Radium Ther. Nucl. Med. **117**:12, 1973.

82. Russell, K.J., and others: Childhood Hodgkin's disease: patterns of relapse, J. Clin. Oncol. **2**:80, 1984.

83. Allen, L.W., and others: Laparotomy and splenectomy in the staging of Hodgkin's disease. Proceeding of the forty-second Annual Meeting of the Society of Laboratory and Clinical Medicine **74**:845, 1969.

84. Glatstein, E., and others: The value of laparotomy and splenectomy in the staging of Hodgkin's disease, Cancer **24**:709, 1969.

85. Lowenbraun, S., and others: Diagnostic laparotomy and splenectomy for staging Hodgkin's disease, Ann. Intern. Med. **72**:655, 1970.

86. Green, D.M., and others: Staging laparotomy with splenectomy in children and adolescents with Hodgkin's disease, Cancer Treat. Rev. **10**:23, 1983.

87. Glatstein, E., Goffinet, D.R.: Staging of Hodgkin's disease and other lymphomas, Clinica Hematol. **3**:70, 1974.

88. Chilcote, R.R., Baehner, R.L., and Hammond, D.: Septicemia and meningitis in children splenectomized for Hodgkin's disease, N. Engl. J. Med. **295**:798, 1976.

89. Ravry, M., and others: Serious infection after splenectomy for the staging of Hodgkin's disease, Ann. Intern. Med. **77**:11, 1972.

90. Rosner, F., and Zarrabi, M.H.: Late infections following splenectomy in Hodgkin's disease, Clin. Sci. Rev. **1**:57, 1983.

91. Chilcote, R.R., Baehner, R.L., and the Investigators of Children's Cancer Study Group (CCSG): The incidence of overwhelming infection in children staged for Hodgkin's disease, Proc. A.S.C.O. **16**:224, 1975.

92. Donaldson, S.S., Glatstein, E., and Vosti, K.L.: Bacterial infections in pediatric Hodgkin's disease: relationship to radiotherapy, chemotherapy, and splenectomy, Cancer **41**:1949, 1978.

93. Hays, D.M., and others: Complications related to 234 staging laparotomies performed in the intergroup Hodgkin's disease in childhood study, Surgery **96**:3, 1984.

94. Reboul, F., Donaldson, S., and Kaplan, H.: Herpes zoster and varicella infections in children with Hodgkin's disease: an analysis of contributing factors, Cancer **41**:95, 1978.

95. Seiber, G.R., and others: Impaired response to pneumococcal vaccine after treatment for Hodgkin's disease, N. Engl. J. Med. **299**:442, 1978.

96. Minor, D.R., Schiffman, G., and McIntosh, L.: Response of patients with Hodgkin's disease to pneumococcal vaccine, Ann Intern. Med. **90**:887, 1979.

97. Addiego, J.E., Jr., and others: Response to pneumococcal polysaccharide vaccine in patients with untreated Hodgkin's disease, Lancet **2**:450, 1980.

98. Peters, M.V.: A study of survivals in Hodgkin's disease treated radiologically, Am. J. Roentgenol. Radium Ther. Nucl. Med. **53**:299, 1950.

99. D'Agio, G.J., and others: The changing management of childhood Hodgkin's disease, Cancer **35**:808, 1975.

100. Sullivan, M.P.: Unpublished data, 1982.

101. DeVita, V.T., Canellos, G.P., and Moxley, J.H.: A decade of combination chemotherapy of advanced Hodgkin's disease, Cancer **30**:1495, 1972.

102. DeVita, V.T., Serpick, A., and Carbona, P.P.: Combination chemotherapy of advanced Hodgkin's disease (HD): the NCI program, a progress report (abstract), Proc. A.A.C.R. **10**:19, 1969.

103. Coltman, C.A., and Delaney, F.C.: Five-drug combination chemotherapy for advanced Hodgkin's disease (abstract), Clin. Res. **21**:876, 1973.

104. Cooper, M.R., and others: A new effective four-drug combination of CCNU (1-[2-chloroethyl]-3-cyclohexyl-1-nitrosourea) (NSC-79038), vinblastine, prednisone, and procarbazine for the treatment of advanced Hodgkin's disease, Cancer **46**:654, 1980.

105. Bonadonna, G., and others: Adriamycin, bleomycin, vinblastine, and imidazol carboxamide (ABVD): a new combination effective in advanced Hodgkin's disease (abstract), Proceedings of the XI International Cancer Congress, Florence, Italy, **1**:271, 1974.

106. Krikorian, J.G., Portlock, C.S., and Rosenberg, S.A.: Treatment of advanced Hodgkin's disease with adriamycin, bleomycin, vinblastine, and imidazole carboxamide (ABVD) after failure of MOPP therapy, Cancer **41**:2107, 1978.

107. Porzig, K.J., and others: Treatment of advanced Hodgkin's disease with B-CAVe following MOPP failure, Cancer **41**:1670, 1978.

108. Rodgers, R.W., and others: ABDIC chemotherapy in MOPP resistant lymphoma, primarily Hodgkin's disease (HD), proc. A.S.C.O. **20**:30, 1979.

109. Schier, W.D., Jr., Wong, R.D.I., and Aisenberg, A.C.: Vinblastine in the treatment of advanced Hodgkin's disease, Cancer **22**:467, 1968.

110. Kaplan, H.S.: Role of intensive radiotherapy in the management of Hodgkin's disease, Cancer **19**:356, 1966.
111. Donaldson, S.S., Berberich, F.R., and Kaplan, H.S.: A program of low dose ratiation and MOPP chemoctherapy for pediatric Hodgkin's disease, Proc. A.S.C.O. **22**:22, 1981.
112. Sullivan, M.P., Ramirez, I., and Bronell, P.: Breaking varicella-zoster virus latency in children with Hodgkin's disease: the triggering effect of postradiotherapy chemotherapy, Proceedings 75th Annual Meeting, American Association Cancer Research **25**:767, 1984.
113. Reboul, F., Donaldson, S., and Kaplan, H.: Herpes zoster and varicella infections in children with Hodgkin's disease, Cancer **41**:95, 1978.
114. Culbert, S.J., and Pickering, L.K.: Principles of total care-physiologic support. In Sutow, W.W., Fernbach, D.J., and Vietti, T.J., editors: Clinical pediatric oncology, ed. 3, St. Louis, 1984, The C.V. Mosby Co.
115. Johnson, M.T., and others: Treatment of varicella-zoster infections with adenine arabinoside, J. Infect. Dis. **131**:225, 1975.
116. Whitley, R.J., and others: Adenine arabinoside therapy at herpes zoster in the immunosuppressed, N. Engl. J. Med. **294**:1193, 1976.
117. Balfour, H., and others: Acyclovir halts progression of herpes zoster in immunocompromised patients, N. Engl. J. Med. **808**:1448, 1983.
118. Perez, C.A., and Thomas, P.R.M.: Radiation Therapy: Basic concepts and clinical implications. In Sutow, W.W., Fernbach, D.J., and Vietti, T., editors: Clinical pediatric oncology, ed. 3, St. Louis, 1984, The C.V. Mosby Co.
119. Frank, R.M., Herdly, J., and Philippe, E: Acquired dental defects and salivary gland lesions after irradiation for carcinoma, J. Am. Dent. Assoc. **70**:868, 1965.
120. Dreizen, S., and others: Radiation-induced xerostomia in cancer patients: effect on salivary and serum electrolytes, Cancer **38**:273, 1976.
121. Hutchinson, G.B.: Survival and complications of radiotherapy following involved and extended field therapy of Hodgkin's disease, Stages I and II, Cancer **38**:288, 1976.
122. Wilimas, J., Thompson, E., and Smith, K.: Long-term results of treatment of children and adolescents with Hodgkin's disease, Cancer **46**:2123, 1980.
123. Exelby, P.R.: Method of evaluating children with Hodgkin's disease, CA **21**:95, 1971.
124. Kaplan, H.S., and Rosenberg, S.A.: Current status of clinical trials: Standford experience 1962-1972, Natl. Cancer Inst. Monogr. **36**:363, 1973.
125. Donaldson, S.S., and others: Pediatric Hodgkin's disease. II. Results of therapy, Cancer **37**:2436, 1976.
126. Ramsey, N., and others: Thyroid dysfunction in pediatric patients after mantle field radiation therapy for Hodgkin's disease, Proc. A.S.C.O. **19**:389, 1978.
127. Shalet, S.M., and others: Thyroid dysfunction following external irradiation to the neck for Hodgkin's disease in childhood, Clin. Radiol. **28**:511, 1977.
128. Constine, L.S., and others: Thyroid dysfunction after radiotherapy in children with Hodgkin's disease, Cancer **53**:878, 1984.
129. Green, D.M., and others: Thyroid function in pediatric patients after neck irradiation for Hodgkin's disease, Med. Pediatr. Oncol. **8**:127, 1980.
130. Li, F.P., Cassady, J.R., and Jaffe, N.: Risk of second tumors in survivors of childhood cancer, Cancer **35**:1230, 1975.
131. daCunha, M.F., and others: Recovery of spermatogenesis after treatment for Hodgkin's disease: limiting dose of MOPP chemotherapy, J. Clin. Oncol. **2**:577, 1984.
132. Chapman, R.M., Sutcliffe, S.B., and Malpas, J.: Cytotoxic-induced ovarian failure in women with Hodgkin's disease. I. Hormone function, JAMA **242**:1877, 1979.
133. Arsenau, J.C., and others: Nonlymphomatous malignant tumors complicating Hodgkin's disease, possible association with intensive therapy, N. Engl. J. Med. **287**:1119, 1972.
134. Canellos, G.P., and others: Second malignancies complicating Hodgkin's disease in remission, Lancet **1**:947, 1975.
135. DeVita, V.T., Canellos, G.P., and Moxley, J.H.: A decade of combination chemotherapy of advanced Hodgkin's disease, Cancer **30**:1495, 1972.
136. Borum, K.: Increasing frequency of acute myeloid leukemia complicating Hodgkin's disease: a review, Cancer **46**:1247, 1980.
137. Griffin, J.Q.: Physical illness in the family. In Miller, J.R., and Janosik, E.H., editors: Family-focused care, New York 1980, McGraw-Hill, Inc.
138. Caplan, G.: Principles of preventive psychiatry, New York: Basic Books, 1964.
139. Shannon, I.L.: Fluoride treatment program for high-caries-risk patients, Clin. Prev. Dent. **4**:11, 1982.
140. Nelson, N.E., Behrman, R.E., and Vaughan, V.C., editors: Nelson textbook of pediatrics, ed. 12, Philadelphia, 1983, W.B. Saunders Co.

CHAPTER 5

Wilms' tumor

PAT STANFILL and ALEXANDER GREEN

Wilms' tumor, or nephroblastoma, is a rapidly growing tumor arising from the renal parenchyma of the kidney. The tumor is encapsulated by a fibrous, fragile capsule that helps to maintain it locally. Rupture of the capsule leads to dissemination of tumor cells throughout the peritoneal cavity. The vascularity of the tumor lends itself to hematogenous spread, particularly to contiguous organs or the lungs, the primary site of metastasis.[1] A Wilms' tumor may vary in size with some weighing over 1 kg. The tumor may be necrotic or hemorrhagic in nature.[2]

INCIDENCE

The tumor, although described before his classic monograph in 1899, is named for Max Wilms.[2] The most common primary renal tumor in children, Wilms' tumor accounts for about 10% of all malignant tumors in childhood with approximately 500 new cases in the United States annually.[3] Thirty percent of Wilms' tumors occur in children less than 1 year of age with 70% of all tumors occurring before the age of four. Wilms' tumors rarely occur in children past the age of seven.[2]

The distribution of cases is equal in all countries and appears stable over time.[1] There is no sexual predominance, but familial cases have been reported, including rare instances in successive generations and in twins.[4] The left kidney is affected slightly more often than the right, and bilateral tumors occur in about 5% of the cases.[1]

ETIOLOGY

The three principal components of Wilms' tumors are undifferentiated blastemal cells, epithelial tissue, and tumor connective tissue. Although disagreements exist, the prevailing concept is that Wilms' tumor arises during intrauterine life from undifferentiated embryonic tissues. Bove and McAdams[5] postulate, however, that classic Wilms' tumor arises in a hamartomatous metanephric precursor, which exists in a stable state until exposed to a carcinogenic event. They argue that their theory is supported by the increased number of tumors being diagnosed at 3 to 4 years of life and later. Knudson and Strong[6] suggest germinal mutation may be present.

Wilms' tumor is often associated with congenital anomalies, particularly of the genitourinary tract suggesting a correlation between oncogenesis and teratogenesis.[2,7] In a review of 547 patients, 24 had genitourinary anomalies such as hypospadias, cryptorchidism, and fusion anomalies of the kidney.[7] Other anomalies such a aniridia, hemihypertrophy, umbilical hernias, and mental and growth retardation have also been noted. Although the cause of Wilms' tumor is still under debate, patient groups with specific congenital anomalies can now be identified to be at risk to develop this tumor.

CLINICAL PRESENTATION

The most common presenting symptom of Wilms' tumor is a large abdominal mass, which is seen in 68% of all cases; but pain, hematuria, fever, or anorexia may be the first sign of the tumor. The mass often appears suddenly because of hemorrhage within the tumor or cystic degeneration. It may first be noticed by the parent during bathing or dressing of the child or may be detected by routine physical examination. Large tumor masses can sometimes be felt on both sides of the abdomen.[2]

Approximately one third of all patients initially have microscopic hematuria, dysuria, urinary frequency, and/or pain.[8] Anorexia, weight loss, and general malaise also may be evident. Mild to severe hypertension is present in as many as 75% of all patients. The increased blood pressure is caused by elevated plasma renin levels presumed to be a result of renin production of neoplastic cells or from normal renal parenchyma whose blood flow is impaired by the tumor.[2]

Metastases are present at initial diagnosis in 15% of cases. One third of the patients go on to develop metastases usually within 24 months of the diagnosis.[8] The most common site of metastasis is the lungs with single or multiple lesions occurring (Fig. 5-1).

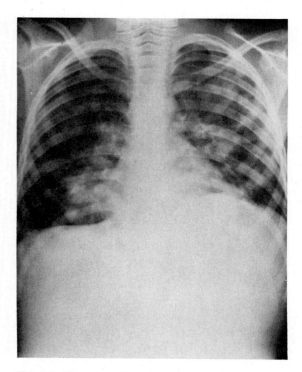

Fig. 5-1. Chest x-ray film of a patient with Wilms' tumor showing multiple metastatic nodules.

DIAGNOSTIC EVALUATION

The primary goal of the diagnostic evaluation is a thorough, rapid diagnosis so that appropriate interventions may occur. Since the patient with Wilms' tumor generally has a visible or palpable abdominal mass, special emphasis is placed on the physical examination and patient history. Evidence of recent weight loss, changes in blood pressure, anemia, hematuria, and dysuria are noted. The presence of congenital abnormalities and a family history of renal problems is also important information to obtain. After a history and physical examination are completed, radiographic, hematologic, and biochemical studies are done.

Radiographic studies may include abdominal and chest films, an abdominal ultrasound, an intravenous pyelogram (IVP), computed tomography (CT), and organ and bone scans. An inferior venacavagram may be indicated to determine tumor involvement of the vena cava. The abdominal roentgenogram will demonstrate a soft tissue density and may also demonstrate organ displacement, particularly of the intestines. Chest films primarily indicate the presence of pulmonary metastases but may demonstrate tumor involvement of the vena cava or right atrium if the tumor is massive.

The IVP usually demonstrates intrinsic distortion of the collecting system with compression or elongation of the calyces (Fig. 5-2).[8] Injected dye may not clear the affected kidney if the renal vein is obstructed by the tumor. The IVP also assists in defining radiation ports postoperatively. If the IVP is not definitive in confirming the diagnosis, arteriography may be used. Abdominal CT scans and bone and liver scans are used to document the existence of metastases (Fig. 5-3). Ultrasonography, although not definitive in children, differentiates between a solid and cystic mass and helps to determine tumor extension in the inferior vena cava.

Hematologic studies are done as a part of the diagnostic evaluation and are useful in determining the patient's physical condition in anticipation of surgery if the diagnosis of Wilms' tumor is supported. A complete blood count, peripheral smear, and platelet count evaluate the degree of anemia

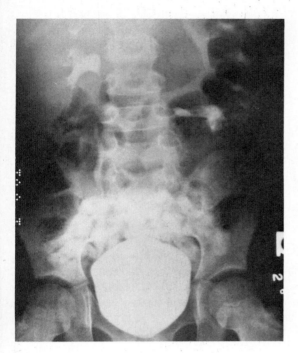

Fig. 5-2. IVP of a patient with Wilms' tumor showing a normal right kidney with displacement of the left kidney and abnormal renal blood flow.

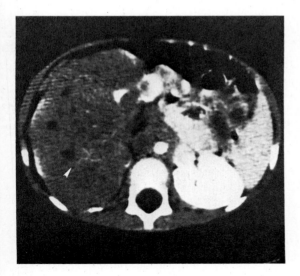

Fig. 5-3. A large mass in the area of the left kidney *(arrow)* with metastasis to the liver.

and determine evidence of polycythemia caused by tumor secretion of erythropoietin.[9] A bone marrow aspirate is sometimes done to rule out metastasis, although rare, or in questionable cases to differentiate between Wilms' tumor and neuroblastoma.

Electrolytes, blood urea nitrogen (BUN), serum and urine creatinine, and liver and renal function studies including urinalysis are done preoperatively. Abnormalities are corrected before surgery, and values obtained are recorded as baseline measurements. Liver and renal function are assessed in preparation to use antineoplastic agents, to remove the affected kidney, and to determine if a preexisting abnormality is evident. Urine levels of vanillylmandelic acid (VMA) may be obtained to rule out neuroblastoma. The definitive diagnosis is made at the time of surgery, but the sophistication of evaluation techniques means an almost certain diagnosis preoperatively.

Staging of the disease is the final evaluative phase of diagnosis. The disease is staged according to surgery findings, pathology findings, and the presence or absence of metastatic disease. There is one major staging system in current use recommended by the National Wilm's Tumor Study Group.[10] Other staging systems in use are consistent with that of the study group although some variations exist. The clinical grouping from the National Wilms' Tumor Studies (NWTS) 1 and 2 is as follows[10]:

The patient's group is decided by the surgeon in the operating room, and is confirmed by the pathologist. If the histological diagnosis and grouping will take more than 48 hours, the surgical grouping stands, the patient is registered and started on treatment.*

Group I: Tumor limited to kidney and completely resected. The surface of the renal capsule is intact. The tumor was not ruptured before or during re-

---

*For National Wilms' Tumor Study 3, this system has been slightly modified. Groups I-V are now called Stages I-V. However, the following changes should be noted: (1) All patients with biopsy-proven positive lymph nodes are Stage III; (2) Children with biopsy of tumor or localized tumor ''spills'' are Stage II. (Children with gross tumor ''spills'' are still Stage III.)

moval. There is no residual tumor apparent beyond the margins of resection.

Group II: Tumor extends beyond the kidney but is completely resected. There is local extension of the tumor; i.e., penetration beyond the pseudocapsule into the peri-renal soft tissues, or peri-aortic lymph node involvement. The renal vessels outside the kidney substances are infiltrated or contain tumor thrombus. There is no residual tumor apparent beyond the margins of resection.

Group III: Residual nonhematogenous tumor confined to abdomen. Any one or more of the following occur: (1) The tumor has been biopsied or ruptured before or during surgery; (2) there are implants on peritoneal surfaces; (3) there are involved lymph nodes beyond the abdominal peri-aortic chains; (4) the tumor is not completely resectable because of local infiltration into vital structures.

Group IV: Hematogenous metastases. Deposits beyond Group II; e.g., lung, liver, bone and brain.

Group V: Bilateral renal involvement.

PROGNOSTIC FACTORS

Survival rates have improved since Farber and his colleagues introduced the use of actinomycin D in the mid-1950s. Continued research has provided further insight into prognostic factors and therapy modifications.[11] Disease stage was the initial prognostic factor seen to influence the course of disease and has evolved from the first system suggested by Garcia and colleagues to current, sophisticated systems such as that developed by the National Wilms' Study Tumor Group.[2] For example, patients with a stage I tumor may expect 2-year survival rates of 95% whereas patients with pulmonary metastases as found with stage IV tumors may expect only a 30% survival rate.[12]

Recent research has indicated that histology plays a significant role in prognosis. Tumors are grouped by cytohistologic patterns into two categories termed "favorable histology" and "unfavorable histology."[13,14] Two relatively uncommon variants of Wilms' tumor, with anaplasia or sarcomatous features, have an unfavorable prognosis. These variants comprised only 11.5% of tumors studied by Beckwith and Palmer[14] and yet accounted for greater than 50% of deaths in NWTS-1. Future therapies should be aggressive for patients whose tumors exhibit anaplasia or sarcomatous features. Patients without anaplasia or sarcomatous features in their tumors have sufficiently low relapse rate and mortality to allow a consideration of less aggressive therapy. Continued refinement of histopathologic techniques and staging systems may further increase their prognostic value.

TREATMENT AND MANAGEMENT

The treatment of Wilms' tumor represents one of the first unified multimodal approaches to solid tumor therapy and has resulted in a high proportion of cures. Disease-free survival has improved from 32% with surgery alone to 80% to 90% with surgery, radiation, and chemotherapy in combination.[10,11] Gross and Neuhauser introduced postoperative irradiation in the early 1950s soon after the transabdominal surgical approach was implemented.[8] In 1956 Farber added the modality of chemotherapy with the use of actinomycin D.[2] With multimodal therapy, disease free survival can occur even in the presence of pulmonary metastases.[15]

The surgical objectives of Wilms' tumor management are to remove the primary tumor even if metastases are present and to provide tissue for pathologic examination. If the mass is unusually large or initial diagnostic workup has indicated contraindications for immediate surgery, chemotherapy and irradiation may be used before surgery or alone to decrease tumor bulk. A transabdominal incision is made to allow adequate visualization of the tumor and surrounding areas. The incision must provide adequate visualization to inspect the uninvolved kidney, abdominal cavity, and inferior vena cava and surrounding nodes; to biopsy and/or remove suspected nodes; and to remove the tumor without disrupting the capsule.

The use of radiation therapy and/or chemotherapy postoperatively depends on the stage and histology of the tumor. The goal of radiation therapy is the control of microscopic residual disease[8] and the treatment of metastases, particularly those in the lungs. Radiation doses to the treatment field usually range from 2000 to 2600 rad delivered over 2 to 3 weeks. Dosages are varied by age and size of the child, stage of disease, and amount of residual or suspected residual tumor. Current trends in radiotherapy include attempts to decrease dosages in an effort to minimize the recognized late effects of irradiation, including growth retardation, organ damage, sterility, and second malignancies.[8,16,17]

Actinomycin D, in combination with vincristine, and doxorubicin (Adriamycin) are the agents of choice to obliterate evidence of microscopic disease, residual tumor remaining after surgery, and metastases. Chemotherapy dosages and schedules are based on stage of disease in the National Wilms' Tumor Study 2. All patients receive actinomycin D and vincristine, and some are later randomized to also receive doxorubicin (Adriamycin).[18] With the trend to decrease irradiation doses because of late effects, the role of chemotherapy in Wilms' tumor therapy is increasing. Since the acute effects of chemotherapy are often manageable, dosage escalations and new combinations are being explored to further impact disease while decreasing the amount of irradiation. There is concern, however, regarding the possible late effects of chemotherapy, such as cardiotoxicity secondary to doxorubicin.

Progression toward more chemotherapy and less radiotherapy has been noted in the evolution of the National Wilms' Tumor Study Group protocols and in other cooperative group or independent agency investigations.[13] NWTS-3, which began in 1979, attempts to refine therapy for those at low risk while determining a more effective therapy for patients at high risk.[18] Patients are carefully staged with histology being considered and are then randomized among differing chemotherapy and radiotherapy regimens. An evaluation of the late effects of NWTS-1 and NWTS-2 therapies is also a part of NWTS-3.

Since a high percentage of patients with Wilms' tumor attain disease-free survival, the ultimate aim of therapy is to maintain or increase survival time while decreasing toxicities of treatment. The success of Wilms' tumor management in children is an excellent model of cooperative group efforts and scientific research leading to a dramatic improvement in survival rates.

CASE STUDY

A.C. is a 28-month-old white female who was well until she was brought to her local physician with bloody urine and a urinary tract infection. Physical examination revealed a mass in the right flank distinguishable from the liver since no movement was noted with respiration. Blood pressure was 118/68, apical pulse was 136, and respirations were 32. History was unremarkable except for confirmed urinary tract infections at 12 and 24 months of age. Family history reveals father has a single kidney. Growth and development were age appropriate. Workup revealed a right renal mass by IVP and confirmed by CT scan that also demonstrated a stag-horn calculus of the left kidney. Right pulmonary nodules were identified by chest roentgenogram, and CT of the chest showed the inferior vena cava and right atrium to be free of tumor.

A right nephrectomy was done. At surgery a nodule was removed from the left kidney and a double renal artery and partial duplication was noted. Multiple lymph nodes were sampled. Pathologic findings of the right kidney revealed Wilms' tumor of favorable histology, changes indicative of long-term pyelonephritis, and areas of metanephric hamartoma and papillary adenoma. Lymph nodes were negative for tumor. Because of the pulmonary metastasis and bilateral disease, she was staged as a group V according to the National Wilms' Tumor Study Group Staging System. She was placed on vincristine, actinomycin D (Dactinomycin), and doxorubicin (Adriamycin) and received 1250 rad total abdominal radiation and 1200 rad to both lungs. A.C. tolerated therapy with minimum toxicity and discontinued therapy 2 years later in complete remission. Soon after, she developed three pulmonary nodules. The pathologic condition was that of Wilms' tumor. Chemotherapy was begun with high-dose vincristine and dactinomycin. Additional chemotherapy, consisting of *cis*-platinum (Cisplatin) and VP-16 was begun after poor response to high-dose chemotherapy. At present, A.C. continues receiving chemotherapy without difficulty but with poor response.

NURSING CONSIDERATIONS

Wilms' tumor may present with no physical symptoms other than a palpable abdominal mass, which is often discovered by the parent. This discovery may create feelings of guilt for not finding it sooner and anger for its occurrence in the child. Once the mass is established, surgery is scheduled within 1 to 2 days after admission to the hospital. The family and child must be prepared for the immediacy of the situation.

The child's abdomen should not be palpated once the diagnosis of Wilms' tumor is suspected. Manipulation of the tumor may cause malignant cells to spread. When inexperienced personnel are caring for the child, it is not inappropriate to post a sign that enforces no manipulation of the abdomen.

Careful assessment of vital signs is essential for the child with Wilms' tumor. Hypertension, secondary to increased renin production, may occur.

Preoperative teaching must involve the parents and the child. Since 70% of the children who develop Wilms' tumor are under age 4,[2] the child may have limited understanding of the situation. The use of hospital play will allow the child to grasp some understanding of the surgery. The use of equipment that the child can touch (such as an operating room gown and mask, nasogastric tube, intravenous tubing) creates a nonthreatening situation from which the child can learn about the operation. This play period, when observed by the parents, can also assist in decreasing their fears of the operation. Through visualization of the procedure many of their questions are answered.

Preparation for the size of the incision and dressing must be included in the preoperative teaching. An extensive incision is needed to adequately assess extent of disease. Again, the use of play, through use of a doll, can help the parents and child visualize the incision. Discussion of the necessary tubes such as a nasogastric tube and intravenous lines should be included in the preoperative teaching session.

Postoperatively, the nurse must be able to assess for complications following abdominal surgery. Vital signs, urinary output, and the presence of bleeding are crucial areas of concern. Any change in the patient's status may be indicative of intestinal obstruction, perforation, or peritonitis. Radiation therapy and chemotherapy are usually begun immediately after surgery, increasing the child's risk for intestinal obstruction from a vincristine-induced ileus. Radiation therapy may induce edema, and postsurgical adhesions are not uncommon. The nurse must be able to closely assess gastrointestinal function by evaluating bowel sounds, bowel movements, and observing for distention or the presence of vomiting and pain.

The initial diagnostic period is often very frightening for the parents. The diagnosis is often established quickly and surgery is scheduled before the parents realize the impact of the diagnosis. Treatment is also instituted rapidly, making it difficult for even the most intelligent parent to comprehend the seriousness of the diagnosis. During this initial period of diagnosis and treatment, parents should not be expected to retain all information given to them. Frequently, the trauma of surgery is all they are able to deal with at the time. It is this period after the child has recovered from surgery when parents are able to fully comprehend the treatment plan. At this time side effects of chemotherapy and radiation therapy should be addressed in detail (see Chapters 20 and 21). Before discharge, the parents must understand the risk of infection for a child on chemotherapy and know what to do should fever occur. Parents need reassurance that their child will be able to return to a life-style comparable to that before diagnosis. Treatment schedules should attempt to accommodate appropriate treatment with daily activities of the child and family.

NURSING CARE PROTOCOL FOR THE CHILD WITH WILMS' TUMOR

Nursing diagnoses (problems/needs)	Goals/objectives (patient/family will:)	Interventions (nurse will:)
1. Knowledge deficit (related to diagnosis and diagnostic workup)	Receive information related to diagnosis verbally and/or in printed material	Assist with and teach regarding procedures (physical examination, laboratory work, urine testing, chest x-ray examination, IVP, CT scan and other scans, ECG, echocardiogram)
	Verbalize purpose of and methods for tests	Encourage questions pertaining to workup
		Give available teaching resources
2. Anxiety (emotional distress related to diagnosis, testing, possible hospitalization, treatment and side effects)	Demonstrate decreased level of anxiety	Provide information related to workup, disease, protocol, and nursing care
	Share feelings with support persons	Refer to other services such as chaplain, social worker, counselor as available
		Encourage verbalization through active listening, empathetic attitude, and providing time for communication
		Use therapeutic play with patient to encourage expression of fears and to prepare for procedures
3. Knowledge deficit (need for information related to preoperative preparation)	Verbalize general understanding of surgery	Participate in and reinforce explanation of surgery; obtain signature on consent forms according to hospital policy
	Be able to state preoperative and postoperative procedures	Provide information about preoperative and postoperative routines (i.e., NPO, IV, preoperative medications, safety measures, turn, cough, deep breath, Foley catheter, NG tube) and other nursing interventions as appropriate

Continued.

NURSING CARE PROTOCOL FOR THE CHILD WITH WILMS' TUMOR—cont'd

Nursing diagnoses (problems/needs)	Goals/objectives (patient/family will:)	Interventions (nurse will:)
4. Injury: potential for post operative complications	Recover from surgery without postoperative complications	Implement preventive measures; identify complications and initiate prompt treatment as indicated
Fluid and electrolyte imbalance and possible alterations in nutritional state	Exhibited balanced intake and output, elastic skin turgor, laboratory work within acceptable limits, and stable weight	Maintain IV and fluid therapy; observe for signs and symptoms of imbalance; encourage PO intake as able to tolerate; monitor weight, I & O, laboratory work; give antiemetics p.r.n. as ordered
Hemorrhage	Have minimum blood loss, stable vital signs, consistent decrease in gross hematuria	Observe for and record amount of hematuria; notify physician if hematuria increases; check dressings frequently; monitor vital signs; note other signs and symptoms related to shock; pertinent laboratory work (Hgb, Hct)
Comfort, alterations in: pain	Verbalize comfort; demonstrate relaxed facial expression; increase mobility gradually; decrease request for pain medications	Initiate comfort measures such as positioning, therapeutic touch, diversion, medication, emotional support
Other common postoperative complications (immobility, alterations in gas exchange, impaired elimination, delayed healing)	Gradually increase participation in activities of daily living; have chest clear, skin intact with healing incision, bowel sounds present	Implement preventive measures (turn, cough and deep breath; ambulation and mobility if possible); identify complications and initiate prompt treatment
5. Knowledge deficit (related to chemotherapy)	Be able to state name of drugs and their general purpose Identify potential side effects and their management	Assess level of understanding and teach accordingly; document teaching and evaluation Discuss potential side effects of each drug, management at home, and when to contact the nurse or physician Provide written information regarding management of side effects

NURSING CARE PROTOCOL FOR THE CHILD WITH WILMS' TUMOR—cont'd

Nursing diagnoses (problems/needs)	Goals/objectives (patient/family will:)	Interventions (nurse will:)
		Provide 24-hour telephone availability in case of emergency or questions
	Experience minimum complications resulting from side effects	Prophylaxis and treatment per nursing and physician orders related to side effects of specific drugs used (see Chapter 20)
	Develop minimum late side effects; comply with follow-up for prompt recognition and treatment of late side effects	Teach importance of return visits for follow-up; observe carefully for potential late effects and refer for treatment when appropriate.
6. Knowledge deficit (related to radiation therapy)	State purpose of therapy Identify expected side effects of radiation and follow-up appropriately Recognize postradiation syndromes	Provide information related to therapy, side effects, and post-therapy syndromes and document Provide information and discuss potential side effects of radiation therapy (i.e. diarrhea, anorexia, nausea and vomiting, and skin sensitivity) Discuss postradiation syndromes
Potential side effects	Have side effects within expected limits and control and will not develop complications resulting from side effects	Provide interventions per nursing or physician orders related to: Diarrhea—bland diet, increased fluids, medications to decrease bowel motility Anorexia, nausea and vomiting—antiemetics, bland, small feedings Skin sensitivity—water-based lotion or cream (Tegaderm, Vigilon, Aquafor)
	Have minimum late side effects; comply with follow-up	Reinforce importance of follow-up; observe for late effects such as sterility and liver damage

Continued.

NURSING CARE PROTOCOL FOR THE CHILD WITH WILMS' TUMOR—cont'd

Nursing diagnoses (problems/needs)	Goals/objectives (patient/family will:)	Interventions (nurse will:)
7. Injury: potential for (recurrence and or metastasis of tumor)	Identify signs and symptoms and notify health team immediately	Provide information related to signs and symptoms of recurrence of metastasis, such as abdominal mass, urinary problems, respiratory distress
	Verbalize understanding of individualized treatment of recurrence or metastasis	Teach importance of notifying health team immediately if recurrence or metastasis is suspected
	Obtain remission or comfort during terminal phase	Discuss rationale, goal, delivery, and side effects of proposed treatment should recurrence or metastasis occur
		Deliver nursing care specific to treatment and patient needs
8. Coping, ineffective family: compromised	Be able to cope with adjustments needed for functioning at home, at school, and with friends	Provide emotional support and teaching; refer to other health care professionals as needed
	Maintain positive self-concept; return to activities of daily living if survivor	Communicate with school and community professionals to facilitate adjustment outside of hospital
		Encourage continued contacts with the health care institution

REFERENCES

1. Schweisguth, O.: Solid tumors in children, New York, 1982, John Wiley & Sons, Inc.
2. DeVita, V.T., Jr., & others: Cancer, principles and practice of oncology, Philadelphia, 1982, J.B. Lippincott Co.
3. Aron, B.: Wilms' tumor: a clinical study of 81 children, Cancer **33:**637,1974.
4. Brown, W.T., and others: Wilms' tumor in 3 successive generations, Surgery **72:**756, 1972.
5. Bove, K.E., & McAdams, A.J.: The nephroblastomatosis complex and its relationship to Wilms' tumor: a clinico-pathologic treatise. In Rosenberg, H.S., and Bolande, R.P., editors: Perspectives in pediatric pathology, vol 3, Chicago, 1976, Year Book Medical Publishers, Inc.
6. Knudson, A.G., and Strong, L.C.: Mutation and cancer: a model for Wilms' tumor of the kidney, J. Natl. Cancer Inst. **48:**313, 1972.
7. Pendergrass, T.W.: Congenital anomalies in children with Wilms' tumor, a new survey. Cancer 37:403, 1976.
8. Cassady, J.R., and others: Considerations in the radiation treatment of Wilms' tumor, Cancer **32:**598, 1973.
9. Waley, L.F., and Wong, D.L.: Nursing care of infants and children, St. Louis, 1983, The C.V. Mosby Co.
10. D'Angio, G.J., and others: The treatment of Wilms' tumor: results of the National Wilms' Tumor Study, Cancer **38:**633 1976.
11. Farber, S.: Chemotherapy in the treatment of leukemia and Wilms' tumor, JAMA **198:**826, 1966.
12. Cassady, J.R., and Jaffe, N.: Wilms' tumor: controversies on current forms of management. In Carter, S.K., Glatstein, E., and Livingston, R.B.: Principles of cancer treatment, New York, 1983, McGraw-Hill, Inc.
13. D'Angio, G.J., and others: Wilms' tumor: an update, Cancer **45:**1791, 1980.
14. Beckwith, J., and Palmer, N.: Histopathology and prognosis of Wilms' tumor, Cancer **41:**1937, 1978.
15. Breslow, N.E., and others: Wilms' tumor: prognostic factors for patients without metastases at diagnosis, Cancer **41:**1577, 1978.
16. Robert, J.C., Parker B.R., and Kaplan, H.S.: Growth retardation in children after megavoltage irradiation of the spine, Cancer **32:**634, 1973.
17. Littman, P., and others: Pulmonary function in survivors of Wilms' tumor, Cancer 37:2773, 1976.
18. D'Angio, G.J., and others: The treatment of Wilms' tumor, Cancer **47:**2302, 1981.

CHAPTER 6

Neuroblastoma and related tumors

PAT STANFILL and F. ANN HAYES

DEFINITION

Neuroblastoma, ganglioneuroblastoma, and ganglioneuroma are tumors of the sympathetic nervous system. Neuroblastoma, a malignant tumor arising from sympathetic ganglion cells or the adrenal medulla, is often considered the most challenging form of malignant disease in childhood.[1] Because of its unpredictable biologic behavior, neuroblastoma presents a complex and frustrating puzzle in pediatric oncology.[2] The primary tumor is most commonly seen in the adrenal glands or adjacent sympathetic ganglia of the abdomen and pelvis but can also occur in the chest, neck, and head. The tumor is very cellular with broad sheets and clusters of cells that invade adjacent structures or encase surrounding organs, often making surgical excision complicated.[3] Common metastatic sites are the bone, bone marrow, lymph nodes, skin and liver. Neuroblastoma has the highest rate of spontaneous remission of any neoplasm, occurring in 1% of cases.[3]

Ganglioneuroblastoma and ganglioneuroma are more differentiated maturational manifestations of neuroblastoma. As the least differentiated, neuroblastoma contains primitive neuroblasts that resemble the fetal adrenal medulla. Ganglioneuroblastoma, or differentiating neuroblastoma, exhibits both primitive neuroblasts and maturing ganglion cells. Both neuroblastoma and ganglioneuroblastoma are considered as malignant and are discussed together since clinical treatments are similar. Ganglioneuroma, a fully differentiated tumor, is benign in nature and requires only conservative therapy.[4]

INCIDENCE

Neuroblastoma is the third most common malignancy of childhood, accounting for 11% of malignant tumors seen in the first 14 years of life.[3,5] It represents 25% to 50% of all neonatal malignancies and up to 14% of all malignancies in the older child.[5] Neuroblastoma occurs at a rate of 1/10,000 live births. Infants, at a rate of 1/200 deaths for other causes, harbor a small focus of "neuroblastoma in situ" in the adrenal gland at autopsy.[4] Whether this is related to neuroblastoma is unknown.

Among white children, neuroblastoma is the second most common malignant solid tumor after tumors of the central nervous system.[2] A lower incidence is seen in black children. The ratio of males to females is 1.25:1 according to several large series.[2,4-6] The age distribution indicates that approximately one half of all neuroblastomas are diagnosed by 2 years of age, and 90% are diagnosed by 5 years of age.[2,5] Cases are rarely seen in adults.

ETIOLOGY

The etiology of neuroblastoma is unknown. Neuroblastomas and related tumors evolve from primordial neural crest cells that migrate from the developing spinal cord to populate the primordia of the sympathetic ganglia and adrenal medulla.[4] Spontaneous mutations and genetic factors are considered important in the etiology of neuroblastoma. Knudson and Strong[7] estimated that as many as 22% of all neuroblastomas could be hereditary. Exposure to environmental factors in the causation of neuroblastoma is thought to be of less significance than genetic factors, but the tumor has been associated with a prenatal exposure to hydantoins, drugs used in the treatment of grand mal and psychomotor seizures.[8]

Children with neuroblastoma often have an increased incidence of congenital anomalies, yet no pattern of specific defects is evident. Neuroblastoma has also been associated with neurofibromatosis and aganglionosis of the colon, suggesting that it might be an expression of neurocristopathy or diseases arising from a maldevelopment of the neural crest.[9] Knudson and Amromin[9] infer that neuroblastoma is a dominant mutation that may be inherited in a similar fashion to retinoblastoma.[8] If their inferences are accepted, offspring of survivors should be observed closely for tumor presentation.

CLINICAL PRESENTATION

The clinical manifestations of neuroblastoma are related to the site of the primary tumor as illustrated in Fig. 6-1 with their relative frequency. Symptomatology may be nonspecific, often masquerading as common pediatric conditions, and may include low-grade fever, weight loss, anorexia, intermittent hypertension, anemia, and pain.[10]

The most common site of neuroblastoma is the abdomen. The tumor may extend across the midline and is usually firm, nodular, and nontender to palpation. Renal ballottement and dullness caused by fluid accumulation do not occur with neuroblastoma of the abdomen and pelvis.[11] Other signs and symptoms occur secondary to pressure or compression of adjacent organs. A dumbbell type tumor that invades the spinal column may cause

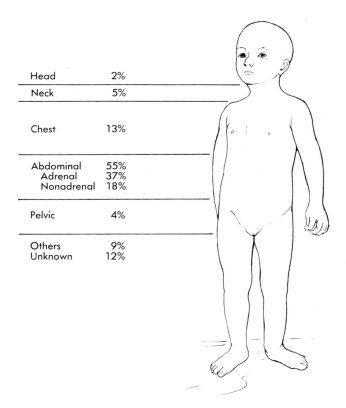

Head	2%
Neck	5%
Chest	13%
Abdominal	55%
Adrenal	37%
Nonadrenal	18%
Pelvic	4%
Others	9%
Unknown	12%

Fig. 6-1. Frequency of primary sites for occurrence of neuroblastoma.

paresis or paralysis of the lower extremities or bladder and bowel incontinence resulting from compression of nerves by tumor growth.[12] An abdominal or pelvic tumor may be missed on routine examination of the abdomen, especially in an irritable or uncooperative child. In many cases, a parent identifies a mass during routine daily care and then brings it to the attention of the pediatrician. A neuroblastoma is generally slow growing, but a rapid increase in size may result from intratumor hemorrhage. Fig. 6-2 demonstrates an abdominal presentation of neuroblastoma.

The thorax is the second most frequent site of neuroblastoma. The primary tumor arises in the posterior mediastinum and may become massive

before it manifests clinically. In many instances the tumor is detected on a chest x-ray film done for other reasons. Symptoms usually present as an upper respiratory infection, although respiratory distress requiring immediate tracheostomy has been documented with a rapidly growing tumor.[13] Horner's syndrome, involving ptosis of the eyelid, constriction of the pupil, and flushing of the affected side of the face may occur if the tumor arises in the stellate ganglion in the upper thorax or lower neck. Posterior mediastinal neuroblastoma may be of the dumbbell type. Compression of the dorsal nerve roots or the spinal cord can lead to pain in the back and neck region and eventually weakness in the lower extremities with bowel and bladder dysfunction. If treatment is not instituted, the compression can lead to paraplegia. Fever, loss of appetite, and weight loss are uncommon findings in children with mediastinal neuroblastoma.

Neuroblastoma of the neck is the primary site in 2% to 7% of all neuroblastoma in children. Patients initially have a unilateral neck mass that may be confused with branchial cleft cyst or enlarged lymph nodes. Symptoms depend on the structure involved and may include facial paralysis, ptosis, earache, dysphagia, and hoarseness.[14]

Metastatic disease is present at diagnosis in 70% of patients over 1 year of age and in 40% to 50% of those less than 1 year of age.[5] Disseminated disease leads to site-specific symptoms and may include limping and refusal to walk, proptosis, masses in the skull, fever, and weight loss.

Signs and symptoms of neuroblastoma in infants include a rapidly enlarging liver, subcutaneous nodules, anemia, feeding difficulties, vomiting, weight loss, and dyspnea.[10] The skin and subcutaneous lesions give the appearance and feel of a blueberry muffin; hence, this term is applied to these lesions. Hydrocephalus, although rare, has been described in infants as a presenting sign of neuroblastoma.[15] Flaccid paralysis of lower extremities at birth can be mistaken for birth trauma when in fact tumor may compress the spinal cord. Urinary dysfunction, including distention and dribbling, may also be indicative of neuroblastoma.

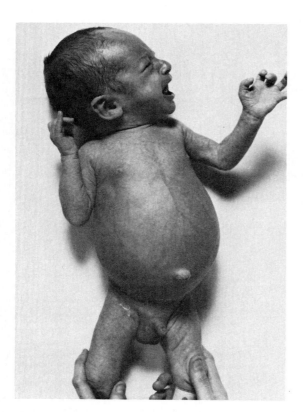

Fig. 6-2. Young infant with abdominal neuroblastoma.

Some neuroblastomas produce large amounts of catecholamines, including epinephrine, norepinephrine, dopa, dopamine, vanillylmandelic acid (VMA), and homovanillic acid (HVA). Catecholamine degradation occurs in three main stages. The tumor cells may synthesize norepinephrine, which ultimately is eliminated in the urine as VMA while other cells synthesize dopamine. Synthesized dopamine may be excreted in this form or further degraded into HVA. Excessive catecholamines may lead to hypertension, excessive sweating, bounding pulse, pallor, polyuria, and polydipsia.

Very rarely, neuroblastoma is associated with a syndrome consisting of chronic diarrhea and failure to thrive, much like that seen in celiac disease.[16] The diarrhea subsides rapidly following excision of the tumor.

DIAGNOSTIC EVALUATION

The diagnostic evaluation for neuroblastoma involves an extensive clinical history, physical examination, blood and urine studies, radiologic studies, and ultrasound. The following list indicates essential diagnostic studies in the evaluation of neuroblastoma:

Clinical history: Increasing irritability, loss of weight, anorexia, difficulty sleeping, abdominal pain, constipation, incontinence, weakness of lower extremities, pain, (dependent on site of primary tumor)

Physical examination: Asymmetry of pupils, weakness in extremities, flaccid paralysis, increased blood pressure, abdominal mass, dyspnea, facial paralysis, proptosis, dysphagia, hoarseness (dependent on site of primary tumor)

Pathology (from biopsy): Broad sheet and clusters of undifferentiated primitive neuroblasts that resemble the fetal adrenal medulla

Complete blood count and bone marrow aspirate: Abnormal if bone marrow involvement; bone marrow aspirate at diagnosis essential

Chemistry panel: Demonstrates renal involvement with elevated blood urea nitrogen, creatinine, liver functions; may be elevated secondary to liver involvement

Urinalysis: Evidence of renal impairment and kidney invasion; creatinine clearance may be done

Urine catecholamines: VMA and HVA elevated

Chest x-ray examination: Occurrence in the superior or posterior mediastinum, localized to one side

Skeletal survey and bone scan: Evidence of bony metastasis by bone destruction or skeletal survey and "hot spots" on bone scan (see Fig. 6-3)

Intravenous pyelogram: Evidence of kidney displacement by effect of tumor mass in abdomen and pelvis

Ultrasound: Evidence of abdominal mass and subsequent organ function

Computerized tomography (CT) scan: Evidence of mass in brain, spine, neck, thorax, and abdomen when specific symptoms are present in these sites (see Fig. 6-4 for massive abdominal neuroblastoma)

Liver scan: Evidence of liver metastasis

A history of altered bowel and bladder patterns, anorexia, weight loss, difficulty sleeping, neurologic changes, and pain contributes to the suspected diagnosis of neuroblastoma. A complete physical examination is indicated, focusing attention to the variety of sites that can be affected by neuroblastoma. Asymmetry of pupils and weakness in extremities point to altered central nervous system integrity. Changes in vital signs, particularly blood pressure, should be noted.

Laboratory studies include measurement of urinary catecholamines, including VMA and HVA, which are elevated in the urine of approximately 80% of affected patients.[4] VMA screening may be done with a spot test or using a 24-hour urine collection. A complete blood count with differential and platelets, renal and liver function studies, and a coagulation screen should be obtained.[5] A bone marrow aspirate is also necessary to rule out marrow involvement.

Radiologic studies define the tumor, its location, and size. A chest roentgenogram will frequently detect the presence of tumor, whereas an abdominal film will rarely detect a tumor unless it is calcified. Skeletal metastasis is seen in at least 50% of children at diagnosis, thus bone scans and skeletal surveys are essential components of the diagnostic workup. Bone scans may show lesions that are imperceptible by the usual skeletal survey.[4,17] Fig. 6-3 shows a bone scan indicating skeletal metastasis. Intravenous pyelogram (IVP) or ultrasonography is standard in determining the presence of

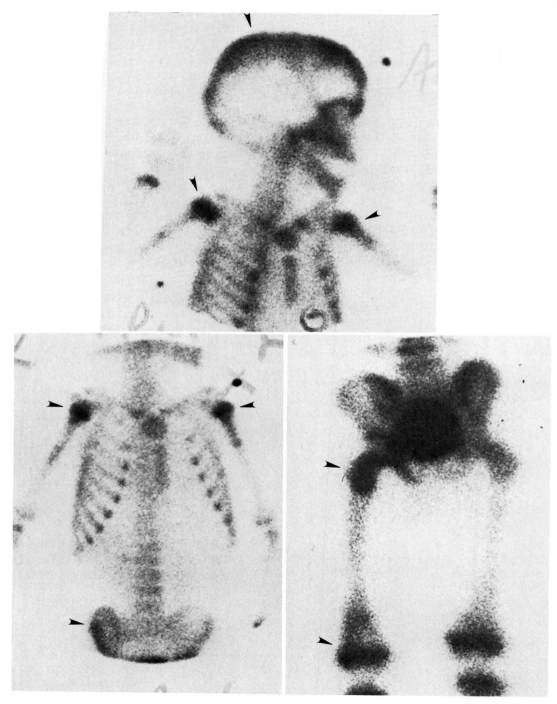

Fig. 6-3. Bone scan of patient with neuroblastoma showing metastasis to both humerus, right femur, posterior ribs, right ileum, and skull as shown by arrows.

an abdominal neuroblastoma.[17,18] A suprarenal neuroblastoma characteristically displaces the kidney downward and laterally, whereas retroperitoneal tumors cause anterior, lateral, and downward displacement.[4,17,18]

Ultrasonography has been accepted as a method to evaluate abdominal masses. CT scan is another noninvasive imaging method that is of particular use in evaluation of the patient with neuroblastoma. Fig. 6-4 demonstrates the results of a CT scan showing massive abdominal neuroblastoma. A liver scan may be indicated in some instances of suspected neuroblastoma to rule out liver metastases if a CT scan is not done. A myelogram may be indicated if cord compression, such as that seen with dumbbell tumors, is evident. Although a variety of diagnostic measures are available to evaluate the possibility of neuroblastoma, only those pertinent to the suspected location and extent of the tumor should be used.

Once the tentative diagnosis of neuroblastoma is made, the role of surgery is determined. Frequently, the diagnosis of neuroblastoma can be made by the presence of characteristic tumor in the marrow, elevated catecholamines, and clinical findings. In these patients no diagnostic surgery is necessary. The initial surgical procedure, depending on results of diagnostic evaluations, may range from simple biopsy to total removal of the tumor. When confirmation of neuroblastoma is made and when the presence or absence of metastases is determined, the disease is staged. The following list outlines the staging system used by St. Jude Children's Research Hospital; other staging systems are available in the literature[3,5,18-21]:

Stage I: Localized tumor completely resected
Stage IIA: Localized tumor completely resected but with pathologic evidence of microscopic tumor through the capsule
Stage IIB: Localized tumor unresectable or partially resected
Stage IIIA: Disseminated disease with no bone or bone marrow involvement
Stage IIIB: Disseminated disease with one localized bone lesion but no bone marrow involvement
Stage IIIC: Disseminated disease with bone marrow and/or generalized bone involvement

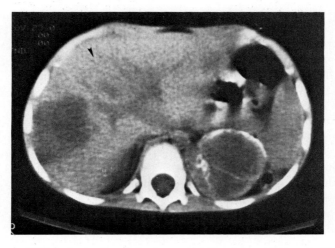

Fig. 6-4. Abdominal CT scan revealing extensive metastasis of neuroblastoma to liver as indicated by left arrow.

PROGNOSTIC FACTORS

The survival rate for patients with neuroblastoma is about 30% at the 2-year follow-up stage.[18] There are two primary prognostic indicators in neuroblastoma.[2] The age of the child impacts on prognosis, with patients under 1 year of age having a greater chance of cure than older children.[2,18] The stage of the disease is the most important prognostic indicator. Children who have a localized tumor or grossly resected or unresected tumor and infants who have stage IV S tumor according to Evans' staging system have a favorable prognosis.[18,21,22] The survival rate decreases as the stage increases, except in stage IV S disease with the localized and resected survival rate being over 90% and localized, unresected survival rate greater than 75%.[18] Disseminated neuroblastoma has a grave prognosis with a survival rate of less than 10% in children over 1 year of age.

Histopathologic grading may also correlate with prognosis. Beckwith and Martin[23] documented a definite correlation between the degree of differentiation (maturation) of neuroblastoma and prognosis. Hughes, Marsden, and Palmer[20] concur that a high level of histologic differentiation correlated with improved survival. Sources differ on whether the presence of lymphoid infiltrates correlates with a poor prognosis.[2,20]

TREATMENT AND MANAGEMENT

Surgery, chemotherapy, and irradiation are used in a variety of combinations in the treatment of neuroblastoma. The stage of the tumor determines the therapeutic approach.

The three primary objectives of surgery are to obtain tissue for diagnosis, stage the disease, and resect the tumor. Biopsies of lymph nodes in drainage areas and liver biopsies with abdominal neuroblastomas are indicated. Surgery alone may effect a cure in children with totally resectable localized disease (stage I and IIA) resulting in a greater than 90% chance of cure.[3,24] In the child with metastatic disease the value of surgical resection of the primary tumor has not been established.[5] Second look surgery after an initial tumor response

to chemotherapy may result in a complete resection of the remaining tumor. When neurologic signs are present, a surgical decompression of the spinal cord may be done to prevent permanent damage although Hayes and others[26] at St. Jude Children's Research Hospital report the use of chemotherapy alone for dumbbell tumors.[16,25]

The goal of chemotherapy in neuroblastoma is to contribute to the attainment of complete remission and to maintain that remission for sufficient time to ensure cure. The decision to employ chemotherapy depends on the stage of the disease and the age of the child.

The rationale for treatment of children with neuroblastoma is stage and age dependent. Children with stage I and IIA disease are managed by surgery alone, since regardless of age they have a greater than 90% cure rate when treated with this single modality therapy. Children with stage IIB disease are given low-dose, sequential cyclophosphamide and doxorubicin (Adriamycin) for 4 months, followed by delayed surgery. Stage III treatment is age dependent with infants under 1 year experiencing a 65% complete remission rate with 4 months of cyclophosphamide and doxorubicin, whereas children over 1 year of age require significantly different therapy. Four agents, cyclophosphamide, doxorubicin, *cis*-platinum (Cisplatin), and VM-26, are used during induction on the premise that multiple agents delivered in a short period of time is the most effective way to prevent the emergence of resistant clones.[24] Other treatment plans employ similar approaches to treatment using comparable regimens.

The role of radiation therapy in the management of neuroblastoma is controversial. Irradiation has been shown to be effective in achieving tumor regression, but the impact on cure rate in metastatic disease has not been significant.[3,27] When irradiation is employed, prescribed dosages depend on the volume of tumor to be treated and the age of the patient.

CASE STUDY

M.S. is a 5-year-old child who was well until 4 weeks before admission to the hospital when she began having fever at night, a decreased appetite, and leg pain. She was seen several times by local physicians with diagnoses of viral illness and anemia. On arrival to the treatment center her physical examination revealed tachypnea, muscle spasms in the lumbar spine area, and positive Kernig's and Brudzinski's signs. A bony mass to the left of the vertex of the skull, and a 1-cm by 1-cm left supraclavicular node were found. No abdominal masses were palpable.

Workup revealed neuroblastoma of the left adrenal gland with metastases to the bone marrow and bone. M.S. was entered on protocol and received three courses of cyclophosphamide and doxorubicin, followed by three courses of *cis*-platinum. She developed an allergy to VM-26 and only received one course. Re-evaluation revealed complete healing of her bones and clearing of her bone marrow. The abdominal tumor had decreased by greater than 50%. M.S. was considered a partial remission and admitted for laparotomy for resection of the remaining mass approximately 5 months after diagnosis. Review of the pathologic findings of the laparotomy revealed a normal liver biopsy, residual minimum ganglion neuroblastoma in the center of the excised adrenal tumor, and one lymph node in the renal hilar area that still contained some metastatic neuroblastoma. M.S. continues receiving maintenance chemotherapy and 18 months after diagnosis remains free of evidence of disease.

NURSING CONSIDERATIONS

A neuroblastoma may compress other structures such as vessels and nerves, decreasing their ability to function; push against organs causing functional problems; or surround areas of tissues causing necrosis. Tumor involvement causes different signs and symptoms depending on the primary site of occurrence. The nurse must be aware of these differences in symptoms to make careful observations.

Children with an abdominal mass require specific assessment. Vital signs must be observed closely for increased blood pressure and pulse. Complaints of pain may indicate compression of nerves. Careful assessment of leg weakness, bladder and bowel habit, and edema or cyanosis must be made. Pain may be severe, requiring use of narcotic analgesics. Even young children may need large amounts of pain medications (see Chapter 25 on management of pain for discussion of common narcotics for control of pain).

Tumor presentation in the thorax frequently causes cough, dyspnea, chest pain, dysphagia, and arm weakness. Dyspnea necessitates prompt attention, often requiring oxygen and the potential for intubation. The mass may cause dysphagia, and close observation of the child's ability to swallow is essential. Pain medication is necessary to provide comfort while not compromising the child's respiratory status.

Head and neck involvement of neuroblastoma can present with a variety of signs and symptoms. Invasion of the retrobulbar soft tissues may cause proptosis of the eye, periorbital swelling, and ecchymosis. These manifestations can be very frightening to the child and family by drastically altering the child's appearance. The nurse must be aware of these changes and be able to assist the family in accepting the child's altered appearance. Invasion of other vital structures may cause cranial nerve palsy, edema of the face, or nasal obstruction. Lymphadenopathy may occur from a tumor located in the neck. Observation for increased intracranial pressure must be made. All these signs and symptoms must be addressed by the nurse through support and education of the family and through implementation of comfort measures and management of pain.

As previously discussed, metastasis occurs predominantly in the bone and bone marrow, with other sites including the liver, skin, and lymph nodes. Bone metastasis occurs predominantly in the skull, femur, and humerus but can spread to the entire skeleton. Bone metastasis creates severe pain that is exacerbated by movement. Pain management is of paramount importance, frequently requiring the use of methadone or morphine. The family must be taught how to care for the child with bone metastasis, including positioning for comfort and administration of pain medication.

The diagnosis of neuroblastoma in a child is a major nursing challenge. Knowledge of the disease, its mass involvement, treatment, and control is essential for the nurse to provide comprehensive care.

NURSING CARE PROTOCOL FOR THE CHILD WITH NEUROBLASTOMA

Nursing diagnoses (problems/needs)	Goals/objectives (patient/family will:)	Interventions (nurse will:)
1. Knowledge deficit (related to diagnosis and diagnostic workup and proposed plan of treatment)	Receive information related to diagnosis verbally or in printed material	Give support during workup by explaining routines and by being available to answer questions
	Verbalize purpose of tests	Explain each test during the workup phase; evaluate and record (i.e., scans, CXR, blood work, IVP, echocardiogram, urine tests)
	Verbalize basic understanding of disease and planned treatment	Stay with family when physician talks with them about stage of disease and protocol
		Give any available teaching resources
		Encourage questions
2. Anxiety (emotional upset related to diagnosis, testing, possible hospitalization, treatment, and side effects)	Share feelings with support persons; have decreased level of anxiety	Provide information related to disease, workup, treatment plan, and nursing care
		Assist with referrals to other services (i.e., chaplain, social worker)
		Encourage verbalization through active listening, empathetic attitude, and providing time for communication
		Use therapeutic play with patient to encourage expression of fears and to prepare for procedures
3. Knowledge deficit (need for presurgical preparation—biopsy and/or resection based on stage)	Verbalize general understanding of surgery	Participate in and reinforce explanation of surgery
	Be able to state preoperative and postoperative routines and their purpose	Obtain signature on consent forms according to hospital policy
		Provide information about preoperative and postoperative routines (i.e., NPO, IV, preoperative medication, safety measures, turn, cough and deep breathe) and other measures as appropriate and document evidence of understanding

NURSING CARE PROTOCOL FOR THE CHILD WITH NEUROBLASTOMA—cont'd

Nursing diagnoses (problems/needs)	Goals/objectives (patient/family will:)	Interventions (nurse will:)
4. Injury: potential for (post-operative complications—based on stage, site and extent of surgery, overall clinical conditions)	Recover from surgery without postoperative complications	Implement preventive measures, identify complications, initiate prompt treatment
Fluid and electrolyte imbalance and possible alterations in nutritional state	Exhibit balanced intake and output, elastic skin turgor, lab work within acceptable limits, and stable weight	Maintain IV and fluid therapy; observe for signs and symptoms of imbalance; encourage PO intake as able to tolerate; monitor weight, I & O, laboratory work; give antiemetics p.r.n.
Hemorrhage	Have minimum blood loss, stable vital signs	Check dressings frequently; monitor vital signs; note other signs and symptoms related to shock; pertinent laboratory work (Hgb, Hct)
Comfort, alterations in: pain	Verbalize comfort. Demonstrate relaxed facial expression. Increase mobility gradually. Decrease request for pain needs	Initiate comfort measures such as positioning, therapeutic touch, diversion, medication; emotional support
Other common postoperative complications—immobility, alterations in gas exchange, impaired elimination, delayed healing	Increase participation in activities of daily living gradually; have chest clear, skin intact with healing incision, bowel sounds present	Implement preventive measures; identify complications and initiate prompt treatment
5. Knowledge deficit (related to chemotherapy)	Be able to state name of drug and broad purpose	Evaluate level of understanding and teach accordingly; evaluate and document
	Identify expected side effects and proper methods of follow-up	Teach, evaluate, and document
	Manage side effects within expected limits and control; experience absence of complications resulting from side effects	Prophylaxis and treatment per nursing and physician orders related to chemotherapy (see Chapter 20)

Continued.

NURSING CARE PROTOCOL FOR THE CHILD WITH NEUROBLASTOMA—cont'd

Nursing diagnoses (problems/needs)	Goals/objectives (patient/family will:)	Interventions (nurse will:)
6. Knowledge deficit (related to radiation therapy)	Have minimum late side effects; comply with follow-up care to allow for prompt recognition and treatment of late effects; recognize indications of possible late side effects and seek help	Provide information related to importance of return visits for follow-up and basic recognition of problems; observe carefully for late effects
	State broad purpose of therapy; identify expected side effects of radiation and follow-up appropriately; recognize postradiation syndromes	Provide information related to therapy, side effects, and posttherapy syndromes and document information by evidence of understanding by patient/family
	Have side effects within expected limits and control; experience absence of complications resulting from side effects; have minimum late side effects; comply with follow-up	Provide interventions per nursing and physician orders related to constipation, anorexia, nausea, and vomiting; reinforce importance of follow-up; observe for late effects; treat skin reactions with Tegaderm or Vigilon
7. Injury: potential for (reoccurrence and/or metastasis of tumor)	Identify signs and symptoms of relapse and notify health team immediately	Provide information related to signs and symptoms of relapse such as abdominal mass, loss of function or sensation, bone pain, respiratory distress and document
	Verbalize understanding of individualized treatment Obtain remission or comfort during terminal phase	Deliver nursing care specific to patient needs
8. Coping; ineffective family: compromised	Be able to cope with adjustments needed and return to maximum functioning	Provide emotional support and teaching; refer to other health professionals as indicated Encourage continued contacts with the health care institutions
	Maintain positive self-concept, work through grief process, return to activities of daily living, if survivor	

REFERENCES

1. Schimke, R.N.: The neurocristopathy concept: fact or fiction? In Evans, A.E., editor: Advances in neuroblastoma research, New York, 1980, Raven Press.
2. Sutow, W.W.: Malignant solid tumors in children: a review, New York, 1981, Raven Press.
3. Carter, S.K. & Glastein, E.: Neuroblastoma. In Carter, S.K.: Principles of cancer treatment, New York, 1982, McGraw-Hill, Inc.
4. Enzinger, E.M., and Weiss, S.W.: Soft tissue tumors, St. Louis, 1983, The C.V. Mosby Co.
5. Hayes, F.A., and Green, A.A.: Neuroblastoma. In Kelley, V.C.: Practice of pediatrics, vol. 5, Philadelphia, 1984, Harper & Row, Publishers, Inc.
6. Young, J.L., Jr., and Miller, R.W.: Incidence of malignant tumors in U.S. children, J. Pediatr. **86:**254, 1975.
7. Knudson, A.G., and Strong, L.C.: Mutation and cancer: neuroblastoma and pheochromocytoma, Proc. Natl. Acad. Sci. USA **24:**514, 1972.
8. Brodeur, G.M.: Genetics and cytogenetics of human neuroblastoma. In Pochedly, C., editor: Neuroblastoma, clinical and biological manifestations, New York, 1982, Elsevier Science Publishing Co., Inc.
9. Knudson, A.G., Jr., and Amromin, G.D.: Neuroblastoma and ganglioneuroma in a child with neurofibromatosis, Cancer **19:**1032, 1966.
10. Bond, J.V.: Neuroblastoma in infants. In Pochedly, C., editor: Neuroblastoma, clinical and biological manifestations, New York, 1982, Elsevier Science Publishing Co., Inc.
11. Delamerens, S.A.: Neuroblastoma of the abdomen and pelvis. In Pochedly, C., editor: Neuroblastoma, clinical and biological manifestations, New York, 1982, Elsevier Science Publishing Co., Inc.
12. Rothner, D.: Congenital "dumbbell" NB with paraplegia, Clin. Pediatr. **10:**235, 1971.
13. Fuller, R.M., and others: Favorable outlook for children with mediastinal NB, J. Pediatr. Surg. **7:**136, 1972.
14. Szymula, N.J., and Lore, J.M.: Neuroblastoma of the head and neck. In Pochedly, C., editor: Neuroblastoma, clinical and biological manifestations, New York, 1982, Elsevier Science Publishing Co., Inc.
15. Bar-Ziv, J. and Nogrady, M.B.: Mediastinal neuroblastoma and ganglioneuroblastoma, the differentiation between primary and secondary involvement on the chest roentgenogram, Ann. J. Roentgenol. **125:**380, 1975.
16. Omenn, G.S.: Ectopic hormone syndromes associated with tumors in childhood, Pediatrics **47:**613, 1972.
17. Sty, J.R.: Radiographic imaging and special radiographic studies in neuroblastoma. In Pochedly, C., editor: Neuroblastoma, clinical and biological manifestations, New York, 1982, Elsevier Science Publishing Co., Inc.
18. Schweisguth, O.: Solid tumors in children, New York, 1982, John Wiley & Sons, Inc.
19. Jaffe, N.: Neuroblastoma: review of the literature and an examination of factors related to prognosis and clinical staging, Cancer Treat. Rev. **3:**61, 1976.
20. Hughes, M., Marsden, H.B., and Palmer, M.K.: Histologic patterns of neuroblastoma related to prognosis and clinical staging, Cancer **34:**1706, 1974.
21. Evans, A.E., D'Angio, G.I., and Randolph, J.: A proposed staging for children with NB, Cancer **27:**374, 1971.
22. Bond, J.V.: Familial neuroblastoma and ganglioneuroma, JAMA **236:**561, 1976.
23. Beckwith, J.B., and Martin, R.F.: Observations on the histopathology of neuroblastoma, J. Pediatr. Surg. **3:**106, 1968.
24. Hayes, E.A., Green, A.A., and Meyer, W.: Therapy for patients with neuroblastoma, Memphis, 1984, Treatment Protocol, St. Jude Children's Research Hospital.
25. Punt, J., and others: Neuroblastoma: a review of 21 cases presenting with spinal cord compression, Cancer **45:**3095, 1980.
26. Hayes, E.A., and others: Surgicopathologic staging of neuroblastoma: prognostic significance of regional lymph node metastases, J. Pediatr. **102:**59, 1983.
27. Jereb, B., and Tefft, M.: Radiotherapeutic management of neuroblastoma. In Pochedly, C., editor: Neuroblastoma, clinical and biological manifestations, New York 1982, Elsevier Science Publishing Co., Inc.

CHAPTER 7

Bone tumors

PAT STANFILL and CHARLES PRATT

Malignant bone tumors are relatively rare, representing less than 1% of malignant neoplasms.[1] There are two primary types: osteogenic sarcoma and Ewing's sarcoma.

OSTEOGENIC SARCOMA

Osteogenic sarcoma, often referred to as osteosarcoma, is a highly malignant tumor derived from specialized connective tissue that forms neoplastic osteoid and osseous tissue.[2] The tumor generally arises in the metaphysial region of the long bones but may occur in the diaphysis. The medullary canal is replaced by tumor that destroys the cortex and then invades the soft tissue surrounding the bone. Diverse types of differentiating cells, including osteosarcomatous, chondrosarcomatous, and fibrosarcomatous elements, may exist within the same tumor.[2,3] Eighty percent of all lesions occur around the knee and shoulder.[1] The most common site is the distal femur.

Pathologic classification subdivides osteogenic sarcoma into four types:

1. *Central osteosarcoma* originates in the medullary canal. The malignant cells within the tumor produce osteoid. Chondroblastic and osteoblastic differentiation are also evident.[4,5]
2. *Telangiectic osteosarcoma* also originates in the medullary canal. Blood and anaplastic cells evident in the cystic spaces allow histologic differentiation from central osteosarcoma.[4,5]
3. *Parosteal osteosarcoma* is a large, dense, lobulated mass attached to the underlying bone but with no involvement of the bone.[5,6]
4. *Periosteal osteosarcoma* occurs as a small lesion on the surface of the bone with spicules of bone perpendicular to the shaft. There is no evidence of pathologic extension into the medullary canal.[4-6]

Incidence

Osteosarcoma is the most frequently diagnosed malignant primary tumor of the bone, occurring at the rate of 4 cases/1 million people under the age of 20 years.[1,2] There are 2500 newly diagnosed cases in the United States annually, and the disease accounts for a mortality of 11.97 deaths/1 million people between the ages of 15 and 19.[1,4] There is a slight male-to-female preponderance with a ratio of 2:1.[3] The majority of osteogenic sarcomas, up to two thirds in some references, occur between the ages of 10 and 20 years.[1,2] The median age is 15 years.

Etiology

Although the cause of osteogenic sarcoma is unknown, there are numerous theories. In adults osteosarcoma is associated with Paget's disease. The tumor is infrequently a complication of previous irradiation for other malignancies.[2] Workers who paint radium dials are also at risk for osteogenic sarcoma.[7] Familial evidence has presented, consisting of several tumors within a family or a familial association of osteosarcoma and cerebral tumors.[8]

Clinical presentation

Pain over the area of the tumor is usually the earliest presenting symptom of osteogenic sarcoma. The pain is of insidious onset and may be intermittent in nature. Often this pain is interpreted as excessive fatigue in an active adolescent.[9] A swollen area or a palpable mass appears over the involved bone. As the tumor impinges on muscles, nerve endings, and blood vessels, edema and increased pain occur.[9] A limp may develop if a weight-bearing extremity is involved, and with further bony destruction from tumor growth, a pathologic fracture may occur. If an upper extremity is involved, diminished strength and/or function may be evident.

A pulsation or bruit may occur in areas of the tumor as a result of an increase in the size and number of blood vessels.[9] As tumor size increases, the skin is stretched and becomes glossy, demonstrating an almost translucent appearance with dilated veins visible beneath the surface.

Metastatic disease is often evident at diagnosis or presents soon after diagnosis. The primary route of spread is hematogenous, with the most common site of metastasis the lungs. Spontaneous pneumothorax or hemothorax as a complication of lung metastases has been reported. Bony metastases occur in approximately 5% to 15% of patients.[3,4] Lymph node involvement in osteogenic sarcoma is rare.

Diagnostic evaluation

The diagnosis of osteogenic sarcoma requires a pathologic confirmation from biopsy of the involved site, but support for the diagnosis is evident before biopsy in many instances. A complete history should include questions about the presence, onset, type, and duration of pain; appearance of a mass or swollen area; and any compromise in use of the involved site. The physical examination includes a visual examination of the site, gentle palpation, auscultation to determine if bruit(s) is(are) present, and comparison measurements of girth in the involved and uninvolved extremities as appropriate.[8]

Radiologic investigation before biopsy should be performed in all children who complain of bone pain without an obvious etiology. Approximately one half of all osteosarcomas may be evident with two roentgenograms of the affected area taken at right angles to each other.[9,10] A periosteal spur, evidence of osteolysis with osteocondensation in the bone and soft tissue, and localization in an adolescent's long bone metaphysis are almost always indicators of the presence of osteosarcoma.[10]

Since bone reacts to all stimuli with bone destruction and/or formation of new bone, radiologic changes in the site are readily apparent.[11] The formation of new bone is irregular and creates a "sunburst" pattern (see Fig. 7-1) that is characteristic of osteosarcoma. An "onion skin" appearance occurs when layers of new bone growth occur (Fig. 7-1). Codman's triangle is a third radiologic manifestation of osteosarcoma that occurs when a triangular section of periosteum is elevated by the bone lesion (Fig. 7-1).

Radiologic findings may be misleading in some suspected cases of osteogenic sarcoma. The extent of the "sunburst" pattern and the amount of ossification may appear to be Ewing's sarcoma. Lesions may look like a benign tumor or an aneurysmal bone cyst. A traumatic hematoma that has ossified may look like a parosteal or periosteal sarcoma on roentgenogram.[11]

Additional radiologic examinations include chest films to rule out metastasis. If films are suspicious, follow-up tomograms and/or computed tomographic (CT) scans are needed.[10] Technetium polyphosphate bone scans and skeletal surveys may demonstrate asymmetric areas of uptake when bone metastases are present. This uptake is commonly referred to as "hot spots."[2] As yet there are no specific laboratory tests to diagnose osteogenic sarcoma.[9] An increased level of serum alkaline phosphatase may occur in osteosarcoma due to the osteoblastic activity within the tumor. Serial levels of alkaline phosphatase may indicate evolution of the tumor. After the tumor is surgically removed levels return to normal.[12]

Once the diagnostic workup is complete, a biopsy must be performed to confirm the diagnosis of osteogenic sarcoma. The most reliable technique is an incisional biopsy with permanent section. Needle biopsies have been used but only allow for

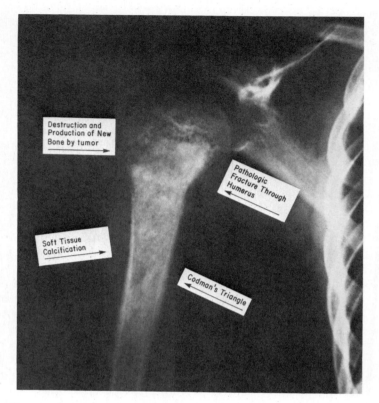

Destruction and
Production of New
Bone by tumor

Pathologic
Fracture Through
Humerus

Soft Tissue
Calcification

Codman's Triangle

Fig. 7-1. Radiograph appearance of changes consistent with osteosarcoma.

a small collection of tumor cells. With the degree of differentiation in the tumor, there is a risk of not obtaining tumor cells in the biopsy. Needle biopsy may also encourage blood-borne dissemination of tumor cells if the vascular structure of the tumor is interrupted.[3]

Prognostic factors

The overall survival rate of osteogenic sarcoma is 30% to 50%.[3] Survival rates may be higher with more distal lesions. In the years before the use of adjuvant chemotherapy the 5-year survival rate was only 17%. Telangiectatic osteosarcoma has the poorest survival rate at not more than 5%.[2] Central osteosarcoma has a 20% survival rate, peri-

osteal sarcoma has a 40% survival rate, and parosteal sarcoma has a survival rate of 80%.[4] Survival rates for patients treated with limb preservation rather than amputation are similar.[13] There is disagreement in the literature as to whether histopathology is an important prognostic factor.[3,14] Rosen and others[14] reports that histologic grading of a resected tumor after preoperative chemotherapy can be used to determine dosage amounts and schedules of chemotherapy.

Treatment and management

There are two challenges in the treatment of osteogenic sarcoma: (1) the local control of the primary tumor and (2) the prevention of metastases.[3]

Metastases generally occur during the first year following diagnosis, and with local treatment alone, occur in 80% of patients.[2,3] Treatment of osteosarcoma is determined by evaluating the site and extent of the tumor, whether metastases are present, and the age of the patient. The objectives of treatment are to eliminate the primary tumor, prevent the development of metastases, and return the patient to an optimum level of function.

The surgical removal of the tumor is the first step in the treatment of osteogenic sarcoma. Amputation or disarticulation have been the usual surgical approaches for tumors of the extremities, but recent advances in limb preservation have been equally successful. If the tumor is located in a flat bone such as the skull or vertebra, surgical intervention involves decreasing tumor bulk. Amputation is usually the treatment of choice in younger patients who have not achieved their full growth potential. The limb is removed approximately 10 cm above the lesion. Disarticulation is practiced in some instances to remove possible tumor foci above the level of the lesion but has disadvantages in the use of a prosthesis.

Limb preservation involves the removal of the affected portion of bone and surrounding soft tissues and the insertion of a prosthetic bone replacement (Fig. 7-2). This procedure is not performed unless the growth of the patient after puberty is greater than the 75th percentile for age for preservation of the lower extremity and greater than the 50th percentile for preservation of the humerus.[2]

Chemotherapy as an adjuvant therapy was introduced in the early 1970s. When amputation alone was the treatment for osteosarcoma, survival rates ranged from 5% to 20%. With the addition of chemotherapy, improvement was noted. The theoretic assumptions on which adjuvant chemotherapy is based include (1) microscopic disease exists at the time of diagnosis, (2) chemotherapy is more effective against smaller amounts of tumor, and (3) drugs effective against clinically evident disease are also useful with microscopic disease.[15]

Before limb preservation surgery, chemotherapy

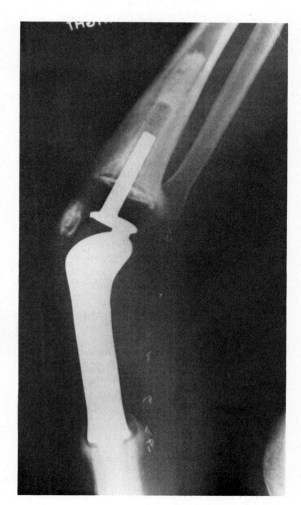

Fig. 7-2. Insertion of prosthetic bone replacement after removal of bone lesions in osteosarcoma.

with multiple agents such as vincristine, high-dose methotrexate, and doxorubicin (Adriamycin) are used in an attempt to shrink the primary tumor and allow time to build the prosthesis.[15] Memorial Sloan-Kettering Cancer Center employs multiple agents before limb preservation and reports that 90% of patients achieve satisfactory intratumoral destruction of viable cells and are thus long-term survivors.[13] Most other reports of long-term survival employing multiple-agent chemotherapy report survival rates of 50%.[13]

The Mayo Clinic initiated a randomized prospective study in which patients received no post-surgical treatment versus patients who received adjuvant chemotherapy. The 2-year disease-free survival rate was 52% in both groups and overall survival was 74% in both groups.[14]

The Pediatric Oncology Group is also attempting to determine the benefits of adjuvant chemotherapy. Patients are randomized to receive initial chemotherapy after surgery or to receive chemotherapy after the appearance of metastases. Doxorubicin, high-dose methotrexate, bleomycin, cyclophosphamide, actinomycin D (Dactinomycin), and *cis*-platinum (Cisplatin) are administered over a 42-week period.[13]

The clinical toxicity of multiple-agent chemotherapy must be considered. With the increasing numbers of agents integrated into treatment protocols, side effects such as nausea, vomiting, skin changes, mucositis, alopecia, the potential for chemical burns, and infection complicate therapies. Anemia, leukopenia, and thrombocytopenia result from the administration of antineoplastic agents. Hepatic and renal function impairment and electrocardiogram and echocardiogram changes may also be noted.

Despite varying reports on the benefits of adjuvant chemotherapy in the treatment of osteogenic sarcoma, it is still an integral part of the accepted treatment program in most centers. Long-term follow-up of patients receiving treatment will be the ultimate answer to the effectiveness of adjuvant chemotherapy.

Radiation therapy has not contributed to the improvement of survival rates in osteogenic sarcoma. Irradiation is useful in decreasing tumor bulk (particularly in unresectable primary lesion), in controlling metastatic disease, and decreasing the pain of the disease. Prophylactic irradiation to the lungs does not decrease the incidence of metastatic disease and in fact damages normal lung tissue, since

dosages greater than 2000 rad create fibrosis and 6000 rad are needed to eradicate tumor-bearing areas.[2]

Cryotherapy, the freezing of the tumor to retard growth, is being investigated but is not considered an integral part of therapy to date. If further investigation proves its benefit, cryotherapy will be especially useful in head and neck osteogenic sarcoma. Immunotherapy is another type of therapy with no clearly defined role in the treatment of osteosarcoma.

The treatment of metastatic disease depends on the site and extent of the involved area. Thoracotomy and wedge resection of involved lung tissue are used in the treatment of pulmonary metastatic disease.[16] Chemotherapy has previously been described as useful in preventing and treating metastatic disease. A new protocol at St. Jude Children's Research Hospital is evaluating ifosfamide in the treatment of children with unresectable primary or metastatic osteosarcoma.[17]

The treatment of osteogenic sarcoma has become an example of a multimodal approach to disease control. Surgery, chemotherapy, and radiation therapy each assume a role in the management of osteosarcoma.

EWING'S SARCOMA

Ewing's sarcoma is also a malignant tumor involving bone. Histologically, the tumor consists of small round cells, but the cell of origin is unknown. They may affect any bone of the skeleton but are less common in the long bones. The tumor widely infiltrates the soft tissues around the involved bone focus. Ewing's sarcomas have a friable, hemorrhagic appearance that is often necrotic.[3]

Incidence

Ninety percent of all cases of Ewing's sarcoma present in patients under the age of 30, with 70% occurring in patients less than 20 years of age.[18] The ratio of occurrence in males to females is 1.6:1. It is a rare malignancy and accounts for 30% of bone tumors occurring in children.[18]

Clinical presentation

The clinical presentation of Ewing's sarcoma is quite similar to the presentation of osteogenic sarcoma. Pain and a soft tissue mass are the usual presenting symptoms. Other symptoms may occur depending on the site of the tumor. For example, vertebral lesions may result in neurologic symptoms and signs as a result of spinal cord compression. A rib tumor, intrathoracic in nature, presents with a respiratory syndrome.

Diagnostic evaluation

Again, the diagnostic evaluation of Ewing's sarcoma is similar to that of osteosarcoma, and a differential diagnosis is often necessary. Biopsy of the lesion is required for a definitive diagnosis.

Prognostic factors

The 5-year, disease-free survival rate for patients with Ewing's sarcoma has been 10% to 15%, with 50% of patients developing metastasis during the first year following diagnosis.[3,18] The prognosis is best for patients with distal lesions and no metastases at diagnoses. Hayes and Thompson[18] project 50% survival rates for 5 years in patients with localized disease and no metastases at diagnosis.[18]

Treatment and management

Like osteosarcoma a multimodal approach is the therapy of choice for Ewing's sarcoma. Radiotherapy with high dosages of 5000 to 7000 rad will control the primary tumor and relieve pain.[18] Surgery is used primarily to resect residual disease after irradiation. Patients generally die from metastatic disease, so extensive surgical attempts to remove the tumor as in osteosarcoma are not warranted.

Micrometastases are present at diagnosis in the majority of patients. Chemotherapy consisting of cyclophosphamide, doxorubicin, daunorubicin, BCNU, vincristine, and actinomycin D are used in varying combinations, dosages, and schedules in an attempt to control metastatic disease.

The use of radiation therapy and chemotherapy

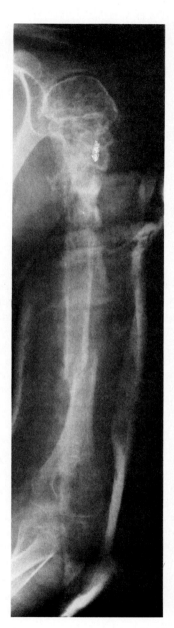

Fig. 7-3. Development of osteoporosis and fracture after radiation therapy consisting of 5000 rad for treatment of Ewing's sarcoma.

in combination is the most promising therapy for Ewing's sarcoma. Long-term side effects of radiation therapy and adjuvant chermotherapy are now being investigated as treatment regimens for Ewing's sarcoma become more effective. Radiation therapy of 5000 to 7000 rad to an affected limb stops bone growth and causes permanent damage to the bony architecture. Osteoporosis may develop, as shown in Fig. 7-3. Patients who have not completed their growth may be considered for amputation because of radiation effects on the growth plate. Chapter 31 discusses late effects of radiation in more detail. Emphasis in the future must focus on eradication of the tumor with minimum functional impairment of the child.

CASE STUDY

L.P. is a 17½-year-old white female who was well until 1981 when she began to have pain and swelling in the left knee. She saw her local physician who treated her conservatively without resolution of her symptoms. One month later she saw another physician who did a joint aspiration, which showed cloudy fluid. No treatment was given. Three months after the aspiration, an orthopedic surgeon was consulted, and on x-ray examination a lytic lesion of the left distal femur was noted. She was referred to a cancer treatment center. She complained of pain, especially with weight bearing, and a 2-month history of decreased appetite.

The initial physical examination showed a young girl in no acute distress but with a moderately wasted appearance. The remainder of the examination was normal with the exception of a 10 cm in circumference swelling over the left knee. Laboratory values included a white blood cell count of 6000/mm³, hemoglobin of 9.8 g/dl, serum alkaline phosphatase of 259 IU/L, LDH of 423 IU/L, and serum phosphorus 4.8 mg/dl. The remaining chemistries were normal. Bone scan demonstrated increased uptake about the left knee involving the left distal femur and proximal tibia. On CT scan of the left leg, a soft tissue mass with bony involvement consistent with a malignant tumor was observed. No metastases were evident. Biopsy of the femur was positive for osteosarcoma.

A high above-the-knee amputation of the left femur was done. She was entered on protocol and randomized to receive 44 weeks of chemotherapy including bleomycin, actinomycin D (Dactinomycin), cyclophospha-mide, high-dose methotrexate, doxorubicin (Adriamycin), and *cis*-platinum (Cisplatin).

Approximately 4 years after diagnosis, L.P. is in the eleventh grade making average grades and with a normal social life. She requires periodic adjustments of her prosthesis, continues to come to amputee clinic every 4 to 6 months, and remains free of evident disease.

NURSING CONSIDERATIONS

The approach to care for the child with a malignant bone tumor is developmental in nature. A consideration of the expected level of growth and development and the developmental tasks of the patient is mandatory. This approach is particularly important in the adolescent. Erikson identifies the adolescent's need for self-identity and the creation of a healthy self-image.[19] In the patient with osteogenic sarcoma this need may be poorly met, particularly if amputation is the treatment employed in disease. The need for peer acceptance and conformity is also threatened. Amputation, hair loss, and other physical changes as a result of therapy create a poor body image that negatively impacts on the adolescent with a bone tumor. Other age groups are also affected in a developmental sense. The preschool child has a fear of castration and mutilation. When the fear is realized, the psychologic impact may be devastating. A recognition of the developmental impact of the disease coupled with physical, emotional, and rehabilitative support is vital.

The nursing care of the child being treated for a bone tumor must take into consideration the extent of surgical intervention. Preparation for the postoperative period should include realistic explanations of the expected surgical outcomes, emphasis on maintaining adequate oxygenation, and a brief discussion of the need for pain control. Turning, coughing, and deep breathing are reinforced to prevent atelectasis and development of pneumonia. Morphine is the most effective drug in the immediate postoperative period.

The child undergoing an amputation requires preparation related to loss of the limb. Even the youngest child must be told that the limb will be removed, and there is no easy way to do this. Frequently, the patient wants to know the details of the amputation such as the technique for removing the limb, how it is disposed of, and what it looks like. Honest, straightforward answers help the child work through his or her fears.

Elevation and wrapping of the stump assists in decreasing swelling and pain for the first 24 hours. When ambulation begins, the stump should be elevated for 30 minutes after ambulation only. Elevating the stump routinely should be avoided after the first postoperative day to prevent contractures. The stump wound must be assessed for signs of infection and bleeding.

Management of phantom pain, an increase in sensation of the amputated limb that actually causes the patient to feel that the limb is still attached, may require long-term care. Patients may experience this pain for up to 6 months after amputation. The use of oral pain medications such as meperidine (Demerol) or codeine may be necessary. It is essential to reinforce that phantom pain decreases and eventually resolves over time.

Rehabilitation begins during the initial hospitalization for the amputation. The physical therapist is consulted to begin teaching basic concepts of mobilization and gait training. The patient is fitted for a prosthesis when healing is complete, usually 6 weeks to 3 months after the amputation. A temporary prosthesis may be used early in the rehabilitative process but, if used excessively, may delay healing of the stump. Once a prosthesis has been fitted, an intensive program of gait training must be instituted to teach the patient proper techniques in using the limb. Physical therapy for gait training is continued until the patient feels comfortable with the prosthesis.

The limb preservation procedure is an option when the tumor is not adjacent to or invading a joint. A 10 cm margin between the tumor and the joint is adequate.[4] The age of the patient must also be considered. The young child may not be a candidate for a lower extremity preservation because of discrepancy in leg length as growth occurs.

Postoperatively, the wound must be assessed for signs of infection and bleeding. Careful evaluation of limb function includes sensation, pulses, color, warmth, and movement. Restriction of mobility is enforced to provide adequate time for healing and stabilization of the prosthetic bone replacement. Weight bearing is limited initially to further ensure healing. After healing has occurred, physical therapy is initiated to strengthen the limb through range of motion exercises. The use of crutches or a cane may be necessary until the muscles surrounding the prosthetic bone are strengthened. The implanted rod can splinter or dislodge when excessive stress is applied to the limb. The child and family must understand activity limitations to prevent trauma to the limb.

Patients may have lung metastases at initial diagnosis or may subsequently develop them during or after therapy. The most effective treatment of metastases is surgical removal by wedge resection. Occasionally, a lobectomy or pneumonectomy is required if the lesions are numerous or unable to be removed by wedge resection.[4] The patient having a thoracotomy must understand what a chest tube is and why it is used. Importance of measures to prevent atelectasis and pneumonia must be stressed. Turning, coughing, and deep breathing are done every 2 hours for at least the first 24 hours. Mobilization of the patient 24 hours after surgery is essential.

Chemotherapy either in the preoperative or postoperative period is an integral part of most protocols, and a brief explanation of the agents and side effects prepares the child and family. Aggressive antiemetic therapy is recommended for the side effects of the agents administered. Adequate fluid and electrolyte balance and nutritional state are priorities. Alopecia should be discussed in conjunction with the presentation of available head coverings including wigs.

The treatment of bone tumors is aggressive and may significantly alter the child's body image. A period of time is needed for the child and family to adjust to the diagnosis and treatment. Emotional support and a realistic discussion of the impact of the disease will facilitate the acceptance process.

NURSING CARE PROTOCOL FOR THE CHILD WITH OSTEOSARCOMA

Nursing diagnoses (problems/needs)	Goals/objectives (patient/family will:)	Interventions (nurse will:)
1. Knowledge deficit (related to diagnostic workup, disease, and treatment)	Verbalize purpose of and methods for tests

Verbalize basic understanding of disease and treatment | Assist with and teach regarding procedures (bone marrow, urine tests, x-ray examinations, blood work, scans, ECG); ensure that teaching is age appropriate
Encourage questions
Provide patient with approved teaching material (i.e., pamphlets); encourage follow-up with questions
Evaluate, document, record:
  Teaching done
  Areas of need for further teaching
  Observations of patient behaviors |
| 2. Anxiety (related to diagnosis, testing, possible hospitalization, treatment, and side effects) | Have decreased level of anxiety | Teach (workup, disease protocol)
Assist with referrals to chaplain, social worker, counselor |
| 3. Knowledge deficit (need for presurgical preparation—amputation or limb sparing procedure) | Verbalize general understanding of surgery
Verbalize understanding of preoperative and postoperative routines | Assist with explanation of surgery; obtain signature on permits
Teach preoperative and postoperative routines (i.e., NPO, IV, preoperative medication, safety measures, turn, cough, deep breath, Foley catheter, NG); incorporate therapeutic play when age appropriate as an adjunct to teaching
Assist patient/family to explore feelings/expectations related to postoperative body image and mobility; teach as specifically as possible what to expect, what rehabilitative measures that will take place; recognize that denial can be a healthy coping mechanism initially in some instances |

NURSING CARE PROTOCOL FOR THE CHILD WITH OSTEOSARCOMA—cont'd

Nursing diagnoses (problems/needs)	Goals/objectives (patient/family will:)	Interventions (nurse will:)
4. Injury: potential for (possible postoperative complications)	Have absence of postoperative complications	Implement preventive measures, identify complications, initiate prompt treatment
5. Mobility, impaired physical	Maintain ROM; chest clear; respirations within normal range; skin intact and without reddened areas; steadily increasing strength and mobility	Encourage bed activities as status permits Provide care for the amputee: Position q.2h. 1st 24 h Elevate stump for 24 h only ROM exercises to unaffected limbs beginning 24-48 hr postoperatively ROM and strengthening exercises to affected limb as soon as possible Stump wrapping and prosthesis fitting as soon possible Consult follow-up for prosthesis training, crutch, walking Monitor respiratory status rate, quality, lung sounds Administer O_2 as ordered Turn, cough, and deep breathe q.2h. Physical therapy consult Turn q.2h. Support unaffected extremities with pillows Elevate stump for 45 minutes after exercise; do not keep stump elevated at other times Lotion/massage Q shift Obtain air mattress
	Need for specialized care of limb-spared extremity	Care of patient who has undergone a limb sparing procedure: Immediate postoperative period in ICU

Continued.

NURSING CARE PROTOCOL FOR THE CHILD WITH OSTEOSARCOMA—cont'd

Nursing diagnoses (problems/needs)	Goals/objectives (patient/family will:)	Interventions (nurse will:)
		Have the following items set up before the patient returns from surgery:
		Air flow mattress on bed
		Overhead trapeze
		IV pole, and bed cradle for support of limb-spared extremity
		Arm care:
		Be sure arm is abducted from body
		Take care not to drop arm; manipulate as little as possible
		Check pulses (radial; brachial if possible), finger warmth, and capillary refill every 1 hr
		Ask patient to move fingers every 1 hr to check for sensation and wrist drop
		Place hemovac to wall suction at 60-80 cm; aspirate hemovac using sterile technique every 4 hr
		Dressing is bulky; check for bleeding every 1-2 hr
		Explain need for immobility of limb to patient
		Provide emotional support and comfort measures to patient/family as indicated
		Enlist adequate assistance from other staff when moving patient to ensure comfort and safety of limb
		Ensure respiratory support as with amputee
		Leg care:
		Keep foot elevated on pillow form
		Take care not to drop or manipulate leg
		Check posterior tibial, dorsal pedal pulses, color, warmth and nailbed capillary refill every 1 h

NURSING CARE PROTOCOL FOR THE CHILD WITH OSTEOSARCOMA—cont'd

Nursing diagnoses (problems/needs)	Goals/objectives (patient/family will:)	Interventions (nurse will:)
		Ask patient to move his toes every 1 h to check for sensation and movement
		Check dressing for bleeding
		Place hemovac to 60-80 cm suction
		Aspirate hemovac every 4 hr using sterile technique
		Enlist adequate assistance from other staff when moving patient to ensure comfort and safety of limb
		Provide emotional support to patient/family and comfort measures as indicated
		Ensure respiratory support as with amputee
		Initial dressing change for limb-sparing procedure:
		Provide psychologic support and preparation regarding the appearance of the limb at the initial dressing change.
		Gather following equipment:
		Scissors—Mayo-bandage-fine iris, Addison
		Betadine swab (×2 boxes) ointment (tubes), scrub (×1)
		Large vaseline gauze
		6 boxes 4 × 4 gauze
		2 boxes ABD dressings
		Sterile towels and drapes
		6-in Kurlex ×6
		4 to 6 6-in ace bandages (appropriate width for smaller children)
		Sterile gloves
		2-in paper or silk tape
		Premedicate for pain and anxiety as indicated
		Enlist the aid of 4-6 people who can assist with the dressing change

Continued.

NURSING CARE PROTOCOL FOR THE CHILD WITH OSTEOSARCOMA—cont'd

Nursing diagnoses (problems/needs)	Goals/objectives (patient/family will:)	Interventions (nurse will:)
6. Nutrition, alteration in: less than body requirements	Develop understanding of increased nutritional needs postoperatively Experience relief from nausea and vomiting; weight stable; PO intake return to usual range	Obtain order for antiemetics and administer p.r.n. Arrange consultation with dietitian Offer small, frequent appetizing meals Mouth care before all meals High-protein, high-carbohydrate diet; well balanced meals Monitor I & O carefully Eliminate unpleasant sights and smells Obtain order for topical mouthwash anesthetic Encourage fluids
7. Comfort, alteration in: pain	Experience relief from pain; able to participate in ADL and diversion activities	Obtain order for pain medication and administer p.r.n. Reposition q.2h. Offer diversional activities—play Administer individualized comfort measures
8. Injury: potential for (infection)	Afebrile; absence of signs and symptoms of infection	Observe strict handwashing aseptic technique with all procedures Monitor temperature—obtain order for p.r.n. Tylenol and blood cultures T >38.5 Monitor surgical site for drainage and odor and culture wound if abnormal
9. Self-concept, disturbance in: body image	Adaptation to body image	Explain all aspects of therapy program and procedures to patient; allow patient/family to participate in the care Encourage therapeutic play in young patients and age-appropriate diversional activities in older children Provide opportunity for verbalization of feelings concerning body image

NURSING CARE PROTOCOL FOR THE CHILD WITH OSTEOSARCOMA—cont'd

Nursing diagnoses (problems/needs)	Goals/objectives (patient/family will:)	Interventions (nurse will:)
		Use resource personnel for counseling (e.g., MD/PNP as directed, pastoral service, social services) Encourage adaptation to new self with prothesis and wig Rehabilitation program in hospital and at home—PT, OT referrals
10. Injury: potential for (complications of chemotherapy) Hemorrhage	Minimum bleeding; laboratory work within acceptable range; vital signs stable	Monitor laboratory work (Hgb, Hct, RBC) Monitor for signs and symptoms of shock Frequent checks of surgical site
Electrolyte imbalance (secondary to N & V, chemotherapy, diarrhea, tumor)	Electrolyte balance	Monitor daily lab work Observe for signs and symptoms hyper/hypokalemia, hyper/hyponatremia, hypomagnesemia Reduce causative factors—nausea and vomiting (N & V), diarrhea Arrange for dietary modifications/supplements as needed
Bone marrow suppression	Counts within expected range and under control	Monitor laboratory values daily (WBC, CBC, and platelet counts) Observe for signs and symptoms of infection, bleeding Instruct to avoid trauma Apply pressure to venipuncture sites Guard against infection/exposure
11. Knowledge deficit Related to chemotherapy	Be able to state name of drug and broad purpose Identify expected side effects (early) and proper methods of follow-up	Evaluate level of understanding and teach accordingly; document teaching and evaluation Teach, evaluate, and document in relation to: Doxorubicin (Adriamycin)

Continued.

NURSING CARE PROTOCOL FOR THE CHILD WITH OSTEOSARCOMA—cont'd

Nursing diagnoses (problems/needs)	Goals/objectives (patient/family will:)	Interventions (nurse will:)
	Have (early) side effects within expected limits and control; absence of complications resulting from side effects	*cis*-Platinum (Cisplatin) Cyclophosphamide Methotrexate Bleomycin Actinomycin D
	Have minimum late side effects; compliance with follow-up care to allow for prompt recognition and treatment of late side effects	Initiate prophylaxis and treatment per nursing and physician orders related to chemotherapy
Related to radiation therapy	Be able to state broad purpose of therapy; identify expected side effects of radiation and follow-up appropriately; recognize postradiation syndromes	Teach, evaluate, and document
	Have side effects within expected limits and control, absence of complications resulting from side effects	Initiate prophylaxis and treatment per nursing and physician orders related to N & V, constipation, anorexia
	Have minimum late effects; compliance with follow-up	
12. Injury: potential for (recurrence and/or metastasis)	Identify signs and symptoms of relapse, metastasis (especially to lung)	Teach, evaluate, document
	Verbalize understanding of individualized treatment	Teach, evaluate, document (see protocol)
	Obtain remission or comfort during terminal phase	Implement nursing care specific to patient needs
13. Coping, ineffective family: compromised	Be able to cope with adjustments needed and return to maximum function	Provide emotional support, teaching, and referral as needed

NURSING CARE PROTOCOL FOR THE CHILD WITH EWING'S SARCOMA

Nursing diagnoses (problems/needs)	Goals/objectives (patient/family will:)	Interventions (nurse will:)
1. Knowledge deficit (related to diagnostic work-up)	Verbalize purpose of and methods for testing	Assist with and teach regarding workup procedures, (PE, laboratory work, scans, ECG, skin tests, bone marrow) Encourage questions pertaining to workup Give any available teaching resources
2. Anxiety (emotional upset related to diagnosis, testing, possible hospitalization, treatment and side effects)	Have decreased level of anxiety; share feelings with support people	Teach (workup, disease, protocol) Assist with referrals to other services (chaplain, social worker, psychologist) Use active listening, use of play, TLC, offer self
3. Knowledge deficit (need for initial surgery biopsy to establish definite diagnosis; need for tumor resection if no evidence of metastatic disease is found)	Verbalize general understanding of surgery Be able to state preoperative and postoperative routines	Assist with explanation of surgery; obtain signature on permits Teach preoperative and postoperative routines (NPO, IV, preoperative medication, safety measures, turn, cough, deep breath, Foley catheter, NG, tour of ICU preoperatively)
4. Injury: potential for (possible postoperative complications)	Have absence of postoperative complications	Implement preventive measures, identify complication, initiate prompt treatment of complication
Infection	Have clean, dry surgical incision that heals without any complications	Keep incision area dry, clean; observe for infection and report; teach how to care for wound and what to report; monitor laboratory work
Hemorrhage	Have minimum blood loss, stable vital signs	Monitor vital signs; note other signs and symptoms related to shock and pertinent laboratory work (Hgb, Hct); frequent dressing checks; observe for increase in drainage of fresh blood from any drainage tubes

Continued.

NURSING CARE PROTOCOL FOR THE CHILD WITH EWING'S SARCOMA—cont'd

Nursing diagnoses (problems/needs)	Goals/objectives (patient/family will:)	Interventions (nurse will:)
Comfort, alteration in: pain	Verbalize comfort; relaxed facial expression; progressive increase in mobility; decreasing request for pain medications	Initiate comfort measures—positioning, touch, diversion, medication, emotional support
Mobility, impaired physical	Have progressive increased participation in activities of daily living; chest clear, skin intact, bowel sounds present, tolerates PO intake, healing incision	Implement preventive measures; identify complications, initiate prompt treatment of complications
5. Knowledge deficit Related to chemotherapy	Be able to state name of drug and broad purpose; be able to state how long therapy will be given	Evaluate level of understanding and teach accordingly; have permits and consent forms signed
	Identify expected side effects (early) and proper methods of follow-up; have early side effects within expected limits and control—absence of complications resulting from side effects	Teach, evaluate, document related to drugs Initiate prophylaxis and treatment per nursing and physician orders related to chemotherapy.
	Have minimum late side effects; compliance with follow-up care to allow for prompt recognition and treatment of late side effects	(See Chapter 20 for further nursing implications) Teach importance of return visits for follow-up; observe carefully for possible late effects
Related to radiation therapy	Be able to state broad purpose of therapy; identify expected side effects and follow-up appropriately; recognize postradiation syndrome	Teach, evaluate, and document
	Have side effects within expected limits and control; absence of complications resulting from side effects	Initiate prophylaxis and treatment per nursing and medical orders related to N & V, constipation, anorexia, stomatitis, skin breakdown

NURSING CARE PROTOCOL FOR THE CHILD WITH EWING'S SARCOMA—cont'd

Nursing diagnoses (problems/needs)	Goals/objectives (patient/family will:)	Interventions (nurse will:)
	Have minimum late side effects; compliance with follow-up	Teach importance of follow-up; observe for late effects—sterility, liver damage
6. Nutrition, alteration in: less than body requirements	Relief from N & V; Weight stable; PO intake return to usual amount	Initiate measures to prevent nutritional problems: Obtain order for antiemetics Arrange consultation with dietition Offer small, frequent appetizing meals Provide mouth care before all meals Offer high-protein, high-carbohydrate diet; well-balanced meals Monitor I & O carefully Eliminate unpleasant sights and smells Obtain order for topical mouth wash anesthetic Encourage fluids
7. Injury: potential for (recurrence and/or metastasis; potential for treatment failure)	Identify signs and symptoms of recurrences—tissue mass; identify signs of treatment failure—progression of primary disease, obvious increase in muscle tumor mass	Teach, evaluate, document
	Verbalize understanding and individualized treatment	Teach, evaluate, and document (see protocol)
	Obtain remission or comfort during terminal phase	Implement nursing care specific to patient
8. Coping, ineffective family: compromised	Be able to cope with adjustments needed and return to maximum functioning	Provide emotional support and teaching and refer as needed
	Maintain positive self-concept, return to activities of daily living	Follow patient as needed

REFERENCES

1. Carter, S.K.: Adjuvant chemotherapy of osteosarcoma. In Carter, S.K.: Principles of cancer treatment, New York, 1982, McGraw-Hill, Inc.
2. Pratt, C.B.: Osteosarcoma. In Kelley, V.C.: Practice of pediatrics, Philadelphia, 1984, Harper & Row, Publishers, Inc.
3. Schweisguth, O.: Solid tumors in children, New York, 1982, John Wiley & Sons, Inc.
4. Eilber, F.R.: Surgical management of osteogenic and Ewing's sarcoma, In Carter, S.K.: Principles of cancer treatment, New York, 1982, McGraw-Hill, Inc.
5. Rosenburg, S.A., and others: Sarcomas of the soft tissue and bone. In Devita, V.T., Hellman, S., and Rosenberg, S.A.: Cancer, principles and practice of oncology, Philadelphia, 1982, J.B. Lippincott Co.
6. Unni, K.K., and others: Intraosseous well differentiated osteosarcoma, Cancer **40:**1337, 1977.
7. Bubis, J.J.: Pathology of osteosarcoma. In Katznelson, A., and Nerubay, J.: Osteosarcoma, new finds in diagnosis and treatment, New York, 1982, Alan R. Liss, Inc.
8. Mulvihill, J., and others: Multiple chldhood osteosarcomas in an American Indian family with erythroid macrocytosis and skeletal anomalies, Cancer **40:**3115, 1978.
9. Katznelson, A., and Nerubay, J.: The clinical picture of osteosarcoma. In Katznelson, A., and Nerubay, J.: Osteosarcoma, new trends in diagnosis and treatment, New York, 1982, Alan R. Liss, Inc.
10. Rubenstein, Z., and Morag, B.: The role of radiology in the diagnosis and treatment of osteosarcoma. In Katznelson, A., and Nerubay, J.: Osteosarcoma, new finds in diagnosis and treatment, New York, 1982, Alan R. Liss, Inc.
11. Unni, K.K., and others: Parosteal osteogenic sarcoma, Cancer **37:**2466, 1976.
12. Levine, A.M., and Rosenberg, S.A.: Alkaline phosphatase levels in osteosarcoma tissue as related to prognosis, Cancer **44:**2291, 1979.
13. Pratt, C.B.: Chemotherapy of osteosarcoma: an overview. In Van Oosterom, Muggia, F.M., and Cleton, F.J., editors: Therapeutic progress in ovarian cancer, testicular cancer and sarcomas, The Hague, 1980, Martinus Nijhoff Publishers.
14. Rosen, G., and others: Chemotherapy and thoracotomy for metastatic osteogenic sarcoma: a model for adjuvant chemotherapy and the rationale for the timing of thoracic surgery, Cancer **41:**841, 1978.
15. Tichler, T.E., Bar Am, Y., and Brenner, H.J.: Chemotherapy in osteogenic sarcoma. In Katznelson, A., and Nerubay, J.: Osteosarcoma, new finds in diagnosis and treatment, New York, 1982, Alan R. Liss, Inc.
16. Shah, A., and others: Thoracotomy as adjuvant to chemotherapy in metastatic osteogenic sarcoma, J. Pediatr. Surg. **12:**938, 1977.
17. Pratt, C.B., and others: Protocol for evaluation of ifosfamide in children with neuroblastoma and unresectable primary or metastatic osteosarcoma: a phase II study, SJCRH, Memphis, Tennessee, November 1983.
18. Hayes, F.A., and Thompson, E.T.: Ewing's sarcoma. In Kelley, V.C.: Practice of pediatrics, Philadelphia, 1984, Harper & Row, Publishers, Inc.
19. Erikson, E.H.: Childhood and society, ed. 2, New York, 1963, W.W. Norton & Co., Inc.

CHAPTER 8

Central nervous system tumors

DEBORAH K. COODY and JAN VAN EYS

Tumors of the central nervous system (CNS) include those of the brain and the spinal cord. These are a mixed group of neoplasms histologically, ranging from benign to highly malignant. For the clinician, distinguishing a tumor's histologic features often becomes secondary to identifying its particular location. A histologically benign tumor may rapidly destroy vital areas of the brain such as the hypothalamus or pituitary, whereas a histologically malignant tumor located in less vital areas may cause less physically disabling destruction. Approximately 60% of childhood tumors arise in the posterior fossa, unlike the situation in adults where the majority are supratentorial. Of the supratentorial tumors in childhood, 10% to 15% are midline in the suprasellar, hypothalamic, and pineal regions. The remaining 25% of the supratentorial brain tumors in children are located in the cerebral hemispheres.[1]

INCIDENCE AND ETIOLOGY

CNS tumors comprise the second most common neoplasm of childhood.[2,3] The incidence rate in the United States is 2.4 per 100,000 children under 15 years of age.[4] The incidence is the same for both black and white children and for boys and girls. However, there is a male preponderance of about 3:2 in medulloblastomas and intracranial germ cell tumors. CNS tumors occur most frequently between the ages of 5 and 10 years, yet age-specific incidence rates depend on histologic type.[2] Astrocytomas peak at age 3 years, whereas medulloblastomas and glioblastomas peak at ages 5 and 7, respectively.[5]

The cause of brain tumors is unknown, but both heredity and environment are contributing factors. The familial and hereditary syndromes associated with the development of brain tumors include neurofibromatosis, tuberous sclerosis, von Hippel-Lindau disease, Sturge-Weber disease, and nevoid basal cell carcinoma syndrome.[2,3,5] The major environmental factor implicated in the etiology of brain tumors is radiation exposure. MacMahon[6] reported that cancer mortality was approximately 40% higher in children exposed prenatally to x-rays than in children not exposed. Modan[7] reported a higher incidence of meningiomas in children who had received radiation for tinea capitis. Impaired immunologic status of a host may also influence the risk of developing a CNS tumor. Brain tumors have been associated with immunologic diseases such as telangiectasia and Wiskott-Aldrich syndrome[3] There is an increased risk of intracranial reticulum cell sarcomas and other lymphomas in immunosuppressed patients receiving renal transplants.[8]

HISTOLOGIC CLASSIFICATION

Classification of CNS tumors is difficult as there is no universally accepted nomenclature. It is useful to look at the different sites of origin. Brain tumors can arise from glial cells, primitive neuroectodermal cells, ependymal linings, and embryonal rests of similar structures. Tumors may arise from the brain, the meninges, or sympathetic ganglia and pineal body.

Tumors of glial origins are gliomas and astrocytomas. Astrocytomas are often graded, though the system of grading according to malignancy is highly controversial. Some individuals speak of astrocytoma grade I through IV, whereas others prefer to use more descriptive terms. When more descriptive terms are used, tumors such as fibrillary astrocytoma, pilocytic astrocytoma, or pleomorphic astrocytoma are tumors that correspond to low grades (I or II); whereas spongioblastomas correspond to astrocytomas grade III, and glioblastoma multiforme or anaplastic astrocytoma correspond to astrocytoma grade IV.

Primitive neuroectodermal tumors are represented in a wide variety of tumors. The most common of these are medulloblastoma and intracranial neuroblastoma, often called specifically primitive neuroectodermal neoplasm.

Embryonic rests include malignant teratomas. Teratomas are mixed tumors containing all germ layers. Teratomas can show a variety of subtypes of malignancies such as embryonal carcinoma, choriocarcinoma, or seminoma. Similar tumors, which almost always occur in the pineal or suprasellar regions, are seminomas (dysgerminoma) and craniopharyngiomas, an embryonal tumor that occurs around the pituitary stalk.

Ependymomas and more malignant ependymoblastomas occur anywhere from embryonic rests or established ependymal cell structures. As is the case for astrocytomas, ependymomas can occur in a wide grading sequence.

It is frequently thought that some tumors are truly malignant whereas others are benign. For instance, a craniopharyngioma is not a malignancy. Yet it is a potentially rapidly growing, space-occupying lesion. There are other tumors, such as hemangiomas arising from blood vessels, neurofibromas arising from peripheral nerves within the cranium, choroid plexus papillomas, and ganglioneuromas that are all benign tumors. However, the enclosed nature of the cranial vault makes it impossible to clinically distinguish benign from malignant.

In addition to these primary CNS tumors, there are occasionally metastatic tumors to the CNS. CNS metastases are most frequently seen in lymphoid malignancies such as lymphoma and leukemia (see Chapters 2 and 3). Occasionally solid tumors of childhood such as neuroblastoma, rhabdomyosarcoma, and Ewing's sarcoma metastasize to the CNS.[1]

FUNCTIONAL CLASSIFICATION OF BRAIN TUMORS

Each major anatomic area of the brain and spinal cord has its own symptomatology when invaded by a tumor. Grouping lesions most commonly seen in these anatomic areas enables the clinician to develop a working classification of CNS tumors. Van Eys[2] presents the following functional classification of CNS tumors:

Supratentorial (above the roof of the cerebellum)
  Hemispheres—astrocytoma, sarcoma, meningioma
  Midline tumors—craniopharyngioma, optic glioma, pinealoma, ependymoma
Infratentorial (below the roof of the cerebellum)
  Cerebellar and fourth ventricular—astrocytoma, medulloblastoma, ependymoma
  Brainstem—brainstem glioma
Spinal cord tumors—ependymoma, astrocytoma
Generalized disease with brain tumor components—neurofibromatosis, tuberous sclerosis, Sturge-Weber disease, von Hippel-Lindau disease, ataxia-telangiectasia, nevoid basal cell carcinoma syndrome
Metastatic tumors

Symptomatology of CNS tumors is discussed in relation to this functional classification.

SIGNS AND SYMPTOMS

Symptomatology of CNS tumors results from both general and focal effects. General effects of lesions are caused by increased intracranial pressure, whereas focal effects are caused by direct involvement of tissues.

General effects

Most manifestations of brain tumors are the result of increased intracranial pressure.[2] Increased intracranial pressure may be caused by cerebral edema surrounding the tumor itself or hydrocephalus secondary to tumor obstruction of cerebrospinal fluid flow. Gradually increasing intracranial pressure causes varying degress of headache, vomiting, impaired vision, cranial enlargement, mental disorders, and convulsions.[2]

Headache. Increased intracranial pressure almost invariably causes headaches in adults, yet in children headaches may not accompany an increase in pressure. A headache is difficult to assess in the child. It may present as restlessness and irritability in a baby or young child.[2,9] The headache caused by increased intracranial pressure characteristically occurs in the morning and is often accompanied by malaise, somnolence, and projectile vomiting without preceding nausea.[2,3] Irritability and vomiting may disappear temporarily in babies after skull sutures separate, allowing for expansion of the head (Fig. 8-1).

Impaired vision. Brain tumors may impair vision in two ways. First, diplopia, or double vision, may be caused either by direct tumor compression of the oculomotor nerves or by generalized increased intracranial pressure. The abducens (cranial nerve VI) nerve, because of its long intracranial course and its proximity to bony structures, may become compromised before any other cranial nerve.[3] Therefore, a sixth cranial nerve palsy, or inability to move the eyes laterally, occurs. Secondly, papilledema, or choked optic disc, may cause transient and intermittent blurred vision. Early papilledema is sometimes mistaken for structural blurring of the disc margins. Fully developed papilledema is more easily identified by a marked elevation at the disc margin and large, distended veins. Papilledema is indicative of increased pressure and is considered a medical emergency.

Cranial enlargement. Increased head circumference is characteristic of increased intracranial pressure in infants and young children whose sutures have not completely closed.[2] Expansion of the skull sutures occurs most completely in very young children but can occur in children of all ages. In addition to cranial enlargement, a bulging fontanel in babies is indicative of increased intracranial pressure.

Mental disturbances. Somnolence, restlessness, irritability, and personality changes can be seen in children with brain tumors.[2] Attentiveness may drop and school performance may deteriorate. These findings may initially be very subtle and of little concern to the parents. Only after the findings progress and are accompanied by physical findings may parents seek medical advice.

Seizures. Seizures are rarely an early sign of a brain tumor and have been reported to occur only in about 15% of children with intracranial lesions.[10] Seizures associated with brain tumors tend to be focal, suggesting specific areas of abnormal neuronal discharge in the brain.[1] Tumors of the temporal lobe cause the highest frequencies of seizures.

Focal effects

Focal effects result from tumor invasion or pressure on a specific area of the brain. Each area of the brain lends itself to a complex of localizing symptoms.

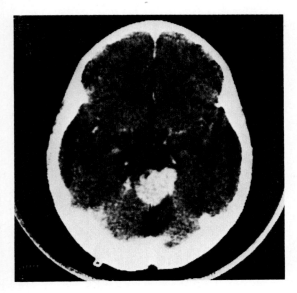

Fig. 8-1. Computerized tomographic (CT) scan of brain with medulloblastoma of posterior fossa *(arrow)*.

Supratentorial tumors, hemisphere location.
The symptoms of a brain tumor in a hemisphere
depend on its exact location. For example, a lesion
in the left hemisphere may interfere with speech
processing. Tumors occuring in the frontal and oc-
cipital lobes are more difficult to assess, since these
are "silent" areas of the brain. However, papilledema is present in about 80% of these patients,
and headache is a common complaint. Children
with supratentorial tumors may exhibit psychomotor and generalized seizure activity, especially
when the tumor is localized in the temporal lobes.[2]
Hemiparesis and sensory deficits are uncommon.

Midline tumors. Abrupt personality changes
may occur as the first symptom of a midline tumor.[2]
Interference with the optic pathways can cause visual field disturbances, and pituitary or hypothalamic involvement can cause endocrine changes
such as diabetes insipidus and precocious puberty.
Most midline tumors cause an insidious onset of
increased intracranial pressure. A child under the
age of 3 years with a hypothalamic tumor may
present with a diencephalic syndrome, which involves sudden failure to thrive followed by severe
emaciation despite adequate oral intake. Eventually, optic atrophy occurs and leads to blindness.
Searching nystagmus can be caused by the impending blindness.[2]

Infratentorial tumors. Cerebellar fourth ventricle tumors and brainstem tumors are included in
the infratentorial category. Obstruction of the ventricular system by an infratentorial tumor causes
increased intracranial pressure, leading to headaches and vomiting. Disturbances in gait and balance and slow, coarse nystagmus are also common
manifestations of infratentorial tumors.[2] Diplopia
may occur secondary to increased intracranial pressure or to direct compression of one of the oculomotor nerves. Head tilt may occur in an effort
to compensate for diplopia.

Spinal cord tumors. Spinal cord tumors may
be intramedullary (in the cord itself) or extramedullary (outside of the cord). Intramedullary tumors
tend to cause symmetric muscle weakness and atrophy, whereas extramedullary tumors tend to cause
specific nerve root effects.[2]

DIAGNOSTIC EVALUATION
History and physical examination

A complete history and physical examination are
fundamental to the evaluation of a child with a
suspected CNS tumor. Duration and severity
of symptoms and past medical history are documented. Specific physical findings, with emphasis
on the neurologic and ophthalmologic examinations, are noted.

Computerized tomographic scan

Computerized tomography (CT) is the primary
diagnostic tool in the evaluation of a child with a
suspected intracranial lesion.[1,11] In recent years the
use of CT scans has almost eliminated the need for
invasive procedures such as pneumoencephalog-
raphy or ventriculography. The unenhanced scan,
which is taken without intravenous contrast material, indicates whether a lesion is solid or cystic
and whether it is calcified or hemorrhagic.[12] The
extent of cerebral edema and dilatation and obstruction of the ventricular system are identified.
Following an unenhanced CT scan, the patient usually receives an intravenous injection of contrast
material. Enhancement of the lesion by contrast
material indicates the degree of tumor invasion,
and in the case of supratentorial malignant tumors,
the degree of enhancement is related to the degree
of malignancy[13] (Fig. 8-1).

Angiography

Angiography defines the vascular supply of a
tumor and in conjunction with the CT scan allows
inferences concerning the degree of malignancy of
certain tumors.[3] Angiography may identify an arteriovenous malformation incorrectly interpreted as
a mass lesion by CT scan. It may also assist the
neurosurgeon in planning the operative approach.

Electroencephalogram

The electroencephalogram (EEG) is often helpful in localizing supratentorial tumors but is of little
value in the diagnosis of infratentorial tumors.[1,2]
Specific EEG techniques such as brainstem-evoked
potentials are useful in evaluating brainstem and
hypothalamic lesions.[14]

Skull radiographs

Skull x-ray films document increased intracranial pressure by demonstrating suture separation, digital markings, calcifications, specific bony erosions at the base of the skull, cranial asymmetry, and changes of the sella turcica[2] (Fig. 8-2).

Cerebral spinal fluid examination

A lumbar puncture in patients with a suspected intracranial lesion should be deferred if there is increased intracranial pressure and should be performed with great caution even when there is no evidence of elevated pressure. Examination of the cerebrospinal fluid documents the presence of tumor cell seeding along the spinal meninges. Such seeding occurs most frequently in medulloblastomas, germinomas, and ependymomas.[2] Spinal fluid examination may not always reveal abnormalities in protein, cell count, or cytology in children with active CNS tumors.[12] The presence of markers associated with tumor cell proliferation has been used as an ancillary indicator of active or recurrent CNS tumors. Spinal fluid polyamine levels are very useful as tumor cell markers for tumors in proximity to the spinal fluid system, especially medulloblastomas.[15]

Nuclear magnetic resonance

In recent years new scanning modalities have arisen. Among these the most promising and most rapidly developing is nuclear magnetic resonance (NMR). The principle of NMR is fundamentally different from that of radiography. In NMR a strong magnetic field is applied, and the change in orientation of certain atoms is recorded. A NMR scan can be applied theoretically to hydrogen, nitrogen, phosphorus, and other atoms. The clinically useful machines at this time are tuned for hydrogen and therefore accentuate structures through the measurement of different hydrogen and specially altered water content. The pictures show magnificent detail (Fig. 8-3). Tumors are often well delineated and better defined than in standard CT scans, with or without contrast. The scanning is in its infancy, and at this time the pictures tend to be overinter-

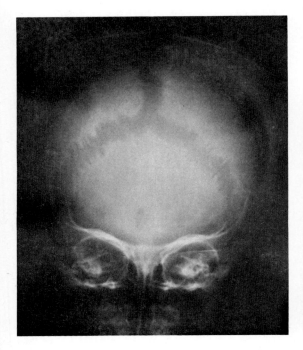

Fig. 8-2. Skull x-ray film demonstrating suture separations and digital markings.

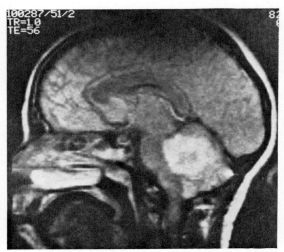

Fig. 8-3. NMR scans often define and delineate tumors better than CT scans.

preted, whereas CT scans are often underinterpreted. For the next few years simultaneous CT scan and NMR scans need to be done to fully learn the capabilities and limitations of both.

Positron emission tomography

Positron emission tomography (PET) is another new scanning modality. In this scan a short-lived radioactive isotope is injected and incorporated into a molecule that may be differently metabolized by tumor cells and normal cells or by living cells as opposed to dead cells. An image is created from the emissions of the decay of the radioactive atoms in the molecule. Through this scanning, differential function can be deduced. This can become a powerful tool in discerning the degree of viability of a defined tumor area.

Stereotactic biopsy

It has become possible through the combined use of CT scanning and careful biopsy techniques to place biopsy needles with great accuracy.[16] By doing such stereotactic biopsies, it is now possible to approach lesions that were once considered inoperable. Because current therapies are being refined and are becoming histology specific, accurate pathologic diagnosis is extremely important. Until recently, it was occasionally necessary to treat on the basis of a diagnosis derived by imaging. It may soon be possible to obtain specific pathologic diagnoses for all patients.

TREATMENT

Approaches to treatment vary depending on the specific goals of treatment and behavior and location of the tumor. Currently, cerebellar astrocytomas, giant cell tumors, and craniopharyngiomas may be treated with surgery alone. Medulloblastomas, ependymomas, and brainstem glioma tumors are best treated with a combination of surgery, radiation, and more recently, chemotherapy.

Surgery

Total removal of the tumor is the goal of surgery but is not always possible without subjecting the patient to residual neurologic damage.[2] Improved surgical techniques and supportive care during and after surgery allow for removal of brain tumors that were previously considered inoperable. Surgery is clearly not curative in all cases. However, if radiation therapy or chemotherapy is to be effective, the tumor to be treated should be as small as possible.

Before the removal of a tumor, a shunting procedure may be done to reduce intracranial pressure. The shunt allows for free flow of cerebrospinal fluid from the ventricles of the brain to another body cavity, such as the peritoneum (Fig. 8-4). Placement of a shunt may allow spread of certain tumor cells to other sites of the body. There have been reports of the development of distant metastases by this mechanism in patients with medulloblastoma and glioblastoma.[17,18]

Radiotherapy

Although all cells are sensitive to radiation, sensitivity is directly related to their mitotic activity. Since most brain tumors grow slowly and the mitotic activity is low, large doses of radiation are required to destroy them. Radiation therapy for brain tumors is in the range of 4500 to 5000 rad over a 6- to 8-week period.[2,19] Since medulloblastomas seed both the spinal and the cranial subarachnoid spaces early, high-dose radiation is delivered to the tumor site with an additional boost to the whole head and spinal cord (Fig. 8-5).

Children under the age of 2 years have incomplete brain maturation, and cranial radiation therapy is detrimental to this maturation process. Radiation to the spinous processes also leads to permanent and severe spinal growth impairment. Therefore cranial irradiation is rarely administered to children under 2 years of age.[1]

Side effects of cranial radiation therapy include temporary or permanent loss or thinning of hair, skin sensitivity, headaches, nausea, vomiting, and fatigue. Headaches, nausea, and vomiting may be caused by cerebral edema resulting from the radiation. Steroids such as dexamethasone (Decadron) are often administered to prevent cerebral

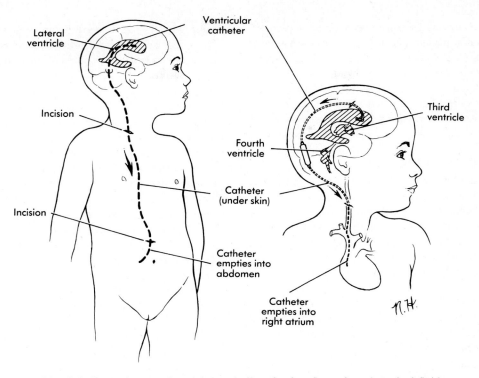

Fig. 8-4. Shunts bypass obstruction and allow for free flow of cerebrospinal fluid.

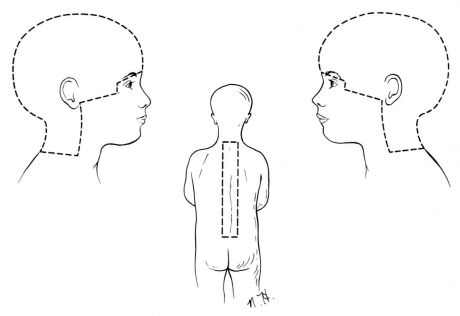

Fig. 8-5. Craniospinal axis radiation therapy field.

edema. Temporary fatigue and sleepiness from cranial irradiation can occur during or up to several weeks after completion of therapy[20] (see Chapter 21). Craniospinal axis radiation results in severe myelosuppression because a large volume of bone marrow is irradiated. In addition, severe pharyngitis can result because the pharynx receives a significant amount of radiation through scatter.

Electron beam irradiation

Radiotherapy can be delivered by a variety of techniques. Different energy beams have different physical characteristics. The photons, such as generated by a cobalt 60 irradiation, have the properties of reaching maximum energy below the skin and therefore tend to be relatively skin sparing. However, they have a rather broad depth of biologic effect so that much surrounding tissue is influenced by the irradiation. Electron beams have the property of very rapid falloff at a depth that can be predetermined. There is more skin reaction, but through careful dosimetry, it is possible to avoid much radiation to the vertebral bodies and pharynx. The result is far less myelosuppression and pharyngitis with its consequent malnutrition. The availability of electron beam radiotherapy depends on the availability of the equipment and the capability for the needed dosimetry which is far more complicated than is that for standard radiotherapy.

Chemotherapy

Chemotherapy as an adjunct to surgery and radiation therapy is still being evaluated yet is becoming more widely accepted.[21] The location of a tumor, rate of its growth, and rate of a drug's entrance into the CNS are all factors that influence the choice of agents and their route of administration.

Since most brain tumors have a low mitotic index, chemotherapeutic agents are believed to be effective in any stage of the cell cycle. A major therapeutic consideration has been the blood-brain barrier and its potential role in preventing drugs from achieving concentrations sufficient to affect tumor growth.[1] In general, compounds that are highly lipid soluble (lipophilic) with a low molecular weight are more effective than water-soluble substances.

The most effective drugs to date against brain tumors include alkylating agents, spindle poisons, antimetabolites, and steroids for control of edema.[2] Nitrogen mustard and the alkylating agents are cell cycle–nonspecific and lipophilic. Except for chloro-ethyl-methyl-cyclohexyl-nitrosourea (CCNU), most are given parenterally. Methotrexate, a cell cycle–specific antimetabolite, is hydrophilic (water soluble) and has poor penetration into the CNS. For this reason, it is given in high doses systemically or by intrathecal administration. Vincristine, a spindle poison, is to some extent lipophilic and is given parenterally. Procarbazine, a methylhydrozine, is lipid soluble in its oxidative form and is believed to have alkylating properties. MOPP combination chemotherapy (nitrogen mustard, vincristine, procarbazine, prednisone) has proven to be effective in salvage therapy for brain tumors in children who failed radiotherapy.[22] This regimen has recently been used in infants in an effort to postpone radiotherapy.[23]

cis-Platinum (Cisplatin), antibiotics, AZQ (a quinine-alkylating agent), and PCNU (a nitrosourea), and dibromoducitol are presently undergoing clinical trials.[2,20] Severe ototoxicity and renal toxicities have prevented prolonged use of *cis*-platinum. Myelosuppression has been a major complicating factor in the use of AZQ.

Historically, chemotherapy in the treatment of brain tumors has been used to combat recurrent or gross residual disease after surgery and radiation. The delivery of chemotherapy immediately after surgery or in conjunction with radiotherapy may offer a higher degree of effectiveness against some of the malignant intracranial neoplasms in the children.

Evaluation of treatment effectiveness involves assessment of tumor size by CT scan and clinical neurologic findings. Additionally, spinal fluid examination may be done in the follow-up of children with medulloblastomas. Brainstem-evoked potential studies may be done in the follow-up of children with brainstem or hypothalamic tumors.

The late effects of brain and spinal tumor therapy can include impaired intellectual function, endocrine abnormalities, scoliosis, and CNS deterioration.[3,21,22,24,25] These are discussed in detail in Chapter 31.

SPECIFIC TUMOR MANAGEMENT
Infratentorial tumors

Medulloblastoma. Medulloblastoma is the most common brain tumor in children, with 80% of the cases occurring during the first 15 years of life.[2] The median age at diagnosis is 5 years. The tumor occurs more frequently in males (4:1).[2] Medulloblastoma is a cerebellar tumor that usually arises in the vermis and may extend into the fourth ventricle and cerebellar hemispheres. It is a highly malignant and rapidly growing tumor that can seed the spinal subarachnoid space and metastasize to other tissues in the body.

The average duration of symptoms to diagnosis is short, usually 1 to 2 months.[3] The children may present with classic signs of increased intracranial pressure (caused by early obstruction of the fourth ventricle) and truncal ataxia. Because of its rapid growth and invasive nature, medulloblastoma is difficult to remove completely at surgery. However, surgery allows for tissue diagnosis, debulking of the tumor, and re-establishment of the free flow of cerebrospinal fluid. Aggressive radiation is the treatment of choice after surgical debulking. This treatment has resulted in significant prolongation of life with 5-year survival of 35% and 10-year survival of 25%.[2,26] Prognosis is poorer for younger patients and boys.[1] Late recurrences do occur.[27]

Several studies suggest that medulloblastoma is sensitive to chemotherapy, yet no specific chemotherapy regimen has proved to be outstanding.[28,29] Combination chemotherapeutic regimens include CCNU, vincristine, and intrathecal methotrexate; CCNU, vincristine, and procarbazine; nitrogen mustard, vincristine, procarbazine, and prednisone (MOPP); and BCNU, another nitrosourea, vincristine, and intrathecal methotrexate. Although results have shown improvement in disease, no single regimen is superior.

Medulloblastoma is known to metastasize outside the CNS to bones and lymph nodes. The most common sites of skeletal involvement include the vertebrae, long bones, and skull.[3] Lymph node involvement is generalized. Soft tissue metastases can be seen in the liver, pancreas, or thymus.

Cerebellar astrocytoma. Cerebellar astrocytomas are considered the most favorable and clinically benign of all brain tumors.[3] They account for approximately 20% of brain tumors in children.[2] Males and females are affected equally; the mean age is 6 to 7 years.[30] The astrocytoma is classically described as being located laterally in the cerebellum yet can arise from the midline region. Midline tumors are seen more frequently in younger children, whereas lateral tumors are seen more frequently in older children. If the lateral cerebellum is involved, symptoms include horizontal nystagmus, clumsiness of one hand, and an awkward gait marked by stumbling to the side of the tumor. There may be no signs of increased intracranial pressure if the ventricular system is not blocked. A midline astrocytoma often blocks the ventricular system, subsequently causing headaches, vomiting, truncal ataxia, and papilledema.

The cerebellar astrocytoma is usually well encapsulated with a tendency to form large cysts with nodules inside and/or small microcysts throughout the tumor. It is generally of low-grade malignancy. Gjerris and Klinken[31] described two types of cerebellar astrocytomas: juvenile, which accounts for 70% of the cases, and diffuse, which accounts for the remaining 30%. The treatment of choice is surgical removal.[32] If the tumor can be excised completely, cure is possible without further treatment. If complete excision is not feasible, recurrence is usually slow, and additional surgery can be performed. Radiation to the posterior fossa in recurrent, diffuse, and more rare malignant varieties of astrocytoma have been used. Prognosis for the juvenile astrocytoma is excellent, with a 25-year survival rate of 95% after surgery alone.[32] However, the 25-year survival rate for the diffuse astrocytoma is 38%.

Ependymoma. Ependymomas represent approximately 9% of brain tumors in children.[33] They can arise anywhere in the neuraxis where ependymal cells are found and within the cerebral hemispheres not contiguous with any ependymal tissue. The majority of intracranial ependymomas occur between 2 to 6 years of age, whereas the majority of spinal ependymomas occur during the teenage years.[12] Most of the intracranial ependymomas in children occur in the posterior fossa. The signs and symptoms vary with location. Any ependymoma originating near the fourth ventricle may mimic a medulloblastoma and present with headache, vomiting, and truncal ataxia.

The prognosis for ependymomas varies according to tumor location, pathologic grade, and treatment regimens.[3] The overall 5-year survival rate is estimated to be 25%.[12] Very few cases of metastatic disease are reported.

Surgery has been the mainstay of treatment but is rarely curative. Postoperative radiotherapy has improved the results of surgery significantly, but there is still controversy about whether local irradiation versus total craniospinal irradiation is preferred. High-grade infratentorial tumors are more likely to seed the spinal cord; thus entire CNS axis irradiation is recommended. Salazar and others[34] recommend that low-grade infratentorial ependymomas are approached with whole brain irradiation to the fifth cervical vertebra and that low-grade supratentorial tumors receive only elective radiation to the whole brain.[35] Chemotherapy has been used in patients with recurrent disease. However, the results have been disappointing.[36]

Brainstem tumors

Brainstem tumors comprise 10% to 15% of all CNS tumors of children.[2,3] Presenting symptoms are variable and can include gait disturbance, facial cranial nerve (VII) paralysis, and nystagmus.[37]

Hemiparesis is often seen contralateral to the cranial nerve palsies. Signs of increased intracranial pressure can be seen if the tumor is located high in the brainstem, causing distortion of the aqueduct and obstruction of cerebrospinal fluid.

The diagnosis of a brainstem tumor is usually made by CT scan alone. The fear of postoperative swelling and injury to vital brainstem structures, plus the concern of gaining correct information from the small amount of tissue obtained at biopsy, has limited the role of surgery in the past. Improved surgical techniques may allow certain patients to benefit from biopsies, evacuation of cysts, or debulking of tumor. The treatment of choice is radiation therapy at a dose of 4000 to 6000 rad to the brainstem.[3] There is often a lag of several weeks between initiation of radiation therapy and signs of improvement. Patients may deteriorate rapidly after initiation of radiation therapy if swelling of the brainstem occurs. High-dose steroids are administered to prevent this. Chemotherapy is sometimes used for recurrent disease, but there is no evidence that it is beneficial. The Children's Cancer Study Group completed a randomized trial of radiation therapy plus vincristine and CCNU.[12] No significant benefit of chemotherapy was observed. Although long-term remissions have occasionally been obtained with radiotherapy and with chemotherapy, the median survival is 15 months.[12] The prognosis of brainstem tumors is partly dependent on the pathologic grade of the tumor and duration of symptoms before diagnosis. The best prognosis is for low-grade tumors with long durations of symptoms, and the worst prognosis is for malignant gliomas. The overall 5-year survival rates are reported as 20% to 30%.[12,38]

Supratentorial tumors

Tumors of the hemispheres. Hemispheric tumors give rise to a wide variety of symptoms, depending on the exact location.[39] Seizures, rarely seen in children with infratentorial tumors, are seen in approximately 40% of the children with tumors of a hemisphere.[1] They are usually partial sensorimotor seizures and may appear years before the tumor is diagnosed. The parietal area is the most common site of hemispheric tumors. Tumors may be of either low- or high-grade malignancy. In one series of 115 hemispheric tumors in children, 46% were astrocytomas, 12% glioblastomas, 12% oligodendrogliomas, and 8% ependymomas.[37] Low-grade tumors are treated primarily by surgery. However, if total excision is not always possible, postoperative local irradiation may be required. Highly malignant tumors are treated by surgery followed by local irradiation. The use of chemotherapy in children with recurrent hemispheric tumors has been limited in the past. Therefore its effectiveness has not been determined.

Prognosis of hemispheric tumors depends on histology. Mean survival time from diagnosis is 14.5 months.[3]

Craniopharyngioma. The most frequent midline tumor in children is the craniopharyngioma. The incidence is between 5% and 11% of all brain tumors.[3] Craniopharyngioma is of developmental origin yet can occur at any age. They are often benign and slow growing yet cause impressive symptomatology because of their proximity to the pituitary. Visual impairment, endocrine abnormalities, and signs of intracranial pressure can be seen. The majority of children with craniopharyngiomas have evidence of calcification seen either on plain skull films or CT scan.

Treatment of craniopharyngiomas varies. Total surgical resection alone, subtotal removal or biopsy plus irradiation, and radiation therapy alone have all been advocated.[2,40-42] Total surgical removal invariably leads to endocrine abnormalities, including panhypopituitarism and hyperphagia.[3] However, there is a high recurrence rate after less than radical surgery. The use of microsurgery has increased the success rate of total removal, thereby averting the problems of recurrence after radiation alone. Radiation therapy alone is considered when total surgical removal is impossible. The usual recommended dose is 4500 to 5500 rad to the tumor over a 5- to 6-week period.[3] Most tumor recur-

rences occur within 3 years. Patients with craniopharyngiomas treated with conservative surgery and radiotherapy have a 10-year survival rate of 72%.[1]

Optic glioma. Optic gliomas occur most frequently between 1 and 5 years of age.[1] They usually arise at the optic chiasm, but other parts of the optic nerve may be involved.[43] They can be associated with neurofibromatosis. Optic gliomas may cause the diencephalic syndrome, but more commonly cause visual defects. They are often slow growing, and prolonged survival is seen following incomplete surgical removal. The effectiveness of radiation therapy and/or chemotherapy in prolonging survival is undetermined at this time.

Pineal tumors. Pineal tumors include gliomas, pinealoblastomas, endodermal sinus tumors, germinomas, and teratomas.[2] Presenting symptomatology includes endocrine abnormalities, impairment of ocular function (especially paralysis of upward gaze) and pupillary reaction, ataxia, and signs of increased intracranial pressure. Treatment consists of relief of hydrocephalus through surgical shunting, followed by radiation therapy. If radiation therapy is not effective in shrinking the tumor, surgical removal may be attempted. Chemotherapy is seldom used, and its effectiveness has not yet been determined. Pinealoblastomas have a tendency to seed the cerebrospinal fluid. The 5-year disease-free survival rate ranges from 31% to 78%.[2]

Spinal cord tumors

Spinal cord tumors are rare, but can occur in children of all ages.[2] Many spinal cord tumors are not primary neoplasms, but are extensions of tumor outside the spinal cord. The most common primary spinal cord tumors include astrocytomas and ependymomas. They often involve the lower portion of the spinal cord (cauda equina). Symptomatology of an intraspinal tumor may include vertebral pain, spinal stiffness, progressive scoliosis, leg paralysis, and anal sphincter paralysis. The neurologic picture is determined by the level of cord compression. Cervical tumors may cause respiratory distress and quadriplegia, which may be severe and sudden in onset. Tumors of the cauda equina lead to abnormalities of sphincter function. Diagnosis is based on radiologic examination of the spine, where paravertebral calcifications and enlargement of the spinal canal can be seen. Myelography, an x-ray examination of the spinal cord after injection of a contrast medium, is helpful in identifying the exact tumor site. Treatment involves immediate surgery in efforts to decompress the spinal cord and remove the tumor. Surgery is often followed by radiation therapy, although cystic astrocytomas can be aspirated with significant palliative effect. The long-term prognosis of intraspinal tumors is variable, depending on tumor histology, degree of extension, and effectiveness of treatment. The functional sequelae depend on the degree of nerve destruction caused by the tumor and aggravated by the duration of cord compression. The progression of spinal cord tumors is usually very slow. Late relapses do occur, and the functional prognosis is poor.

CASE STUDY #1: MEDULLOBLASTOMA

A.B. is a 7-year-old white male who was well until March 16, 1982, when he was brought to his local pediatrician with headaches and vomiting. The history revealed that the headaches began 3 weeks before the visit and had worsened progressively. They were more severe in the morning. After vomiting, they were relieved for a short time but returned. He was not noticeably nauseated before vomiting. Physical examination revealed an irritable and restless child who preferred to sit still in a dark and quiet examination room. Fine lateral nystagmus, papilledema, and ataxia were noted. The remainder of the examination was normal. An emergency CT scan showed a posterior fossa mass and hydrocephalus. A craniotomy was performed, and pathology revealed medulloblastoma. After a 6-week postoperative recovery, craniospinal radiation therapy was delivered at a dose of 5000 rad to the posterior fossa and 3000 rad to the entire craniospinal axis. He did well until 2 years later, when he began to experience lower back pain. A spinal x-ray examination revealed tumor metastasis to the cauda equina. A complete bone survey showed no other sites of metastasis. Chemotherapy with MOPP (nitrogen mustard, vincristine, procarbazine, and prednisone) was ini-

tiated. After 3 months, the bone survey showed arrest of the spinal metastasis, and no further metastases were noted. MOPP chemotherapy was continued for 2 full years without recurrence of metastases.

CASE STUDY #2: CRANIOPHARYNGIOMA

W.E. is an 8-year-old white male who was referred to a pediatric endocrinologist for evaluation of short stature. The history was unremarkable except for two severe headaches over the previous few weeks. Physical examination revealed a height of 4 cm below the 3rd percentile for age and a weight at the 75th percentile for age. An eye examination revealed left homonymous hemianopsia (blindness on the left halves of both eyes). The remainder of the examination was normal. A lateral skull x-ray film showed suprasellar calcification, and a CT scan of the brain showed a suprasellar cystic tumor. A frontal craniotomy was performed. The capsule of the tumor was incised, 15 cc of fluid was drained, and the total capsule was then removed. The tumor was diagnosed to be a craniopharyngioma. Postoperatively, W.E. developed diabetes insipidus, which was treated with vasopressin (Pitressin). One month after surgery, a full endocrine workup indicated panhypopituitarism. He was placed on thyroid, cortisone, antidiuretic hormone (DDAVP), and growth hormone replacement. Three years after surgery, a CT scan revealed no tumor recurrence.

NURSING CONSIDERATIONS

The diagnosis of a brain tumor in a child is psychologically and emotionally devastating. Brain tumors have historically been equated with very little hope for survival, and the physical effects can quickly alter the child's ability to function normally within his environment. He may appear or behave differently to family and friends, who may have difficulty understanding and accepting the change. Physical dependency may increase because of deterioration of motor function, and alteration in body image can occur secondary to disease and treatment.

Diagnosis

The family must understand the reality and meaning of the diagnosis before treatment is discussed. In presenting the diagnosis, it may be helpful for family members to view the CT scan or a three-dimensional model of the brain. Symptomatology can then be presented in relation to the tumor's location, and hydrocephalus or other findings can be better defined. The nurse may need to interpret and reiterate for the family the physician's statements regarding diagnosis. Neurologic signs and symptoms can be very confusing to parents, and the nurse can help decipher what the findings mean. Since shocked and grief-stricken parents may retain very little information in the initial discussions, it may be helpful to jot down the most salient points of the discussions to give them. The child's primary health care providers must initiate introduction of their roles early on so that the family can direct questions and concerns appropriately. The purpose of diagnostic procedures, such as a CT scan of the brain or lumbar puncture, should be discussed in detail with the child and family. If the child is allergic to iodine, intravenous contrast material should not be given for the CT scan. The importance of lying still during the scan cannot be overemphasized to the child. Babies and younger children may require sedation or general anesthesia if they are unable to undergo a CT scan without moving. Education and preparation for a lumbar puncture is of utmost importance. This procedure is frightening for the child, since he is unable to see what is happening behind his back. The child should lie flat for 1 hour after a lumbar puncture to allow for equalization of cerebrospinal fluid and to prevent headaches.

Treatment

The child and parents must understand the rationale behind treatment, the expected side effects, the anticipated outcomes, and the possible alternatives if the treatment should fail. The nurse plays an integral role in presenting such information in understandable terms. During therapy, the child should be encouraged to function at maximum potential in school and in extracurricular activities, despite side effects of treatment and possible impairment of fine or gross motor skills, vision, or speech. Contacting the child's school nurse and

teachers to discuss his diagnosis and treatment is crucial to a smooth transition from hospital to school. Special provisions may need to be made for children with visual problems, behavior changes, limb weakness, articulation difficulties, ataxia, urinary or bowel incontinence, or perceptual alterations. School personnel often welcome a site visit from the child's oncology nurse. The nurse invests and shares emotionally in the child's daily triumphs and setbacks during treatment and becomes acutely aware of the subtle changes in the child's physical and mental performance. Documentation and follow-up of subtle findings is important.

If a craniotomy is planned, the child and parents should be aware that part or all of the hair will be shaved and that bruising around the eye orbits may occur following surgery. Craniotomies may take many hours to complete, depending on the location and behavior of the tumor, and frequent operating room progress reports can help alleviate parents' anxiety. Most children recover in an intensive care unit before transfer to their hospital rooms. Neurologic vital signs are monitored closely during the first few days after surgery. Sudden deterioration in neurologic vital signs may indicate hemorrhage at the operative site. The child's physician should be notified immediately if neurologic deterioration occurs. Children who experience no complications recover amazingly quickly from neurosurgery.

The child with a tumor requiring postoperative radiation therapy, such as medulloblastoma, is usually given 4 to 6 weeks to recuperate from surgery before radiation therapy is initiated. Before therapy, the family may benefit from touring the radiation therapy department and meeting the staff members. An oral steroid, such as dexamethasone (Decadron), is usually started at the beginning of therapy to alleviate clinical deterioration. The child should be instructed to avoid salt intake while on steroids to prevent fluid weight gain, edema, and hypertension. The parents should be aware that steroids can cause a voracious appetite, temporary cushingoid appearance, and irritability. The steroids are tapered toward the completion of radiation therapy. If craniospinal radiation is given, complete blood counts should be checked once or twice a week, since thrombocytopenia and neutropenia can result from bone marrow destruction in the vertebral bodies. If the blood counts drop to unacceptable levels, therapy may be discontinued for a short time to allow for marrow recovery. The child should be instructed to avoid large crowds and ill people during the nadir of myelosuppression. Radiation therapy leads to temporary hair loss, which can be frustrating for the child who just begins to notice hair regrowth after surgery. The skin may become darkly pigmented, dry, and irritated in the radiation field. Care of the radiated skin involves the use of water-based creams and protection from outdoor sun. The radiation fields are usually delineated with red lines and should not be washed off throughout treatment. It is important to inform the child that radiation therapy causes only temporary hair loss but may cause permanent hair thinning. Pharyngitis, a common side effect of craniospinal radiation, leads to an inability to tolerate swallowing solid foods. The patient should be referred to a dietitian for management of adequate caloric intake. Several palatable liquid dietary supplements are available for children until the pharyngitis resolves (see Chapter 26).

Chemotherapy

Nursing management of a child with a brain tumor receiving chemotherapy does not differ greatly from children with other tumors. The mixing and delivery of drugs and specific side effects of each drug are discussed in Chapter 20. The use of antiemetics must be used very wisely in children with severe neurologic impairment, since these drugs can cause sedation, possibly leading to aspiration should vomiting occur. Children with hemiparesis may have poor circulation in the paralyzed limbs. These limbs should be avoided for intravenous entry sites, especially for delivery of extravasational agents, since the child is unable to feel the usual sensation of infiltration. If infiltration should occur, healing may be delayed in a paralyzed limb with impaired circulation.

The specific nursing interventions during diagnosis and treatment of CNS tumors are presented in the nursing care protocol.

NURSING CARE PROTOCOL FOR THE CHILD WITH BRAIN/CNS TUMOR

Nursing diagnoses (problems/needs)	Goals/objectives (patient/family will:)	Interventions (nurse will:)
1. Knowledge deficit (related to diagnosis and diagnostic workup)	Verbalize purpose of methods for tests	Assist with and teach regarding procedures (physical examination, laboratory work, skull x-rays films, CT scan of brain, lumbar puncture) Note allergy to iodine and notify CT department of allergy Encourage questions pertaining to workup
	Receive information related to diagnosis verbally and/or in printed material	Give available teaching resources

NURSING CARE PROTOCOL FOR THE CHILD WITH BRAIN/CNS TUMOR—cont'd

Nursing diagnoses (problems/needs)	Goals/objectives (patient/family will:)	Interventions (nurse will:)
2. Anxiety (emotional distress related to diagnosis, testing, possible hospitalization, treatment, and side effects)	Demonstrate decreased level of anxiety Share feelings with support persons	Provide information related to workup, disease, protocol, and nursing care Refer to other services such as chaplain, social worker, counselor as available Encourage verbalization through active listening, empathetic attitude, and providing time for communication Use therapeutic play with patient to encourage expression of fears and to prepare for procedures
3. Knowledge deficit (need for information related to preoperative preparation)	Verbalize general understanding of surgery Be able to state preoperative and postoperative routines	Participate and reinforce explanation of surgery Provide information about preoperative and postoperative routines (i.e., NPO, IV, preoperative medication, safety measures, deep breathing, NG tube, Foley catheter, shaving of hair, surgical site dressing)
4. Injury: potential for (postoperative complications) Hemorrhage at the operative site	Recovery from surgery without postoperative complications Have minimum blood loss, stable vital signs, and stable neurologic status	Check dressings frequently for drainage of blood; monitor vital signs and neurologic vital signs; notify physician immediately if sudden clinical deterioration occurs
Comfort, alterations in: pain	Demonstrate a decrease in pain perception through verbalization, facial expressions, increased mobility, and decreased request for pain medication	Initiate comfort measures such as positioning, therapeutic touch, diversion, medications, and emotional support; propping into a sitting position can help to alleviate head pain; narcotics interfere with neurologic status and are given only when absolutely necessary

Continued.

NURSING CARE PROTOCOL FOR THE CHILD WITH BRAIN/CNS TUMOR—cont'd

Nursing diagnoses (problems/needs)	Goals/objectives (patient/family will:)	Interventions (nurse will:)
Increased intracranial pressure caused by tissue swelling and blockage of CSF flow	Have no signs of increased intracranial pressure (severe headache, vomiting, papilledema)	Monitor neurologic vital signs closely; if signs of increased intracranial pressure occur, notify physician immediately; have intravenous dexamethasone (Decadron) and mannitol available; prevent overhydration
Fluid and electrolyte imbalance (especially with craniopharyngiomas)	Exhibit balanced intake and output and electrolytes within normal limits	Monitor intake and output and urine/serum chemistries; if excessive thirst and large quantities of unconcentrated urine occur, notify physician; diabetes insipidus is common immediately postoperatively in craniopharyngiomas—treat with vasopressin (Pitressin) or DDAVP
Other common postoperative complications, (immobility, alterations in gas exchange, impaired elimination, delayed healing)	Gradual increase in participation in activities of daily living; have chest clear, skin intact with healing incision, bowel sounds present	Encourage mobility, ambulation; implement preventive measures (deep breathe, ambulation if possible, movement); identify complications and initiate prompt treatment
5. Knowledge deficit (related to therapy)	State purpose of therapy	Provide information related to radiation therapy
	Identify potential side effects of therapy and appropriate treatment	Provide information and discuss potential side effects of radiation therapy (i.e., skin sensitivity and peeling, headaches, nausea, vomiting, alopecia)
	Recognize postradiation fatigue and sleepiness	Discuss possibility of postradiation fatigue and sleepiness, and reinforce that it is a temporary phenomenon
	Have side effects within expected limits and control, and will not develop complications resulting from side effects; have minimum late side effects	Provide interventions per nursing and physician orders related to: Skin sensitivity and peeling—teach to avoid sun exposure to head, give water-based cream (Tegaderm, Vigilon, Aquafor)

NURSING CARE PROTOCOL FOR THE CHILD WITH BRAIN/CNS TUMOR—cont'd

Nursing diagnoses (problems/needs)	Goals/objectives (patient/family will:)	Interventions (nurse will:)
		Headaches, nausea, vomiting—verify that patient starts taking dexamethasone before or at initiation of treatment; verify that shunt is functional; notify physician if patient has severe headaches, vomiting, and neurological deterioration; have intravenous dexamethasone available
		Alopecia—reinforce that alopecia is usually temporary; offer scarves, caps, if child is self-conscious
		Reinforce importance of long-term follow-up; observe for late effects such as decreased intellectual performance, endocrine abnormalities, scoliosis, CNS deterioration
6. Knowledge deficit (related to chemotherapy)	Be able to state name of drugs and their general purpose	Assess level of understanding and teach accordingly; document teaching and evaluation; provide written information on each drug
	Identify expected side effects and their management	Discuss potential side effects of each drug, management at home, and when to contact the nurse/physician
	Experience minimum complications resulting from side effects	Provide written information regarding management of side effects; provide 24-hr telephone availability in case of emergency or questions
	Develop minumum late side effects; comply with follow-up for prompt recognition and treatment of late side effects	Prophylaxis and treatment per nursing and physician orders related to side effects of specific drugs used
		Teach importance of return visits for follow-up; observe carefully for potential late effects and refer for treatment when appropriate

Continued.

NURSING CARE PROTOCOL FOR THE CHILD WITH BRAIN/CNS TUMOR—cont'd

Nursing diagnoses (problems/needs)	Goals/objectives (patient/family will:)	Interventions (nurse will:)
7. Injury: potential for (recurrence and/or metastasis of tumor)	Identify signs and symptoms of recurrence or metastasis and notify health team immediately Verbalize understanding of individualized treatment of recurrent or metastasis Obtain remission of disease or comfort during terminal phase	Provide information related to signs and symptoms of recurrence of metastasis such as recurrence of original symptoms at initial diagnosis, bone pain (medulloblastoma), or paresis from spinal involvement (medulloblastoma, ependymoma) Teach importance of notifying health care team immediately if recurrence or metastasis is suspected Discuss rationale, goal, delivery, and side effects of proposed treatment should recurrence or metastasis occur Deliver nursing care specific to treatment and patient needs
8. Coping, ineffective family: compromised	Be able to cope with adjustments necessary for maximum functioning at home, at school, and with friends Maintain positive self-concept, return to activities of daily living	Provide emotional support and teaching; refer to other health care professionals as needed Communicate with school and community professionals to facilitate adjustment outside of hospital Encourage continued contacts with the health care institution

REFERENCES

1. Schweisguth, O.: The central nervous system. In Schweisguth, O., editor: Solid tumors in children, New York, 1982, John Wiley & Sons, Inc.
2. van Eys, J.: Malignant tumors of the central nervous system. In Sutow, W.W., Fernbach, D.J., and Vietti, T.J., editors: Clinical pediatric oncology, ed. 3, St. Louis, 1984, The C.V. Mosby Co.
3. Cohen, M., Duffner, P., and Tebbi, C.: Brain tumors in children: diagnosis and management. In Tebbi, C., editor: Pediatric and adolescent oncology, Boston, 1980, G.K. Hall & Co.
4. Young, J., and Miller, R.: Incidence of malignant tumors in U.S. children, J. Pediatr. **86:**254, 1975.
5. Schoenberg, B., Schoenberg, D., and Christine, B.: The epidemiology of primary intracranial neoplasms of childhood, Mayo Clinic Proc. **51:**51, 1976.
6. MacMahon, B.: Prenatal x-ray exposure and childhood cancer, J. Natl. Cancer Inst. **28:**1173, 1982.
7. Modan, B., and others: Radiation-induced head and neck tumors, Lancet **1:**277, 1974.
8. Schneck, S., and Penn, I.: De-novo brain tumors in renal transplant recipients, Lancet **1:**983, 1971.

9. Honig, P., and Charney, E.: Children with brain tumor headaches, Am. J. Dis. Child. **136:**121, 1982.

10. Critchley, M.: Brain tumors in children, their general symptomatology, Br. J. Child. Dis. **22:**251, 1925.

11. Houser, O., and others: Evaluation of intracranial disorders in children by computerized tomography: a preliminary report, Neurology **25:**607, 1975.

12. Walker, R., and Allen, J.: Pediatric brain tumors, Pediatr. Ann. **12:**5, 1983.

13. Butler, A., and others: Computerized tomography in astrocytomas, Radiology **129:**443, 1978.

14. Nadar, R., Hahan, J., and Levine, H.: Brain stem auditory evoked potential in determining site of lesion of brain stem gliomas in children, Laryngoscope **90:**1980.

15. Marton, L., and others: CSF polyamines: a new and important means of monitoring patients with medulloblastoma, Cancer **47:**757, 1981.

16. Conway, L.: Stereotactic biopsy of deep intracranial tumors. In Schmidek, H., and Sweet, H., editors: Current techniques in operative neurosurgery, New York, 1977, Grune & Stratton, Inc.

17. Makeever, L., and King, J.: Medulloblastoma with extracranial metastasis through a ventriculovenous shunt, Am. J. Clin. Pathol. **46:**245, 1966.

18. Wakumatsu, T., and others: Glioblastoma with extracranial metastasis through ventriculopleural shunt, J. Neurosurg. **34:**697, 1971.

19. Sheline, G.: Radiation therapy of tumors of the central nervous system in childhood, Cancer **35:**957, 1975.

20. Freeman, J., Johnson, P., and Voke, J.: Somnolence after prophylactic cranial irradiation in children with acute lymphoblastic leukemia, Br. Med. J. **4:**523, 1973.

21. Fewer, D., Wilson, C., and Levin, V.: Brain tumor chemotherapy, Springfield, 1976, Charles C Thomas, Publisher.

22. Cangir, A., and others: Combination chemotherapy with MOPP in children with recurrent brain tumors, Med. Pediatr. Oncol. **4:**253, 1978.

23. van Eys, J., and others: MOPP regimen as primary chemotherapy for brain tumors in infants, J. Neuro. Oncol. **3:**237, 1985.

24. Samaan, N., and others: Hypopituitarism after external irradiation, Ann. Intern. Med. **83:**771, 1975.

25. Shalet, S., and others: Pituitary function after treatment of intracranial tumors in children, Lancet **2:**104, 1978.

26. Bloom, H., and Walsh, L.: Tumors of the central nervous system. In Blood, H., and others, editors: Cancer in children, Berlin, 1975, Springer-Verlag.

27. King, G., and Sagerman, R.: Late recurrence in medulloblastoma, Am. J. Roentgenol. Radium Ther. Nucl. Med. **123:**7, 1975.

28. Cangir, A., and others: Combination chemotherapy with MOPP in children with recurrent brain tumors, Med. Pediatr. Oncol. **4:**253, 1978.

29. Edwards, M., Levin, V., and Wilson, C.: Chemotherapy of pediatric posterior fossa tumors, Childs Brain **7:**252, 1980.

30. Griffen, T., Beaufait, D., and Blasko, J.: Cystic cerebellar astrocytomas in childhood, Cancer **44:**276, 1979.

31. Gjerris, F., and Klinken, L.: Long-term prognosis in children with benign cerebellar astrocytoma, J. Neurosurg. **49:**179, 1978.

32. Geisinger, J., and Bucy, P.: Astrocytomas of the cerebellum in children, Arch. Neurol. **24:**125, 1971.

33. Dorhmann, G., Farwell, J., and Flannery, J.: Ependymomas and ependymoblastomas in children, J. Neurosurg. **45:**273, 1976.

34. Salazar, O., and others: Improved survival of patients with intracranial ependymomas on irradiation: dose selection field extension, Cancer **35:**1563, 1975.

35. Sheline, G.: Radiation therapy of CNS tumors, Cancer **35**(suppl.):957, 1975.

36. Evans, A., and others: Adjuvant chemotherapy for medulloblastoma and ependymoma. In Paoletti, P., and others, editor: Multidisciplinary aspects of brain tumor therapy, New York, 1979, Elsevier North-Holland, Inc.

37. Panitch, H., and Berg, B.: Brain stem tumors of childhood and adolescence, Am J. Dis. Child. **119:**465, 1970.

38. Littman, P., and others: Pediatric brainstem gliomas, Cancer **45:**2787, 1980.

39. Low, N., Correll, J., and Hammill, J.: Tumors of the cerebral hemispheres in children, Arch. Neurol. **13:**547, 1965.

40. Katz, E.: Late results of radical excision of craniopharyngiomas in children, Neurology **42:**83, 1964.

41. Mori, K., and others: Results of treatment for craniopharyngioma, Childs Brain **6:**303, 1980.

42. Richmond, I., Wara, W., and Wilson, C.: Role of radiation therapy in the management of craniopharyngiomas in children, Neurosurgery **6:**513, 1980.

43. Chutorian, A., and others: Optic gliomas in children, Neurology **14:**83, 1964.

CHAPTER 9

Rhabdomyosarcoma

RALPH VOGEL and CHARLES PRATT

Rhabdomyosarcoma is a malignancy of striated (skeletal) muscle cells that presents in four major histologic types plus recently recognized special groups. It is the most common soft tissue malignancy in children and can present at any age from birth through adolescence. It also can present anywhere in the body, causing a wide variety of symptoms. These tumors often are misdiagnosed, causing a delay in referral and treatment.

Planning treatment and parent/patient teaching must be individualized because of the diversity of age, site, stage, and histology—all of which affect prognosis.

INCIDENCE

Rhabdomyosarcoma accounted for 78 malignancies of 1000 children with malignant disease (7.8%) in one major study[1] and 121 of 1200 solid tumors (10%) in another major cancer center.[2] A male-to-female predominance of 1.4:1 was reported in 554 cases of rhabdomyosarcoma in the Intergroup Rhabdomyosarcoma Study I (IRS-I).[3] This is similar to the experience at St. Jude Children's Research Hospital where 95 to 158 cases were male (M:F = 1.21:1).

IRS-I found 67% of children with rhabdomyosarcoma were under 10 years of age, 24% were between 11 and 15 years, and 9% were 15 to 20 years of age. The single most common age group was between 3 and 5 years (33%).[4]

HISTOLOGY

Histologically, rhabdomyosarcoma is characterized as a small, round cell tumor, as is neuroblastoma, Ewing's sarcoma, some types of non-Hodgkin's lymphoma (NHL), and acute lymphocytic leukemia (ALL). The individual malignant rhabdomyoblasts usually have a large, immature nucleus and irregular, vacuolated cytoplasm and may give the appearance of myeloblasts such as those seen in acute myelocytic leukemia (AML). These similarities can make the final diagnosis of rhabdomyosarcoma difficult.

There are four major histologic types of rhabdomyosarcoma classified as embryonal, alveolar, pleomorphic, and mixed. The most common type of rhabdomyosarcoma is embryonal; it accounted for 57%[3] to 71%[5] of identified cases in the Intergroup Rhabdomyosarcoma Study and at St. Jude Children's Research Hospital.[5] The rhabdomyoblasts in this histologic group resemble fetal cells at about 6 to 8 weeks of development. Sarcoma botryoides is a variety of embryonal rhabdomyosarcoma distinguished by a clinical presentation that includes (a) growth of a mass with a cystic "cluster of grapes" appearance; (b) presentation within a hollow organ, most commonly the vagina, bladder, or occasionally the head and neck region; and (c) peak incidence in children under age two. Fig. 9-1). Embryonal rhabdomyosarcoma has the best prognosis among the histologic varieties.

Alveolar rhabdomyosarcoma correlates with fetal rhabdomyoblasts at about 10 to 12 weeks of development. It has accounted for 14.6%[5] to 18%[3] of identified cases and is more commonly seen at a later age, especially in adolescents.[6] This histologic type is more likely to metastasize to lymph nodes or distant organs and therefore has a significantly poorer prognosis.

Other subtypes of rhabdomyosarcoma include

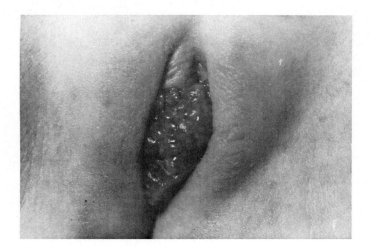

Fig. 9-1. Embryonal rhabdomyosarcoma (sarcoma botryoides) presenting in the vagina.

pleomorphic, which is rarely seen in children but not uncommon in adults, and "mixed," which contains elements of both embryal and alveolar histologic types.

Recently the Intergroup Rhabdomyosarcoma Study has identified new subtypes that arise within or near bone.[3] Special undifferentiated cell type I is a small cell tumor that is found in soft tissue adjacent to bone. The cells have a typical appearance of Ewing's sarcoma, but only soft tissue and not bone is involved. Special undifferentiated cell type II has larger cells that present in soft tissue adjacent to bone and may also be related to Ewing's sarcoma.

To assist in the final diagnosis the pathologist may examine the malignant cells with an electron microscope where cells of striated muscle have a characteristic Z band appearance with thin filaments or striations. Special stains may also help distinguish rhabdomyosarcoma from other small, round cell tumors. Because muscle cells are high in glycogen, this tumor will be periodic acid–Schiff (PAS) positive, whereas neuroblastoma, malignant fibrous histiocytoma, fibrosarcoma, and synovial sarcoma are usually negative.[7]

ETIOLOGY

Grufferman, and others[8] examined environmental factors in a case-control study of childhood rhabdomyosarcoma involving 33 diagnosed cases and 99 controls. They concluded that there were statistically significant correlations among cigarette smoking in fathers (but not mothers), fewer immunizations, children born past their due date, and diets high in organ meats and pork. Li and Fraumeni[9] found a higher incidence of rhabdomyosarcoma in children with a family history of breast carcinoma or other sarcomas.

CLINICAL PRESENTATION

Rhabdomyosarcoma may present in any site, although in both the IRS and the St. Jude Children's Research Hospital experience, the head and neck area accounted for over 30% of all cases (Table 9-1).

The single most common symptom for rhabdomyosarcoma is the presence of a mass. The mass is usually very hard and nontender unless it is causing pressure on surrounding tissue (Fig. 9-2). Other signs and symptoms are related to the site of origin (Table 9-2).

Table 9-1. Sites of presentation

Site	Percentage
Intergroup rhabdomyosarcoma study through 1978 (554 patients)	
Orbit	10
Head and neck	28
Trunk	7
Extremity	18
Genitourinary tract	21
Intrathoracic	3
Perineum/anus	2
Retroperitoneum	7
Gastrointestinal and hepatic	3
Other	1
St. Jude Children's Research Hospital Study 1962-1981 (144 patients)	
Head and neck (including orbit)	31
Trunk (including intrathoracic, and retroperitoneum)	37
Extremity	16
Genitourinary tract	15
Unknown	1

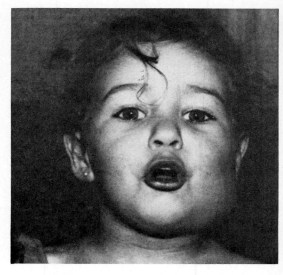

Fig. 9-2. Four-year-old girl with rhabdomyosarcoma of the left cheek. After three courses of doxorubicin (60 mg/m^2) and DTIC (250 mg/m^2 × 5 days) given every 3 weeks, there was no palpable mass by physical examination.

Table 9-2. Relationship between site of origin and symptoms

Site of presentation	Associated symptoms
Head and neck	
Orbit	Pain, swelling, ptosis, visual disturbances, and changes in cranial nerves III, IV, VI
External auditory canal	Earache, ear drainage, hearing loss unilaterally, poor visualization of tympanic membrane with suspected foreign object (tumor)
Surface muscle primary	Swelling, mass not associated with injury, changes in cranial nerves—especially VII, enlarged firm cervical lymph nodes with lymphatic metastasis
Nasopharyngeal	Chronic sinusitis with purulent or clear discharge, chronic unilateral otitis media unresponsive to antibiotics, dizziness, headaches, mastication or feeding difficulty, epistaxis
Central nervous system (CNS)	Thirty-five percent of patients with nasopharyngeal primary rhabdomyosarcoma develop direct meningeal extension within 6 months of diagnosis;[10,11] presenting symptoms may include headaches, vision changes, cranial nerve change, gross motor changes, and presence of malignant cells in spinal fluid; rhabdomyosarcoma cells in the spinal canal may also develop into "drop" metastasis along lower areas of the cord, causing compression with associated paralysis or neurologic symptoms such as "shooting" pain or numbness
Trunk	
Chest wall	Swelling, respiratory distress, pleural inflammation; usually asymptomatic until mass very large
Retroperitoneal, pelvis, perineum	Flank or back pain, renal obstruction, constipation, hematuria (rare), hypertension with hydronephrosis and increased renin secretion
Extremity	Changes in gait, decreased use of limb, enlarged lymph node proximal to lesion, enlarging mass
Genitourinary	
Bladder, urinary tract, prostate	Urinary obstruction, hematuria, dysuria, progressive regression in toilet training, urinary tract infection
Vagina	Vaginal bleeding, vaginal drainage, protruding mass

Rhabdomyosarcoma most commonly metastasizes to lymph nodes, lung, bone, bone marrow, and occasionally the liver. Nasopharyngeal rhabdomyosarcoma has a high rate of parameningeal involvement,[10,11] whereas alveolar rhabdomyosarcoma in adolescent females may metastasize to the breast.[12] When this malignancy disseminates and invades major organs or systems, the prognosis is greatly reduced, with long-term survival less than 20%.[13,14]

DIAGNOSIS AND STAGING

Once rhabdomyosarcoma is confirmed by biopsy or surgical resection the child will need a complete evaluation to determine the extent or stage of disease. Since the most common sites for metastasis include lungs, bone, bone marrow, lymph nodes, central nervous system (CNS), and liver, the evaluation is focused on these areas. Diagnostic workup begins with complete blood counts (CBC) and chemistry profile. These are usually normal unless metastatic disease results in decreased hemoglobin from bone marrow disease, elevated serum calcium from bone disease (less than 10%), or abnormalities not associated with the malignancy.

Radiologic studies include chest x-ray films and/or computerized tomography (CT) scan of the chest to detect metastasis to the lungs, bone scan to evaluate for bone metastasis, liver-spleen scan, and CT scan of the primary site and adjacent areas. An excretory urogram is performed for abdominal or genitourinary tract primary tumors and can be done with the CT scan in most cases. Abdominal and pelvic ultrasound may provide additional information for tumors in these sites, particularly with the clinical presentation of sarcoma botryoides.

Echocardiogram and ECG are usually done as baseline studies to rule out cardiac abnormalities before use of doxorubicin and for comparison with later evaluations.

Special procedures include bone marrow biopsy and/or bone marrow aspirate and lumbar puncture for head and neck primaries.

After all diagnostic studies are completed, the tumor is assigned a "stage" that will determine the type of chemotherapy regimen to be used and whether radiation therapy is indicated. Staging also allows the physician or nurse to give the family and patient an estimate for the overall prognosis. The two most common staging systems are presented as follows:

Intergroup Rhabdomyosarcoma Study I

Group I Localized disease, completely resected

Group II a) Grossly resected localized disease with microscopic residual
  b) Regional disease extending into adjacent organ or lymph nodes resected with no microscopic residual
  c) Regional disease resected with microscopic residual

Group III Regional disease with incomplete resection and gross residual disease

Group IV Metastatic disease to lung, liver, bone, bone marrow, CNS, brain or distant muscle, or lymph nodes

St. Jude Children's Research Hospital Protocol RMS IV, V

Group I Localized disease, completely resected

Group II a) Localized to site of origin, resected with microscopic residual disease
  b) Localized to site of origin, unresected or resected with gross residual disease
  c) Local/regional disease with involvement of contiguous organs or regional lymph nodes

Group III a) Disseminated disease without marrow involvement
  b) Disseminated disease with bone marrow involvement

TREATMENT

The primary treatment of choice for rhabdomyosarcoma is wide local surgical excision (Fig. 9-3). However, radical surgical procedures such as pelvic exenteration or amputation have not been shown to substantially improve prognosis and are generally only performed as "salvage" procedures in patients who have developed tumor relapse.[15-17]

Chemotherapy schedules or dosages may vary depending on the institution, protocol, or stage of the disease. However, vincristine, actinomycin D (Dactinomycin), cyclophosphamide, and doxoru-

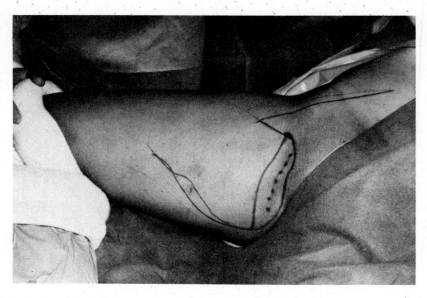

Fig. 9-3. Outline for surgical resection of synovial sarcoma demonstrates the extensive surgical approach used for rarer soft tissue sarcomas.

bicin are commonly used for rhabdomyosarcoma and are usually the most effective agents. More recently, dimethyl-triazeno-imidazole-carboxamide (DTIC)[18-20] has been shown to be very effective against soft tissue sarcomas in general and rhabdomyosarcoma specifically. *cis*-Platinum may have a synergistic effect when used in combination with doxorubicin but appears to have little activity on its own.[21-23] Melphalan (L-PAM)[24] has excellent tumorcidal properties in vivo studies but has not been as successful in phase II studies.

Except for patients with localized disease, radiation therapy is used in all patients with rhabdomyosarcoma. Because of the great variation in sites of presentation, age of the child, and extent of disease, the radiation therapy plan must be specific in each patient. Therefore parent/patient teaching needs to be individualized based on (1) the child's age, (b) dosage of radiation, (c) site to be irradiated and organ systems likely to be affected, and (d) method used to irradiate (linear accelerator, cobalt 60, implantation).

Surgically unresectable gross residual disease may be treated with radiation therapy in two ways.

First, the tumor mass may be irradiated before any attempt at surgical resection in the hope that enough shrinkage will be obtained to allow less radical surgery or a complete surgical resection. Secondly, if surgery is not feasible the tumor may be treated with radiation and chemotherapy in combination.

Microscopic residual disease can be controlled effectively with 3000 to 4000 rad[25-27] if used in combination with chemotherapy. Gross residual disease must be treated with greater than 4000 rad to be effective, greatly increasing the short- and long-term side effects.

PROGNOSIS

With rhabdomyosarcoma most relapses occur within 2 years of diagnosis and during therapy. The relapse rate between 2 and 5 years in patients having completed therapy without evidence of disease is less than 20%. The survival curves generally remain consistent after 5 years, with first relapses rare after this time. Therefore we do not consider a child "cured" until 5 years from diagnosis with no evidence of disease (NED) and no previous relapses.

The single most important prognostic indicator is stage, since it measures the extent to which the disease has spread. In general, children with stage I rhabdomyosarcoma have an 80% chance of cure; stage II, 60% to 70%; stage III, approximately 40%; and stage IV (metastatic disease) less than 20% chance of cure.[5]

Other factors affecting prognosis include (a) the age at diagnosis with children under age five, and especially under age three, having a greater chance for cure; (b) histology,[6] since alveolar rhabdomyosarcoma tends to spread more rapidly and reoccur more frequently; and (c) site of disease,[2,3,5,16] with genitourinary and superficial head and neck lesions having the best prognosis. Overall, the cure rate for rhabdomyosarcoma is approximately 50%.

CASE STUDY

B.A. is a 4-year-old white boy who acutely developed abdominal pain and anuria. He was taken to a local emergency room where the physician noted his bladder was distended and attempted catheterization, which was unsuccessful because of urethral blockage. A urologist was immediately consulted, who ordered a pelvic ultrasound, which demonstrated a solid mass in the area of the prostate. Therefore he was referred to the nearest pediatric oncology center.

Biopsy through a cystoscope revealed embryonal rhabdomyosarcoma of the prostate. Staging studies included a CT scan of the chest, abdomen, and pelvis with an IVP that revealed a 3- by 5-cm mass causing a 90% obstruction of the urethra but no other evidence of disease; a 2-cm left inguinal lymph node was noted. Bone scan, liver-spleen scan, and bone marrow aspiration were also normal. Lumbar puncture was not done, since CNS disease was anticipated only with head and neck primaries or rhabdomyosarcoma of the chest or trunk that invades the spinal cord.

Surgical resection was not felt to be possible without cystectomy, partial bowel resection, and rendering the child impotent. Therefore therapy was initiated with doxorubicin and DTIC, to be given for three courses 3 weeks apart. Evaluation by CT scan then revealed a 60% reduction in tumor size. This was followed by three courses of vincristine, cyclophosphamide, and actinomycin D given at 3-week intervals; these further reduced the mass so that it was undetectable by CT scan.

Radiation therapy by cobalt 60 to 3500 rad then was given to the tumor bed, followed by a 1000-rad boost to the prostate by linear accelerator. Biopsies to determine if further radiation was needed were negative, and the patient was maintained disease free with alternating courses of doxorubicin and DTIC and cyclophosphamide, vincristine, and actinomycin D.

NURSING CONSIDERATIONS

Rhabdomyosarcoma presents a teaching challenge to the nurse and all medical professionals because each case must be approached individually, based on patient age, site of presentation, state of disease, and anticipated behavior of the histologic type.

Families must first be made aware that comparisons between this malignancy and malignancies seen in adults are not valid—neither are comparisons between rhabdomyosarcoma and other sarcomas seen in the pediatric age group including the rarer soft tissue sarcomas.

Further complicating teaching and understanding of the therapy plan for rhabdomyosarcoma is the fact that surgical approaches and radiation therapy ports and doses vary according to the location of the tumor, the extent of disease at the primary site, and the morbidity associated with aggressive approaches with these treatment modalities. Teaching should include explanations that extreme surgical approaches such as amputation have not shown significant changes in overall prognosis whereas radiation therapy must be in higher dose ranges (3500 rad or greater) to be effective.

The one consistency is the chemotherapeutic approach where the only variation may be a shorter duration of therapy for stage I disease. However, the family may have unrealistic, preconceived ideas of toxicity related to chemotherapy, and this should be explored.

When teaching of side effects is initiated for the patient with rhabdomyosarcoma, as in most solid tumors, the difference between relative risks of infections between a patient with a healthy hematopoietic system and the child with leukemia should be emphasized. Because therapy is not aimed at the bone marrow, the ability to recover from chemotherapy-related neutropenia with solid tumors is greater and occurs more rapidly. Therefore prolonged or repeated hospitalizations from therapy are the exception, and the child will usually be able to maintain much of his normal life-style including school, group activities, and in some cases noncontact sports.

Four drugs are considered "standard" therapy and include vincristine, actinomycin D, cyclophosphamide, and doxorubicin. Other agents likely to be included in the treatment protocol include DTIC, melphalan (L-PAM), or *cis*-platinum. Recent trends in both the IRS-III study and St. Jude Children's Research Hospital study are for greater variation of treatment approaches depending on prognostic variables and the addition of newer agents, so six- or seven-drug combinations may not be unusual in the future.

NURSING CARE PROTOCOL FOR THE CHILD WITH RHABDOMYOSARCOMA

Nursing diagnoses (problems/needs)	Goals/objectives (patient/family will:)	Interventions (nurse will:)
1. Knowledge deficit (related to diagnostic workup)	Verbalize purpose of and methods for testing	Assist with and teach regarding workup procedures (PE, laboratory work, scans, ECG, echocardiogram, skin tests, bone marrow) Encourage questions pertaining to workup Give any available teaching resources
2. Anxiety (emotional upset related to diagnosis, testing, possible hospitalization, treatment and side effects)	Have decreased level of anxiety; share feelings with support people	Teach (workup, disease, protocol) Assist with referrals to other services (chaplain, social worker, psychologist) Active listening, use of play, TLC, offer self
3. Knowledge deficit (need for initial surgery biopsy to establish definite diagnosis; need for tumor resection if no evidence of metastatic disease is found)	Verbalize general understanding of surgery Be able to state preoperative and postoperative routines	Assist with explanation of surgery; obtain signature on permits Teach preoperative and postoperative routines (NPO, IV, preoperative medication, safety measures, turn, cough, deep breath, Foley catheter, NG)
4. Injury: potential for (possible postoperative complications) Infection	Have absence of postoperative complications Have clean, dry surgical incision that heals without any complications	Implement preventive measures, identify complication, initiate prompt treatment of complications Keep incision area dry, clean; observe for infection and report; teach how to care for wound and what to report; monitor laboratory work

NURSING CARE PROTOCOL FOR THE CHILD WITH RHABDOMYOSARCOMA—cont'd

Nursing diagnoses (problems/needs)	Goals/objectives (patient/family will:)	Interventions (nurse will:)
Hemorrhage	Have minimum blood loss, stable vital signs	Monitor vital signs; note other signs and symptoms related to shock and pertinent laboratory work (Hgb, Hct); frequent dressing checks; observe for increase in drainage of fresh blood from any drainage tubes
Comfort, alteration in: pain	Verbalize comfort; relaxed facial expression; progressive increase in mobility; decreasing request for pain medication	Comfort measures—positioning, touch, diversion, medication, emotional support
Mobility, impaired physical	Have progressive increased participation in activities of daily living; chest clear, skin intact, bowel sounds present, tolerates PO intake, healing incision	Implement preventive measures, identify complications, initiate prompt treatment of complications
5. Knowledge deficit (related to chemotherapy)	Be able to state name of drug and broad purpose; be able to state how long therapy will be given	Evaluate level of understanding and teach accordingly; have permits and consent forms signed
	Identify expected side effects (early) and proper methods of follow-up; have early side effects within expected limits and control—absence of complications resulting from side effects	Teach, evaluate, document understanding related to drugs; prophylaxis and treatment per nursing and physician orders
6. Knowledge deficit (related to radiation therapy)	Be able to state broad purpose of therapy; identify expected side effects and follow-up appropriately; recognize postradiation syndromes	Teach, evaluate, and document

Continued.

NURSING CARE PROTOCOL FOR THE CHILD WITH RHABDOMYOSARCOMA—cont'd

Nursing diagnoses (problems/needs)	Goals/objectives (patient/family will:)	Interventions (nurse will:)
	Have side effects within expected limits and control; absence of complications resulting from side effects	Prophylaxis and treatment per nursing and medical orders related to N & V, constipation, anorexia, stomatitis, skin breakdown
	Have minimum late side effects; compliance with follow-up	Teach importance of follow-up; observe for late effects—sterility, liver damage
7. Nutrition, alteration in: less than body requirements	Relief from nausea and vomiting (N & V); weight stable; PO intake return to usual amount	Obtain order for antiemetics Arrange consultation with dietician Offer small, frequent appetizing meals Mouth care before all meals High-protein, high-carbohydrate diet; well balanced meals Monitor I & O carefully Eliminate unpleasant sights and smells Obtain order for topical mouth wash anesthetic Encourage fluids
8. Injury: potential for (recurrence and/or metastasis; potential for treatment failure)	Identify signs and symptoms of recurrences—tissue mass; identify signs of treatment failure—progression of primary disease, obvious increase in muscle tumor mass; notify health team	Teach, evaluate, document
	Verbalize understanding and individualized treatment	Teach, evaluate, and document (see protocol)
	Obtain remission or comfort during terminal phase	Nursing care specific to patient
9. Coping, ineffective family: compromised	Be able to cope with adjustments needed and return to maximum functioning	Provide emotional support and teaching; referral as needed
	Maintain positive self-concept, return to activities of daily living	Follow-up as needed

REFERENCES

1. Sutow, W.W.: General aspects of childhood cancer. In Sutow, W.W., Fernbach, D.J., and Vietti, T.J., editors: Clinical pediatric oncology, St. Louis, 1973, The C.V. Mosby Co.
2. Pratt, C., and others: Protocol III for the treatment of childhood rhabdomyosarcoma and other soft tissue sarcomas with surgery, chemotherapy, and radiotherapy, Memphis, 1977, St. Jude Children's Research Hospital.
3. Maurer, H.M., and others: The Intergroup Rhabdomyosarcoma Study: a preliminary report, Cancer **40:**2015, 1977.
4. Sutow, W.W.: Rhabdomyosarcoma. In Sutow, W.W.: Malignant solid tumors in children: a review, New York, 1981, Raven Press.
5. Etcubanas, E., and others: Protocol IV for the treatment of childhood rhabdomyosarcoma, Memphis, 1981, St. Jude Children's Research Hospital.
6. Hays, D., and others: Mortality among children with rhabdomyosarcomas of the alveolar histologic subtypes, J. Pediatr. Surg. **18:**412, 1983.
7. Enzinger, F.M., and Weiss, S.W.: General considerations. In Enzinger, F.M., and Weiss, S.W.: Soft tissue tumors, St. Louis, 1983, The C.V. Mosby Co.
8. Grufferman, S., and others: Environmental factors in the etiology of rhabdomyosarcoma in childhood, J. Natl. Cancer Inst. **68**(1):107, 1982.
9. Li, F.P., and Fraumeni, J.F.: Soft tissue sarcomas, breast cancer, and other neoplasms: a familial syndrome, Ann. Intern. Med. **71:**747, 1969.
10. Tefft, M., and others: Incidence of meningeal involvement by rhabdomyosarcoma of the head and neck in children, Cancer **42:**253, 1978.
11. Berry, M.P., and Jenkin, R.D.T.: Parameningeal rhabdomyosarcoma in the young, Cancer **48:**281, 1981.
12. Howarth, C.B., Caces, J.N., and Pratt, C.B.: Breast metastases in children with rhabdomyosarcoma, Cancer **46:**2520, 1980.
13. Lawrence, W., and others: Lymphatic metastasis with childhood rhabdomyosarcoma, Cancer **39:**556, 1977.
14. Ruymann, F.B., and others: Bone marrow metastasis at diagnosis in childhood rhabdomyosarcoma, Proc. Am. Assoc. Cancer Res. **20:**194, 1979.
15. Fleming, I.D., and others: The role of surgical resection when combined with chemotherapy and radiation in the management of pelvic rhabdomyosarcoma, Ann. Surg. **199:** 509, 1984.
16. Hays, D.M., and others: Extremity lesions in the Intergroup Rhabdomyosarcoma Study (IRS-I), Cancer **48:**1, 1982.
17. Kumar, A.P.M., and others: Combined therapy to prevent complete pelvic exenteration for rhabdomyosarcoma of the vagina or uterus, Cancer **37:**118, 1976.
18. Cangir, A., and others: Combination chemotherapy with Adriamycin and dimethyl triazeno imidazole carboxamide in children with metastatic solid tumors, Med. Ped. Oncol. **2:**183, 1976.
19. Saiki, J.H., and others: Adriamycin and single dose DTIC in soft tissue and bone sarcomas: a Southwest Oncology Group study (abstract C-703), Proc. Am. Soc. Clin. Oncol. **1:**181, 1982.
20. Gottlieb, J., and Benjamin, R.: Role of DTIC in the chemotherapy of sarcomas, Cancer Treat. Rep. **60:**199, 1976.
21. Pratt, C., and others: Pharmacokinetic evaluation of Cisplatin in children with malignant solid tumors: a phase II study, Cancer Treat. Rep. **65:**1021, 1981.
22. Pratt, C., and Crom, B.: Cisplatin and doxorubicin for locally recurrent and metastatic childhood rhabdomyosarcoma, Chemotherapy **11:**18, 1984.
23. Brenner, J., and others: Phase II trial of cisplatin in previously treated patients with advanced soft tissue sarcomas, Cancer **50:**2031, 1982.
24. Houghton, J., and others: L-phenylalanine mustard: a potential new agent in the treatment of childhood rhabdomyosarcoma, Cancer Treat. Rep. (in press).
25. Tefft, M., Lindberg, R., and Gehan, E.: Radiation of rhabdomyosarcoma in children combined with systemic chemotherapy: local control in patients enrolled into the Intergroup Study, Int. J. Radiat. Oncol. Biol. Phys. **4** (suppl.):82, 1978.
26. Tefft, M., and others: Pelvic rhabdomyosarcoma in children: is radiotherapy necessary to regional nodes? Int. J. Radiat. Oncol. Biol. Phys. **5**(suppl.):43, 1979.
27. Jereb, B., and others: Local control of embryonal rhabdomyosarcoma in children by radiation therapy when combined with chemotherapy, Int. J. Radiat. Oncol. Biol. Phys. **5**(suppl.):44, 1979.

CHAPTER 10

Retinoblastoma

PAT STANFILL and CHARLES PRATT

DEFINITION

Retinoblastoma is a rare, congenital tumor of the eye found only in children. The tumor may be unilateral with several areas of tumor foci in the same eye or bilateral. There are two presentations of retinoblastoma, the endophytic form and the exophytic form. When the tumor spontaneously arises from the retina and develops anteriorly into the vitreous humor, the configuration produced is referred to as endophytic. The mass is nodular with a white or light pink color and a well-vascularized surface.[1,2] In the exophytic form the tumor invades the subretinal space, causing retinal detachment but no ophthalmoscopically visible nodule in the vitreous cavity.[1,2] Local extension of the tumor may occur along the optic nerve leading to the subarachnoid space or may invade the orbital cavity.[1] Metastases may be found in the lymph nodes after invasion of the orbit or in the bone because of hematogenous dissemination. Invasion of the meninges can occur, resulting in retinoblastic meningitis.[1]

The tumor is most often composed of small, round, undifferentiated cells with hyperchromatic nuclei and scant cytoplasm.[2] Necrosis is often evident and may cause an inflammatory response. Spontaneous regression of tumor, if tumor necrosis progresses, has been reported.[2] The treatment of retinoblastoma in an interdisciplinary (multimodal) fashion has improved function and survival rates in children.[3]

INCIDENCE AND ETIOLOGY

Retinoblastoma accounts for approximately 1% to 3% of all childhood malignancies, occurring at the rate of 1/20,000 to 30,000 live births.[3,4] There are 300 cases reported annually in the United States. The mean age at diagnosis is 18 months, and rarely are the tumors seen after the age of eight. Bilateral retinoblastomas usually present at a younger age than do unilateral tumors. There is no sexual or racial preponderance. Retinoblastoma is responsible for almost 5% of childhood blindness.[4]

Retinoblastoma may be transmitted from generation to generation with the gene being transmitted by the parent or acquired as the result of mutation.[5,6] The transmitted gene may be for unilateral or bilateral disease. About 30% of the tumors are bilateral, which is thought to represent the congenital form of retinoblastoma.[7] Bilateral tumors are considered to be dominantly inherited and should be counted as hereditary, since almost 50% of children of patients with bilateral disease develop retinoblastoma.[7] Not all people who inherit the gene for retinoblastoma develop the disease, but they may transmit the gene to their offspring.

The D-deletion syndrome involving chromosome 13, a chromosome abnormality characterized by eczema, microcephaly, malformed ears, cleft palate, and mental deficiency is associated with retinoblastoma.[8] Retinoblastoma has also been observed in monozygotic twins.[1] Strong and others,[9] in a series of 95 patients at M. D. Anderson Hos-

152

pital and Tumor Institute, found that relatives of retinoblastoma patients are at an increased risk to develop cancer.

CLINICAL PRESENTATION

Two classic signs of retinoblastoma, often noticed first by the parents, are the cat's-eye reflex and strabismus. The cat's-eye reflex is characteristically described as a white light noticed in the pupil that is glimpsed only with certain angles or lighting. The cat's-eye reflex is caused by the alignment of the anterior pole of the tumor with the dilated pupil.[1] The eye is blind. Strabismus may be the only clue to blindness in the infant. All squints in infancy deserve an ophthalmoscopic examination to rule out tumor. As the tumor increases in size, the eye may take on a red, inflamed appearance. Conjunctivitis and glaucoma may develop.[1]

Other presenting symptoms that may lead to the need for a differential diagnosis include pseudoglioma, inflammatory disease, glaucoma, and/or detached retina.[1,2] Failure to respond to conservative treatment generally leads to further evaluation and finally to a correct diagnosis.

The remainder of the child's physical examination is usually normal, although poor vision, a strange facial expression, and/or anorexia or failure to thrive have also been seen as presenting signs of retinoblastoma.[2]

DIAGNOSTIC EVALUATION AND STAGING

The diagnostic evaluation of retinoblastoma includes computed tomography (CT) scans, echograms, and an examination of the optic fundus under general anesthesia. Scans define the volume, site, and density of the tumor, whereas examination of the optic fundus allows visualization of the whole retina in both eyes to determine extent of the tumor and observe for other tumor foci. Ophthalmologic evaluation may include fluorescein angiography and isoenzyme determinations of the aqueous humor.[10] All patients should be examined for metastatic disease with a bone marrow aspirate,

skeletal survey, and lumbar puncture.

A classic grouping of retinoblastoma for treatment is defined by Reese and Ellsworth[10]:

Group I: Very favorable prognosis
A. Solitary tumor, less than 4 disc diameters (dd)* in size, at or behind the equator
B. Multiple tumors, none over 4 dd in size, all at or behind the equator

Group II: Favorable prognosis
A. Solitary lesion 4 to 10 dd in size, at or behind the equator
B. Multiple tumors 4 to 10 dd in size, behind the equator

Group III: Doubtful prognosis
A. Any lesion anterior to the equator
B. Solitary tumors larger than 10 dd behind the equator

Group IV: Unfavorable prognosis
A. Multiple tumors, some larger than 10 dd
B. Any lesion extending anteriorly to the ora serrata

Group V: Very unfavorable prognosis
A. Massive tumors involving over half the retina
B. Vitreous seeding

Unfortunately, more than 85% of unilateral tumors and more than 90% of bilateral retinoblastomas are in the least favorable group at the time of diagnosis. Howarth and others[11] devised a staging system based on histologic and ophthalmologic criteria to better define differences in prognosis:

Stage I: Tumor (unifocal or multifocal) confined to retina
A. Occupying 1 quadrant or less
B. Occupying 2 quadrants or less
C. Occupying more than 50% of retinal surface

Stage II: Tumor (unifocal or multifocal) confined to globe
A. With vitreous seeding
B. Extending to optic nerve head
C. Extending to choroid
D. Extending to choroid and optic nerve head
E. Extending to emissaries

---

*One disc diameter = 1.6 mm.

Stage III: Extraocular extension of tumor (regional)
    A. Extending beyond cut end of optic nerve (including subarachnoid extension)
    B. Extending through sclera into orbital contents
    C. Extending to choroid and beyond cut end of optic nerve (including subarachnoid extension)
    D. Extending through sclera into orbital contents and beyond cut end of optic nerve (including subarachnoid extension)
Stage IV: Distant metastases
    A. Extending through optic nerve to brain
    B. Blood-borne metastases to soft tissues and bone
    C. Bone marrow metastases

PROGNOSTIC FACTORS

Stage is the single most important prognostic indicator in retinoblastoma. The higher the stage, the poorer the prognosis. Vitreous seeding, tumor invasion of the choroid and emissary vessels, optic nerve involvement, and extraocular extension to the orbit and subarachnoid impact negatively on survival.[11] Redler[12] correlated an increased mortality with the extent of choroidal involvement.

The overall survival rate of retinoblastoma is 80% to 90%, up from less than 25% at the beginning of the century.[3,11] Almost all patients in stage I are assured of cure, and approximately 85% with stage II disease survive. Only 9% of children with macroscopic disease will survive, and metastatic disease is uniformly fatal.[3] If relapse occurs, retreatment is rarely successful.

TREATMENT

The treatment of retinoblastoma is based on the extent of the disease or stage[6]:

Stage I
    A,B. Cryotherapy, photocoagulation, or radiotherapy and systemic chemotherapy for 1 year*

C. Enucleation (unilateral tumor) or radiotherapy and systemic chemotherapy for 1 year
Stage II
    A. Enucleation (unilateral tumor) or radiotherapy and systemic chemotherapy for 1 year
    B. Enucleation only
    C,D,E. Enucleation and systemic chemotherapy for 1 year
Stage III
    A,C. Enucleation and radiation to cranium, intrathecal chemotherapy,* and systemic chemotherapy for 1 year
    B. Enucleation or exenteration, radiation to orbit, and systemic chemotherapy for 1 year
    D. Enucleation or exenteration, radiation to orbit and cranium, intrathecal chemotherapy, and systemic chemotherapy for 1 year
Stage IV
    A. Treatment as for IIIA and C
    B,C. Enucleation, systemic chemotherapy for 1 year, and radiotherapy for painful or disfiguring masses

The goal of therapy is to eradicate the tumor and preserve vision without compromising survival.[3] The therapy for retinoblastoma is an excellent example of an interdisciplinary approach with surgery, radiation therapy, chemotherapy, and local nonradiologic procedures.

Each tumor must be carefully evaluated on an individual basis by an ophthalmologist to determine if conservative treatment such as irradiation, cryotherapy, or light coagulation is indicated or if enucleation of the eye is necessary.[10] Systemic chemotherapy is indicated in all patients judged at risk for micrometastases. Agents of choice are vincristine and cyclophosphamide. Tumor extension into the central nervous system is treated with intrathecal methotrexate and cranial irradiation at a dose of 2500 rad.[10]

Enucleation with removal of the longest possible segment of the optic nerve offers the best chance for local control.[3] It is the treatment of choice for patients whose vision cannot be preserved. Removal of the optic nerve segment minimizes access

---

*Vincristine: 1.5 mg/m^2 IV weekly for 6 doses, then 1 mg/m^2 IV weekly to 1 year. Cyclophosphamide: 300 mg/m^2 IV weekly for 6 doses, then 200 mg/m^2 IV weekly to 1 year.

---

*Methotrexate: 12 mg/m^2 IT weekly for 6 doses.

to the meninges and central nervous system by tumor cells.

The most important advance in the use of irradiation to treat retinoblastoma came with the development of techniques and megavoltage beams with small focal spot size (linear accelerator or betatron). These allow treatment of the retina without direct irradiation of the lens.[3] If the lens is irradiated, cataract formation is almost certain.

Retinoblastoma, stage I, may be managed with local treatment of only a portion of the retina. Radioactive applicators, cryotherapy, and light coagulation are useful in early, local disease management.[11-13] Cryotherapy also may assume a role in the management of recurrent disease. Cryotherapy involves freezing and thawing the retinal tumors through an external probe. Because this therapy allows maintenance of useful vision, greater use of cryotherapy is predicted. Light coagulation is a laser treatment that destroys the vascular supply of a tumor.

Genetic counseling is considered part of the treatment plan for retinoblastoma. Patients with bilateral tumors should be followed for life, since they are at risk for second malignancies.[3,14] Nonradiation-induced neoplasms, osteosarcoma, fibrosarcoma, and skin cancers in irradiated patients and a risk for leukemia are possible.[15] Because of the hereditary nature of retinoblastoma, counseling of the patient and family should also be a priority. Siblings of patients with retinoblastoma should be examined for 5 years. As the number of survivors increases, the incidence of bilateral retinoblastoma will increase.

CASE STUDY

B.J., a 15-month-old white female, had been in good health until February 1971 when her parents noted a deviation of the right eye medially with failure to follow consensual movements. An ophthamologic examination of the globes revealed a mass filling the posterior chamber of the right eye. On arrival at the treatment center, a careful history and physical examination was done. The family history for retinoblastoma was negative, and there was one instance of cancer in a distant relative. The physical examination was essentially normal except for esotropia involving the right eye, within which a

large gray-white mass could be seen, and several gray-white areas were seen on fundoscopic examination of the left eye.

B.J was examined by an ophthalmologist and carefully evaluated. Enucleation of the right eye was done. The tumor involving the right globe was described as filling 75% to 80% of the vitreous. The choroid and optic nerve were found not to be involved. One hundred percent of the retinal surface was involved. Examination of the left globe revealed an endophytic type retinoblastoma in two areas with a small superior nasal lesion. A larger lesion in the inferior temporal quadrant was present with vitreous seeding.

Radiotherapy was directed to the right globe through a single anterior port. Chemotherapy consisting of vincristine and cyclophosphamide was administered.

B.J. is currently a 15-year-old adolescent with a right eye prosthesis and useful vision in her left eye. Her course was complicated by a radiation cataract that was surgically removed in 1974. Since that time she has done well.

NURSING CONSIDERATIONS

The impact of the malignant disease process and the potential risk for loss of vision may be overwhelming for the patient and family experiencing retinoblastoma.[16] Parents may have anger, fear, anxiety, guilt and depression that must be considered in any plan of care. Depending on the age of the child at diagnosis, personal fears or a sense of the parent's fears must be considered.

Once the diagnosis of retinoblastoma is made, the treatment plan is presented to the family. When the plan includes enucleation, obtaining parental consent is often traumatic. Recognizing the importance of vision, parents may fear the future impact on the child's growth and development, the disfigurement resulting from the surgical procedure, and the emotional state of the child as he grows to adulthood. Parents must be given information about the disease, course of treatment, prognosis, and potential complications, so an informed decision can be made. Seeing a prosthesis or perhaps meeting another child with an artificial eye may help to allay anxiety.

Preoperatively, depending on the child's age, therapeutic play may be used to communicate facts about the surgery and resultant loss of vision. Remembering that the goal of therapy is to prevent loss of useful vision if possible, the child and family must have a clear idea of what the treatment plan entails. The child may want to see a prosthesis if possible and may want to have the eye bandaged before surgery so that he can experience the postoperative feeling. Bandaging a doll may also help.

Postoperative care requires close observation for hemorrhage, edema, and evidence of infection. A clear plastic sphere or conformer is placed in the orbit so parental fears of an empty socket are unfounded. The permanent prosthesis is generally fitted 5 to 6 weeks after the enucleation. Normal activity levels may be resumed 1 to 2 days postoperatively.

If bilateral retinoblastoma requires intervention that renders the patient sightless, the situation is even more traumatic. Professional counseling to include resources about schools for the blind should be considered. Emphasizing the potential for cure of a malignant process without giving false hope or misinformation is encouraged. The potential for a long and healthy life even if sightless may be explored with the family.

Genetic counseling or information must be provided. Since almost 90% of patients with retinoblastoma are cured, the potential for living into adulthood and reproduction is increased. Patients should be told of the potential for transmitting the disease to their offspring. Patients surviving retinoblastoma should be informed that in familial and bilateral retinoblastoma, 45% of their offspring will develop the tumor.[15] Careful monitoring of siblings and offspring throughout the years is encouraged.

NURSING CARE PROTOCOL FOR THE CHILD WITH RETINOBLASTOMA

Nursing diagnoses (problems/needs)	Goals/objectives (patient/family will:)	Interventions (nurse will:)
1. Knowledge deficit (lack of understanding of diagnostic workup)	Verbalize purpose of and methods for tests	Assist with and teach regarding procedures (history and physical examination, fundoscopic examination, x-ray of involved bones, ultrasonography, bone marrow aspiration, laboratory work, lumbar puncture, urinalysis, appropriate photographs, fluorescein angiography, CT of skull, orbits) Encourage questions pertaining to workup Give any available teaching resources
2. Anxiety (emotional upset related to diagnosis, testing, possible hospitalization, treatment and side effects, body image alterations, blindness)	Have decreased level of anxiety Share feelings with support people	Teach (workup, disease, protocol) Assist with referrals to other services (chaplain, social worker, counselor, occupational therapist) Use active listening, offer self Use therapeutic play

NURSING CARE PROTOCOL FOR THE CHILD WITH RETINOBLASTOMA—cont'd

Nursing diagnoses (problems/needs)	Goals/objectives (patient/family will:)	Interventions (nurse will:)
3. Knowledge deficit (need for presurgical preparation)	Verbalize general understanding of surgery/treatment	Assist with explanation of the surgery/treatment; obtain signature on permit according to hospital procedure
	Be able to state preoperative and postoperative treatment routines	Teach preoperative and postoperative treatment routine (i.e., NPO, IV, preoperative medication, safety measures, turn, cough, deep breath, Foley catheter, NG)
4. Injury: potential for (surgical complications)	Have absence of postoperative complications	Implement preventive measures, identify complications, initiate prompt treatment for complications
Cryosurgery Stain at surgical site	Absence of hemorrhage or stain at surgical site	Instruct patient (and family) to avoid swimming, lifting heavy objects, bending, stooping, jogging, and other strenuous activity; teach to return in 1 month for postoperative checkup; encourage family to resume usual activities if checkup shows no problems
Potential blindness	Have minimum limitation of sight Adapt to level of sight loss	Provide emotional support to patient and family; refer as needed for adaptation (i.e., counseling, occupational therapy)
Enucleation Self-concept, disturbance in: body image	Maintain positive body image, adapting to changes in appearance	Prepare parents and patient (as appropriate for age) for child's appearance postoperatively Teach regarding care of prosthesis and refer for follow-up as needed
Infection	Will not exhibit signs of infection as demonstrated by a clean, healing surgical site	Keep clean eye patch in place; instruct parents to change patch daily or more frequently if needed; contact physician if elevated temperature or eye drainage occurs
Potential blindness	Adaptation to level of sight loss	Provide emotional support to patient and family; refer as needed for adaptation to sight loss

Continued.

NURSING CARE PROTOCOL FOR THE CHILD WITH RETINOBLASTOMA—cont'd

Nursing diagnoses (problems/needs)	Goals/objectives (patient/family will:)	Interventions (nurse will:)
5. Knowledge deficit (needs related to chemotherapy)	Be able to state name of drug and broad purpose; be able to verbalize how long therapy will be given	Evaluate level of understanding and teach accordingly; have permits and consent forms signed; interventions depend on unilaterality or bilaterality of disease, whether one or both eyes enucleated
	Identify expected side effects and early and proper methods of follow-up; have early side effects within expected limits and control	Teach, evaluate, and document related to drugs; prophylaxis and treatment per nursing and physician orders related to specific chemotherapeutic agents (see Chapter 20)
6. Knowledge deficit (needs related to radiation therapy)	Be able to state broad purpose of therapy; identify expected side effects of radiation and follow-up appropriately; recognize postradiation syndromes	Teach, evaluate, and document
	Have side effects within expected limits and control; absence of complications resulting from side effects	Initiate prophylaxis and treatment per nursing and physician orders related to radiation dermatitis and/mucositis, bone marrow aplasia or hypoplasia at site of radiation, radiation cataract, retinopathy, alopecia, phthisis bulbi
	Have minimum late side effects; compliance with follow-up	Teach importance of follow-up; observe for late effects (see above)
7. Injury: potential for (recurrence and/or metastasis)	Identify signs of metastasis and notify health team Verbalize understanding of individualized treatment	Teach, evaluate, and document; be alert for evidence of conversion to second malignancies
8. Coping, ineffective family: compromised	Be able to cope with adjustments needed and return to maximum functioning	Provide emotional support and teaching and referral as needed
9. Knowledge deficit (need for genetic counseling for patient and family)	Verbalize understanding of genetic implications	Teach and refer as necessary regarding role of genetics in this disease; emotional support for any guilt expressed by parents

REFERENCES

1. Sweisguth, O.: Solid tumors in children. New York, 1982, John Wiley & Sons, Inc.
2. Nicholson, D.H., and Green, W.R.: Tumors of the eye, lids and orbit in children. In Harley, R.D., editor: Pediatric ophthalmology, Philadelphia, 1975, W.B. Saunders Co.
3. Cassady, J.R.: Retinoblastoma: questions in management. In Carter, S.K., editor: Principles of cancer treatment, New York, 1982, McGraw-Hill, Inc.
4. Howard, R.O., and others: Retinoblastoma and chromosome abnormality, Arch. Ophthalmol. **92:**490, 1974.
5. Knudson, A.G., Hethcote, N.W., and Brown, B.W.: Mutation and childhood cancer: a probalistic model for the incidence of retinoblastoma, Proc. Natl. Acad. Sci. USA **72:**5116, 1975.
6. Vogel, F.: Genetics of retinoblastoma, Genetics **52:**1, 1979.
7. Pratt, C.B.: Retinoblastoma. In Kelley, V.C.: Practice of pediatrics, Philadelphia, 1985, Harper & Row, Publishers, Inc.
8. Knudson, A.G., Jr. and others: Chromosomal deletion and retinoblastoma, N. Engl. J. Med. **295:**1120, 1976.
9. Strong, L.C., and others: Cancer mortality in relatives of retinoblastoma patients, J. Natl. Cancer Inst. **73**(2):303, 1984.
10. Reese, A.B., and Ellsworth, R.N.: The evaluation and-current concept of retinoblastoma therapy, Trans. Am. Acad. Opthalmol. Otolaryngol. **67:**164, 1963.
11. Howarth, C., and others: Stage-related combined modality treatment of retinoblastoma, Cancer **45**(5):851, 1980.
12. Redler, L.D., and Ellsworth, R.M.: Prognostic importance of choroidal invasion in retinoblastoma, Arch. Ophthalmol. **90:**294, 1973.
13. Sheilds, J.A., and Augsburger, J.J.: Current approaches to the diagnosis and management of retinoblastoma, Surv. Ophthalmol. **25:**347, 1981.
14. Ellsworth, R.M.: Tumors of the eye. In Holland, J.F., and Frei, E., editors: Cancer medicine, ed. 2, Philadelphia, 1982, Lea & Febiger.
15. Meadows, A.T., and others: Bone sarcoma as a second malignant neoplasm in children: influence of radiation on genetic predisposition, Cancer **46:**2603, 1980.
16. Crom, D.B., Pratt, C.B.: Care of retinoblastoma patients and their families, J. Ophthalmic Nurs. Technol. **1**(2):16, 1982.

CHAPTER 11

Rare tumors of childhood

RALPH VOGEL

Most rare tumors of childhood are soft tissue sarcomas other than rhabdomyosarcoma. Rare tumors individually account for less than 1% of all childhood malignancies. Statistically valid numbers of children treated for these tumors and results of therapy are not available, and therefore they either are not treated by established protocols or are treated by protocols for rhabdomyosarcoma. Of the rare soft tissue sarcomas, synovial sarcoma and fibrosarcoma appear to be the most common. Malignant schwannoma (neurofibrosarcoma), leiomyosarcoma, liposarcoma, and malignant fibrous histiocytoma are occasionally reported. Hepatomas, including hepatoblastoma and hepatocarcinoma, comprise the single most common rare tumors of childhood confined to a single organ or site and account for 1% to 2% of childhood malignancies.

FIBROSARCOMA

Fibrosarcoma is a malignancy of fibrous tissue that is graded based on degree of differentiation as follows[1]:

Grade 1: Well differentiated
Grade 2: Moderately well differentiated
Grade 3: Moderately poorly differentiated
Grade 4: Poorly differentiated

This tumor most commonly presents in the extremities although it may also arise in the trunk or head and neck area.[2] The lower extremities are more frequently involved than the upper extremities.[3]

Soule and Pritchard[4] reviewed 110 cases of fibrosarcoma and found 36% were diagnosed at birth and 62% presented before age five. However, Exebby and others[5] in a small series of 22 found 80% were older than 6 years, and none of their cases were congenital with the youngest being 18 months of age. Their data may be skewed by the fact that only four of their cases were originally diagnosed at their institution and the remaining 18 were referred.

This malignancy has been associated with previous treatment with ionizing radiation and as a second malignancy with retinoblastoma.[6-8] It has also been reported as a second malignancy in several adult tumors and in five of 24 patients treated for Hodgkin's disease who developed a sarcoma of bone or soft tissue.[9]

The treatment of choice is wide surgical excision, since local control of the tumor affords the best prognosis. Fibrosarcoma tends to recur locally, usually within 2 years, with an average length of time after surgery being 8 months.[2] Metastases are uncommon but most frequently involve the lungs or bone.[3,10,11]

Radiation therapy may be effective in doses over 6000 rad; however, the sequelae of high-dose irradiation in a child often makes this mode of treatment unfeasible. Fibrosarcoma responds to vincristine, cyclophosphamide, actinomycin D, doxorubicin, and DTIC and in most institutions is treated with chemotherapy regimens similar to those for rhabdomyosarcoma.[10,12]

Prognosis is difficult to predict although the grade of the fibrosarcoma is considered to be an important factor. Grades 1 and 2 are less aggressive and therefore have a significantly better prognosis than grade 3 or 4. With adequate surgical procedures grades 1 and 2 have an overall 70% survival rate at 5 and 10 years whereas grades 3 and 4 have 40% and 30%.[1]

SYNOVIAL SARCOMA

Histologically, this malignancy has characteristics of synovial tissue; however, it is almost never found in the joint capsules or areas where synovial cells are commonly found. Synovial sarcoma most frequently presents in the extremities and is the most common malignancy of the hand or foot in children.[13,14]

The second and third decade of life are the peak age groups, but 40% of the cases occur between age 10 and 19.[14,15] Pain and inflammation have been reported as early symptoms in this malignancy as opposed to the usual presentation of a painless swelling or mass commonly seen with other soft tissue sarcomas.[16]

Local recurrence may develop several years after initial diagnosis. Synovial sarcoma may also metastasize with 80% of metastatic lesions involving the lungs, 23% involving regional lymph nodes, and 20% involving bone.[13]

Aggressive surgery including amputation is the treatment of choice. Wide local excision may be successful; however, the response of this tumor to either radiation therapy or chemotherapy has not been documented, and microscopic residual disease may lead to recurrence. Chemotherapy usually consists of combinations similar to those used in other soft tissue sarcomas including vincristine, cyclophosphamide, actinomycin D, doxorubicin, and DTIC. Radiation therapy may be effective in higher dose ranges (greater than 5000 rads); however, extremity lesions may lead to soft tissue fibrosis, reducing function and mobility of the limb, or pathologic stress fractures from bone damage secondary to irradiation.

MALIGNANT SCHWANNOMA (NEUROFIBROSARCOMA)

Malignant schwannoma, also known as neurofibrosarcoma, accounted for 3% of all soft tissue sarcomas in the third National Cancer Survey.[17] It involves the peripheral nerves or develops from neurofibroma. The exact diagnostic criteria for this tumor remains vague and makes statistical comparisons difficult.[18]

There is no reported age preference in the pediatric population although this malignancy is probably more common in the older child. Clinically, the most important feature is this malignancy's strong association with neurofibromatosis (von Recklinghausen's disease).[19-21] From 3% to 13% of persons with neurofibromatosis will develop malignant schwannoma, usually after a long latent period of greater than 10 years.[18] It has also been reported that as high as two thirds of the patients with malignant schwannoma will also have signs of neurofibromatosis.[19]

Malignant schwannoma is an aggressive tumor that can have either local recurrence or metastatic spread, usually to the lungs.[19-21] Wide local excision or amputation can significantly improve the prognosis, especially since the sensitivity of this tumor to either radiation or chemotherapy has not been established.

Following surgical resection residual disease is usually treated with radiation and/or chemotherapy with the treatment plan being similar to protocols for rhabdomyosarcoma. When complete surgical excision is possible, the 5-year survival rate is 60%.[20,21] The prognosis appears to be significantly less, approximately 30%, in patients where the malignancy is associated with neurofibromatosis.[21]

LEIOMYOSARCOMA

Leiomyosarcoma is a malignancy of smooth muscle that may arise in the gastrointestinal tract, genitourinary tract, respiratory tract or from smooth muscle found in blood vessels throughout the body. It may be difficult to distinguish from leiomyomas, and the diagnosis of malignancy is based on the number of mitotic figures present in a high-power field (HPF), with less than five favoring a more benign lesion. However, Enzinger and Weiss[18] caution that tumors with less than five mitotic figures may eventually metastasize, especially if they are large and have areas of necrosis. In one series, 39% of leiomyosarcomas had a mitotic count below five on HPF, and in the small intestine leiomyosarcomas, 65% (13/20) were below five.[22]

Symptoms are related to the site of origin with abdominal primaries of the gastrointestinal tract or retroperitoneum causing swelling, pain, bowel obstruction, hematemesis and anemia in 88% of patients in one series.[23]

Leiomyosarcoma arising in the genitourinary tract may cause urinary retention, urinary frequency, hematuria, vaginal bleeding, and pain. The mass can sometimes be palpated by rectal examination if in the area of the prostate; however, caution should be taken not to induce tumor rupture and bleeding.

Respiratory lesions may be asymptomatic or may mimic other childhood respiratory diseases with cough, wheezing, and shortness of breath. Chest pain and hemoptysis may also be present.

Leiomyosarcoma arising from blood vessels in peripheral soft tissue usually presents as a mass that may or may not have associated pain.

Treatment of leiomyosarcoma should include wide surgical excision in an attempt to remove all tumor. If the HPF mitotic count is below five, further therapy may not be necessary although the patient should be closely followed for recurrence that may develop several years after initial surgery.

If the mitotic count is above five per HPF or if surgical resection is not possible, the child should receive further therapy. The value of radiation therapy is questionable although recent reports indicate it can be effective in controlling microscopic residual disease, especially presenting in the uterus.[24,25] However, since uterine primaries have not been seen in the pediatric age group, this malignancy is still generally felt to be radioresistant in children.

Good responses have been seen with the agents normally used for other soft tissue sarcomas including vincristine, cyclophosphamide, actinomycin D, doxorubicin, and DTIC.[26]

Metastasis of abdominal primaries to the regional lymph nodes and the liver is common. Leiomyosarcoma has also been reported to metastasize to the lung.[27] Prognosis is guarded even with complete surgical excision of the tumor because of the tendency for low-grade leiomyosarcomas to develop late relapses. With slower growing tumors, repeated surgeries may be adequate for disease control, and this malignancy may become a chronic illness while maintaining the risk for distant metastasis.

LIPOSARCOMA

Liposarcoma is the most common soft tissue sarcoma in adults but is rare in the pediatric age group and extremely rare in the young child or infant. Most cases in children present between the age of 10 and 15 years and are derived from primitive mesenchymal cells.

Enzinger classified liposarcomas under five histologic categories: well differentiated, myxoid, round cell type, pleomorphic, and mixed. These classifications are considered important prognostic indicators, with more mature (well-differentiated) types having a significantly better prognosis than immature classes such as round cell type or pleomorphic. Shmookler found 13 of 17 cases of liposarcoma in children to be of the myxoid classification, whereas Evans found well differentiated to be more common. Both are considered to have good prognosis.[28]

Liposarcoma arises from adipose tissue and therefore can present in any area of the body. However, the thigh (29.6%) and knee (11.8%) were the most common sites in Shmookler's experience, and this is consistent with other reports.[29,30] Both a male and female predominance have been reported.[28,31]

Some of the confusion about the clinical patterns of this malignancy may arise from statistical inferences being drawn from reports based on the experience with adults with liposarcoma. In a review of over 2500 cases on file at the Armed Forces Institute of Pathology (AFIP), Shmookler found only 17 occurred under 15 years of age.[28]

Local surgical excision is the treatment of choice

and can be effective for local recurrences.[28] The role of radiation therapy is unclear although it is probably effective if given in higher dose ranges (6000 rads or greater).[28,32-34] The responsiveness of liposarcoma to chemotherapy is unclear, and it is generally only used if surgery and radiation therapy are not effective or not feasible. Cyclosphosphamide, vincristine, actinomycin D, doxorubicin, and DTIC may be used in regimens similar to those for rhabdomyosarcoma.

The prognosis in children may be significantly better than adults. Shmookler and Enzinger[28] found only 3/17 children relapsed and only one eventually died of disease. In their review of previously reported cases in children only 3/22 died of disease. Metastases in children are not documented but can be anticipated in any child with the poorer prognostic histiologic types (i.e., round cell type, pleomorphic, or mixed). The most common sites in these groups are lung and liver.

MALIGNANT FIBROUS HISTIOCYTOMA

Malignant fibrous histiocytoma (MFH), also called malignant histiocytoma and malignant xanthoma, is a malignancy of histiocytic origin distinct from histiocytosis X.

Of 167 cases reviewed by Kearney, Soule, and Ivins,[35] only seven occurred below age 19 and only one below age ten years. Weiss and Enzinger[36] reported nine patients under age 20 of 200 cases reviewed.

The histopathologic classification of this malignancy is confusing, since it may contain fibrocyte type cells, histiocytes, or giant cells. This malignancy may present in soft tissue or bone.[37] MFH has been reported as a second malignancy.[9]

The most common sites of presentation are extremity sites varying from 48% to 65% of reported cases in different series. The trunk is the second most common site.[35,36,38,39]

Complete surgical resection is essential to ensure disease-free survival. Of 138 patients thought to have complete surgical removal of tumor, 70 (51%) recurred, and 39 (28%) had more than one local recurrence after surgical removal was believed

complete.[35] This malignancy is felt to be radiotherapy resistant even at high-dose ranges. Chemotherapy responses in 39% of patients treated (7/18) have been reported, but no complete responders were observed. The median time of response was 10 months with no difference seen between cyclophosphamide, vincristine, doxorubicin, and DTIC and cyclophosphamide, vincristine, doxorubicin, and actinomycin D.[38] Two patients at St. Jude Children's Research Hospital have shown dramatic response to doxorubicin at a dose of 60 mg/m^2 with complete resolution of tumor by radiologic examination. However, when doxorubicin was stopped because the total dosage was approaching cardiotoxic levels, the tumor rapidly returned, and both patients died of progressive local disease.

Pulmonary metastasis occurred in 82% of patients with the second most common site being lymph nodes.[36] Other reported metastatic sites, usually rare cases, include liver, pancreas, spleen, cerebrum, bone, kidney, and gastrointestinal tract.

Prognosis without complete surgical resection is poor because of lack of effective adjuvant therapy for even microscopic disease.

HEPATIC TUMORS

Liver tumors account for approximately 1.5% of all malignancies in children with hepatoblastoma and hepatocarcinoma being the most common types. There is no male-female predominance; however, most reported cases are in white children.[40,41] Hepatoblastoma usually occurs under age 3 years and is rare after age 5 years, whereas hepatocarcinoma usually presents after age 5 years.[42]

Clinical symptoms include upper abdominal swelling, pain, weight loss, vomiting, and anorexia. Jaundice is seldom seen, although elevations of liver enzymes or serum bilirubin may be seen, especially in hepatocarcinoma.[43,44] Local recurrences are common, and both tumors have the ability to metastasize, usually to the lungs, lymph nodes, and central nervous system.

Treatment should include an aggressive surgical approach including lobectomy for tumors confined to one lobe. Complete resection is often not possible because of multifocal disease, but the patient must be made surgically free of disease to have a chance of cure.

Chemotherapy may be used in conjunction with radiotherapy or alone. The most effective agents include vincristine, cyclophosphamide, and 5 fluorouracil with methotrexate[44] and doxorubicin.[44,45] *cis*-Platinum has also been used. Although chemotherapy is believed to be effective in controlling localized or microscopic disease. Dramatic responses with gross residual or metastatic disease are rare. Local recurrences are common, and both tumors have the ability to metastasize, usually to the lungs, lymph nodes, and central nervous system.

NURSING CONSIDERATIONS

The rare sarcomas of childhood individually account for only a small percentage of pediatric malignancies yet collectively account for almost 25% of all soft tissue malignancies and 1.6% of all malignancies in childhood.[17]

Surgery is generally the treatment of choice; because of the questionable value of adjuvant radiation and chemotherapy, surgery is likely to be more aggressive than the approaches used for rhabdomyosarcoma. Therefore both short- and long-term postsurgical complications are more prevalent and should be the major focus of nursing care plans and parent-patient education. Referrals to physical therapy, orthopedics, vocational therapy, and social work should be made early to allow preventive teaching and to help the patient and family know what recovery of functions to expect and where to find resources.

Psychologically, the patient or family may have a feeling of isolation because they are often the only ones with these diagnoses. They may have difficulty relating to patients with more common tumors and feel less peer support. Since treatment of rare tumors is not established and no written parent education material or protocol is available for parents, they may feel very confused about

data presented and treatment plans and never feel they truly have an understanding of the disease or treatment. This can enhance the feeling of isolation, and if trust and support systems are not established early, the ability to cope may become strained.

It is important to children with rare tumors to be honest about the lack of understanding of these malignancies. It should be emphasized that the treatment plan proposed is felt to be the most likely effective regimen but may not be the only alternative. Any prognosis given may not be based on adequate statistical numbers to be totally valid but may only represent trends.

REFERENCES

1. Pritchard, D.L., and others: Fibrosarcoma: clinicopathologic statistical study of 199 tumors of the soft tissues of extremity and trunk, Cancer **33**:888, 1974.
2. Bizer, L.S.: Fibrosarcoma: report of 64 cases, Am. J. Surg. **121**:586, 1971.
3. Castro, E.B., Hajdu, W.I., and Fortner, J.G.: Surgical therapy of fibrosarcoma of the extremities, Arch. Surg. **107**:284, 1973.
4. Soule, E.H., and Pritchard, D.J.: Fibrosarcoma in infants and children: a review of 100 cases, Cancer **40**:1711, 1977.
5. Exebby, P.R., and others: Soft tissue fibrosarcoma in children, J. Pediatr. Surg. **8**:415, 1973.
6. Goldstein, H.I.: Sarcoma of the tongue, Med. Times **49**:158, 1921.
7. Soloway, H.B.: Radiation-induced neoplasms following treatment for retinoblastoma, Cancer **19**:1984, 1966.
8. Ferlito, A., Recher, G., and Tomazzoli, L.: Radiation-induced fibrosarcoma of the mandible following treatment for bilateral retinoblastoma, J. Laryngol. Otol. **93**:1015, 1979.
9. Halperin, C., Greenberg, M.S., and Suit, H.D.: Sarcoma of bone and soft tissue following treatment of Hodgkin's disease, Cancer **53**:232, 1984.
10. Hays, D.M., and others: Fibrosarcoma in infants and children, J. Pediatr. Surg. **5**:176, 1970.
11. Jeffree, G.M., and Price, C.H.: Metastatic spread of fibrosarcoma of bone: a report on forty-nine cases and a comparison with osteosarcoma, J. Bone Joint Surg. **58**(4): 418, 1976.
12. Gottlieb, J.A., and others: Chemotherapy of sarcomas with a combination of adriamycin and dimethyl triazeno imidazole carboxamide, Cancer **30**:1632, 1972.
13. Cadman, N.L., and others: Synovial sarcomas: an analysis of 134 tumors, Cancer **18**:613, 1965.

14. Buck, M.D., Mickelson, M.R., and Bonfiglio, M.: Synovial sarcoma: a review of 33 cases, Clin. Orthop. **156:**211, 1981.
15. Crocker, D.W., and Stout, A.P.: Synovial sarcoma in children, Cancer 12:1123, 1959.
16. Schinose, H., and others: The early clinical presentation of synovial sarcoma, Clin. Orthop. **142:**185, 1979.
17. Young, J.L., and Miller, R.W.: Incidence of malignant tumors in U.S. children, J. Pediatr. **86:**254, 1975.
18. Enzinger, F.M., and Weiss, S.W.: Malignant tumors of peripheral nerves. In Enzingerg F.M., and Weiss, S.W.: Soft tissue tumors, St. Louis, 1983, The C.V. Mosby Co.
19. White, H.R.: Survival in malignant schwannoma: an 18 year study, Cancer 27:720, 1971.
20. D'Agostino, A.N., Soule, E.H., and Miller, R.H.: Primary malignant neoplasms of nerves in patients without manifestation of multiple neurofibromatosis (Von Recklinghausen's disease), Cancer 16:1003, 1963.
21. Ghosh, B.C., and others: Malignant schwannoma: a clinicopathologic study, Cancer 31:184, 1973.
22. Ranchod, M.B., and Kempson, R.L.: Smooth muscle tumors of the gastrointestinal tract and retroperitoneum, Cancer 39:255, 1977.
23. Wurlitzer, F.P., and others: Smooth muscle tumors of the stomach in childhood and adolescence, J. Pediatr. Surg. 8:421, 1973.
24. Gilbert, H.A., and others: The value of radiation therapy in uterine sarcoma, Obstet. Gynecol. 35:468, 1970.
25. Badib, A.O., and others: Radiotherapy in the treatment of sarcoma of the corpus uteri, Cancer 24:724, 1969.
26. Ragab, A.H., and others: Malignant tumors of soft tissues, In Sutow, W.W., Fernbach, D.J., and Vietti, T.J., editors: St. Louis, 1984, Clinical pediatric oncology, The C.V. Mosby Co.
27. Enzinger, F.M., and Weiss, S.W.: Leiomyosarcoma. In Enzinger, F.M., and Weiss, S.W.: Soft tissue tumors, St. Louis, 1983, The C.V. Mosby Co.
28. Shmookler, B.M., and Enzinger, F.M.: Liposarcoma occurring in children: an analysis of 17 cases and review of the literature, Cancer 52:567, 1983.
29. Celik, C., and others: Liposarcomas: prognosis and management, J. Surg. Oncol. 14:245, 1980.
30. Evans, H.L.: Liposarcoma: a study of 55 cases with reassessment of its classification, Am. J. Surg. Pathol. 3:507, 1979.
31. Kaufman, S.L., and Stout, A.P.: Lipoblastic tumors of children, Cancer 12:912, 1959.
32. Kinne, D.W., and others: Treatment of primary and recurrent retroperitoneal liposarcoma: twenty-five year experience at Memorial Hospital, Cancer 31:53, 1973.
33. Edland, R.W.: Liposarcoma: a retrospective study of 15 cases: a review of the literature and discussion of radiosensitivity, Am. J. Roentgenol. 103:778, 1965.
34. Castleberry, R.P., and others: Childhood liposarcoma: report of a case and review of the literature, Cancer 54:579, 1984.
35. Kearney, M.M., Soule, E.H., and Ivins, J.C.: Malignant fibrous histiocytoma: a retrospective study of 167 cases, Cancer 45:167, 1980.
36. Weiss, S.W., and Enzinger, F.M.: Malignant fibrous histiocytoma: an analysis of 200 cases, Cancer 41:2250, 1978.
37. Feldman, F., and Norman, D.: Intra- and extraosseous malignant histiocytoma, Radiology 104:497, 1972.
38. Leite, C., and others: Chemotherapy of malignant fibrous histiocytoma, Cancer 40:2010, 1977.
39. Towfik, H.H., and others: Postirradiation malignant fibrous histiocytoma, J. Surg. Oncol. 16:199, 1981.
40. Young, J.L., and Miller, R.W.: Incidence of malignant tumors in U.S. children, J. Pediatr. 96:254, 1975.
41. Young, J.L., and others: Cancer incidence, survival and mortality for children under 15 years of age (ACS Professional Educational Publication), New York, 1978, American Cancer Society.
42. Shende, A., and Valderrama, E.: Miscellaneous childhood tumors. In Lanzkowsky, P., editor: Pediatric oncology, New York, 1983, McGraw-Hill, Inc.
43. Exelby, P.R., Filler, R.M., and Grosfield, J.L.: Liver tumors in children in particular reference to hepatoblastoma and hepatocellular carcinoma, J. Pediatr. Surg. 10:329, 1975.
44. Ishak, K.G., and Glunz, P.R.: Hepatoblastoma and hepatocarcinoma in infancy and childhood: report of 47 cases, Cancer 20:396, 1967.
45. Falkson, G.: Therapeutic approaches to hepatoma, Cancer Treat. Rev. 2:73, 1975.

PART II

HEMATOLOGIC DISORDERS OF CHILDREN

CHAPTER 12

Introduction to hematology

THOMAS R. KINNEY

Blood is the originating cause of all men's diseases (the Talmud, Baba Bathrra III. 58a).

Hematology may be defined as the science of blood, including its nature, its functions, and its diseases.[1] Pediatric hematology is that branch of hematology focused on diseases of blood affecting the fetus, infant, child, and adolescent. The clinical practice of this discipline requires a knowledge derived from the basic physical and medical sciences, including chemistry, pathology, biochemistry, physiology, genetics, pharmacology, and anatomy. Similarly, the clinical practice of pediatric hematology requires knowledge of each of the clinical sciences because of the protean manifestations that blood disorders may express and because of the multitude of hematologic abnormalities that may accompany dysfunction of a specific organ.

The subsequent chapters of this section discuss the more common blood disorders of infants, children, and adolescents. The material highlights the more typical clinical presentations of each disease, discusses the pathophysiology of the disease and its relationship to the patient's signs and symptoms, and provides the authors' therapeutic recommendations. During the presentations of the material, the relationships between the basic and clinical sciences will be obvious, as will the application of this knowledge to the care of the patient.

This chapter, however, is intended to provide a brief overview of the development of hematology and to provide reflections on this subspeciality that may be of interest to the nurse preparing for a career in this field.

Mankind always has been fascinated by blood. Blood has been referred to throughout history as the essence of life, and a myriad of physical and psychiatric disturbances have been attributed to abnormalities within the blood. With the development of the microscope, it became possible to define and study the morphology of the cellular components of blood. In the seventeenth century, Antonj van Leeuwenhoek first described the red cells. In the eighteenth century, the leukocytes were described in detail by William Hewson, who has been called the father of hematology for this work and that involving the lymphatic system. Platelets, the smallest of blood's particles, were described several years after the white cells when microscopes with better resolution were developed. Dr. Paul Ehrlich (1854-1915) subsequently developed techniques to stain blood cells, which had important implications for the study of blood and the changes that occur in its cellular elements as a consequence of disease.

From these beginnings the discipline of hematology took its origins. Within this century the rapid accumulation of knowledge gathered from the use of the scientific method has produced dramatic advances in our understanding of blood disease, the hematologic abnormalities that accompany diseases of other organ systems, and our ability to provide care to children with disorders of the blood. Multiple examples may be cited to attest to this statement's accuracy, and it is only possible to highlight a few of these instances. The interested reader is referred to the excellent book entitled *Blood, Pure and Eloquent* edited by Dr. Maxwell M. Wintrobe for an in-depth discussion of the fascinating history of hematology and many of the key developments in the field that have resulted in our current understanding of the blood and the treatment of its diseases.[2]

Two of the more dramatic examples that illustrate the interrelationships between the basic sciences and the clinical sciences are found in the areas of the hemoglobinopathies and the thalassemia syndromes. Sickle cell disease is a most notable example in the area of the hemoglobinopathies. In 1910 the original clinical description of sickle cell disease appeared in the medical literature.[3] Subsequent investigations centered about the structure of the hemoglobin from patients with similar morphologic abnormalities of their red cells led to the characterization of the amino acid abnormality in the beta chain of hemoglobin S. With the characterization of this abnormality, sickle cell anemia was heralded as the first "molecular disease," since its myriad of signs and symptoms were related to the single amino acid substitution of valine for glutamic acid at the sixth position of the beta chain. Later, it was shown that this abnormality was the result of a single abnormality in the DNA of the beta globin gene. Today our understanding of the mechanisms that produce the sickle cell come from the use of a variety of sophisticated techniques employing principles of physical chemistry and x-ray crystalography.

Likewise, studies of the thalessemia disorders have led to an explosive increase of knowledge in the fields of protein synthesis and molecular genetics. The understanding of gene structure and function that has come through research in thalassemia is also being applied to other genetic disorders. These investigations undoubtedly will result in major breakthroughs that should make possible the curing of a multitude of diseases by specific gene replacement therapy. For example, by providing the person with beta thalessemia major or sickle cell anemia with a normal beta globin gene that is capable of normal function, that person's respective illness could be cured. Likewise, it should be possible to cure any genetic illness by providing the patient with a normal gene to correct the basic defect.

In the coagulation disorders, basic science investigations in the field of biochemistry made possible an understanding of the events culminating in the formation of a blood clot. This knowledge coupled with advances in blood transfusion, storage, and extraction of specific coagulation proteins from the plasma has dramatically improved the fate of children with coagulopathies.

In a similar vein, advances in blood banking techniques have made major contributions to the current practice of medicine and surgery. Recognition of the blood group antigens made red cell transfusion a relatively safe procedure. The development of the technology to harvest white cells and platelets from single blood donors has made possible modern day aggressive chemotherapy and bone marrow transplantation by enabling patients to be supported during periods of marrow aplasia. Likewise, the development of rapid methods to detect the presence of infectious agents in donor blood products has reduced the infectious hazards of blood transfusions.

Advances in biochemistry and physiology have contributed to the understanding of the disorders of white cells. Recently, it has become possible to ascribe specific biochemical defects to many of these previously poorly understood disorders—a first step toward finding a cure.

At present the field of pediatric hematology remains one of the most exciting in modern medicine. It presents significant challenges for both the physician and the nurse who are asked to care for the child affected by a blood disease. For example, clinical skills in the areas of history taking and physical assessment are required to extract the relevant information from the patient's history. The health care provider must be knowledgeable of the clinical laboratory and its ability to provide results, which are germane to establishing a diagnosis or providing information relevant to the patient's total care. Similarly, the health care provider must be able to interpret the clues provided by examination of the peripheral blood smear or bone marrow.

The clinician needs to be both empathic to the patient and objective. Empathy is required to enable the patient to speak freely with the care provider. Without a free exchange of information, it often is not possible to meet the total needs of the patient and family as they apply to both physical and mental well-being. Without objectivity, the clinician may not be able to make an accurate assessment of the problem or evaluate the patient's response to therapy.

Many of the diseases encountered by the pediatric hematology practitioner are not curable, and many of them have important genetic implications. The chronic nature of these illnesses provides an additional set of challenges. The clinician must be knowledgeable about the various stages of the diseases and be able to provide the patient and family with anticipatory guidance regarding the natural history of the specific disease. The clinician must also understand the normal physical and emotional patterns of children so that age appropriate counseling can be provided.

The genetic implications for many of the more serious hematologic disorders also present challenges to the clinician. Parents of children with such genetic diseases as thalassemia or hemophilia are obviously often severely stressed by the guilt feelings for "having caused their child to be sick." Likewise, affected children may "blame" their parents for causing the disease. The clinician must be attuned to these potential feelings of the parents and the affected child and be able to provide support to them as they attempt to cope with these issues.

Diligence is required to provide the necessary long-term care needed to ensure that the patient's full potential is maximized. The clinician must be attuned to subtle changes in the patient's condition and must anticipate potential problems if possible. Likewise, the clinician must seek out new knowledge as it develops in the field so that the most current therapeutic information and techniques can be made available to the patient.

In summary, the practice of clinical pediatric hematology is both challenging and rewarding. Its challenges stem from the complex nature of many of the diseases of blood and the therapeutic challenges that they provide. The rewards are produced not only by establishing the correct diagnosis and providing effective therapy but also by being able to provide comfort and support to the patient and family affected by the illness. The continued rapid advances in both the understanding of the various blood diseases and the ability to provide effective therapy enhances the rewards associated with this area of pediatrics.

REFERENCES

1. Hoerr, N.L., and Osol, A., editors: Blakiston's new Gould medical dictionary, ed. 2, New York, 1956, McGraw-Hill, Inc.
2. Wintrobe, M.M., editor: Blood, pure and eloquent: a story of discovery, of people, and of ideas, New York, 1980, McGraw-Hill, Inc.
3. Herrick, J.B.: Peculiar elongated and sickle-shaped red corpuscles in a case of severe anemia, Arch. Intern. Med. **6:**517, 1910.

CHAPTER 13

Childhood anemias

MARILYN J. HOCKENBERRY and WILLIAM KEITH HOOTS

CLASSIFICATION OF ANEMIAS

Reduction of red cell mass or hemoglobin concentration below normal ranges is defined as anemia. When there is a reduction in circulating hemoglobin, there is a resultant decrease in the oxygen-carrying capacity of the red blood cell. Profound physiologic problems usually do not occur unless the hemoglobin falls below 7 to 8 g/dl.[1] Physiologic and morphologic classifications of anemia are clinically helpful in assessing a patient with anemia. Characterization of anemias according to functional disturbances giving rise to a decrease in red cell mass is very helpful as a first step in determining its cause. There are three generic disturbances (or a combination thereof) which will produce anemia: impaired or decreased production of red cells, nutritional deficiencies or metabolic disturbances, or increased erythrocyte destruction. Any of the three may occur in combination and are therefore not exclusive of one another. The physiologic causes of anemias most commonly found in children as classified by different functional disturbance are as follows[2]:

Anemias caused by inadequate production
  Aplastic anemia
    Acquired
    (Constitutional)
  Pure red cell aplasia
    Diamond-Blackfan anemia
    Congenital
    Transient erythroblastopenia of childhood
Anemias caused by nutritional deficiencies or metabolic abnormalities
  Iron deficiency

Folic acid deficiency
Vitamin B_{12} deficiency
Lead poisoning
Copper deficiency
Anemias of chronic disease
Sideroblastic anemia
Vitamin dependency
Anemias caused by increased destruction (hemolysis)
  Hereditary spherocytosis, elliptocytosis, stomatocytosis
  Paroxysmal nocturnal hemoglobinuria
  Liver disease
  Glucose 6 phosphate dehydrogenase deficiency (G6PD)
  Pyruvate kinase deficiency
  Hemoglobinopathies
  Acquired hemolytic anemia
    IgG-induced hemolytic anemia
    IgM-induced hemolytic anemia

Red blood cell indices: tool for classification of anemias

Red blood cell indices are based on ratios of red blood cell volume, count, and hemoglobin concentration. They provide a useful means of designating different types of childhood anemias by size and hemoglobin content. Normal values for mean corpuscular volume (MCV) and mean corpuscular hemoglobin (MCH) do not remain constant during infancy and childhood, whereas mean corpuscular hemoglobin concentration (MCHC) values are much more constant.[1]

Mean corpuscular volume. MCV indicates the average volume of a red cell. Normal MCV ranges from 80 to 94 fl.[1] MCV indicates the size of the red blood cell itself. A normal MCV defines the cells as normal, termed normocytes. A low MCV less than 80 fl indicates small cells, labeled microcytes. A high MCV, greater than 94 fl, creates large red cells, called macrocytes. Fig. 13-1 expresses MCV percentile curves for age in boys and girls.

Mean corpuscular hemoglobin. MCH is defined as the quantity of hemoglobin per red blood cell. Normal MCH ranges from 27 to 32 pg.[1] A decreased MCH closely parallels the MCV. A cell with a normal MCH is normochromic and will stain with the normal red color on Wright stain of the peripheral blood smear (PBS). A low MCH indicates the cell to be low in hemoglobin, or hypochromic. These cells have a large area of central pallor on stained PBS examination. A high MCH indicates the cell to have excessive hemoglobin or hyperchromia. The latter cells have little central pallor and are usually spheroid rather than biconcave disc shaped.

Mean corpuscular hemoglobin concentration. MCHC indicates the amount of hemoglobin in the individual red blood cell. This finding is calculated from the amount of hemoglobin in 100 ml of red blood cells rather than that in whole blood. The MCHC usually remains constant throughout infancy and childhood at about 33 g/dl.[2]

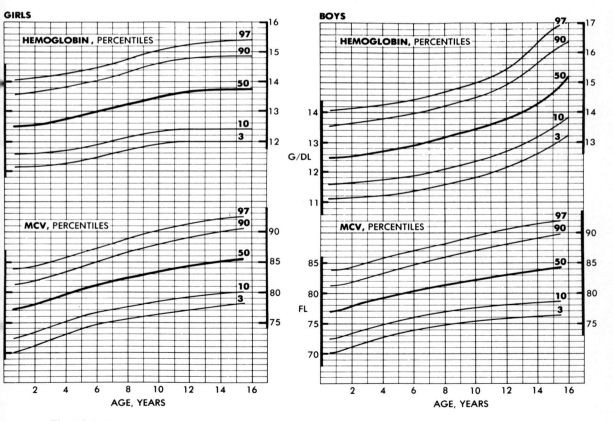

Fig. 13-1. Hemoglobin and MCV percentile curves for girls and for boys. (From Dallman, R.R., and Siimes, M.A.: Percentile curves for hemoglobin and red cell volume in infancy and childhood, J. Pediatr. **94:**26, 1979.)

Normal erythrocyte regulation and function.
Red blood cell homeostasis is dependent on the
balance between regulation of red blood cell production and destruction. This provides for the tissue oxygenation and normal blood viscosity that
allows for free flow throughout the vessels. Erythrocyte production is believed to be controlled by
tissue demands. Erythropoiesis, or production of
red blood cells, is essential to maintain homeostasis
and is dependent on a number of factors essential
for maintaining production. First, hematopoietic
stem cells must be present in the bone marrow. In
early embryonic and fetal life, red blood cells are
made primarily in the liver and spleen. By birth,
production of red blood cells is located almost exclusively in the bone marrow. Second, specific hormone regulation must be present to stimulate red
blood cell production. The hormone erythropoietin, which is largely excreted by the kidneys, is
responsible for stimulating the bone marrow to produce new red blood cells. Erythropoietin not only
affects the rate of release of red blood cells from
the bone marrow but also influences red blood cell
maturation. Third, the microenvironment of a red
blood cell must be able to support maturation from
stem cell to committed erythroid precursor. Normal
red cell production is dependent on several substances. Iron, amino acids, copper, and vitamin B
compounds serve as substituents to form new red
blood cells. In addition to these substances, intrinsic factor from the gastric mucosa is necessary for
absorption of vitamin B_{12}. The latter is essential
for cell division of red blood cell precursors.[3]

Promotion of red blood cell homeostasis
Gastric mucosa
↓
Intrinsic factor
↓
Promotes absorption of vitamin B
    (extrinsic factor)
↓
Necessary for cell division of red blood cell
    progenitors
↓
Dividing progenitors develop into mature
    red blood cells

The normal erythrocyte goes through several
stages of development. First, the stem cell develops
into erythroblasts, followed by normoblasts, then
reticulocytes, and finally into mature non-nucleated
red blood cells.[1] The stimulated bone marrow, because of the signal indicating an increased need for
red blood cells, may discharge into the peripheral
system immature red blood cells, identified as nucleated red cells on the peripheral blood smear.
Mature erythrocytes have no nucleus. Ordinarily,
the complete maturation sequence to mature red
blood cells takes 4 to 6 days, but when a bone
marrow is stimulated, these immature red cells appear in the peripheral blood much earlier.[3]

Maturation of the erythrocyte
Hemocytoblast (stem cell)
↓
Erythroblast
↓
Normoblast
↓
Reticulocyte
↓
Mature erythrocyte

The reticulocyte count is an important indicator
of bone marrow function. The reticulocyte count
is the percentage of reticulocytes present in the
circulating red cell mass. When elevated, it is an
indicator of increased red blood cell production.
Normally, the reticulocyte count is between 0.5%
to 2%; however, it may increase to 20% to 30% in
a marrow stimulated to produce and release cells
in response to anemia.[4] Once demands of tissues
are met, production of the hormone erythropoietin
decreases, and red blood cell production and reticulocyte count both return to normal.

Under normal conditions, an erythrocyte survives 120 days following its release from the bone
marrow. As the red blood cell grows old, its membrane ruptures (lyses), and the cell remnants are
phagocytized by the reticuloendothelial cells of the
spleen, liver, and bone marrow. Hemoglobin is broken down into protein-bound iron (ferritin and hemosiderin) and bile pigments. Ferritin supplies iron
for production of new red blood cells by the bone

marrow. Hemosiderin is a storage form of iron that is less available for bone marrow use and may be increased in states in which excessive iron is present. Bile pigments are excreted by the liver.

HISTORY AND PHYSICAL FINDINGS IN ANEMIA

A detailed history and physical examination are as important as any laboratory findings in evaluating causes for childhood anemia. They should be performed before any laboratory tests are ordered. The anemia must first be established as an acute versus chronic episode. Duration of symptoms must be evaluated. Rate of growth in a child is a crucial finding to establish chronicity of the disease. An adequate history must review numerous factors that will assist in diagnosing the cause of anemia.

Family

Family and social history play major roles in the diagnostic evaluation. Ethnic and geographic origins often help establish the diagnosis. For example, thalassemia syndromes occur most commonly among patients of Mediterranean or oriental descent; G6PD deficiency is also observed in these ethnic groups but also is quite common in blacks. Hemoglobin S and C are also more common in blacks, whereas beta thalassemia is seen more frequently in whites. Alpha thalassemia trait is more frequently carried among nonwhites. Family members must be tested along with the child when there is suspicion of a defect in hemoglobin synthesis or structure.

The presence of jaundice, anemia, splenomegaly, or gallstones in any family member should be addressed.[5] It is important to inquire about family members who may have died, especially siblings, whom the family may not readily discuss.

Diet

Dietary intake is an essential component of the history. Sources of iron and vitamins, quantities of milk and meat ingestion, and food fads should be carefully documented. A 24-hour dietary history should be included in the workup. History of pica should be noted, especially when there is suspicion of iron deficiency.

Drugs

Numerous drugs can induce or aggravate hematologic disease. For example, phenytoin (Dilantin) is closely associated with development of megaloblastic anemia. Numerous toxic chemicals have been linked to the onset of aplastic anemia.[6] The child's daily activities should be carefully reviewed, since many exposures to toxic chemicals occur incidentally.

Age

The child's age is an important variable in the differential diagnosis of anemia. Inquiry about a history of prematurity should be made. Iron deficiency caused by malnutrition is not seen in term infants less than 6 months of age although in premature infants it may occur after the infant doubles his or her birth weight.[2] Anemia occurring during the neonatal period is usually secondary to blood loss, isoimmunization, infection, or manifestation of a congenital hemolytic anemia.[2] Anemia detected before 6 months of age is often indicative of a congenital disorder of hemoglobin synthesis or structure.

Infection

Any history of recent infection should be evaluated and carefully documented. Infections can be strongly linked to development of red cell aplasia or hemolytic anemia.[3] Hepatitis should be considered, especially in a child who has bone marrow hypoplasia.

REVIEW OF SYSTEMS

Signs and symptoms resulting from hematologic disease are important findings that will aid in determining its cause. A general review of systems includes numerous symptoms resulting from anemia that should be closely documented[6]:

General: Change in behavior, easy fatigability, inactivity, malaise

Skin: Onset of pallor, jaundice, petechiae, ecchymoses, rashes, ulcerations

Head: Headaches, dizziness, trauma

Eyes: Scleral jaundice, diplopia, blurring, spots, cataracts

Ears: Tinnitus, vertigo

Nose: Epistaxis

Mouth and throat: Stomatitis, swelling, bleeding of gums, ulcerations of buccal mucosa, change in texture of tongue

Neck: Adenopathy

Cardiopulmonary: Palpitations, dyspnea, edema, dizziness

Gastrointestinal: Bleeding, diarrhea, melena, vomiting, anorexia

Genitourinary: Hematuria, menstrual irregularities, urinary frequency

Musculoskeletal: Muscle pain or cramps, joint pain, swelling, stiffness, weakness, numbness, coldness, discoloration of extremities

Nervous system: Loss of consciousness, syncope, paresthesia, seizures, decreased mental concentration

Endocrine: Temperature intolerance, polyuria, polydipsia, polyphagia

PHYSICAL EXAMINATION

A complete assessment should be performed with detailed examination of each organ to establish the general health of the child. Certain systems are more affected by hematologic disease and are evaluated more completely in the following outline:

General: Performance status, mental activity and concentration, general appearance, height and weight for age, rate of growth for past year

Skin: Color of skin/pallor, jaundice, pigmentation, pinkness of palmar creases, nailbeds, conjunctiva, mucous membranes and lips; petechiae, ecchymoses, leg ulcers

Head and neck: Head circumference, shape of skull, ecchymoses, bumps, hair texture and pattern

Eyes—scleral jaundice, eye grounds (pallor of retina, tortuous vessels, hemorrhages and exudates, edema of eyelids, cataracts)

Nose—bleeding

Mouth—pallor of mucosa, ulcerations, bleeding, hematoma

Tongue—texture and color, swelling

Neck—adenopathy, thyroid enlargement

Heart and lungs: Tachycardia, increased pulsations, bruits, gallop S_3-S_4, systolic heart murmur at apex, arrhythmia, abnormally shaped chest; respirations—increased rate and depth

Abdomen: Splenomegaly, hepatomegaly

Genitalia: Inflammation, ulcerations, bleeding, edema, Tanner stage

Rectum: Ulcerations, bleeding, inflammation, hemorrhoids

Musculoskeletal: Painful swollen joints, stiffness, discoloration of extremities, triphalangeal thumbs, spoon nails, ulceration of lower extremities

Lymph nodes: Swollen, tender

Nervous system: Paresthesias, decreased mental concentration

LABORATORY FINDINGS

Appropriate laboratory studies should initially begin with a complete blood cell count, red blood cell indices, reticulocyte count, and review of the peripheral smear.[4] The logical approach to the evaluation of anemia can be made simple at any child's age if close attention is made to the initial laboratory studies.

Hemoglobin and hematocrit

Hemoglobin is a true indicator of the physiologic potential of blood to transport oxygen to the tissue. Hematocrit indicates percentage volume of circulating packed red cells of the total blood and normally is approximately three times the concentration of hemoglobin in g/dl. Hemoglobin and hematocrit, under normal conditions, are in a fixed relationship with each other and vary according to the child's age.

From 6 months of age through schoolage, a hemoglobin of 11 g/dl may be regarded as the absolute lowest level of normal.[4] Hemoglobin level gradually rises until puberty when adult values are

Table 13-1. Average normal blood values in infancy and childhood

Age	Hemoglobin (gm/dl)	RBC (× 10¹²/liter)	Hematocrit (%)	MCV (fl)	MCH (pg)	MCHC (%)	Reticulocytes (%)
Cord blood	16.8	5.25	63	120	34	31.7	3.2
1 day	19.0	5.14	61	119	36.9	31.6	3.2
3 days	18.7	5.11	62	116	36.5	31.1	3.8
7 days	17.9	4.86	56	118	36.2	32.0	0.5
2 weeks	17.3	4.80	54	112	36.8	32.1	0.5
3 weeks	15.6	4.20	46	111	37.1	33.9	0.8
4 weeks	14.2	4.00	43	105	35.5	33.5	0.6
2 months	10.7	3.40	31	93	31.5	34.1	1.8
3 months	11.3	3.70	33	88	30.5	34.8	0.7
6 months	12.3	4.60	36	78	27	34	1.4
8 months	12.1	4.6	36	77	26	34	1.1
10 months	11.9	4.6	36	77	26	34	1.0
1 year	11.6	4.6	35	77	25	33	0.9
2 years	11.7	4.7	35	78	25	33	1.0
4 years	12.6	4.7	37	80	27	34	1.0
6 years	12.7	4.7	38	80	27	33	1.0
8 years	12.9	4.7	39	80	27	33	1.0
10-12 years	13.0	4.8	39	80	27	33	1.0
Adult men	16.0	5.4	47	87	29	34	1.0
Adult women	14.0	4.8	42	87	29	34	1.0

From Miller, D.L., and others: Blood diseases of infancy and childhood, St. Louis, 1984, The C.V. Mosby Co.

established. Precise relationships between age and values for hemoglobin and hematocrit results are shown in Table 13-1. It should be realized that normal hemoglobin levels in black children may be slightly lower than white children. Reasons for racial variations in hemoglobin are as yet unknown. Hemoglobin and MCV percentile curves are shown in Fig. 13-1 comparing age and sex.

Reticulocytes

A reticulocyte is a large, purplish-appearing red blood cell very recently released from the bone marrow synthetic pool. The percentage of reticulocytes indicate the percentage of red blood cells formed within the last 24 to 48 hours.[1] Increased reticulocytes indicate hyperactivity of the bone marrow, whereas a low count indicates decreased production. A normal reticulocyte count ranges from 0.5% to 2.0%.[7] A reticulocyte count is a simple yet sensitive indicator of bone marrow activity.

Peripheral smear

Examination of the peripheral smear may help establish the type of anemia and certainly suggests the next appropriate diagnostic test to perform. Estimation of red blood cell size should be established first by comparing red cell size to a normal lymphocyte, since many are similar in size.[4] Shape of the red cells should be evaluated. Characteristic alterations in shape may lead to a direct diagnosis as in hereditary spherocytosis where cells seen on the smear appear small and round and lack central pallor. Color of the red cells should be observed. Red cells should be evaluated for the presence of other features within the cells. For example, Howell-Jolly bodies, which are small, rounded areas of dense RNA in the cell, are seen in many

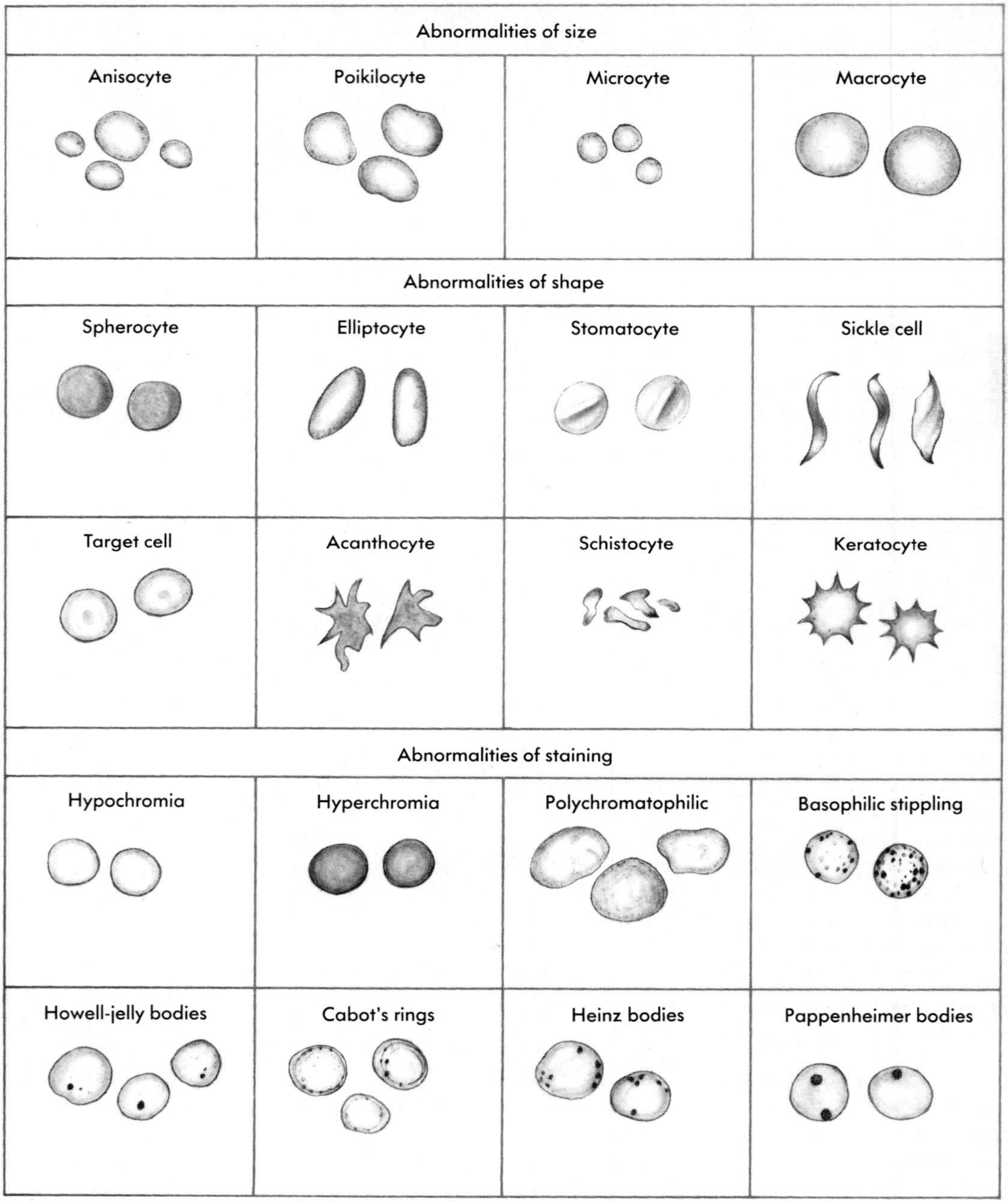

Fig. 13-2. Abnormalities in shape, size, and staining of red blood cells.

anemias with splenic dysfunction or agenesis under normal conditions.[1] The spleen "pits" remove these RNA deposits from maturing reticulocytes. Terms defining size, shape, and staining of red blood cells are listed below and illustrated in Fig. 13-2:

Abnormalities of size
Anisocytes: Excessive variation in size
Poikilocyte: Irregular shape
Microcyte: Small cell, less than 6.5 m
Macrocyte: Large cell, greater than 8.5 m

Abnormalities of shape
Spherocytes: Globular, thick, and round without centralized pallor
Elliptocytes: Oval, vary in shape
Stomatocytes: Oval with linear, slitlike area across center of cell
Sickle cells: Elongated and narrow, half-moon shaped
Target cells: Bull's-eye center, round
Acanthocytes: Spherocytes with equal spiny projections
Schistocytes: Fragmented cells
Keratocyte: "Burr cell," large irregular horny projections

Abnormalities of staining
Hypochromia: Increased central pallor
Hyperchromia: Lack central pallor
Polychromatophilic: Nucleus not visible but still bluish in color
Basophilic stippling: Round, fine bluish granules in cytoplasm
Howell-Jolly bodies: Small, rounded densely stained nuclear material
Cabot's rings: Circular, twisted "figure-eight" rings
Heinz bodies: Blue, irregular shaped granules at periphery of cell
Pappenheimer bodies: Blue-stained double granules or dots

Bone marrow examination

Bone marrow aspiration and biopsy are useful tools in determining types of cells present and their numbers being produced (Fig. 13-3). Wright- or Giemsa-stained smears of bone marrow aspirations can be evaluated for determination of the myeloid cell total as compared to the erythroid cell total (normal is 3:1), differential count, detection of abnormal cells, evaluation of iron stores, and kinetic studies.

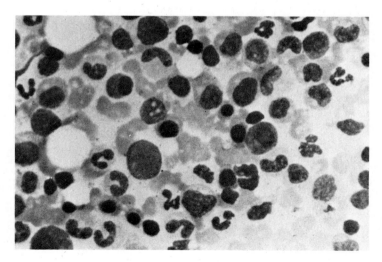

Fig. 13-3. Bone marrow film demonstrating normal cellular constituents.

Bone marrow biopsy may be necessary when hypoplasia or infiltration is suspected. Touch preparations are made on slides and stained with Wright or Giemsa stain to assist in cell identification along with the biopsy attained.

Evaluation of the cause of anemia in a child can be performed in a simple step-by-step process once initial history, physical, and laboratory tests have begun. Three major questions allow for further identification of the cause (Fig. 13-4). First, are there characteristic abnormalities in the shape and size of the cells shown by the MCV and MCH? Second, is there reduced cell production or in-creased production indicated by the reticulocyte count? Third, are white blood cells and platelets affected as observed on the total blood count?[8]

A rational approach to anemia involves the combination of a thorough clinical history, physical examination, and initiation of simple laboratory tests. Through use of these tools a correct diagnosis can be established in most cases, or appropriate further diagnostic tools can be recommended. This introduction to the classification of anemias and initial evaluation for diagnosis gives an appropriate background from which to discuss the specific anemias according to their classification.

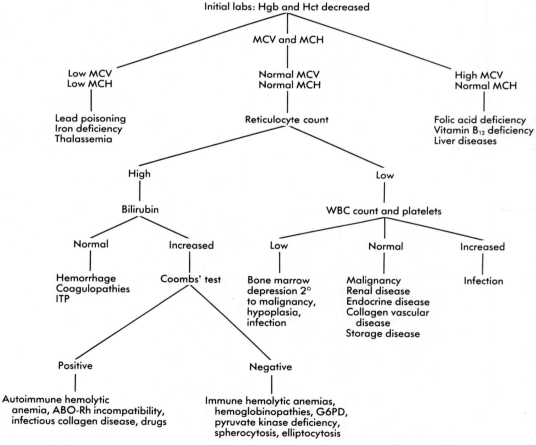

Fig. 13-4. Differentiation of anemia. (Adapted from Emerg. Med. **15**(2):64, Nov. 30, 1983.)

Major childhood anemias are now presented according to their etiology, clinical manifestations, diagnostic criteria, and mode of treatment. Anemias of the newborn period will not be specifically addressed. *Blood Diseases of Infancy and Childhood*[1] is recommended for reading on anemias in the newborn period.

ANEMIA CAUSED BY INADEQUATE PRODUCTION
Acquired aplastic anemia

The disorder characterized by reduction or absence of red blood cells, granulocytes, and platelets in the bone marrow is known as aplastic anemia. Absence of marrow elements results in peripheral pancytopenia. Severe disease constitutes at least two of the following: reticulocyte count less than 1%, platelet count below 20,000/mm³, and granulocyte count below 500/mm³.[9] Children typically have a complication secondary to the underlying absence of a marrow element.

The overall incidence of acquired aplastic anemia is approximately 1000/year in the United States.[1]

Forty to fifty percent of children developing aplastic anemia have no underlying etiology. Known causes are most frequently identified as exposure to drugs, chemicals, or toxins. Aplastic anemia caused by agents or conditions other than drugs or chemicals are infrequent and occur in only 10% to 15% of all cases.[10] Less than 10% of all cases spontaneously recover from aplasia. The median survival for patients with severe disease is 3 months. One year survival rate ranges around 20%.[11]

Onset of aplastic anemia from drug or chemical pathogenesis affects marrow production by one of two ways. First, the offending agent exerts a direct toxic effect on hematopoietic precursors, causing reduction or absent stem cell production in the bone marrow.[1] This reduction of stem cells, which are to differentiate into circulating red blood cells, granulocytes, and platelets, is the primary mechanism in the development of aplastic anemia. Second, the drug or chemical creates a defective environment in which the stem cell cannot grow and differentiate.[1]

Drugs. Chloramphenicol is one of the most common causes of aplastic anemia. The risk of aplastic anemia is approximately 1/30,000 following the use of this drug.[3] It usually occurs within 10 weeks of the administration and is usually reversible. Chemotherapeutic agents, especially alkylating agents, have been known to cause aplastic anemia although it is usually transitory. Anticonvulsants such as phenytoin (Dilantin) have been associated with onset of aplastic anemia, megaloblastic anemia, and pure red cell aplasia.[1] Onset may occur within 2 weeks after treatment or as late as 6 months. Phenylbutazone is known as one of the most common causes of aplastic anemia but is rarely seen in children because of its uncommon use. Effects on the marrow are often prolonged and may last for years. Quinacrine (Atabrine) is a significant cause in the development of aplastic anemia in countries where malaria is prevalent but is uncommon in the United States.[2]

Chemicals and toxins. Benzene is the most common chemical associated with aplastic anemia.[9] Toxic effects may result from mere inhalation. Numerous individuals developing aplastic anemia secondary to benzene exposure subsequently develop leukemia. Leukemia may occur up to 10 years after benzene exposure and recovery from aplastic anemia.[9] Benzene is a common compound found in organic solvents, model airplane glue, coal derivatives, petroleum products, and insecticides.

Radiation. Radiation therapy damages hematopoietic stem cells. At doses of 1000 to 1200 rad, aplasia occurs and is lethal when bone marrow transplantation is not performed.[2]

Infections. Viral hepatitis has been associated with onset of severe aplastic anemia, occurring within 2 months after onset. Aplastic anemia occurring after hepatitis has a poor prognosis with a 90% mortality.[2] Bacterial and viral illness have been known to cause mild pancytopenia. Mycobacterial infections have been linked to the onset of aplasia. Mononucleosis has also been reported to lead to aplastic anemia.

Others. Systemic diseases such as pancreatic disease have been known to cause aplasia. Pregnancy has been documented to cause aplastic anemia. Paroxysmal nocturnal hemoglobinuria has been complicated by aplasia.[2]

Clinical manifestations. The child typically has complications attributed to the absence of marrow elements causing anemia, granulocytopenia, or thrombocytopenia. These symptoms are also associated with numerous other diseases, which may make the differential diagnosis difficult. Bone marrow biopsy is essential to determine extent of hematopoietic activity. Signs and symptoms of anemia can be caused by bone marrow infiltration of leukemia, lymphoma, and other malignancies and must be ruled out as a cause for bone marrow failure.

Thrombocytopenia may cause the child to bruise more easily. Bleeding of the mucous membranes of the mouth and nose occur frequently; however, major bleeding complications are rare initially. Granulocytopenia increases the child's susceptibility for infections. The child may have fever and no known etiologic findings. Bacterial infections are common initially.

The child frequently is seen clinically with severe anemia with hemoglobin findings ranging from 3 to 7 g/dl.[10] Pallor and fatigue are common with severe anemia, leading to tachycardia and even heart failure. Physical findings other than those brought on by absence of marrow elements may be indicative of other underlying diseases such as leukemia or lymphoma. Adenopathy is not found in aplastic anemia. Hepatosplenomegaly is usually absent, except in children with congestive heart failure.

Laboratory findings. Severity of aplasia is based on the absolute granulocyte count, platelet count, reticulocyte count, and extent of hypocellularity of the bone marrow. Severe aplasia is described as a granulocyte count less than 500/mm³, platelets below 20,000/mm³, and a reticulocyte count less than 1%. The bone marrow presents as hypocellular with greater than 85% lymphocytes.[9]

Neutropenia is a constant finding in this disease and is less than 1800 in 90% of the cases at diagnosis. Thrombocytopenia occurs consistently with a count less than 100,000 and less than 20,000 in 50% of the cases. Initially, patients may have abnormalities of only one cell line and then subsequently develop abnormalities with other marrow elements months later.

Fetal hemoglobin is frequently increased to as high as 15%. Coomb's test is negative. Vitamin B_{12} and folate levels are normal. Immunoglobulins are normal with B and T cell lymphocyte ratio being proportionately normal. Blood lymphocyte chromosomes are also normal. Serum iron levels are elevated with iron-binding capacity saturated. There is prolonged iron clearance with decreased turnover and use of iron, demonstrating erythroid hypoproliferation. Bone marrow biopsy reveals hypoplasia with reduction of hematopoietic precursors. Fat, empty spicules, reticulum cells, mast cells, lymphocytes, and plasma cells may be the only nucleated cells present[9] (Fig. 13-5).

Treatment

Bone marrow transplantation. Bone marrow transplantation is the treatment of choice in children with severe aplastic anemia.[3] All children with compatible donors should be transplanted as soon as possible to minimize exposure to blood products. Family members should be typed for histocompatibility immediately on confirmation of the diagnosis. Transfusions of red blood cells and platelets should be withheld if the child has not presented with a life-threatening situation from anemia or thrombocytopenia. If transfusions are essential to maintain support, blood products from relatives should not be used until eligibility of transplantation is known. Under no situation should blood products from relatives be used in a child undergoing bone marrow transplantation. Eligibility for bone marrow transplantation is discussed at length in Chapter 22. Survival rate of transplantation for aplastic anemia using a sibling donor is increasing and now reaches 50% to 70%.[11] Bone marrow transplantation has considerably higher survival rates than any other current treatment mo-

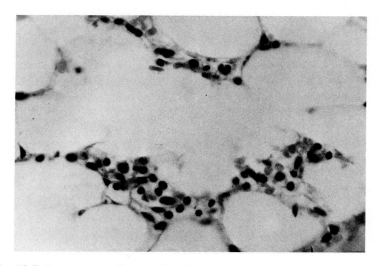

Fig. 13-5. Bone marrow film revealing hypoplasia secondary to aplastic anemia.

dality. The continued obstacle of chronic graft versus host disease remains the greatest side effect of transplantation in aplastic anemia.

Androgens. Androgen therapy is used to increase erythropoiesis.[3] Improvement usually occurs within 6 to 7 weeks after initiation of therapy, although periods up to 3 months have been reported before detecting adequate responses. Oxymetholone is used most frequently at a dose of 2 to 6 mg/kg/day orally. Other agents include testosterone propionate, methandrostenolone (Dianabol), fluorymesterone (Halotestin), nandrolone decanoate, or methyltestosterone (Metandren).[1,2] Major side effects of androgen therapy include virilization causing skin flushing, acne, voice changes, and growth of pubic hair. Virilizing effects, excluding growth of pubic hair, are reversible when the drug is terminated. Liver toxicity may result from using androgens, most frequently being mild with the presence of hyperbilirubinemia. In a small group of children, hepatocellular carcinoma has developed. Low-dose prednisone at 0.5 to 1 mg/kg is used concomitantly to prevent maturation of growth centers caused by the androgens.[2,10]

Effectiveness of androgens remains controversial. It is hoped that children with a constitutional form of aplastic anemia will demonstrate success with improvement of erythropoiesis by the use of androgens. To date, no prospective studies have been reported.

Immunosuppression. Immunologic mediated stem cell destruction has been identified as the cause of severe aplastic anemia in numerous cases.[11] Marrow recovery has been reported following the use of various immunosuppressive regimens alone or with allogeneic bone marrow transplantation. Cyclophosphamide, antithymocyte globulin and antilymphocyte globulin have been used in patients demonstrating severe aplastic anemia secondary to immunologic incompetence.[11] Most patients have demonstrated only a partial, gradual response associated with a marked decrease in clinical symptoms over a period of months.

Toxicities of antithymocyte globulin and antilymphocyte globulin vary from patient to patient and include fevers, joint swelling, rashes and dermatitis, serum sickness, and rarely anaphylaxis.[11]

Further immunosuppression in a patient already demonstrating neutropenia places them at even greater risk for a life-threatening infection.

Supportive care. Infusion of red blood cells, platelets, and at times white blood cells must be used for supportive care. Administration should be planned carefully to ensure immediate benefits and not jeopardize future therapy. Sensitization of donor blood cells is the most crucial limitation to effective transfusion therapy. Anemia, bleeding, and infection are the major side effects of aplasia and must be dealt with continuously to prevent the development of life-threatening illnesses. The child with aplastic anemia is at risk for numerous problems related to the reduction of normal red blood cells, white blood cells, and platelets. Chapter 23, on blood products, discusses in detail transfusion therapy and its side effects. The following sections outline supportive care specific to the child with aplastic anemia.

Anemia. Reduction of red blood cells resulting in anemia produces weakness and malaise. Red blood cell transfusion should be used to maintain a hemoglobin above 7 g/dl.[1] Signs and symptoms of anemia do not usually develop when the hemoglobin is maintained above this level.

Washed, frozen red blood cells should be given to avoid sensitization and febrile reactions. Children will often need transfusions every 2 to 4 weeks. There is no evidence that withholding blood transfusions will stimulate the marrow to produce erythroid precursors.[2] Children who have undergone a bone marrow transplant or who have received immunosuppressive therapy such as antithymocyte globulin should receive irradiated blood products only to prevent graft versus host disease.

There are several precautions that can be taken to minimize the onset of symptoms caused by anemia:

1. Frequent rest periods throughout the day
2. Small frequent meals with a well balanced diet
3. Adequate rest at night (as much as 12 hours)
4. No participation in strenuous sports that require more energy

Bleeding. Bleeding may occur under the skin and from the nose, gastrointestinal tract, kidneys, bladder, lungs, optic fundi, and brain.[1] Episodes of bleeding may increase during infections requiring more frequent transfusions. Prophylactic platelet transfusions for counts less than 20,000 remain controversial. Two absolute indications for platelet transfusions are the presence of signs and symptoms of a life-threatening bleed or surgery.

Single donor platelet transfusions are preferable because they decrease exposure to platelet antigens and should be used when available. Human-leukocyte antigen (HLA)-matched platelets may be needed when patients fail to respond to single donor units. HLA-matched platelets should not be used in candidates for bone marrow transplantation as previously discussed.

There are several precautions in patients with thrombocytopenia that can prevent or control bleeding:

1. No aspirin compounds
2. No intramuscular shots (give immunizations SQ)
3. No contact sports
4. Oral contraceptives or hormonal suppression when there is increased bleeding with menses
5. High-fiber diets
6. Use stool softeners

Infection. A neutrophil count less than 500/mm^3 places the child at high risk for an overwhelming infection.[1,2] Common infections include *Staphylococcus aureus, pseudomonas, coag negative staphylococcus, Candida* and *Klebsiella*.[12] Onset of fever in a child with aplastic anemia may warn of a life-threatening illness. Sepsis may progress rapidly, and frequently no specific underlying etiologic factors are identified. Viral and bacterial cultures of the blood, throat, urine, and stool should be obtained and broad-spectrum antibiotics should be administered immediately. The child should be watched closely during the first 24 hours for signs and symptoms of septic shock, which can occur within a matter of hours in a neutropenic patient.

Children with aplastic anemia generally tolerate

viral infections better than bacterial and fungal infections.[10] Fungus should be suspected in a child with persisting fever while continuing on broad-spectrum antibiotics. Viral and bacterial cultures should be performed, and amphotericin B may be essential to treat for fungus. White blood cell transfusions are not routinely administered; their use and documented effectiveness continue to be controversial. When used, they follow the unsuccessful treatment regimen of broad-spectrum antibiotics and amphotericin B.[12]

Development of overwhelming infection is often not preventable. However, the following precautions can be taken to decrease the risk of infections in the child with aplastic anemia:

1. Wear shoes at all times to prevent scrapes and cuts that may develop into infection
2. Maintain stringent oral mouth care to prevent ulcerations
3. Avoid large crowds in closed areas
4. Separate the child from individuals with obvious infection
5. Protect from sunburn that can develop into subsequent infection.
6. Clean open lesions or cuts with hydrogen peroxide solution and apply topical antibiotics

Constitutional aplastic anemia

Constitutional aplastic anemia is defined as either congenital, with the child being born with it, or inherited, with a family propensity for bone marrow failure.[9] Incidence of congenital or inherited aplasia is 30% that of acquired aplastic anemia.[1] The most common type of constitutional aplasia is Fanconi's anemia. Dyskeratosis congenita, constitutional aplastic anemia Type II, and Estren-Dameshek anemia without congenital anomalies are included in this classification. Constitutional aplasia is characterized by pancytopenia, a hypoplastic bone marrow, and the presence of congenital defects or familial history of occurrence.

Fanconi's anemia may be associated with numerous anomalies that are recognized early in infancy.[13] These anomalies are usually detected before any hematologic abnormality is observed. Presentation of aplasia is rare before 17 months of age and may not develop until around the age of 10.[1] Average age of onset is 6 to 8 years of age with male:female ratio of occurrence being 14:1.[11] Fanconi's anemia is an autosomal recessive disorder with variable penetrance. Table 13-2 compares Fanconi's anemia with acquired aplastic anemia.

Clinical manifestation. *Skin* hyperpigmentation is frequently associated with Fanconi's anemia. Areas of involvement are commonly the neck, axilla, abdomen, umbilicus, and genitalia. Cafe au lait spots may be present. *Skeletal* anomalies are seen, especially of the hands and forearms, with absent thumbs and radii (Fig. 13-6). Short stature occurs from a short trunk although legs are normal length. Hypoplasia of the thumbnail may be present. *Renal* anomalies including horseshoe kidneys, hydronephrosis, double ureters, or absence of a kidney may be seen. *Central nervous system* (CNS) abnormalities are frequent and may include microencephaly, low birth weight, microphthalmia, mental retardation, deafness, ptosis, strabismus, and nystagmus. Hyperreflexia is the most common CNS symptom observed. Hypogenitalism may also occur.

Children with dyskeratosis congenita also initially have pancytopenia.[11] Differences in clinical presentation of a child with dyskeratosis congenita include ectodermal dysplasia, with skin pigmentations consisting of cutaneous telangiectatic erythema and atrophy. Dystrophic nails, dental dysplasia, sparse hair, blocked lacrimal ducts, and possible esophageal dysplasia may occur. Skeletal, chromosomal, and renal abnormalities are absent as compared with Fanconi's anemia.

Constitutional aplastic anemia type II is present at birth with a clinical presentation of thrombocytopenia. Congenital anomalies and chromosome aberrations are absent.

Laboratory findings. Pancytopenia may take months to years to develop in Fanconi's anemia. Thrombocytopenia is observed initially, with the bone marrow in the early stages presenting with erythroid hyperplasia and megaloblastosis.

Onset of aplasia with Fanconi's anemia presents

Table 13-2. Characteristics of acquired aplastic anemia and Fanconi's aplastic anemia

	Acquired aplastic anemia	Fanconi's aplastic anemia
Inheritance	Not inherited	Autosomal recessive with variable penetrance
Onset	Rapid	Gradual
Age	Variable	Less than 10 years
Response to androgens	Not common	Frequent
Birth weight	Normal	Low
Stature	Normal	Short
Skeletal deformities	Rare	Rare
Frequent		
Skin pigmentation	Rare	Frequent
Renal anomalies	Rare	Frequent
Platelet	20,000-100,000	20,000-100,000 (usually occurs first)
Hemoglobin	3-7 g/dl	3-7 g/dl
White blood cells	$<1.8 \times 10^9$/liter	$<1.8 \times 10^9$/liter
Fetal hemoglobin	15%	10%
Coomb's test	Negative	Negative
Vitamin B_{12} and folate	Normal	Normal
B & T cell lymphocyte rates	Normal	Normal
Peripheral chromosomes	Normal	Abnormal
Serum iron	Elevated	Elevated
Iron clearance	Prolonged	Prolonged
Iron-binding capacity	Saturated	Saturated
Bone marrow	Hypoplastic with reduction of all hematopoietic precursors	Hypoplastic with reduction of all hematopoietic precursors

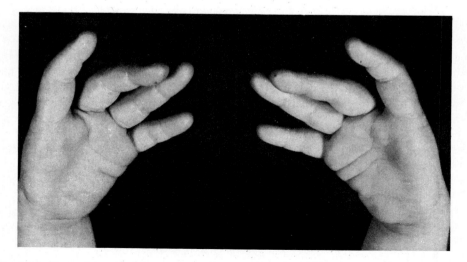

Fig. 13-6. Fanconi's syndrome, showing bilateral absence of thumbs. (From Miller, D.L., and others: Blood diseases of infancy and childhood, St. Louis, 1984, The C.V. Mosby Co.)

Table 13-3. Red cell aplasias

Signs and symptoms	Diamond-Blackfan anemia	Transient erythroblastopenia of childhood	Pure red cell aplasia
Age of onset	Less than 1 year	1-4 years	Unknown in childhood; Adolescence and adult onset
Etiology	Congenital—autosomal recessive	Acquired—after onset of viral illness	Secondary to autoimmune deficiency
Physical examination	25%-30% have congenital anomalies	Normal	Presence of thymomas in 50% of patients
Hemoglobin	2-4 g/dl	3-9 g/dl	3-9 g/dl
White blood cell	Normal	Normal	Normal
Platelet count	Normal or increased	Usually increased	Normal
Hgb F	Increased	Normal	Normal
i antigen	Present	Absent	Absent
Response	60%-80% response with corticosteroids	Spontaneous recovery	25% response with thymoma removal alone
Prognosis	Long-term survival seen; effects of chronic transfusion therapy cause complications	—	Autoimmune disorder usually causes patient's demise

similarly to acquired aplasia. The bone marrow reveals hypoplasia with few normal precursors seen. Differentiation of constitutional versus acquired aplasia is based on the physical examination, skeletal survey, intravenous pyelogram, and chromosome analysis. Chromosome anomalies are seen as breaks, gaps, constrictions, and even translocations in patients with Fanconi's anemia.[3]

Treatment. Treatment of constitutional aplasia is similar to that of aplastic anemia. There has been a good response noted with administration of androgens and steroids. Long-term remission is now reaching 50% since the use of androgens and steroids. Bone marrow transplantation is now considered a treatment of choice when the child becomes unresponsive to androgen and steroid therapy.

The child with Fanconi's anemia is at higher than normal risk for the development of a malignancy. As many as 10% will develop a malignancy later on in the illness.[1] Myelomonocytic leukemia, myelocytic leukemia, solid tumors, and hepatocarcinomas have been seen in patients with Fanconi's anemia.[11]

Supportive care is of utmost importance. Considerations previously identified in the management for acquired aplasia are also crucial in the management of the child with constitutional aplastic anemia.

Pure red cell aplasia

Several disorders have been identified in which only red cell production is affected (Table 13-3). Congenital red cell aplasia known as Diamond-Blackfan anemia and transient erythroblastopenia of childhood are unique in children. Acquired pure red cell anemia is found most commonly in adults and has been also noted in a small number of patients with malignancies.

Aplasia occurs in various diseases and hemolytic disorders. Hereditary spherocytosis, immune hemolytic anemia, and sickle cell disease have all been known to produce aplastic crises thought to be produced by viral infections.[1] Drugs and chemicals have been associated with the onset of red cell aplasia. Malnutrition has been known to cause cessation of erythropoiesis.[2]

Congenital pure red cell aplasia. Congenital hypoplastic anemia, known as Diamond-Blackfan anemia, is a rare disorder identified as failure of erythropoiesis with normal platelet and leukocyte production. Onset develops early in childhood, most commonly before 6 months of age.[14]

Approximately 200 cases of Diamond-Blackfan anemia have been reported. Exact etiology is uncertain although hereditary transmission is postulated as being an autosomal dominant disorder.[2] Most evidence tends to reveal that the erythroid stem cell is defective. There is an equal distribution among sexes.

One-fourth of these children have congenital anomalies. The most frequent anomaly identified is triphalangeal thumbs. Short stature is commonly seen. Other anomalies such as webbed neck, strabismus, hypertelorism, hypotelorism, cleft lip and palate, retinopathy, ventricular septal defect, microcephaly, mental retardation, and renal malformation have been identified although their relationship to erythroid hyperplasia remains uncertain.

At the time of diagnosis, all patients display a normocytic, normochromic anemia with a hemoglobin ranging between 2 to 4 g/dl.[14] The reticulocyte count is decreased or nonexistent. The platelet count and white blood cell count are normal. Fetal hemoglobin levels are elevated along with antigen levels. Bone marrow examination reveals absence of erythroid precursors with normal production of granulocytes, platelets, and their precursors. Myeloid-erythroid ratio often appears as high as 50:1.[15]

Serum iron is high or at high normal finding with an increased iron-binding capacity. Erythropoietin is elevated. Folic acid and vitamin B_{12} are normal. Peripheral blood chromosomes are normal in patients with Diamond-Blackfan anemia.

Therapy for patients with Diamond-Blackfan anemia consists of corticosteroids, transfusions, and rarely splenectomy.[15] Corticosteroids are known to be successful in the majority of cases if started immediately after diagnosis is confirmed. A dosage of 2 mg/kg/day of prednisone or pred-

nisolone is initiated. Reticulocytosis appears within 1 to 4 weeks following steroid initiation but may take as long as 4 to 6 months.[2] Once a response is achieved, the steroid is tapered slowly until a maintenance dose is found that will maintain a hemoglobin level near 10 g/dl.

One fourth of the patients may experience a spontaneous remission.[2] Up to 50% of these patients can be controlled on maintenance doses of corticosteroids. Patients not obtaining a response to steroids may be changed to other corticosteroids and/or androgens. Those not responding to steroids or androgens must remain on a chronic transfusion program.

Transient erythroblastopenia of childhood

Idiopathic erythroblastopenia is a benign disorder of unknown cause, occurring in children during the first few years of life.[14] The onset is insidious. It is characterized by anemia, reticulocytopenia, and erythroid hypoplasia of the bone marrow. Most incidences are associated with a viral illness occurring 2 weeks to 2 months before onset of anemia.[2] The anemia is temporary and usually resolves within weeks from the time of onset.

Physical examination is normal except for presence of pallor. Hemoglobin findings range from 3 to 9 g/dl with a reticulocyte count below 1%.[1] White blood cell count and platelet count are normal. Bone marrow examination demonstrates reduction in erythroid precursors. MCV, fetal hemoglobin levels, i antigen levels, and red cell enzyme levels are usually normal.[1]

Most children with transient erythroblastopenia of childhood recover within 1 to 2 months after diagnosis and require no treatment. A number of children have required transfusions during this time because of severe anemia. Prednisone is sometimes used in patients not responding rapidly who may be thought to have Diamond-Blackfan anemia.

Acquired red cell aplasia

Pure red cell aplasia occurs primarily in adults but has been seen at puberty. It is an acquired defect of erythropoiesis, thought to be of autoimmune origin. Up to 50% of these individuals also have a thymic mass.[2]

Onset of anemia is insidious with physical findings similar to those found in congenital anemias. The high prevalence of associated thymoma, radiographic studies including chest computed tomographic (CT) scan and tomograms should be performed.

The anemia is normochromic, normocytic, with reticulocytopenia. The bone marrow is absent of erythroid precursors. Serum iron is increased with reduced iron clearance and low iron use.

Autoimmune disease may be detected by presence of antibodies to red cells. Positive antinuclear antibodies, lupus erythematosis preparations, tests for myasthenia gravis, antibodies to smooth muscles, or intrinsic factors and paraproteins may also be present.[3]

Removal of the thymoma has led to a cure in 25% of these individuals with pure red cell aplasia in the presence of a thymoma. Corticosteroids with or without androgen therapy has been used without a significant response. Splenectomy has had limited success with a few individuals responding to steroids afterward.

Immunosuppressants such as 6-mercaptopurine and cyclophosphamide have been used with some success following splenectomy. Spontaneous remissions are not frequently seen.

Transfusion therapy provides supportive care and is the primary treatment for 75% of the patients who have failed to respond to steroids, androgens, immunosuppressive agents, and splenectomy.[3]

Long-term prognosis is questionable, with patients usually dying from the autoimmune disorders. Those surviving the autoimmune disorder face complications of chronic transfusion therapy.

ANEMIAS CAUSED BY NUTRITIONAL DEFICIENCIES OR METABOLIC DISTURBANCES

Malnutrition remains a major concern for a large portion of the world's population. Anemias caused by nutritional deficiencies are most frequently associated with decreased bone marrow production of red blood cells. Examples include iron, folate, and vitamin B_{12} deficiencies. Although these anemias are characterized by decreased red cell production, there is also indication of increased red cell destruction. A lack of essential nutrients may restrict either cell proliferation or differentiation or both. Numerous substrates are necessary for production and maintenance of red blood cells. Copper plays an essential role in iron and hemoglobin metabolism. Pyridoxine is required for heme synthesis, whereas vitamin E protects the red cell from oxidation. Vitamin B_{12} and folic acid are essential for normal metabolic processes and nucleic acid synthesis. Deficiencies in these essential components result in various forms of anemia. Chronic diseases may impede their absorption or metabolism. Shortened red cell survival secondary to impaired flow of iron to the marrow may exacerbate an anemia of chronic disease. Toxic metals such as lead cause anemia by inhibiting heme synthesis. In the following section specific types of anemia resulting from nutritional deficiencies of metabolic disturbances are discussed.

Iron deficiency anemia

Iron deficiency is the most frequent nutritional deficiency found in children. It occurs most commonly in term infants at 9 to 15 months of age and preterm infants at 4 to 9 months of age.[1] Low iron composition in many diets, interference with iron absorption, rapid growth during infancy, and gastrointestinal blood loss can lead to iron deficiency.[15] Increased growth and poor dietary iron intake are of primary concern.

There are numerous factors associated with iron deficiency. The incidence is higher among lower socioeconomic groups, and the prevalence is greater in black than white children. Diet is also important. Children receiving cow's milk exclusive of other foods during the first year of life are at highest risk for developing iron deficiency anemia. The iron content of cow's milk is low, and what is available is poorly absorbed. Additionally, up to 50% of all infants fed cow's milk develop iron deficiency that is exacerbated by gastrointestinal

Table 13-4. Iron content and absorption of various milks

	Absorption (%)	Iron content
Breast milk	50	0.8 mg/qt
Iron-fortified formulas	5-10	12 mg/qt
Cow's milk	10	0.5 mg/qt

bleeding caused by milk protein.[2] The use of iron-fortified formulas during the first year of life usually prevents development of iron deficiency anemia. Breast feeding also protects against iron deficiency because the iron in breast milk is more readily absorbable by the gut mucosa. Table 13-4 demonstrates iron content and rate of absorption of various forms of milk.[16]

Term infants should take in 1 mg/kg/day of elemental iron beginning at 4 months of age.[2] Iron stores present at birth are sufficient to supply iron needs. A dose of 10 to 15 mg/day of oral iron is sufficient to provide this requirement and maintain a normal hemoglobin, since only 10% of the oral preparation is actually absorbed.[2]

Growth. Rapid growth is characteristic of infancy and adolescence. Therefore the incidence of iron deficiency is greater during these years. During the first year of life, the birth weight of a normal infant will increase by at least 300%. Blood volume and iron stores are proportional to body weight; hence each kilogram of weight gain increases the need for iron by 35 to 45 mg. During the first year of life, approximately 200 mg of iron is needed to infiltrate and maintain adequate iron stores. Rapid growth may lead to depletion of these stores predisposing infants of low birth weight and/or premature infants, twins or multiple births to iron deficiency. Puberty increases iron requirements to 0.5 mg/day of elemental iron for boys and 0.6 mg/day of elemental iron for girls. Adolescent females naturally have higher needs to compensate for menstrual losses.[2]

Blood loss. Blood loss predisposes an individual to the development of iron deficiency anemia. Pre-natal blood loss may occur transplacentally (by twin to twin transfusion), intraplacentally, or retroplacentally.[2] Postnatally, hemorrhage usually does not cause iron deficiency, since the blood from internal bleeding is reabsorbed and the iron reused. However, if bleeding is external, for example from the umbilicus or into the gut, it can lead to iron deficiency during early infancy.

Hemorrhage in later infancy and childhood can be occult or obvious. As noted above, as many as 50% of infants with iron deficiency have guaiac positive stools. Blood loss is thought to be caused by effects of iron deficiency on the mucosal lining cells. This creates a cycle in which dietary deficiency of iron causes mucosal damage that then leads to worsened anemia from gastrointestinal blood loss. Severe iron deficiency may also induce an enteropathy known as the "leaky gut" syndrome in which numerous blood and red blood cells are lost.[15]

Ingestion of cow's milk should be considered as the cause of iron deficiency with any of the following clinical situations[18]:

Consumption of 1 quart or more of cow's milk per day

Iron deficiency anemia coexisting with hypoproteinemia and hypocupremia

Iron deficiency anemia occurring in the absence of low birth weight, poor iron intake, or rapid growth

Iron deficiency anemia recurring after an initial hematologic response

Rapid onset of iron deficiency anemia

A less than optimum response to treatment with iron

Consistently positive guaiac stools in the absence of gross bleeding

Return of gastrointestinal function and alleviation of anemia after discontinuing cow's milk

Pulmonary hemosiderosis, another cause of iron deficiency should be considered when chronic pulmonary disease and hypochromic anemia coexist.[15] In this disease chronic bleeding into the lung parenchyma causes dyspnea, fever, cough, and pallor.

Goodpasture's syndrome has features of pulmonary hemosiderosis, including iron deficiency anemia in association with glomerulonephritis. The diagnosis of Goodpasture's syndrome should be suspected when the symptoms of pulmonary hemosiderosis accompany proteinuria, hematuria, and progressive renal failure.[15]

Clinical manifestations. Iron deficiency anemia is a major system disorder rather than a purely hematologic condition associated with anemia. Early stages of iron deficiency anemia have no clearly identifiable signs and symptoms. Irritability, listlessness, and pallor usually occur only after the hemoglobin drops. Pallor of the skin and mucous membranes with or without splenic enlargement may be the only clinical findings. However, other symptoms of iron deficiency anemia that are not infrequently observed in children with iron deficiency are discussed in the following sections.

Anorexia. Lack of appetite is prevalent in children demonstrating iron deficiency and may occur early in the disease process. Once iron is implemented in the daily diet, a clearly demonstrated improvement in appetite and weight gain follows. The perversion of appetite to purposeful and consistent ingestion of unsuitable substances is known as pica. It is commonly seen with iron deficiency anemia. Numerous etiologic factors (nutritive, psychologic, socioeconomic, cultural, and organic) have been implicated in pica. Numerous studies indicate that pica can be cured with the implementation of iron therapy.

Gastrointestinal effects. A generalized malabsorption syndrome has been seen in iron deficiency anemia. Guaiac positive stools are present in up to 50% of these children. This exudative enteropathy, which leaks red cells, plasma proteins, albumin, immune globulins, copper, and calcium, can be completely corrected by iron administration.

Central nervous system. Weakness, fatigue, and lack of ability to concentrate are hallmarks of iron deficiency anemia. Iron deficiency is thought to impair the development of the CNS and cause behavioral changes in early childhood.[19] It is hypothesized that iron deficiency in early life may impair DNA synthesis, thus impeding normal neuronal growth and myelinization.[18] Also several of the enzymes involved in neurotransmission (e.g.,

monoamine oxidase) are iron dependent. Behavioral observations and observed low performance scores observed in iron-deficient children may be related to a reduction in monoamine oxidase activity. Iron deficiency also leads to a buildup of certain porphyrin precursors of heme, which may cause behavioral changes.[15] Therefore these collective biochemical defects resulting from iron deficiency during the first 2 years of life may greatly jeopardize the child's cognitive development.

Cardiovascular system. Iron deficient children tolerate extremely low hemoglobin levels (<4 g/dl) without apparent clinical symptomatology.[5]

Musculoskeletal system. Roentgenographic changes in the skull and metacarpal bones have been demonstrated in children with iron deficiency. These features vary from moderate widening of the skull to widening of the diploic space with prominent vertical structures.[2] The bony changes of the skull are radiographically identical with the "hair standing on end" appearance seen in children with chronic hemolytic anemias and thalassemias. Such radiologic abnormalities are seen more commonly in infants of low birth weight. Associated protein deficiency may also be a contributing factor in roentgenographic changes seen in iron deficiency anemia.

Laboratory findings. The red blood cells of an iron deficient patient are hypochromic and microcytic. MCHC is less than 30%. MCV, associated with a low serum transferrin saturation is usually less than 70 fl. The MCH is less than 27 pg (Table 13-5).

Microcytes, poikilocytes, elliptical cells, and target cells are present on the smear. Basophilic stippling may occur. The platelet count is variably normal or increased.

Erythroid hyperplasia is seen with an increased number of polychromatophilic normoblasts. There is a decrease of iron granules in the normoblasts and absence of stainable iron in the marrow.

Serum iron represents an equilibrium between iron entering and leaving the circulation.[2] The total iron binding capacity is usually a sensitive indicator of iron status and reflects the capacity of the protein

Table 13-5. Diagnostic tools iron deficiency anemia

Diagnostic tools	Iron deficiency anemia
Blood smear	Hypochromic, microcytic
MCV	<70 fl
MCH	<27 pg
MCHC	<30%
Bone marrow	Erythroid hyperplasia, unstainable iron
Serum iron	Decreased
Iron-binding capacity	Increased
Transferrin saturation	Decreased
Ferritin	Decreased
Erythrocyte porphyrin	Elevated
Iron absorption	Increased
Response to oral iron	Usually with 72 hours

transferrin to bind more elemental iron. With increasing iron deficiency, the serum iron decreases, and the iron binding rises. The serum iron-TIBC ratio reflects the extent of transferrin saturation. When transferrin saturation drops below 15% to 16%, iron shortage inhibits hemoglobin production. Serum iron and transferrin saturation vary widely depending on age, sex, diurnal, and dietary factors.[1] Serum iron levels are usually <16 mcg/dl in a child who has severe iron deficiency (normal level is approximately 120 mcg).[1]

Serum ferritin is an indicator of the level of body iron stores. Plasma ferritin levels from 6 months to 15 years of age, average 30 mg/ml.[15] Ferritin levels may be more indicative of the degree of anemia.

Free erythrocyte porphyrin (FEP) is a measurement of the amount of porphyrin precursors that have not been converted into heme. Therefore disturbances in heme synthesis will cause FEP to be elevated in both iron deficiency and lead poisoning, with the latter having much higher values.[2] The erythrocyte porphyrin—hemoglobin ratio and ferritin-FEP ratio are helpful in identifying iron deficiency anemia. Concentration of erythrocyte porphyrin also correlates with the amount of stainable iron in the marrow.[2]

On establishment of the diagnosis of iron deficiency, iron supplementation should be initiated. A baseline reticulocyte count may be obtained so that a rise in this count early on in therapy can be used to ensure proper response and/or compliance with therapy. Most children will respond to oral ferrous sulfate at a dose of 1.5 mg/kg/dose three times a day.[15] Administration of doses much larger than this increase side effects (constipation, diarrhea, nausea), without furthering a hematologic response.

Administration of iron causes the stools to blacken in color. Liquid preparations of iron may stain the teeth, and instruction should be given to brush the teeth after each administration. Parents should be prepared for these side effects, but it should be emphasized that they are temporary.

Ferrous sulfate or ferrous gluconate tablets may be preferred in older children, since they usually result in fewer side effects (i.e., gastric irritation, nausea, vomiting). The tablets should be taken three times a day at mealtime. When side effects of nausea, vomiting, and diarrhea occur, the parents should be instructed to omit the iron for one day and then resume it to continue treatment.

Therapeutic doses of iron should be continued for 6 to 8 weeks after restoration of hemoglobin to a normal level. Initial response can be observed by a reticulocytosis occurring 2 to 3 days after initiation of iron with a peak rise at 7 to 10 days. Hemoglobin response to iron therapy is brisk, rising at a rate of 0.25 to 0.4 g/dl a day during the first 7 to 10 days of iron therapy.[1]

A substantial increase in hemoglobin should occur within 3 to 4 weeks after initiation of iron. Failure to achieve a level around 11 g/dl indicates a need for further investigation.

Prevention of iron deficiency anemia. Recognition of the numerous factors predisposing to the development of iron deficiency may allow for preventive efforts to be undertaken. Low birth weight infants gain weight more quickly than term infants and therefore have a higher iron requirement. Iron-fortified formulas are needed if the infant is not being breast fed. Cow's milk should not be substituted for formulas during the child's first year of life. Careful examination of children at risk for development of iron deficiency should be performed. Evaluation should include a complete dietary history, assessment of growth patterns, inquiry concerning blood loss or history of pica, and a complete physical examination.

Folic acid deficiency

Folic acid is an essential vitamin for normal hematopoiesis. The minimum daily requirements are 50 to 75 μg for adults and 25 to 50 μg for children.[15] Absorption occurs throughout the small intestine. Folic acid is stored primarily in the liver, but stores are rarely sufficient for more than a few months. Primary causes of folic acid deficiency are inadequate intake, malabsorption, increased requirement of excretion, or inadequate metabolism.

Inadequate intake. Folates are found in numerous foods. A normal diet contains 1 to 1.2 mg/day of folate. Foods high in folic acid include fresh green and yellow leafy vegetables, liver, kidney, legumes, nuts, citrus fruits, and berries. Cow's milk is a poor source of folic acid. Breast milk, however, provides sufficient folate during infancy, since it contains approximately 25 μg folate/liter.[15] Goat's milk is extremely low in folate, causing nutritional folate deficiency in countries where goat's milk is given to infants and children.

Lack of folate in the daily diet often results from a loss of the vitamin during cooking rather than from not eating folate-containing foods. Cooking, canning, or other means of heat processing destroys 50% to 95% of the folate contained in food.

Malabsorption. Intestinal malabsorption caused by chronic diarrheal states such as tropical sprue, gluten intolerance, and idiopathic steatorrhea lead to folic acid deficiency. Folate deficiency also causes changes in the intestinal mucosa, further inhibiting absorption. Active Crohn's disease may create a deficiency of folate as a result of poor intake and increased requirements because of malabsorption.[15] Anticonvulsant medications, especially phenytoin, may cause folate deficiency by unknown mechanisms. Congenital malabsorption

of folate has been described in a few patients. These infants have a defect in folic acid absorption with otherwise normal gastrointestinal absorption.

Increased requirement or excretion. Premature infants are especially at risk for development of folate deficiency, since they have increased requirements for rapid growth and low folate stores. Pregnant women are likewise at risk, since they require three to six times the normal daily folate requirement. Folate deficiency is most commonly seen in patients who are also iron deficient, in twin pregnancies, when serum and red cell folate levels are low in early pregnancy, or in multiparous females.

Hemolytic anemias commonly cause folate deficiency, particularly when there is associated ineffective erythropoiesis. The thalassemias are primary examples. Various infections have also been associated with folate deficiency. Patients with lymphoma and leukemia have an increased demand for folic acid, as do patients with extensive skin diseases. Deficiency in the latter group may be attributable to or be associated with intestinal changes causing malabsorption.

Patients undergoing hemodialysis for renal disease may lose folate from their plasma into the dialysis fluid. Heart disease may also predispose to folate deficiency because of excessive urinary excretion.[2]

Inadequate metabolism. Defects in metabolism producing folate deficiency may be congenital or acquired. Drugs that are folic acid analogues such as antimetabolites interfere with reduction of folate to its metabolically active state and produce acquired folate deficiency. Trimethoprim may also interfere with folate metabolism and in those children with limited folate reserves or poor dietary intake may produce some of the following clinical symptoms.

Clinical manifestations. Signs and symptoms of folic acid deficiency occur because the DNA of red blood cell precursors cannot divide normally. Macrocytic anemia, neutropenia, and thrombocytopenia are the ultimate consequences of this biochemical defect. Folate deficiency most frequently accompanies other superimposed illnesses (e.g., growth failure, diarrhea, or infection). Unlike the situation with vitamin B_{12} deficiency, neurologic findings are not found with folate deficiency.

Laboratory findings. Hematologic changes observed in folate deficiency are identical to those seen in vitamin B_{12} deficiency. Macrocytic anemia, neutropenia and thrombocytopenia parallel the degree of deficiency. Hypersegmentation of neutrophils on the peripheral smear in the presence of macrocytosis strongly indicates a deficiency of either B_{12} or folate or both. An average of more than 4.2 lobes/cell in 100 neutrophils is considered abnormal. Bone marrow aspiration establishes whether megaloblastosis is present.

The serum folate level is the sensitive assay for the presence of folate (folic acid) deficiency. Levels below 3 ng/ml are low, 3 to 5 ng/ml are borderline, and 5 to 6 ng/ml are normal.[15]

Red cell folate, more truly reflective of the hematologic abnormalities, is low in children with folate deficiency (normal range 160 to 640 ng/ml).[15] Red cell folate is also abnormal in about 60% of patients with vitamin B_{12} deficiency, particularly in patients with severe anemia (Table 13-6). Increased red cell folate occurs in patients with reticulocytosis from hemolysis or hemorrhage, since reticulocytes contain more folic acid than mature cells.

Treatment. Treatment of children with established folate deficiency includes correction of the folate deficiency by dietary supplementation, correction of the underlying etiology, if possible (e.g., antibiotic treatment for infection-induced malabsorption) and follow-up evaluation to monitor status.

Treatment with 100 to 200 μg of folic acid daily for 7 to 14 days is usually sufficient to correct the hematologic abnormality. Most commonly, 5 mg orally is used, since commercial tablets are available at this dose. However, to adequately replete folate stores, supplementation for several months may be required. An improved diet is encouraged and improvement of status of the underlying disease is sought. When poor dietary intake is the primary cause of the deficiency, dietary education should be an essential part of treatment.

The individual usually improves within 1 to 2 days as evidenced by improved appetite. Reticulocytosis begins in 2 to 4 days and reaches a peak production by 1 week. Leukocytosis and thrombocytosis parallel the reticulocytosis. Megaloblastic changes in the marrow diminish within 1 to 2 days.

Vitamin B_{12} deficiency

Vitamin B_{12}, essential for a number of biochemical reactions within the body, is present in most foods; hence, dietary insufficiency is rare. Vitamin B_{12} is dependent for its absorption on a glycoprotein (intrinsic factor) secreted by the gastric mucosa. The B_{12}-intrinsic factor complex passes to the terminal ileum where specific absorptive sites exist.[15] In the presence of the intrinsic factor and calcium, vitamin B_{12} traverses the intestinal mucosa and enters the bloodstream. The absorption of B_{12} sets up several potential mechanisms by which B_{12} deficiency can occur:

1. Inadequate intake
2. Inadequate secretion of intrinsic factor by the gastric mucosa
3. Consumption or inhibition of the B_{12}-intrinsic factor complex
4. Abnormalities involving receptor sites in the terminal ileum

Dietary insufficiency. Dietary deficiency is rare unless the individual is a strict vegetarian, since eggs, meat, or other animal products have the chief sources of this vitamin. Infants breast fed by vitamin B_{12} deficient mothers may also develop B_{12} deficiency. This infantile deficiency is characterized by developmental retardation or delay, megaloblastic anemia, and hyperpigmentation of the skin and mucosa. This syndrome is reversible with supplementation of B_{12} only if CNS damage has not occurred.

Defective absorption. Pernicious anemia, which is megaloblastic anemia resulting from absence of intrinsic factor leading to malabsorption of B_{12}, is rare in infants and adults.[20] Congenital pernicious

Table 13-6. Clinical characteristics of dietary B_{12} and folate deficiencies

	Folic acid deficiency	B_{12} deficiency
Etiology	Inadequate intake, defective absorption, increased requirements, disorders of metabolism, increased excretion	Inadequate intake, failure to secrete intrinsic factor, failure of absorption in small intestine, competition for B_{12}, defective transport, disorders of metabolism
Foods	Green and yellow vegetables, legumes, nuts, liver, fruits, cereals	Animal origin only—liver, meat, fish, dairy products
Cooking effect	May destroy completely	Little or no effect
Daily requirement	100 μg	1-2 μg
Normal daily intake	600-700 μg	3-30 μg
Body stores	6-20 mg (4 months)	3-5 mg (2-4 years)
Absorption Site	Duodenum and jejunum	Terminal ileum
Mechanism of absorption	Deconjugation, reduction, and methylation	Gastric intrinsic factor
Clinical findings in deficient patients	Superimposed illnesses, growth failure, diarrhea, infection	Glossitis—("beefy red" tongue), CNS changes; paresthesias; diarrhea; skin pigmentation; fever; palpable spleen
Laboratory findings		
Peripheral smear	Oval macrocytes; variation of size and shape of red cells; Hypersegmentation of neutrophils; leukopenia and thrombocytopenia in proportion to anemia	Oval macrocytes, variation of size and shape of red cells; hypersegmentation of neutrophils; leukopenia and thrombocytopenia in proportion to anemia
Bone marrow	Hypercellular with megaloblastic changes of erythroid cells; lowered myeloid-erythroid ratio; identical to B_{12} deficiency	Hypercellular with megaloblastic changes of erythroid cells; lowered myeloid-erythroid ratio; identical to folate deficiency
MCV	110 to 140 fl	110 to 140 fl
Serum vitamin B_{12}	Low or normal	Less than 100 pg/ml
Serum folate	3 ng/ml or lower	Normal or high >5 ng/ml
Red cell folate	Low	Low in 60% of patients
Schilling test	Normal 10%-35% excretion	<3% excretion in 24 hours

anemia is a rare autosomal recessive disorder manifested by megaloblastic anemia developing before 3 years of age.[15] Gastric mucosa of these patients is normal with no active intrinsic factor being found in gastric secretions. Types of juvenile pernicious anemias include the following: autoimmune pernicious anemia with gastric atrophy, congenital absence of intrinsic factor and low incidence of parietal cell antibody in the serum; autoimmune pernicious anemia secondary to endocrinopathies (e.g., hypoparathyroidism, myxedema, or Addison's disease) and pernicious anemia secondary to IgA deficiency. The latter deficiency persists despite B_{12} therapy and has the classic findings seen in the other types of juvenile pernicious anemias.[21]

Gastric problems which necessitate gastrectomy may also cause vitamin B_{12} deficiency by removing the source of intrinsic factor. Megaloblastic anemia usually occurs 2 to 8 years after the gastrectomy has been performed.

Failure of absorption of the intrinsic factor— vitamin B_{12}. Intrinsic factor receptors exist in the small intestine and play a major role in absorption of B_{12}.[2] Abnormally structured intrinsic factor proteins have been demonstrated in some individuals causing malabsorption of B_{12}. Furthermore, abnormalities in the ileal uptake of vitamin B_{12} have been described in some families. Tests including gastric biopsy, gastric acid, and intrinsic factor secretions are typically normal; yet intrinsic factor– B_{12} complex is not absorbed when an ileal defect is the cause.[15] Ingestion of chelating agents such as EDTA also interferes with vitamin B_{12} absorption in the terminal ileum, since it is a calcium-dependent mechanism.

Small intestinal diseases leading to generalized malabsorption or ileal resection will cause B_{12} deficiencies. Crohn's disease and other inflammatory disorders of the ileal mucosa impair B_{12} absorption and also may necessitate ablative bowel surgery.[2] Severe chronic pancreatitis has also been known to cause vitamin B_{12} absorption by lowering the pH in the ileum.

A disease entitled "blind-loop syndrome" produces symptoms of diarrhea, steatorrhea, weight loss, and cramping associated with vitamin B_{12} deficiency and anemia. This syndrome results from anatomic abnormalities of the small intestine and is thought to be caused in part by intestinal stasis with bacterial overgrowth resulting in use of B_{12} by intestinal bacteria.[21]

TCII (Trancobalamin II), is the principal transport system of vitamin B_{12}. Its deficiency, an autosomal recessive disease, is a potentially fatal cause of malabsorption in infancy. Within 1 month of age, infants with this deficiency demonstrate vomiting and diarrhea, failure to thrive, and pancytopenia with megaloblastic changes. Therapy includes massive doses of vitamin B_{12}.[1]

Once vitamin B_{12} is taken into the cell it must be converted into an active form. Abnormalities at a cellular level may result in alterations of activity of enzymes for the activation. In some patients, these essential enzymes have been absent or unable to be formed.[1]

Clinical manifestations. Onset of vitamin B_{12} deficiency is insidious. Pallor, apathy, fatigue, and anorexia occur early. A common feature is glossitis with the presence of a beefy red sore tongue with papillary atrophy. Diarrhea, episodic or profuse, frequently accompanies these symptoms.

Paresthesias may be present, but the other characteristic CNS symptoms are not as frequently observed in children as in adults. These include difficulty in walking and manual manipulation. The symptoms arise because of the B_{12}-induced peripheral neuropathy that may result in degeneration of the posterior and lateral tracts of the spinal cord.[1] Lower extremities are usually more severely affected than the upper extremities with a noted loss of position and vibration sense, ataxic gait, positive Romberg's signs, and development of a hyperreflex spastic paresis. Flaccid weakness may also occur.

Pigmentation of the skin from mild jaundice when combined with pallor caused by anemia, gives the individual's skin a yellowish tint. Mild fever may be present. The spleen is palpable in approximately 50% of the severely anemic children.

Laboratory findings. Hemoglobin levels may be as low as 4 to 6 g/dl. There is marked variation of size and shape of the red cells with oval macrocytes, cell fragments, and distorted cells being seen most prominently. The MCV is between 110 to 140 fl.[1] The red cells contain normal amounts of hemoglobin for the increased volume; hence, this is usually normal. Leukopenia with hypersegmented neutrophils is common. Thrombocytopenia may be present and is in proportion to the severity of anemia.

Increased numbers of pronormoblasts and myeloblasts are present. Erythoid precursor cells have immature nuclei for the degree of cytoplasm. These are the characteristic changes of megaloblastosis.

The ineffective erythropoiesis results in shortened red cell survival and increased death of cells in the marrow.

The definitive assay for the diagnosis of B_{12}-

induced megaloblastic anemia is naturally the serum assay for the vitamin. In a deficient individual the serum vitamin B_{12} level is less than 100 pg/ml, and serum folate is usually high.[15]

The Schilling test, a urinary secretion test is widely used to establish a differential diagnosis for megaloblastic anemias. Radioactive B_{12} is given orally followed in 2 hours by intramuscular injection of nonradioactive B_{12}. All urine is collected for 24 hours. Normal individuals excrete 10% to 35% of the administered B_{12} whereas those with malabsorption of vitamin B_{12} excrete less than 3%. The Schilling test measures intrinsic factor availability and the intestinal ability to absorb B_{12}. To differentiate between the two causes, the test is repeated with the addition of purified intrinsic factor. Vitamin B_{12} malabsorption will persist despite addition of intrinsic factor if the cause is intestinal malabsorption.

Assays for intrinsic factor and parietal cell antibodies should be performed if deficiency of intrinsic factor is felt to be the source of the B_{12} deficiency. Absence of acid in gastric secretions following histamine stimulation may assist in distinguishing between the types of pernicious anemia found in children.

If intrinsic factor deficiency is ruled out as the cause of B_{12} deficiency, ileal disease should be evaluated by gastointestinal absorption studies and barium roentgenograms.

Treatment. In such conditions known to place the individual at risk for B_{12} deficiency, such as total gastrectomy or ileal resection, vitamin B_{12} should be given prophylactically. Usually B_{12} deficiency requires treatment throughout life. On confirmation of the diagnosis, several daily doses of 25 to 100 μg intramuscularly should be given initially.[1] Afterward, intramuscular injection of 500 or 1000 μg of B_{12} every 1 to 2 months is sufficient to prevent recurrence of the deficiency.

Lead poisoning

Lead is a hematologically toxic metal that continues to be a significant health problem, most commonly in young children from poor urban communities. Major sources of lead poisoning for children include lead in paints, gasoline, and food. Lead causes anemia chiefly by inhibiting the essential enzymes for heme synthesis.

Peeling paint found in old houses is a concentrated source of lead and is the *major* source of exposure in older cities. Iron deficiency–induced pica in children often potentiates this problem.

Ideally, children should have no exposure to lead in their environment! In a practical sense the maximum permissible intake in children is 30 μg/day (blood level <40 μg/dl). However, adverse effects from lead ingestion have been seen even with blood levels less than 40 μg/dl.[1]

CNS symptoms predominate following acute or chronic lead exposure. Acute ingestion results in an encephalopathy that is marked by seizures, coma, and even respiratory arrest.[2] Death may occur within 48 hours. Chronic exposure to lead presents differently, with vague symptoms of abdominal pain, vomiting, general malaise, and alterations in behavior. The transition from general good health to progressing encephalopathy is reason for lead screening in any child. Renal impairment and anemia are also common in severe lead poisoning. Clinical sequelae of lead encephalopathy is often marked with seizure disorders and behavior impairment.

Laboratory findings. A blood lead level measures absorption of excess lead from the environment. As noted, symptoms of lead poisoning can be seen at blood levels less than 40 μg/dl.[1] The encephalopathy of lead intoxication has been seen when blood lead levels are in range from 90 to 800 μg/dl. Blood lead levels over 70 μg/dl are treated as a medical emergency, even in the absence of clinical symptomatology and require chelation therapy.

FEP is reflective of the precursors of heme synthesis. In lead intoxication the enzyme blockade results in marked increase of the protoporphyrin precursors. Hence, markedly increased FEP suggests severe lead intoxication, whereas mildly increased FEP is compatible with either iron deficiency or low-grade iron exposure.

Red blood cells are small on the peripheral blood smear and are often stippled with basophilic inclusions of heme precursors.[2]

Treatment

Symptomatic children. Treatment for symptomatic children includes control of convulsions, maintenance of diuresis, and implementation of chelation therapy. Once lead intoxication is established, chelation therapy should be initiated with BAL and CaNaEDTA.[1] For acute ingestion, BAL is infused intramuscularly as the first line chelation agent at a dose of 4 mg/kg. Once treatment is started, the blood level rapidly falls, and BAL alternating with CaNaEDTA every 4 hours to a dose of BAL equalling 24 mg/kg/day and CaNaEDTA equalling 75 mg/kg/day provides maximum tolerated chelation therapy. CaNaEDTA is administered intramuscularly or intravenously with 2% procaine to avoid local severe pain. Renal toxicity is the major complication of this chelating agent.[1]

When the blood lead level falls below 60 μ/dl, BAL may be discontinued. Additional treatment for 5 days with CaNaEDTA is continued until blood lead levels are less than 40 μ/dl. Levels greater than 70 μ/dl invariably require several courses before substantial lead excretion is obtained. For chronic lead intoxication, several months of treatment with BAL and CaNaEDTA or CaNaEDTA alone may be necessary to stabilize a blood lead level below 40 μg/dl.

Asymptomatic children. Once a diagnosis of lead poisoning has been verified and a blood level is greater than 70 μg/dl, treatment should be the same for asymptomatic as for symptomatic children. Evidence for the treatment's benefit should be evaluated after an initial dose. Those children not responding to CaNaEDTA chelation therapy should be observed, and treatment should consist of removing the source of lead and observation.

Prevention and screening. Prevention of lead poisoning is the single most important treatment to prevent intoxication but will be achieved only when sources of lead are eliminated. The trend toward use of unleaded gas has assisted in decreasing lead in the air, yet most children remain at the highest risk because of family dwellings where they continue to ingest lead paint. Large scale screening programs have prevented numerous cases from becoming severe.

Education programs aimed at informing the public regarding the seriousness of lead ingestion in children remains vital for its prevention.

Copper deficiency

Copper insufficiency (hypocupremia) is seen primarily in iatrogenic dietary circumstances (e.g., intravenous hyperalimentation when copper is omitted from the infusate solution, treatment of patients with powdered milk who have severe nutritional deficiency states, or rarely in association with exudative enteropathy).[2]

Copper stores approximate 100 to 150 mg in an adult and are found primarily in the liver. Copper stores are usually five to ten times greater at birth than in the adult and do not decrease to an adult level until 5 to 15 years. Normal copper intake is 0.04 to 0.15 mg/kg/day in the growing child.

Copper deficiency is frequently seen in combination with other nutritional abnormalities, particularly iron deficiency. A low plasma copper level is the earliest manifestation. Anemia may or may not be found but when present is mild and hypochromic. Leukopenia with marked neutropenia is consistently associated with copper deficiency.

Treatment consists of 0.2 mg/kg/day of copper in the form of 0.5% copper sulfate.[2] This will result in prompt reticulocytosis and resolution of the anemia. Dietary alterations should be made to correct the copper deficiency when possible.

Anemias of chronic disease

Anemia is a common occurrence in chronic disease. Its etiology is not completely understood with potential causes being numerous, depending on the nature and extent of disease. Anemia may occur frequently in any of the following diseases[2]:

Chronic inflammatory illnesses
    Rheumatoid arthritis
    Inflammatory bowel disease
    Systemic lupus erythematosus

Sarcoidosis
Burns
Trauma
Chronic infections
    Tuberculosis
    Pyelonephritis
    Osteomyelitis
    Chronic fungal infections
    Subacute bacterial endocarditis
    Pelvic inflammatory disease
    Empyema
Other chronic disorders
    Renal disease
    Liver disease
    Endocrine disorders
    Malignant neoplastic disease

Factors involved in the pathogenesis of anemia in chronic disease include a shortened red cell survival, impaired marrow response to anemia, and impaired flow of iron to the marrow.[1] The shortened red cell survival has been documented to be caused by extracorpuscular factors. Inadequate erythropoiesis in response to this mild rate of hemolysis potentiates the onset of anemia in chronic disorders. The cause for this ineffective erythropoiesis is unclear.

Anemia of chronic disease is mild to moderate in degree. Hemoglobin ranges between 7 to 10 g/dl. This level of hemoglobin does not in itself create physical symptoms unless complicated by other problems from the underlying disorder. The anemia develops rapidly, during the first 1 to 2 months after onset of the illness. The degree of anemia correlates with the severity of the chronic disease but is usually not progressive.

Laboratory findings. Red blood cells on the peripheral smear are normocytic and normochromic. Hemoglobin is rarely <7 g/dl. Occasionally, hypochromia occurs, but marked microcytosis in the absence of iron deficiency is rarely seen. The reticulocyte count may be normal or slightly elevated but usually is not sufficient to indicate effective erythropoiesis.[22] The bone marrow is normal or has increased cellularity. Erythroid precursors are present in normal numbers.

Serum iron levels and iron-binding capacity are often decreased. Serum ferritin is high in hypochromic anemia secondary to chronic diseases as compared with being low in hypochromic anemia secondary to iron deficiency.[22]

Treatment. Treatment for anemia involves management of the underlying chronic disease. The degree of anemia is generally mild to moderate, and no specific measures should be taken. Blood transfusions are not indicated frequently, since their benefit is transient and potential complications of transfusion are not insignificant. Iron therapy is not recommended. Careful followup of the anemia should continue throughout the illness.

Sideroblastic anemia

Individuals with sideroblastic anemia have severe anemia with microcytosis and hypochromia. Erythropoiesis is essentially ineffective.[15] The anemia is not responsive to iron therapy. In some cases individuals have responded to pyridoxine, and a dose of 50 to 250 mg/day should be used to attempt a response.[2] This type of anemia may be seen in association with malignancies and inflammatory and endocrine diseases.[22] A number of drugs and toxins have been reported to induce sideroblastic anemia, the most important one being lead.

Vitamin dependency states

There is a group of rare inherited disorders that are partially corrected by large doses of vitamins, as much as ten times the normal recommended dosage. These unusual disorders include a microcytic hypochromic anemia that is pyridoxine responsive, a thiamine responsive megaloblastic anemia, and an anemia that is megaloblastic and associated with methylmalonic aciduria that is partially responsive to vitamine B_{12}.[2]

ANEMIAS CAUSED BY INCREASED DESTRUCTION
Hemolytic anemias

The hemolytic anemias consist of several disorders intrinsic to the red cell that include membrane defects, hereditary hemoglobinopathies, and congenital enzyme defects. There are also acquired hemolytic disorders, caused by extrinsic factors such as drugs, bacteria, toxins, warm and cold antibodies, and trauma. Hemolytic anemias have one feature in common: they cause premature or accelerated destruction of red cells. The most common *intrinsic* and *extrinsic* causes of hemolytic anemia are as follows:

> *Intrinsic causes of hemolytic amemia*
> Defects of red cell membrane
> > Hereditary spherocytosis
> > Hereditary elliptocytosis
> > Paroxysmal nocturnal hemoglobinuria (PNH)
> > Liver disease
>
> Enzyme defects
> > G6PD deficiency
> > Pyruvate kinase deficiency
> > Other enzyme deficiencies
>
> Hemoglobinopathies (see chapters 15 and 16)
> > Sickle cell syndromes
> > Other abnormal hemoglobins
> > Thalassemias
>
> *Extrinsic causes of hemolytic anemias*
> Anti–red cell antigen (warm reacting antibodies IgG)
> > Idiopathic acquired autoimmune hemolytic anemia (AIHA)
> > AIHA associated with collagen vascular disease
> > AIHA associated with malignancies
> > AIHA associated with infectious diseases
> > Drug-related AIHA
>
> Anti–red cell antigen (cold reacting antibodies IgM)
> > Idiopathic cold agglutinin disease (CAD)
> > CAD associated with infections
> > CAD associated with lymphoproliferative disorder
> > Toxins, chemicals, animal venoms inducing CAD
>
> Other
> > Turbulent flow over prosthetic heart valves
> > Microangiopathic hemolytic anemia secondary to vascular injury (e.g., disseminated intravascular coagulation, [DIC], TTP, HUS)
> > Hypersplenism
> > Burns

Defects of red cell membrane. The red blood cell has numerous demands placed on it during its 120-day life span. It must maintain its structural integrity and still be able to alter its shape to squeeze through small capillaries. It must survive both the turbulent flow through a beating heart and the labyrinthine splenic red pulp. Inherited disor-

ders of the red cell membrane often cause a shortened red blood cell life span because of susceptibility to hemolysis from these peripheral stresses.

Hereditary spherocytosis. Hereditary spherocytosis, one of the most common inherited hemolytic anemias, is inherited as an autosomal dominant condition with variable degrees of expression. The red blood cell membrane surface is structurally decreased relative to the cell volume, producing an inflexible sphere. This sphere is able to deliver oxygen but is much more easily trapped in the red pulp of the spleen than are normal biconcave discoid red blood cells. So impeded, they are then destroyed by reticuloendothelial cells.

There is a wide variability in the clinical severity of hereditary spherocytosis. The most commonly identified features of hereditary spherocytosis include anemia, jaundice, and splenomegaly. The disease often presents in the newborn period as severe hyperbilirubinemia, often requiring exchange transfusion.[23]

During childhood and adolescence, jaundice is slight and often precipitated by infection. Anemia is usually mild, but the red blood cell volume may fall precipitously from severe hemolysis during periods of splenic sequestration. Modest splenomegaly is often present. Splenic size does not correlate with severity of disease. Many patients with hereditary spherocytosis who have mild anemia may go undetected until adulthood.

Leg ulcers, rare in children, occur commonly in later life. Cholestasis from gallstones is a frequent complication attributable to the chronic hemolytic state.

Aplastic crisis is a serious complication of any congenital hemolytic anemia. This event occurs most commonly in early childhood. It presents as a sudden cessation of red cell production by the bone marrow, which when combined with a shortened red cell survival, results in a rapid drop in hemoglobin and hematocrit, resulting in severe anemia.[15] Onset of aplastic crisis is rapid and often life threatening. The bone marrow arrest may persist for 1 to 2 weeks after onset, necessitating transfusion support and close cardiovascular monitoring of the child.

LABORATORY FINDINGS. The hemoglobin of most children with hereditary spherocytosis is between 7 and 10 g/dl. Hypoplastic crisis can drop the hemoglobin to 2 to 3 g/dl. Reticulocyte count is elevated and ranges from 3% to 15%, correlating inversely with the hemoglobin if bone marrow production is normal. Peripheral blood smear shows a predominance of spherocytes that have a decreased diameter and absence of central pallor. However, in one fourth of patients the smear may appear normal.[24] MCV is usually reduced, and the MCHC is greatly increased from 35% to 38%.

Examination of the bone marrow reveals normoblastic hyperplasia. No spherocytes are seen, since the defect of hereditary spherocytosis is found only in circulating red blood cells.[4] Stainable iron tends to be increased.

The osmotic fragility test is a most useful tool in detecting the presence of spherocytes in the peripheral blood. When whole blood from patients with hereditary spherocytosis is incubated at 37° C (98.6° F) for 24 hours, the red cells will become even more spherocytic. Furthermore, when red blood cells are challenged with a saline solution, the cells lyse more readily than do normal erythrocytes.[25]

For the autohemolysis test, cells are incubated at 37° C for 48 hours in isotonic sodium chloride; 10% to 50% of the erythrocytes from patients with hereditary spherocytosis will lyse, compared to a much smaller percentage of normal red blood cells. With the addition of glucose or adenosine triphosphate (ATP), the extent of abnormal autohemolysis will decrease.[7]

TREATMENT. Splenectomy is the treatment of choice in older children. Following splenectomy, the red cell life span returns to normal, hyperbilirubinemia is resolved (eliminating the risk of gallbladder disease), typical hypoplastic crises cease to exist, the reticulocyte count returns to normal, and the anemia is resolved. In children less than 5 years of age, splenectomy should be delayed if at all possible because of the significant risk of life-threatening bacterial infection after splenectomy in this age group.

All patients should be evaluated for gallstones before surgery even if they are asymptomatic. If gallstones are present, a cholecystectomy is performed at the time of splenectomy. Prophylactic folic acid should be given until the splenectomy is performed because of rapid cell turnover, which results in increased folic acid requirements.

Approximately 3.5% of splenectomized patients with hereditary spherocytosis will develop life-threatening septicemia. Sixty percent of these individuals die from their infection. Immunization with pneumococcal vaccine (Pneumovax 0.5 ml subcutaneously) is essential to prevent development of infections in the splenectomized patients, since the most frequent organism causing sepsis is *Streptococcus pneumoniae*. Hematologists agree that children who undergo a splenectomy before age six should receive prophylactic antibiotics, although there is no data to support this approach. Pen-Vee-K at a dose of 250 mg twice a day is recommended in children under 6 years of age. Emphasis must be placed on the importance of parents seeking immediate medical intervention for their child with hereditary spherocytosis when fever develops. They must be informed that in the presence of fever following splenectomy the child needs immediate assessment to rule out infection.

Hereditary elliptocytosis. Hereditary elliptocytosis is a disorder of the membrane skeleton that results in red cells taking on an oval, pencil or cigar-shaped appearance. The disease appears worldwide and is more common in Europeans and American blacks.[2] The common type of hereditary elliptocytosis is inherited as a dominant autosomal condition with complete penetrance. There is clinical heterogeneity of the disease. Most often, there is little evidence of hemolytic anemia, and individuals are clinically indistinguishable from normal.

As noted, most patients with hereditary elliptocytosis are symptom free with only 12% having clinical evidence for hemolytic anemia. Symptomatic individuals have the same clinical manifestations as those seen in hereditary spherocytosis.

LABORATORY FINDINGS. Elliptocytes, comprising 25% to 90% of the red cells[15] in the blood smear, are elongated or oval cells. MCHC is normal. In the presence of increased hemolysis, spherocytes and fragmented cells may also be seen.

A small percentage of the cells may appear with increased osmotic fragility after incubation. Slightly increased autohemolysis that corrects with the addition of glucose or ATP may also be seen in those patients with clinical hemolysis.

As in patients with hereditary spherocytosis, transfusion, splenectomy, and prophylactic folic acid administration are indicated therapeutic measures for those individuals who have hemolysis.

Hereditary stomatocytosis. Hereditary stomatocytosis is a rare disorder characterized by hemolytic anemia of variable severity. It has an autosomal dominant mode of inheritance and mimics hereditary spherocytosis.

Clinical manifestation of this disease includes mild jaundice at birth and splenomegaly first seen at 6 months of age, becoming increasingly significant by 3 to 4 years of age. Pallor and jaundice are associated with onset of infections as seen with other red cell membrane disorders.

LABORATORY FINDINGS. The peripheral smear indicates an increased number of stomatocytes, which are unusually shaped red cells with a linear slitlike area of central pallor. Reticulocytosis is often present.

There is an increase in osmotic fragility and autohemolysis.

TREATMENT. There is marked variability in severity of anemia, length of red cell survival, and splenic sequestration.[2] Some patients show improvement following splenectomy, whereas others continue to have a mild hemolytic anemia not severe enough to require surgical intervention. Increased occurrence of gallstones may be seen in the latter group.

Paroxysmal nocturnal hemoglobinuria. Paroxysmal nocturnal hemoglobinuria (PNH) is a rare disorder of the hematopoietic stem cell that results in the production of defective red blood cells and platelets. There is a defect of a red cell membrane protein that results in abnormal interaction with serum complement in such a way as to make the membrane susceptible to hemolysis.[2] Because of the effect on the red blood cell membranes, it is often grouped with other diseases of red cell membranes.

Patients may initially have hemoglobinuria that is usually worse at night. A chronic unexplained anemia may occur, and over a period of years some patients develop pancytopenia and marrow aplasia. Hemolysis and iron wasting through the kidneys results in iron deficiency.

Thrombotic or embolic events are commonly seen associated complications. Hepatic, portal, cerebral, or other venous thromboses have occurred. Associated abdominal and back pain is also thought to be secondary to small venous thromboses.

LABORATORY FINDINGS. The disease is characterized by the ability of acidified normal serum to lyse PNH cells known as the Ham's test.[7] Normal cells will not lyse under identical conditions.

Sucrose lyse test is performed by placing cells and small amounts of serum in isotonic sucrose. Sensitive PNH cells lyse, whereas normal red blood cells do not.

TREATMENT. There is no treatment for PNH. Packed red blood cell transfusion may be required; however, washed packed red blood cells should be administered carefully, since transfusions have been known to precipitate hemolytic and thrombotic events.[7] Iron therapy, while necessary, may also induce hemolysis, and caution must be exercised in repleting the iron stores. Androgens, steroids, and splenectomy have been used with varying degrees of success.

Mildly affected patients tend to be asymptomatic, whereas more severely affected patients often suffer morbidity from the noted complications. The majority of these children will survive well into adulthood.

Acanthocytosis: "spur cell anemia." Acanthocytosis or spur cell anemia is caused by abnormal lipid metabolism seen in severe liver disease that results in accumulation of cholesterol and phospholipid on the red cell membrane.[25] A similar congenital acanthocytosis is seen in children with a betalipoproteinemia. Hemolysis in the latter is usually less, and other symptoms referrable to abnormal lipid metabolism usually distinguish this entity from the isolated red blood cell abnormality.

Spur cell anemia in adults is most commonly seen in alcoholic cirrhosis. It also may be associated with metastatic liver disease, hepatitis, and Wilson's disease.[2]

Patients initially have a moderate anemia with a hematocrit from 20% to 30%. Jaundice, while often present, usually is secondary to underlying liver disease. Splenomegaly is a common finding.

There are usually greater than 20% acanthocytes on the peripheral smear. These appear as small red cells with thorny projections. Hyperbilirubinemia is present in conjunction with elevated liver function tests or the primary manifestations of severe hepatic dysfunction. Red cell life span is greatly reduced as a result of splenic sequestration.

Treatment of acanthocytosis caused by severe liver disease remains a dilemma. Splenectomy may present too much of a risk in a patient with liver disease and may not be wise in an already severely debilitated patient. If possible, treatment of the underlying disorder should improve the anemia. Otherwise, support with red cell transfusions may be used as necessary.

Erythrocyte enzyme disorders. Erythrocyte enzyme deficiencies encompass a varied group of red cell disorders, most of which are associated with chronic hemolysis and nonspecific changes in red cell morphology. To understand the pathophysiology of enzyme disorders, one must understand the metabolism of red blood cells. Mature red blood cells lack mitochrondria and are incapable of making protein. Hence, enzymes in circulating red blood cells cannot be repleted.

Enzyme abnormalities are a result of progressive instability as the red cells begin to age. The lack of mitochondria precludes alternative energy production aside from the enzyme-dependent Embden-Meyerhof and hexosemonophosphate shunt pathways. Glucose is the major metabolic substrate for red blood cells in these two major pathways: the glycolytic pathway (Embden-Meyerhof anaerobic pathway) and the oxidant protective pathway (hexosemonophosphate shunt or HMP).[15] Abnormalities in the metabolism of glucose through these two pathways result in hemolytic anemia caused by shortened red blood cell survival.[26] The two most common enzyme disorders resulting in hemolytic anemia are G6PD deficiency (which alters the reduction potential of the cell by decreasing production of nicotinamide adenine dinucleotide phosphate (NADPH)-reduced glutathione that protects intracellular proteins from oxidative assult) and pyruvate kinase deficiency (which impedes the ATP energy–producing pathway that is necessary for fueling vital chemical reactions in the membrane).[26]

Glucose 6 phosphate dehydrogenase deficiency. G6PD is the most common inherited enzyme deficiency of the red cell.[7] The gene for G6PD is sex linked. It is carried on the X chromosome and fully expressed only in hemizygous males and homozygous females. In blacks the defect usually has a mild clinical presentation. Hemolysis usually occurs only following exposure to oxidant stresses such as infections, drugs, or oxidant toxins. Infectious hepatitis has been frequently associated with hemolytic episodes in blacks with G6PD. Individuals of Mediterranean descent have a much more severe course, exhibiting a chronic hemolysis and being predisposed to acute, life-threatening hemolytic anemia when exposed to significant oxidant stresses.

Severity of hemolysis is dependent on the magnitude of the oxidant stress. Heinz bodies, which are accumulations of oxidatively denatured hemoglobin, are often produced in these individuals. They in turn may adversely affect the cell membrane. Hemolysis results from the action of the spleen and reticuloendothelial system on the damaged red cell. Over 100 structural variants of the G6PD enzyme exist.[7]

In most cases, G6PD-deficient individuals are not anemic, and hemolysis is seen only intermittently with infections or drug.[7] The most common cause of hemolysis in this disorder is infection, with virtually every type of infection being implicated.

Drug-induced hemolytic episodes are seen commonly in blacks but also occur in whites. A list of these compounds associated with hemolysis in G6PD deficiency follows. A number of these less active drugs produce hemolysis only in whites, since the deficiency is more severe in this group. Clinical effects of drug ingestion are the appearance of dark urine, pallor, and jaundice. Drugs commonly causing hemolysis in G6PD patients are as follows:

> *Antipyretics and analgesics*
> Acetylsalicylic acid (aspirin)
> Acetanilid
> Acetophenetidin (phenacetin)
> Antipyrine
> Aminopyrine (Pyramidon)
> P-Aminosalicyclic acid (PAS)
> *Antibacterials*
> Sulfanilamide
> N^2- Acetylsulfanilamide
> Sulfapyridine
> Sulfacetamide (Sulamyd)
> Sulfisoxazole (Gantrisin)
> Salicylazosulfapyridine (Azulfidine)
> Sulfamethoxypyridazine (Kynex, Midicel)
> *Nitrofurans*
> Nitrofurantoin (Furadantin)
> Furazolidone (Furoxone)
> Furaltadone (Altafur)
> Nitrofurazone (Furacin)
> *Antimalarials*
> Primaquine
> Aminoquin (Pamaquine)
> Pentaquine
> Plasmoquine
> Quinocide
> Quinacrine (Atabrine)
> Quinine
> *Others*
> Sulfoxone
> Naphthalene (moth balls)
> Methylene blue
> Vitamin K
> Phenylhydrazine
> Acetylphenylhydrazine
> Tolbutamide (Orinase)
> Probenecid
> Fava Bean
> Dimercaprol (Bal)
> Chloramphenicol
> Quinidine
> Chloroquine
> Nalidixic acid (NegGram)

LABORATORY FINDINGS. Special stains of the peripheral blood smears with methylene blue or crystal violet reveal Heinz bodies during hemolytic crises. Spherocytes and cells that are "bitten" by the splenic removal of Heinz bodies are frequently seen.

There are several simple screening tests that measure for a deficiency of G6PD. Cells of an individual with G6PD contain from up to 26% normal enzymatic activity with larger amounts present in the younger red blood cells.[15] Therefore the assay may produce false-negative results when the most deficient cells have been removed by hemolysis. A more representative enzyme assay result can be obtained 2 to 3 months after the hemolytic crisis has occurred.

TREATMENT. There is no specific treatment for individuals with G6PD deficiency. Drugs that could potentially cause hemolysis should be avoided. The most common offending drugs that induce hemolysis in individuals with G6PD deficiency are sulfonamide antibiotics and antimalarial drugs.[26]

Red blood cell transfusion may be required but only in the situation when the anemia is severe enough to cause cardiovascular compromise. Splenectomy is of no benefit. Folic acid supplementation (1 mg/day) to replete folic acid stores used in expanded erythropoiesis is indicated following periods of hemolysis.

Pyruvate kinase deficiency. Pyruvate kinase deficiency is an autosomal recessive enzyme deficiency. This enzyme is responsible for glycolytic reactions necessary in ATP production so that deficiency causes abnormalities in the red cell membrane, leading to decreased deformability.

Children with homozygous pyruvate kinase deficiency may have up to 25% of the red cells exhibiting normal pyruvate kinase levels. Pyruvate kinase deficiency is a relatively rare disease but accounts for more than 90% of all glycolytic enzymopathies.

There is a wide variability in the severity of hemolysis. Generally, the patient exhibits chronic anemia, reticulocytosis, and hyperbilirubinemia.

The anemia is frequently exacerbated with onset of viral infections. When chronic hemolysis occurs, these viral episodes may cause a hypoplastic crises of the bone marrow, manifesting as a decreased reticulocyte count and increased anemia. Hence, individuals with severe pyruvate kinase deficiency are always at risk for aplastic crisis and must be observed closely during all viral infections.

A history of neonatal jaundice is common, with many patients having required exchange transfusions. Kernicterus with pyruvate kinase deficiency has been reported during the newborn period. Other individuals present with much milder symptoms and are not diagnosed until adulthood. Growth and development are frequently delayed, and bone changes characteristic of patients with an erythroblastic bone marrow may be observed.

LABORATORY FINDINGS. Examination of the peripheral smear shows a nonspherocyte anemia with macrocytes, ovalocytes, polychromatophilia, and anisocytes. There are numerous red cells that appear as acanthocytes, with projecting spicules and spines. Numerous fragmented red blood cells are seen as a result of the relative instability of the abnormal cells during their passage through the splenic red pulp.

Osmotic fragility is normal or decreased in unincubated blood samples and increased in incubated blood samples. There is an increased rate of autohemolysis without correction with glucose. When ATP is added, the rate of hemolysis decreases. Definitive diagnosis requires specific assay pyruvate for the kinase enzyme.

TREATMENT. Hemolysis does not cease following splenectomy, but the procedure may decrease its severity. Most individuals require fewer transfusions following splenectomy, and higher reticulocyte count and increased packed cell volume usually follow splenectomy in patients with pyruvate kinase deficiency. Folic acid (1 mg/day) should be administered as in other hemolytic anemias.

Immune hemolytic anemias

WARM REACTING ANTIBODIES, IgG. IgG antibodies against one of the Rh erythrocyte antigens are most commonly implicated as the cause of auto-immune hemolytic anemia.[27] The optimum temperature for activity of the antibody is 37° C (98.6° F) and for this reason this syndrome is termed *warm antibody-induced hemolysis*. These antibodies that are directed against red cell antigens bind complement and thereby induce premature destruction of normal red blood cells in the extravascular circulation (primarily in the spleen).[25]

IgG-induced hemolytic anemia occurs without any discernible underlying disease at the time of diagnosis (termed *idiopathic immune hemolytic anemia*) in 50% of patients. IgG immune hemolytic anemia has been associated with immune proliferative disorders such as lymphocytic leukemia, non-Hodgkin's lymphoma, or systemic lupus erythematosus.[27] Acute and chronic bacterial and viral infections (especially cytomegalovirus infection) have also been circumstantially implicated in IgG-induced hemolytic anemia.[28]

The clinical presentation of patients with immune hemolytic anemia will vary widely. The severity of anemia may relate to an associated disease or syndrome. The typical patient appears weak and pale and has generalized malaise. Most commonly, symptoms will have had an acute onset. Frequently there is history of a viral infection occurring 1 to 2 weeks before the onset of hemolysis. As always with severe hemolysis, jaundice develops. Splenomegaly is common.

Laboratory findings. Microspherocytic cells are frequently observed on the blood smear. The platelet count is usually normal unless there is an associated idiopathic thrombocytopenic purpura (ITP, Evan's syndrome). Erythroid hyperplasia is the hallmark of the bone marrow examination. Reticulocytosis is usually quite prominent, and the MCV from the Coulter counter is usually normal.

Warm antibody (IgG) hemolytic anemia is established by the direct Coombs' test. The Coombs' agglutination test indirectly examines the red blood cell surface for presence of bound antibody or bound complement. The direct Coombs' test uses nonspecific Coombs' antiserum, which is derived from rabbits immunized against human IgG. The Coombs' antiserum will induce agglutination of the red blood cells if there is bound IgG antibody or complement on their surface. A positive direct Coombs' test should be followed by specialized elution procedures in the blood bank to attempt to identify the specificity of the antibody if at all possible.

Treatment. Effective treatment is aimed first at control of the underlying disorder in non-idiopathic AIHA. If such therapy is unsuccessful in controlling the hemolytic process or if the patient has idiopathic AIHA, then therapy for the anemia becomes primary. It may entail any or all of the following: steroids, splenectomy, or immunosuppressive therapy. Transfusions are indicated in those circumstances when the anemia is deemed life threatening. Patients with immune hemolytic anemia are extremely difficult to cross-match, increasing the likelihood that red cells with shortened survival will be required in a condition already problematic because of short red blood cell survival. Identification of the antibody, when possible, allows selection of compatible red blood cells.[29] When such complete compatibility is not possible, least incompatible units of washed red blood cells are administered slowly and concommitantly with high-dose corticosteroids. When hemolysis is occurring rapidly, patients may need blood every 8 to 12 hours.[30]

STEROIDS. Corticosteroid administration is indicated for the treatment of IgG-mediated immune hemolytic anemia. A dose of 1 to 2 mg/kg/day prednisone or its equivalent should be initiated, increasing to 8 to 10 mg/kg/day for 5 to 7 days if necessary. Steroid therapy is thought to effect clinical improvement by decreasing the production of abnormal IgG antibody, by removing IgG antibody from the erythrocyte surface, and by interfacing with macrophage receptors responsible for erythrocyte destruction.

An effective therapeutic response is measured by a gradual rise in hemoglobin without requirement of further transfusion. When such a response is achieved, corticosteroids should be maintained for several weeks with tapering toward withdrawal requiring several months. When chronic administration of steroids are required for hemoglobin sta-

bility, an every-other-day dosing alleviates undue side effects. Many patients will continue to have a positive Coombs' test in light of improved erythrocyte survival.

SPLENECTOMY. Splenectomy is an effective mode of treatment in IgG-induced hemolytic anemia and may be required when response to corticosteroids has been unsatisfactory. Splenectomy has been shown to decrease production of IgG antierythrocyte antibody.[27]

IMMUNOSUPPRESSIVE AGENTS. Immunosuppressive drugs may be used when there has been no response to steroids or splenectomy. Immunosuppressive agents are said to decrease production of the antibody. Cyclophosphamide, azathioprine, and chlorambucil have been used.

COLD-REACTING ANTIBODIES, IgM. The cold agglutinin syndrome is caused by IgM antibody. These large antibodies bind to antigens on the red cell surface best at temperatures well below 37° C (98.6° F). IgM-induced hemolytic anemia is most commonly associated with mycoplasma pneumonia but may also occur in infectious mononucleosis, cytomegalovirus, and mumps.

Cold agglutinin syndrome has also been identified with immunoproliferative disorders, specifically chronic lymphocytic leukemia, non-Hodgkin's lymphoma, and systemic lupus erythematosus. Idiopathic cold agglutinin disease, in which there are no identifiable underlying pathologic findings, is commonly chronic in nature.

The IgM antibody in cold agglutinin disease is usually directed against the I antigen or its related antigens located in the red cell membrane. The IgM antibody is more easily fixed to the red cell antigen in the cold, 0° to 10° C. Most agglutinins have no activity above 20° C.

Signs and symptoms of hemolytic anemia secondary to an IgM antibody are similar to those caused by IgG. Likewise, symptoms associated with the underlying cause are frequently present as well.

Cold agglutinin disease may occur in association with Raynaud's phenomenon, which includes painful swelling of the ears and digits in cold weather.

The anemia is intermittent and precipitated by cold exposure. Jaundice and splenomegaly are less frequent than in IgG-induced hemolytic anemia.[15]

Laboratory findings. Peripheral blood smear findings in IgM-induced hemolytic anemia are similar to IgG induced hemolysis. Spherocytic cells are less likely to be found on the smear as compared to IgG-induced hemolytic anemia. Bone marrow smears demonstrate erythroid hyperplasia.

A cold agglutinin titer is obtained by examining the patient's plasma for agglutinating activity directed against normal erythrocytes containing the I antigen. Cold agglutinin titers in patients with IgM immune hemolysis are usually greater than 1:1000.

The direct Coombs' test is weakly positive in most patients with immune-induced hemolytic anemia.

Treatment. Specific treatment is usually not administered. Steroids, splenectomy, and immunosuppressive therapy are much less effective in cold agglutinin disease. Care must be given to prevent exposure to cold, since extreme hemolytic episodes have been noted with lowered ambient temperature.

Drug-induced hemolytic anemia. Patients with drug-induced immune hemolytic anemia have symptoms indistinguishable from patients with autoimmune hemolytic anemias. Three (3) different pathophysiologic mechanisms may result in drug induced hemolysis.[2]

First, a drug (most commonly penicillin) forms a complex with the erythrocyte surface, resulting in an antibody directed against the red cell drug complex in what is defined as a hapten complex. This response is more frequently IgG mediated and rarely develops unless patients have received more than 20 million units/day of penicillin. Diagnosis is determined by incubating the serum with donor red cells previously incubated in penicillin and examining the red cells for IgG antibody by the Coombs' test.

Second, a number of drugs, when bound to plasma proteins, function as antigens that cross-react with red blood cell antigens. The red cell antigens become innocent bystanders to antibodies directed against quinine, stibophen, chlorpromazine, sulfamides, and phenacetin or some similar drugs. The antidrug antibody reaction causes an antigen-antibody complex in the vincinity of the red cell and may cause subsequent damage to the cell.

Third, a drug-related immune hemolytic state is caused by alpha-methyldopa and dopamine. An antibody is formed against red cell antigens that closely resembles IgG-induced hemolysis. Approximately one fourth of these patients develop a positive Coombs' test for IgG. Few patients develop significant hemolysis.

Drug-induced hemolysis should be treated by discontinuing the drug, which usually results in the disappearance of the antibody. A brief course of corticosteroid therapy may be necessary initially once the drug has been discontinued.

Traumatic hemolytic anemias. Hemolytic anemia, caused by mechanical trauma to the red cell, may result in varying severity of hemolysis depending on the cause.[25] Damage to the red cells may be caused by any of the following: splenectomy, prosthetic heart valves, vasculitis, thrombotic thrombocytopenic purpura, malignant hypertension, disseminated intravascular coagulation (DIC), severe burns, and overwarmed transfused blood.[25]

In DIC and related vascular syndromes, traumatic anemia is referred to as microangiopathic hemolytic anemia and occurs because red blood cells are damaged as they are forced through tiny capillaries partially occluded by fibrin strands. Signs and symptoms vary in severity and are directly related to the underlying disease. Anemia may be intermittent and mild to severe.

The blood smear in microangiopathy hemolytic anemia confirms the diagnosis. The blood smear shows burr cells, schistocytes, helmet cells, and microspherocytes. Thrombocytopenia is present. The marrow indicates erythroid hyperplasia. In some cases elevated serum fibrin degradation products may occur, indicating DIC.

Traumatic hemolytic anemias have fragmented

cells or schistocytes on peripheral blood smear and are associated with loss of hemoglobin and hemosiderin through the urine. Concomitant iron deficiency may exacerbate the anemia and necessitate supplemental iron therapy.

Treatment involves controlling the primary disease. Supportive care is aimed at preventing complications from hemolysis.

CASE STUDY #1: ANEMIA CAUSED BY DECREASED PRODUCTION: ACQUIRED APLASTIC ANEMIA

R.K. is a 4-year-old white female with a 2- to 3-week history of increased bruising. There was no past history of bleeding problems. Past medical history was unremarkable. The admission physical examination revealed multiple areas of ecchymoses and petechiae. The peripheral blood smear revealed a hemoglobin of 6.8; hematocrit 20; white blood cell count of 2.5 with 4% neutrophils, 96% lymphocytes; and a platelet count of 9000. Reticulocyte count was 0.4. Bone marrow aspiration and biopsy was performed, revealing a markedly decreased cellularity with no tumor cells present. There were a small number of lymphocytes noted, but megakaryocytes and other precursors were completely absent. R.K. began receiving prednisone 60 mg/m², and HLA typing was performed on her parents and two brothers. There were no compatible donors. R.K. was discharged after receiving red blood cell transfusions and instructed to remain on prednisone until returning to the clinic in 1 week. At that time she completed 2 weeks of prednisone and another bone marrow aspirate and biopsy was performed. Should the bone marrow again be hypocellular, antithymocyte globulin (ATG) therapy would be considered.

CASE STUDY #2: ANEMIA CAUSED BY NUTRITIONAL DEFICIENCY: IRON DEFICIENCY ANEMIA

L.R. is a 9-month-old black male who came to the pediatric clinic with a month history of irritability, listlessness, and pallor. Significant history revealed L.R. to be receiving cow's milk since 6 months of age. Physical examination revealed pallor of the skin and mucous membranes and splenomegaly. Guaiac stool evaluation indicated the presence of blood. Height and weight for his age revealed him to be less than the 5th percentile. Examination of the peripheral blood smear showed a hypochromic, microcytic anemia with a hemoglobin of 6 g/dl, reticulocyte count of 1%, and an MCV of 71. Serum iron and ferritin levels were low, and the erythrocyte porphyrin level was elevated. The diagnosis of iron deficiency anemia was established. L.R. was begun on oral ferrous sulfate at a dosage of 1.5 mg/kg, three times a day. L.R. was placed on an iron fortified formula, which his mother was instructed to continue until after 1 year of age. L.R. returned to the clinic in 1 week, at which time his hemoglobin was 8.2 g/dl and his reticulocyte count was 12.5%. Oral iron was continued for 2 months after restoration of a normal hemoglobin level.

CASE STUDY #3: ANEMIA CAUSED BY INCREASED RED CELL DESTRUCTION: HEMOLYTIC ANEMIA

M.R. is a 3-year-old white female who was in her usual state of good health until 4 days before her hospital admission. At that time she presented with fever to 105° F (40.56 C) and a viral-like syndrome. She was seen by her family pediatrician who attributed her fever to viral illness and sent her home. The night before admission her parents noticed her urine becoming very dark, and on awakening in the morning, she was pale. Her parents immediately took her to the emergency center, where she presented as an extremely lethargic, pale child with massive hepatosplenomegaly and an S3 gallop. Her hemoglobin was 3.3, and Coombs' test was strongly positive. Her MCV was 257, with review of this extraordinary finding by peripheral smear indicating marked clumping of the red cells. There was marked polychromasia, and many nucleated red blood cells were seen. Because of her life-threatening anemia and cardiac failure, a partial exchange transfusion with 1 unit of the least incompatible type O negative washed red blood cells was performed. Transfusion was performed slowly to closely evaluate for increased hemolysis and to avoid exacerbating compromised cardiac status secondary to high output. She began receiving Solumedrol 10 mg/6 hr that evening.

NURSING CONSIDERATIONS
The child with anemia

Anemia is not a disorder but a symptom caused by an underlying disease process, requiring nursing care to assist in determining its cause, provide supportive care, carry out therapeutic treatments, and decrease tissue oxygen demands.[31] The nurse plays an integral role in establishing the cause of anemia. A careful history taken by the nurse provides additional information that is pertinent to the diagnosis. Preparation for intrusive procedures is essential for the child, since numerous laboratory tests are frequently performed during the initial diagnostic period. The nurse should be able to explain the significance of each diagnostic test, provide support by preparing the child for the test, and be physically present during the procedure to provide comfort to the child.

Minimizing tissue oxygen demands is a primary nursing responsibility with the child who has anemia. The child's ability to perform routine activities of daily living and play should be assessed. The nurse must work with the child and family to establish routine schedules that will minimize physical exertion while allowing for participation in activities essential for the child's growth and development. Close observation of cardiac complications should be made routinely. Signs and symptoms such as tachycardia, palpitations, tachypnea, breathlessness, dizziness, light-headedness, diaphoresis, and change in skin color must be observed.

Bone marrow failure

Specific nursing considerations for the child with anemia caused by bone marrow failure are numerous. The child and family are faced with a life-threatening chronic illness that will alter the entire family life-style. The nurse plays an integral role in initiating a trusting relationship between the family and the hematology team. A knowledge base of the various diseases causing bone marrow failure is essential. Specific tests required in the diagnostic workup must be explained in terms the family and child is able to understand. Reduction of red blood cells, granulocytes, and platelets may cause life-threating situations for the child, which the family must be prepared for. Teaching is a major importance to prevent complications such as infection and bleeding. Discharge planning after the child's initial diagnosis must include numerous discussions of the possible complications caused by bone marrow failure. Supportive care involves the use of blood products when other modes of treatment such as bone marrow transplantation, steroids, or androgen therapy are not effective. Complications are numerous, making it crucial for those providing supportive care to be knowledgeable concerning treatment and its side effects.

Nutritional and metabolic disturbance

Anemias caused by nutritional deficiencies or metabolic disturbances create areas of major concern for the nurse. Dietary deficiencies cause numerous problems previously discussed. Knowledge of essential nutrients and their role in promoting growth and development is of paramount importance in dealing with a child who has anemia caused by inadequate nutritional or metabolic deficiency. Careful evaluation of the child's history frequently reveals the cause of anemia. The nurses's history and assessment frequently assists in establishment of the diagnosis. Education of the family is a major aspect in treatment for anemia caused by nutrition or metabolic disturbances. The nurse must realize this teaching role as crucial and a major factor in successful treatment.

Increased red blood cell destruction

Anemias caused by increased red blood cell destruction may have an acute onset, causing a life-threatening situation within hours. This crisis causes shock and alarm in the parents who may not easily understand what has occurred. The child may be admitted critically ill. The nurse's major role at this time is to stabilize the patient, although understanding of the immediacy of the situation makes it easier for the nurse to perform certain tasks essential to the child's stabilization.

Once the immediate crisis is over, support of the parents is essential in assisting them to understand the child's illness. Anemia secondary to hemolysis is frequently a chronic illness, lending itself to the importance of teaching parents and the child about the illness. Preventive care in the hope of minimizing red blood cell destruction should be pursued by the nurse.

NURSING CARE PROTOCOL FOR THE CHILD WITH ANEMIA

Nursing diagnoses (patient problems)	Goals/objectives (patient/family will:)	Interventions (nurse will:)
1. Knowledge deficit (related to diagnosis and diagnostic workup)	Receive information related to diagnosis; express purpose of tests and their methods	Assist with and teach reasons for performing tests (laboratory tests, bone marrow examination); encourage questions regarding workup; hand out any available written material
2. Knowledge deficit (related to establishment of diagnosis)	Gain trust in the nursing staff; express concerns as to the cause of anemia; ask questions regarding the etiology of anemia	Take careful history regarding common causes of anemia; take a detailed history reviewing the following: Dietary intake Recent infections Ingestion of lead, toxic substances, pica Bowel habits, presence of frank blood or tarry stools Family history of hereditary diseases Be aware of various blood tests and their normal findings
3. Knowledge deficit (related to preparation of laboratory tests)	Demonstrate decreased level of anxiety; verbalize understanding of the importance of various diagnostic tests; be able to state method for the test	Explain the need for repeated venipunctures or fingersticks; allow child to perform venipunctures and fingersticks on dolls during play; allow older children to review slides under microscope; observe closely for decreased Hgb and Hct caused by multiple blood sampling
4. Knowledge deficit (related to specific types of anemia) Bone marrow failure	Develop basic understanding of the severity and its implications; gain knowledge regarding care	Assist in discussing failure of the marrow to produce cells causing anemia thrombocytopenia neutropenia; discuss in detail their implications and review possible

NURSING CARE PROTOCOL FOR THE CHILD WITH ANEMIA—cont'd

Nursing diagnoses (patient problems)	Goals/objectives (patient/family will:)	Interventions (nurse will:)
		complications of infection (discussed in nursing care protocol in chapter on neutropenias) and bleeding (discussed in nursing care plan in chapter on thrombocytopenia)
	Gain knowledge of side effects and requirements for home care	Prepare for discharge planning once diagnosis has been established to allow parents time to feel comfortable with home care; contact public health nurse to assist in monitoring child at home
	Re-establish patterns of daily living	Assist in communicating the child's illness to professionals; reinforce need to inform parents immediately should fever or bleeding develop
Nutritional metabolic deficiencies	Gain understanding of the cause for anemia and its necessary treatment	Assist in discussing cause of the anemia and its severity
	Be able to verbalize treatment necessary for the child (i.e., use of iron-fortified formulas in place of cow's milk in iron deficiency)	Review treatment plan with parents; give out any written information; write schedule for medications to be taken at home; contact home care agencies when necessary to ensure treatment compliance; assist in evaluating treatment plan when child returns
Increased destruction	Verbalize fears and demonstrate decreased anxiety	Assist in discussing cause of hemolysis, allowing parents to express their feelings of fear and anxiety
	Demonstrate awareness of clinical symptoms of hemolysis and ability to cope with assessing the child at home	Review signs and symptoms of rapid hemolysis to assure adequate assessment at home: Change in behavior Lack of appetite Pallor

Continued.

NURSING CARE PROTOCOL FOR THE CHILD WITH ANEMIA—cont'd

Nursing diagnoses (patient problems)	Goals/objectives (patient/family will:)	Interventions (nurse will:)
		Enlargement of spleen (swollen abdomen) Increasing lethargy Stress importance to call physician immediately if any of these symptoms occur once the child is discharged; refer to home care agencies when appropriate for close supervision
	Be able to administer steroids at home	Review schedule for steroid administration and discuss importance of its use
5. Tissue perfusion; (alteration in: cardiopulmonary)	Understand importance of determining the child's physical tolerance; be able to establish a schedule to meet physical requirements and developmental needs; demonstrate minimum side effects from decreased tissue oxygen	Assess child's level of physical tolerance; assist in daily activities the child may not be able to perform; provide play activities that promote development while providing rest and quiet; promote interaction with other children who may also require restricted activity
6. Anxiety (emotional distress related to physical limitations of anemia)	Demonstrate decreased level of anxiety; share feelings with support persons	Discuss child's irritability, short attention span, and changing moods as secondary to anemia; assist with activities before child's mood changes, and becomes fatigued; encourage support from parents while stressing independence
7. Injury: potential for: (infection)	Exhibit awareness of other complications brought on by anemia and underlying disease; demonstrate knowledge of precautions necessary to prevent complications	Observe closely for signs/symptoms of infections, fever, leukocytosis, and presence of infection; practice good hand washing; place child with noninfectious patient; maintain adequate nutrition

NURSING CARE PROTOCOL FOR THE CHILD WITH ANEMIA—cont'd

Nursing diagnoses (patient problems)	Goals/objectives (patient/family will:)	Interventions (nurse will:)
8. Injury: potential for (congestive heart failure)	Be aware of complications caused by anemia; maintain stable vital signs and adequate cardiac output	Assess signs and symptoms of heart failure from increased cardiac demands, decreased blood pressure, tachycardia, palpitations, dyspnea, diaphoresis, change in color; notify physician immediately when these symptoms are present Provide oxygen as ordered when decreased oxygen to tissue creates difficulty breathing; administer blood when ordered (see nursing care protocol on blood transfusion Chapter 24)
9. Coping, ineffective family: compromised	Demonstrate effective coping mechanisms necessary for optimum functioning at home, school, and in the community	Provide emotional support and refer to other health professionals when needed Communicate with other agencies and school to facilitate optimum care at home Stress importance of re-establishing normal life-style

REFERENCES

1. Miller, D.R., and others: Blood diseases of infancy and childhood, St. Louis, 1984, The C.V. Mosby Co.
2. Nathan, P.G., and Osky, F.A.: Hematology of infancy and childhood, vol. 1, Philadelphia, 1978, W.B. Saunders Co.
3. Anthony, C.P., and Kolthoff, N.J.: Textbook of anatomy and physiology, St. Louis, 1971, The C.V. Mosby Co.
4. Piomellin, S.: Diagnostic approaches to anemia, Pediatr. Clin. North Am. **8**(1):199, 1971.
5. Nelson, W.E., and others: Textbook of pediatrics, Philadelphia, 1979, W.B. Saunders Co.
6. Williams, W.J., and others: Hematology, New York, 1983, McGraw-Hill, Inc.
7. Reich, P.R., and Deykin, D.: Hematology and physiopathologic basis for clinical practice, Boston, 1978, Little, Brown & Co.
8. A differential for childhood anemia, Emerg. Med. **15**(2): 64, Nov. 30, 1983.
9. Alter, B.P.: Bone marrow failure in children, Pediatr. Ann. **8**(7):53, 1979.
10. Lipton, J.M., and Nathan, D.G.: Aplastic and hypoplastic anemia, Pediatr. Clin. North Am. **27**(2):217, 1980.
11. Warkentin, P.I. and others: Immunosuppressive therapy for severe aplastic anemia, Am. J. Pediatr. Hematol. Oncol. **2**(4):327, 1980.
12. Hutchinson, M.: Aplastic anemia, Nurs. Clin. North Am. **18**(3):543, 1983.
13. McIntosh, S., Berg, W.R., and Lubiniecki, A.S.: Fanconi's anemia, the preanemic phase, Am. J. Pediatr. Hematol. Oncol. **1**(2): 107, 1979.
14. Alter, B.P.: Childhood red cell aplasia, Am. J. Pediatr. Hematol. Oncol. **2**(2):121, 1980.
15. Lanzkowsky, P.: Pediatric hematology-oncology, New York, 1980, McGraw-Hill, Inc.
16. Oski, F.A.: Anemia in children, Hosp. Pract. **11**:63, 1976.
17. Wolfe, L.C., and Lux, S.E.: Nutritional anemias of childhood, Pediatr. Ann. **8**(7):38, 1979.
18. Oski, F.A., and Stockman, J.A.: Anemia due to inadequate iron sources or poor iron utilization, Pediat. Clin. North Am. **27**(2):237, 1980.
19. Iron deficiency and mental development, Nutr. Rev. **41**(8):235, 1983.
20. Maurer, H.S. and others: Pernicious anemia with persistent malabsorption of vitamin B_{12} in a child, J. Pediatr. **83**(5):832, 1973.
21. Herbert, V.: The nutritional anemias, Hosp. Pract. **68**:21, 1980.
22. Lynch, E.C., and Jackson, D.: Anemia and malignancies, Heart Lung **12**(4):447, 1983.
23. Bellingham, P.J., and Prankard, T.A.: Hereditary spherocytosis, Clin. Haematol. **4**(1):139, 1975.
24. Lux, S.E., and Wolfe, L.C.: Inherited disorders of the red cell membrane skeleton, Pediatr. Clin. North Am. **273**(2):463, 1980.
25. Forget, B.G.: Hemolytic anemias: congenital and acquired, Hosp. Pract. **15**:67, 1980.
26. Sullivan, D.W., and Glader, B.F.: Erythrocyte enzyme disorders in children, Pediatr. Clin. North Am. **27**(2):449, 1980.
27. Schreiber, A.D.: Autoimmune hemolytic anemia, Pediatr. Clin. North Am. **27**(2):253, 1980.
28. Zuelzer, W.W. and others: Autoimmune hemolytic anemia, Lancet **545**, March 6, 1980.
29. Petz, L.D.: Autoimmune hemolytic anemia, Hum. Pathol. **14**(3):251, 1983.
30. Conley, C.L. and others: Autoimmune hemolytic anemia with reticulocytopenia, JAMA **244**(15):1688, 1980.
31. Whaley, L.R., and Wong, D.L.: Nursing care of infants and children, St. Louis, 1979, The C.V. Mosby Co.

ADDITIONAL READINGS

Alter, B.P., Potter, N.U., and Li, F.P.: Classification and etiology of the aplastic anemias, Clin. Haematol. **7**:431, 1978.

Crosby, W.H.: Prescribing iron? Think safely, Arch. Intern. Med. **138**:766, 1978.

Dallman, P.R., and Siimes, M.A.: Percentile curves for hemoglobin and red cell volume in infancy and childhood, J. Pediatr. **94**:26, 1979.

Diamind, L.K., Wang, W.C., and Alter, B.P.: Congenital hypoplastic anemia, Adv. Pediatr. **22**:349, 1976.

Gross, S.J., and others: Malabsorption of iron in children with iron deficiency, J. Pediatr. **88**:795, 1976.

Li, F.P., Alter, B.P., and Nathan, D.G.: The mortality of acquired aplastic anemia in children, Blood **40**:153, 1972.

Pirofsky, B.: Clinical aspects of autoimmune hemolytic anemia, Semin. Hematol. **13**:251, 1976.

Swisher, S.N., and others: Symposium on immune hemolytic anemias, Semin. Hematol. **13**:247, 1976.

Thomas, E.D., and others: Bone marrow transplantation, N. Engl. J. Med. **292**:832, 1975.

Todd, D.: Diagnosis of haemolytic states, Clin. Haematol. **4**:63, 1975.

Worlledge, S.M.: Immune drug-induced hemolytic anemias, Semin. Hematol. **10**:327, 1973.

CHAPTER 14

Sickle cell disease

BECKY PACK and THOMAS R. KINNEY

Sickle cell disease is a generic term applied to a group of inherited hemoglobinopathies characterized by the production of hemoglobin S (Hb S). The most common forms of the disease include sickle cell anemia (Hb SS), hemoglobin SC disease (Hb SC), and the hemoglobin S beta thalassemia syndromes (Hb S beta thal). Uncommon forms of sickle cell disease include hemoglobin SD and Hb SO$_{Arab}$ disease.

Although the production of Hb S is a common feature of the sickle cell disorders, the various forms demonstrate a very wide spectrum of clinical severity. There also exists considerable variability among patients who have the same form of the disease. The impact of the condition on other health-related events such as pregnancy, anesthesia, and surgery is significant. The variability in expression and impact on other health-related events creates significant challenges to the health care provider.

This chapter reviews historic aspects of sickle cell disease and the pathophysiology, diagnostic laboratory findings, and the common clinical complications of the sickle cell syndromes and sickle cell trait. Maintenance health care and nursing considerations applicable to infants, children, and adolescents with sickle cell disease are discussed. Transfusion therapy and its complications, speculations regarding future therapies, and issues surrounding genetic counseling and screening programs also are highlighted.

HISTORICAL PERSPECTIVES

The first descriptive report of sickle cell disease appeared in 1904 and was authored by Dr. James Herrick, a Chicago physician.[1] In 1917 Emmel demonstrated that some of the blood cells sickled when sealed under glass.[2] Ten years later, Hahn and Gillespie speculated that low oxygen tension caused the cell to assume the characteristic sickle form.[3] In 1949 Pauling and Itano developed a technique for hemoglobin electrophoresis.[4] They postulated that the sickling phenomenon was produced by an abnormality within the hemoglobin molecule. It was not until 1927, however, that Ingram defined the structural abnormality in Hb S. This abnormality is a single amino acid substitution, the replacement of glutamic acid at the sixth position of the beta chain by valine.

PATHOPHYSIOLOGY

The cardinal features of most forms of sickle cell disease include chronic hemolytic anemia and organ dysfunction.

The hemolytic anemia and other manifestations of the disease can be traced ultimately to the amino acid substitution. In Hb S, valine replaces glutamic acid normally found at the sixth position of the beta chain. The net effect of this substitution is to reduce the solubility of the deoxygenated Hb S molecule within the red cell. The deoxygenated Hb S molecules polymerize, forming tactoids, which distort the shape of the red cell from a biconcave disc to the shape of a sickle. On reoxygenation, the red cell initially can resume its normal shape. After repeated cycles of sickling and unsickling, however, the cell becomes "irreversibly sickled."[5] The anemia is a consequence of loss of red cell deformability produced by membrane changes secondary to the repeated cycles of sickling and unsickling. In sickle cell anemia, the red cell life span is reduced from a normal length of 120 days to 12 days.

The sickling phenomena is influenced by several factors including the composition of the hemoglobin within the individual red cells and the amount of time that the hemoglobin remains deoxygenated.

There is variability in the hemoglobin composition of red cells within the same individual. For example, some red cells contain more fetal hemoglobin (Hb F) than other red cells. Hb F does not participate in the formation of deoxygenated Hb S polymers. The presence of Hb F within a specific red cell therefore will increase the time for the red cell to sickle or, if the level is high enough, prevent the cell from sickling altogether. Likewise, Hb A also does not participate readily in the polymerization process of deoxygenated Hb S molecules and can provide protection from red cell sickling except under adverse conditions.

On the other hand, hemoglobin C and other abnormal hemoglobins like hemoglobin D or O_{Arab} do participate in the sickling process. When these structural variants are contained within the red cell in addition to Hb S, the red cell will sickle when the hemoglobins of the cell are in the deoxygenated state.

Another important factor related to the sickling of the erythrocyte is the duration of time that the hemoglobin is in the deoxygenated state. Sickling of the cells is more likely to occur in those areas where the flow of blood is relatively slow. The slow flow allows more time for the deoxygenated Hb S molecules to come into contact with each other and initiate the events of polymer formation.

The acute and chronic complications of sickle cell disease are related to the vaso-occlusion produced by erythrocyte sickling. Sickled cells can clump together producing an obstruction to blood flow. The tissue downstream from the occlusion suffers the sequelae of ischemic injury. The extent of the injury is proportional to the duration of the ischemia and the size of the ischemic area. Long-term complications from these ischemic insults relate to the tissue's ability to repair itself.

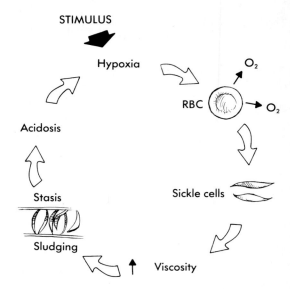

Fig. 14-1. Cycle causing vaso-occlusive episodes in sickle cell anemia. (Redrawn from Sheehy, T.W., and Plumb, V.J.: Treatment of sickle cell disease, Arch. Intern. Med. **137:**779, 1977.)

Fig. 14-1 illustrates the viscous nature of the vaso-occlusive crises. Release of oxygen causes the Hb S molecules to sickle, thereby increasing the local viscosity of the blood and promoting sludging with accompanying local ischemia and acidosis. These events promote further sickling, acidosis, and ischemia in a self-perpetuating cycle.

THE LABORATORY DIAGNOSIS OF SICKLE CELL DISEASE

The requirements for the diagnosis of sickle cell disease include a complete blood count, inspection of the peripheral smear, a hemoglobin electrophoresis and quantitation of the minor hemoglobins A_2 and F, and an assessment of the distribution of Hb F within the red cells. A confirmatory test for the presence of Hb S such as the dithionite test also is recommended.

Table 14-1 lists the results of the complete blood count and the hemoglobin electrophoresis in individuals with the more common types of sickle cell disease.[6] There is considerable variation in results

Table 14-1. Hematologic findings in sickle cell disorders

Diagnosis	Frequency	Severity	Hemoglobin (g/dl) (range)	Hematocrit (%) (range)	Mean corpuscular volume (u)	Percentage of reticulocytes (range)	Red blood cell morphology	Phoresis
Hb SS	1:625	Moderate-severe	7.5 (6-10)	22 (18-30)	93	11 (4-30)	Many ISCs, target cells, nucleated red cells	80-90%S 2-20;-cF 3.6%A
Hb SC	1:833	Mild-moderate	10 (9-14)	30 (26-40)	80	3 (1.5-6)	Many target cells, rare ISCs	45-55%S 45-55%C 0.2-8%F
HbS β^0 thal		Moderate-severe	8.1 (7-12)	25 (20-36)	69	8 (3-18)	Marked hypochromia, microcytosis and target cells, variable ISCs	50-85%S 2-30%F 3.6%A$_2$
HbS β^+ thal	1:1667	Mild-moderate	11 (8-13)	32 (25-40)	76	3 (1.5-6)	Mild microcytosis, hypochromia, rare ISCs	55-75%S 15-30%A 1-20%F >3.6%A$_2$

Modified from Lubin, B., Kleman, K., and Des Pennathur, R.: Lab management **18**:38, 1980.

between patients within the same disease category and overlap among patients within different categories.

Because levels of Hb F are elevated in infancy and because of the similarity between the hemoglobin electrophoresis results in sickle cell anemia and many sickle-thalassemia syndromes, it often is necessary to perform hematologic studies on the child's parents to determine the specific sickle cell syndrome affecting the child. The studies on the parents are identical to those performed on the child.

In some circumstances, it may be necessary to perform special tests on the patient to establish a precise diagnosis of a thalassemic condition in association with Hb S. These tests may include quantification of the alpha (α) globin gene number and studies to determine the rate of alpha (α), beta (β), and gamma (γ) globin chain synthesis.

In the more severe forms of sickle cell disease, there are sickled forms found on the peripheral smear. The classic sickle cell is pointed at both ends and has no central pallor. These sickled cells are irreversibly sickled.

The presence of sickle cells on the peripheral smear is not an absolute requirement for the diagnosis of sickle cell disease. They invariably, however, are found in sickle cell anemia and in the other more severe forms of the disease such as sickle β^0-thalassemia. The number of sickle cells does not correlate with the presence or absence of sickle cell crisis. Rather, there is a general correlation with the patient's hemolytic rate. The greater the number of sickled cells, the greater the rate of hemolysis.[7]

COMPLICATIONS

A myriad of complications have been described in individuals with sickle cell disease. As a general rule, the clinical course of patients with Hb SS or Hb S β^0-thalassemia is more severe than that of patients with milder sickle cell variants such as Hb SC or Hb S β^+-thalassemia. The complications described below are common in the Hb SS patients but also occur in the patients with Hb SC, the Hb S β-thalessemia syndromes and unusual forms of the disease such as Hb SD and Hb SO$_{Arab}$.

Dactylitis

Dactylitis, or the hand-and-foot syndrome, is often the first clinical manifestation of sickle cell anemia. The syndrome is characterized by swelling of the soft tissues over the metacarpals or metatarsals and the proximal phalanges of the hands and feet. The swelling is often symmetric and usually is accompanied by pain and increased temperature over the swollen area. Irritability and fever may accompany this type of vaso-occlusive crisis.

The cause of the hand-and-foot syndrome is not clear. It may be precipitated by nonspecific infections, dehydration, or environmental cold. The syndrome is common after the age of 6 months in Hb SS patients but usually does not occur after the age of 4 years. Initial evaluation of the patient includes a complete blood count and bacterial cultures of the throat, blood, and urine if the child is febrile.

In the initial stages of the syndrome, x-rays of the affected areas are usually normal. After approximately 2 weeks, radiographic findings may include subperiostial new bone formation, irregular areas of radiolucency, cortical thinning, or bone destruction. These changes may suggest a diagnosis of osteomyelitis. Most of the bone changes are reversible although they may persist for 8 months or more.[8,9]

Dactylitis is self-limiting. Treatment is symptomatic and includes fluids and analgesics. If the infant cannot maintain an adequate fluid intake at home, hospitalization may be required. Application of moist heat to affected areas may offer some relief.

Splenic sequestration crisis

Splenic sequestration crisis is a term applied to the sudden pooling of blood in the spleen produced by the total occlusion of venous outflow by sickled cells. Sequestration crisis is a life-threatening emergency requiring immediate intervention. It usually occurs in young children with sickle cell anemia between the ages of 6 months and 4 years of age. It has been reported in older patients with Hb SC and Hb S β$^+$-thalassemia. It is unclear as to what precipitates this crisis although infections have been implicated.

Clinically, the child has a history of acute illness less than 24 hours in duration. The illness is characterized by progressive pallor, irritability, and abdominal distension and pain produced by the enlarging spleen. Examination confirms the pallor. The child may be tachycardic and hypotensive from loss of effective intravascular blood volume. The spleen is markedly enlarged and tender to palpation.

Initial laboratory evaluation should include a complete blood count with a reticulocyte and platelet count. Specimens for cross-match and blood cultures should be obtained. The blood count results reveal worsening anemia in the presence of adequate reticulocytes and often thrombocytopenia secondary to the trapping of platelets within the spleen.

Immediate therapy is the restoration of the effective circulating blood volume by transfusion of packed red cells. If the patient is febrile, antibiotics should be initiated pending the results of the bacterial cultures. As the sequestration crisis reverses, the spleen becomes immediately smaller as the blood returns to the systemic circulation. If simple transfusion does not immediately improve the patient, a double volume exchange transfusion should be performed. If there is still no improvement, splenectomy should be done.

If a patient survives a sequestration crisis without having a splenectomy, the risk of recurrence is high. Two options exist to reduce the risk of recurrence. These options include a splenectomy and a chronic transfusion program. For children under the age of 4 years, we use a transfusion program of 6 to 9 months. This theoretically allows the child to become more immunologically mature while reducing the risk of recurrence. After the transfusion program is stopped, the patient is followed closely for signs of recurrence. The parents are taught to monitor the child's spleen size closely and to come to the hospital immediately if the size increases. If a second episode of sequestration is documented, the spleen is removed.

Aplastic crisis

Aplastic crisis is an infrequent complication of sickle cell disease in children. It is defined as a significant decrease in the total hemoglobin concentration associated with reticulocytopenia. It is caused by a temporary cessation of erythropoiesis. Often it is temporarily related to nonspecific infection. Recently, parvovirses have been shown to cause aplastic crisis.[10]

At presentation the child usually is pale, fatigued, tachycardic, and may be febrile. If anemia is severe, signs of congestive heart failure may be present. Initial laboratory evaluation should include a complete blood count with differential, platelet, and reticulocyte counts. The characteristic peripheral blood findings in aplastic crises include an anemia, normal white cell, differential, and platelet count but a striking reticulocytopenia for the degree of anemia. Bone marrow aspirate reveals reduced or absent red cell precursors.

Treatment is symptomatic. If the patient is symptomatic from the anemia, packed red cell transfusions are indicated. The blood should be given slowly to prevent circulatory overload.

In occasional circumstances, worsening anemia for other reasons than transient erythroid aplasia may occur in children with sickle cell disease. Examples of these types of occurrences include iron deficiency from chronic blood loss or inadequate dietary intake and rarely folic acid deficiency. Inspection of the peripheral smear often provides appropriate clues to the cause of the worsening anemia. Treatment depends on the cause and is similar to those situations when the anemia occurs in individuals without sickle cell disease.

Painful crisis

The painful crisis is the most frequent complication of sickle cell disease. It is characterized by the onset of pain, which may occur anywhere in the body. The patient may describe the pain as burning, gnawing, or crushing. There is often a waxing and waning quality to the pain, and the episode may last anywhere from hours to over a week. The waxing and waning quality of the pain may deceive the health care provider who is unfamilar with the vaso-occlusive pain of sickle cell disease and make the clinician think that the patient is faking or malingering.[11]

The frequency of pain crisis is variable. Generally, those patients with one or two severe episodes per month or 11 to 12 episodes per year requiring hospitalization are considered to have clinically severe disease. Those patients with two to six episodes per year requiring hospitalization have clinically moderate disease. Patients with one or no painful episodes per year have clinically mild disease.[12] There exists, however, tremendous variability in the frequency of painful crisis among patients with specific sickle cell disorders and for the same patient over extended periods of time.

The management of pain in sickle cell disease can present a difficult challenge to the clinician. The first step is to establish the cause of pain. Although many of the other complications of sickle cell disease have specific laboratory criteria that support the diagnosis, the painful episode does not have objective laboratory criteria. Painful crisis is a diagnosis of exclusion. Failure to recognize an underlying condition responsible for the pain can lead to inappropriate treatment, which may jeopardize the patient. Similarly, unnecessary laboratory and radiologic investigations are expensive and may contribute further to the patient's discomfort and parents' anxiety. Fortunately, a thorough history, a high index of suspicion coupled with a firm understanding of the disease and its symptom complex, and careful monitoring of the patient usually results in the correct diagnosis. The following outline summarizes a partial list of considerations for the cause of pain by anatomic location in children and adolescents with sickle cell disease:

Headache
  Tension
  Migraine
  Sinusitis
  Cerebrovascular disease
  Meningitis

Chest Pain
  Sternal or rib pain from marrow infarction
  Pulmonary infarction or emboli
  Pneumonia
  Pericardial disease
  Pleural disease
Abdominal pain
  Hepatobiliary disease
    Hepatitis
    Gallstones
  Intestinal tract disease
    Bacterial or viral gastroenteritis
    Appendicitis
    Intestinal obstruction
  Genitourinary disease
    Pyelonephritis
    Cystitis
    Renal stones
    Papillary necrosis
    Tubal pregnancy

The treatment for the painful episode depends on the cause of the pain. If the patient is felt to have only a painful crisis, treatment includes analgesia and fluids. For mild painful crises, acetaminophen may provide adequate analgesia. For more severe pain, relief may be obtained with mild narcotics such as codeine. For severe pain, opiates may be required.

The preferred route for administration of parental narcotics is intravenous, since this minimizes the anxiety children experience with intramuscular or subcutaneous injections. The route of administration should be decided by the physician, nurse, and patient to ensure optimum comfort. In the initial management of the painful crisis, pain medications should be administered on a scheduled basis rather than adhering to a p.r.n. order.[13]

During painful crises, the patient should increase their daily fluid intake to one and a half times maintenance if cardiac and renal function permit. This may be accomplished by either the oral route or by the use of intravenous fluids. Because the child with sickle cell disease is unable to concentrate the urine, parenteral fluids are indicated if the child is not able to maintain an adequate oral intake. The choice of parenteral fluid is determined by the results of serum electrolyte determinations and the status of the patient's cardiac and renal function. In general, a hypotonic salt solution is recommended with careful monitoring of the patient's weight, pulse, and respiratory rates, serum electrolytes, and daily intake and output.

Priapism

Priapism is a persistent painful erection of the penis unaccompanied by sexual desire. In addition to pain, the patient may experience difficulty with urination. Episodes may occur at any hour but are more frequent in the early morning hours. An episode may last less than an hour or more than a month.

The pathophysiology of this condition is related to occlusion of blood flow within the erectile tissues of the corpora cavernosa. This occlusion prevents detumescence.[14] Priapism may occur after sexual activity or in association with infections of the genitourinary tract or painful crisis. Hematologic values are unchanged from baseline during episodes of priapism.

The goals of therapy for priapism include the relief of the condition and the retention of potency. Impotency may complicate an episode of priapism as a result of fibrosis of the delicate tissues of the corpora cavernosa.

There are two initial approaches to management: medical and surgical.[15] Medical management includes the administration of intravenous fluids at a rate of one and a half to two times maintenance. If no response occurs within 24 hours, red cell transfusions are used to reduce the concentration of Hb S to less than 30% of the total hemoglobin concentration.

If the patient fails to respond to fluids or transfusion, surgical detumescence of the penis is indicated. This can be accomplished by the creation of a shunt between the corpora spongiosum and corpora cavernosa through an incision in the glans. This shunting procedure may also be employed as initial therapy in conjunction with transfusions if the episode has persisted for longer than 48 to 72 hours before presentation. Following this shunting procedure, detumescence usually occurs quickly. The risk of recurrence, however, remains as it does for patients whose episodes are managed medically. Complications of the shunting procedure include infection, fistulae, and impotency.

The pain of priapism is usually exquisite and adequate analgesia is mandatory. Bladder catheterization may be required to promote bladder emptying if the patient is unable to void spontaneously. Patients may experience depression and be embarrassed by the episode. Sensitivity is required in caring for these patients. For those patients who develop impotency after an episode, penile prosthesis may provide a mechanism to allow them to resume sexual intercourse.

Cerebral vascular accidents

Cerebral vascular accidents (CVAs) are estimated to affect 6% to 10% of children with sickle cell disease and are associated with a recurrence rate of 67% for untreated patients.[16] CVAs are more common in Hb SS than Hb SC disease. There are three broad categories of CVA in children with sickle cell disease, which include cerebral infarction, hemorrhage, and fat embolization.

Infarction is the most common in children and arises as a consequence of vaso-occlusion of major vessels. Intracranial hemorrhages may be either the intracerebral or subarachnoid variety and are not all related to erythrocyte sickle cells but may result from other causes such as aneurysms. Intracranial hemorrhage is more common in adults. Fat embolism is rare and occurs as a complication of marrow infarction with subsequent embolization of the marrow to the brain.

Variables such as Hb F levels, blood pressure, previous hospitalizations, and severity of painful crises do not predict the risk for a CVA.[17] Some investigators have felt that a prior history of bacterial meningitis may predispose the child to a CVA.[18]

The clinical symptomatology at presentation of a CVA is variable, depending on the location and extent of the lesion. Common presentations for cerebral infarction include aphasia, hemiplegia, hemiparesis, seizures, and cranial nerve palsies. Coma may develop. Patients with subarachnoid hemorrhage often have severe headache and altered level of consciousness.

In addition to a complete blood count, serum electrolytes, and blood sugar determinations, the patient should have a computed tomography (CT) scan of the brain. The CT may serve to localize the lesion and to determine the risk of lumbar puncture. Cerebral arteriography may be obtained to document the extent of the vascular disease and is indicated to exclude surgically correctable lesions, which are manifest as intracranial hemorrhage on CT scan. Since iodinated contrast material may induce sickling, the patient should be transfused before the arteriogram to reduce the concentration of the Hb S to less than 20% of the total hemoglobin concentration.

Immediate therapy for CVAs includes a double volume exchange transfusion. Many children are subsequently maintained on chronic transfusion programs to reduce the risk of recurrence.[19,20] The goals of the transfusion program include a suppression of the Hb S to less than 30% of the total hemoglobin and the maintenance of the hemoglobin concentration above 11 g/dl. Although subsequent CVAs may occur on transfusion, there appears to be less risk of recurrence while the patient is on a transfusion program. Controversy exists regarding the period of time the transfusions should be maintained.

Rehabilitation of the patient is an important aspect of care. Patients often require extensive physical and speech therapy. Psychometric testing may provide important information for structuring educational programs for the child. The patient should be carefully monitored for signs of progress. Failure to demonstrate improvement over a span of 6 months often indicates that the recovery is complete.

Aseptic necrosis

Aseptic necrosis of bone most commonly involves either the proximal femur or proximal humerus. Few symptoms accompany aseptic necrosis of the humerus but aseptic necrosis of the hip can produce severe pain and limitation of motion.

At present the mainstays of therapy for aseptic necrosis of the hip include bracing to prevent dislocation of the femoral head and relief of pain. The role of transfusion therapy remains to be defined. Some patients may require an artificial hip joint.

Ocular complications

A variety of ocular complications of sickle cell syndromes have been reported. These include proliferative retinopathy, which may be associated with retinal detachment, and with loss of vision. Another complication resulting in vision loss is central retinal artery occlusion. Patients with Hb SS and with Hb SC and the Hb S β-thalassemic disorders are all at risk for ocular complications. All patients beginning in their adolescent years should have annual eye examinations so that abnormalities may be detected before the onset of symptoms.

Treatment of ocular complications is dependent on the nature of the defect and the extent of the lesion. Patients with complications should be referred to an ophthalmologist skilled in the care of sickle cell–related eye disease for complete evaluation and therapy.

Bacterial infection

Bacterial infection is a major problem for patients with sickle cell disease, particularly those with sickle cell anemia. Infants and children have an increased risk of life-threatening bacterial infection.[21] Infections account for a significant proportion of hospitalizations and are responsible for the majority of the deaths under the age of 3 years.[22]

The types of bacterial infections roughly correlate with the age of the patient. Infants between the ages of 6 months and 3 years are more susceptible to bacteremia and meningitis caused by pneumococcal and *Haemophilus influenzae* organisms. Barrett-Conner[23] noted that the incidence of pneumococcal meningitis in children with sickle cell anemia was 600 times that of children in the general population.

In children over the age of 6 years, there is a higher incidence of *Salmonella* infection than is found in the general population. There is a particularly high incidence of salmonella osteomyelitis in sickle cell anemia.

Basic defects in the immune system of children with sickle cell disease contribute to the increased risk of infection. These defects have been best studied in patients with sickle cell anemia. The documented defects include decreased opsonizing activity, decreased to absent splenic function, and reduced antibody synthesis in response to intravenous antigens.

Children with fever and sickle cell disease deserve prompt evaluation at the time of fever. The history and physical examination should be directed to identifying a cause for the fever. Laboratory evaluation should include a complete blood count, bacterial cultures of the throat, blood and urine and a chest x-ray examination if the patient has a cough, tachypnea, or rales. If meningitis can not be excluded by the physical examination, a lumbar puncture is indicated. Bacterial cultures of the stool are indicated in the presence of diarrhea.

The treatment of the child with sickle cell disease and fever must be individualized depending on the immediate situation. If the child appears toxic or has a serious documented infection, hospitalization and intravenous antibiotics are indicated. The initial antibiotic coverage should include appropriate therapy for pneumococcal and ampicillin-resistant *Haemophilus influenzae* infections. If a minor infection is identified during the evaluation and the patient appears stable, outpatient therapy is appropriate, provided that contact is maintained with the family to monitor the child's progress.

Surgery and general anesthesia

Patients with sickle cell disease may require surgical intervention to treat problems both related to their disease and unrelated. Examples of disease-related problems include surgical interventions required for gallstones, priapism, and management of aseptic necrosis of the hip. Other types of surgical interventions include those required to manage traumatic injuries and other problems such as acute appendicitis. The indications for surgery in patients with sickle cell disease are similar to those in the general population. The risk of surgery, however, is greater when general anesthesia is employed. The risks may be reduced by the judicious use of transfusions and meticulous perioperative management.

In those situations where general anesthesia is used, the patient should be transfused to increase the concentration of Hb A to 70% of the total hemoglobin and to increase the hemoglobin concentration to between 12 to 14 g/dl. If the surgery is elective, this may be accomplished by a series of packed red cell transfusions in the outpatient department. If immediate surgery is needed, exchange transfusion may be used. Before surgery, a consult from the anesthesia service should be obtained, alerting them to the special needs of the child. Approximately 12 hours before surgery, intravenous fluids at a rate of one and a half times maintenance should be instituted and continued until the child is tolerating oral fluids well. The fluids are recommended because the patient is at risk for dehydration, since the kidney is unable to concentrate urine. During surgery, it is important to prevent acidosis and hypoxia, which are associated with erythrocyte sickling. The use of tourniquets to create a "bloodless field" should be avoided if possible, since the stasis created by the tourniquet may induce sickling at the site of application. After surgery, it is important to maintain oxygenation and good hydration of the patient.[24,25]

HEALTH CARE MAINTENANCE

Although much of this chapter has concentrated on the pathophysiology and management of complications of the disease, routine health care maintenance, which is required with any child, should not be overlooked. The special needs of these children can be incorporated into the routine well-child evaluations. Children with sickle cell disease face the same developmental hurdles as other children. The problems, however, may be intensified because of their disease. Table 14-2 represents a schedule of routine clinic visits for the child with sickle cell

Table 14-2. Schedule of routine clinic visits for the child with sickle cell disease and suggested approaches for the health care provider

Age	Laboratory examination	Physical examination	Plan
2 months	Complete blood count (CBC), platelet, differential, reticulocyte count	Routine well-baby examination	Review diagnosis and implications of the disease with the parents Review basic infant care including the following: Nutrition Taking temperatures Use of car seats/accidents Sleep/wake patterns Sibling rivalry Begin immunizations #1 DPT/OPV
4 months	CBC, platelet, differential, reticulocyte count	Routine well-baby examination Record developmental gains: height, weight Pay particular attention to the presence/absence of a liver/spleen, swelling of hands/feet Document findings	Review infant care including the following: Nutrition Taking temperatures Accident prevention Sleep/wake patterns Teething/drooling Continue immunizations #2 DPT/OPV

Continued.

Table 14-2—cont'd. Schedule of routine clinic visits for the child with sickle cell disease and suggested approaches for the health care provider

Age	Laboratory examination	Physical examination	Plan
6 months	CBC, platelet, differential, reticulocyte count	Routine well-baby examination Record developmental gains: height, weight Pay particular attention to presence/absence of a palpable liver/spleen, swelling of hands/feet Document findings	Review with parents physical examination findings and discuss physical symptoms they should be concerned about in their child (pallor, weakness, decreased fever, swelling of hands/feet); continue immunizations #3 DPT/OPV
10 months	CBC, platelet, differential, reticulocyte count	Routine well-child examination Record developmental gains: height, weight Pay particular attention to presence/absence of a palpable liver/spleen, swelling of hands/feet Document findings	Review basic infant care including the following: Nutrition Accident prevention (give prescription for Ipecac)
12 months	CBC, platelet, differential, reticulocyte count	Routine well-child examination Record developmental gains: height, weight Pay particular attention to presence/absence of a palpable liver/spleen, swelling of hands/feet Document findings	Review basic infant care including the following: Nutrition Accident prevention Temper tantrums Disciplines Review signs and symptoms of infection Tuberculosis skin test Consider pneumococcal immunization
15 months	CBC, platelet, differential, reticulocyte count	Routine well-child examination Record developmental gains: height, weight Pay particular attention to presence/absence of a palpable liver/spleen, swelling of hands/feet Document findings	Review basic child care including the following: Nutrition Accident prevention MMR immunization Consider H-Flu immunization
18 months	CBC, platelet, differential, reticulocyte count	Routine well-child examination Record developmental gains: height, weight Pay particular attention to presence/absence of a palpable liver/spleen, swelling of hands/feet Document findings	Review basic child care including the following: Nutrition Accident prevention Continue immunizations #4 DPT/OPV
2 years	CBC, platelet, differential, reticulocyte count, urinalysis, blood urea nitrogen (BUN), creatinine, liver function tests	Routine well-child examination Record developmental gains: height, weight Pay particular attention to presence/absence of a palpa-	Review basic child care including the following: Nutrition Accident prevention Temper tantrums/discipline

Table 14-2—cont'd. Schedule of routine clinic visits for the child with sickle cell disease and suggested approaches for the health care provider

Age	Laboratory examination	Physical examination	Plan
		ble liver/spleen, swelling of hands/feet Document findings Observe for effects of anemia: heart murmur (children with sickle cell disease have cardiomegaly and murmur; SEM heard best along LSB with radiation)	Toilet training Review signs and symptoms of infection Primary pneumococcal immunization or pneumococcal booster if immunized at age 12 months
3 years	CBC, platelet, differential, reticulocyte count, urinalysis, BUN, creatinine, liver function tests	Routine well-child examination Record developmental gains: height, weight Pay particular attention to presence/absence of a palpable liver/spleen, swelling of hands/feet, heart murmurs Document findings	Review basic child care including the following: Nutrition Accident prevention Toilet training/bed-wetting Brushing teeth Use of television
4 years	CBC, platelet, differential, reticulocyte count, urinalysis, BUN, creatinine, liver function tests	Routine well-child examination including visual and hearing screens Record developmental gains: height, weight Pay particular attention to presence/absence of a palpable liver/spleen, effects of anemia and hemolysis (e.g., heart murmur, scleral icterus)	Review basic child care including the following: Nutrition School readiness Use of television Schedule readiness Schedule dental evaluation
5 years	CBC, platelet, differential, reticulocyte count, urinalysis, BUN, creatinine, liver function tests	Routine well-child care Record developmental gains: height, weight Observe for the following and record findings: frontal bossing, gnathopathy, scleral icterus, heart murmur hepatosplenomegaly (spleen should not be palpable in the homozygous patient secondary to autosplenectomy, however, may still be palpable in patients on chronic transfusion programs.)	Review basic child care Information should be sent to the child's school via parents and/or medical staff outlining particular needs of the child Discuss with the child the nature of the disease if not already done; answer child's questions Dental evaluation every year Discuss enuresis Booster immunization DPT/OPV
6 years to 10 years	CBC, platelet, differential, reticulocyte count, urinalysis, BUN, creatinine, liver function tests	Routine well-child care Record developmental gains: height, weight Observe for the following and	Review issues regarding normal growth and development; peer relationships are of increasing importance to the child

Continued.

Table 14-2—cont'd. Schedule of routine clinic visits for the child with sickle cell disease and suggested approaches for the health care provider

Age	Laboratory examination	Physical examination	Plan
		record findings: frontal bossing, gnathopathy, scleral icterus, heart murmur hepatosplenomegaly (Spleen should not be palpable in the homozygous patient secondary to autosplenectomy, however, may still be palpable in patients on chronic transfusion programs.)	Encourage participation in group activities, such as boy scouts, girl scouts; health care provider may need to assist parents and child in modifying activities, participation in sports Discuss role and responsibility of child in the family Discuss appropriate use of television Provide anticipatory guidance regarding increasing fluid intake during increased activity or heat
11 years to 13 years	CBC, platelet, differential, reticulocyte count, urinalysis, BUN, creatinine, liver function tests	Routine adolescent examination Record developmental gains: height, weight Observe for the following and record findings: frontal bossing, gnathopathy, scleral icterus, heart murmur hepatosplenomegaly (Spleen should not be palpable in the homozygous patient secondary to autosplenectomy, however, may stilll be palpable in patients on chronic transfusion programs.) Include documentation of Tanner staging	Discuss with the patient the presence or absence of body change (Growth and development may be slower than other peers', but changes will occur.) Discuss issues related to hygiene Begin annual eye examination to check for sickle-related retinopathy
14 years to 18 years	CBC, platelet, differential, reticulocyte count, urinalysis, BUN, creatinine, liver function tests (gynecologic examination for females)	Routine adolescent examination Record developmental gains: height, weight Observe for the following and record findings: frontal bossing, gnathopathy, scleral icterus, heart murmur hepatosplenomegaly (Spleen should not be palpable in the homozygous patient secondary to autosplenectomy, however, may still be palpable in patients on chronic transfusion programs.) Include documentation of Tanner staging	Discuss identity issues including vocational/professional career plans Discuss with teenager issues pertaining to venereal disease, sex education, birth control Discuss the hazards of smoking and drug abuse Review need for increased fluid intake during periods of increased activity and during hot weather Prepare for transfer to adult clinic

disease and suggested approaches for the health care provider. Infants are routinely evaluated at 2, 4, 6, 9, and 12 months of age. Toddlers are seen at 3- to 6-month intervals. Preschool and schoolage children are seen at 6-month intervals. Teenagers are also seen at 6-month intervals or more often if problems occur. The schedule addresses particular age-related physical and psychologic areas and is not exhaustive in the suggested approaches. If additional well-child evaluation material is needed, refer to one of the many tests on pediatric primary care.[26]

SICKLE CELL TRAIT

Sickle cell trait is not a disease and does not progress to sickle cell anemia. Approximately 1: 10 Black Americans have sickle cell trait. The individual with sickle cell trait has a predominance of Hb A compared with Hb S. The red cells contain about 60% Hb A and 40% Hb S. In certain parts of the world endemic for malaria, Hb S is thought to have arisen because it provided some protection against forms of malaria. When an infected mosquito pierces the skin, it deposits the parasite *Plasmodium falciparum* into the host. The parasite penetrates the red blood cell and depletes the cell of nutrients and oxygen. As the red blood cell is destroyed, the parasite is released into the circulatory system for invasion into more red blood cells. When the malarial parasite enters the red blood cell of an individual with sickle cell trait or disease, the severe depletion of oxygen in the cell causes it to be sickled. It is removed from the circulatory system by the reticuloendothelial system before the malarial parasite can complete its growth and multiply.

Individuals with sickle cell trait rarely have symptoms related to the Hb S. Individuals with sickle cell trait are not anemic. Should anemia develop, its cause must be investigated. Individuals with sickle cell trait do not have an increased risk in receiving general anesthesia. They should avoid hypoxia, which may occur in flying in an unpressurized aircraft above 17,000 feet, since the hypoxia may precipitate erythrocyte sickling. They

are prone to hematuria as a consequence of intrarenal sickling because of the high osmolarity of the renal medulla. The bleeding usually responds to medical management, and nephrectomy should be avoided.

Genetic implications of sickle cell trait must be explained to individuals in a nondirected S trait so that they can make informed decisions regarding having children.

TRANSFUSION THERAPY AND ITS COMPLICATIONS

Judicious use of red cell transfusions plays a central role in the management of specific complications of sickle cell disease.[27] Clear indications for transfusion include acute anemic events, such as the splenic sequestration and symptomatic aplastic crises, and the presence of pulmonary disease, which reduces the oxygenation of the blood. Transfusion is also indicated in the management of cerebral vascular accidents and priapism and in preparation for prolonged general anesthesia. Transfusions may also be indicated in the management of pregnancy and in some instances for patients with refractory leg ulcers. Transfusion should not be used for the management of painful crises.

There are several different types of transfusion techniques and red cell products that may be used. Transfusion techniques include simple transfusion, partial exchange transfusion, and exchange transfusion. The latter techniques are used most when it is desirable to reduce the Hb S concentration as rapidly as possible.

Types of red cell products commonly used include packed red cells, washed red cells, and frozen-thawed-washed red cells. For most patients, packed red cells are adequate provided that they are less than 10 days old. The oxygen-carrying capacity of older red cells is reduced because of a decrease in the red cell 2,3,DPG levels during storage. This reduction in 2,3,DPG causes a greater affinity for oxygen of the hemoglobin in stored blood. The decrease in the 2,3,DPG usually corrects itself within 24 hours of transfusion. If the immediate goal of transfusion, however, is to improve tissue oxygenation, this delay may be unacceptable.

For patients without a history of febrile transfusion reactions, packed red cells are the product of choice for most transfusions. If the patient has experienced multiple febrile reactions, washed cells may be substituted. The washing procedure removes white cells, platelets, and plasma proteins, reducing the incidence of febrile reactions. Recent work with filtration of packed red cells with a 40-μ filter immediately before transfusion also appears to be an effective method for reducing the incidence of febrile reactions. This technique is faster and less expensive than washing the red cells. Frozen-thawed-washed red cells should be reserved for those patients who are sensitized to multiple red cell antigens and therefore require blood from rare donors. The freezing procedure permits prolonged storage of these rare blood cells. The freezing and washing procedure is very expensive and contributes little more than does only washing to the reduction of the incidence of febrile transfusion reactions.

It is our practice not to transfuse blood from individuals with sickle cell trait to patients with sickle cell disease. There are no documented adverse effects from the use of blood from trait donors; however, it is not possible to monitor accurately in the patient the endogenous Hb S production by quantitative hemoglobin electrophoresis.

The goals of most chronic transfusion programs are to maintain the Hb S concentration below 30% of the total hemoglobin and to keep the total hemoglobin concentration above 11 g/dl. After a series of initial transfusions, this can be accomplished by transfusions at 3- to 4-week intervals, provided that the patient is not sensitized to the donor units. The transfusions can be performed in the outpatient clinic to reduce cost and to minimize disruption to patient and family.

Before the institution of a transfusion program, the patient's red cell antigen phenotype should be determined. This may assist the blood bank in the identification of an alloantibody, which may arise from subsequent transfusions. The patient should also have determinations made of liver enzymes and for the status of hepatitis B antigen and antibody and iron stores. The latter may be accomplished with a serum ferritin. The hepatitis B status and liver function tests are subsequently monitored at 6-month intervals if the patient is asymptomatic.

A decision to transfuse must always be made in light of the risks and the benefits. Potential risks include the transmission of an infectious disease, sensitization to red cell antigens, and if transfusions are carried out over a prolonged period, the risk of iron overload. The reader is referred to Chapter 23 on blood products for a more detailed discussion of the problems of transmission of infection and red cell sensitization.

Iron overload from transfusion has the potential for being a major complication of transfusion therapy when the transfusions are administered for an extended time. Unlike thalassemia major, however, most sickle cell patients are not transfusion dependent. In those uncommon instances, such as in the treatment of CVAs where transfusions may be administered for many years, iron overload may become a significant problem. In these situations, treatment with desferrioxamine is indicated as described in Chapter 15.

FUTURE THERAPY FOR SICKLE CELL DISEASE

Despite the advances that have been made in the diagnosis and management of sickle cell disease in the past 50 years, a practical curative therapy does not exist at present. This is, however, an area of active research.

Although sickle cell disease is curable by bone marrow transplantation, this procedure is not a reasonable approach because at present the morbidity and mortality from the transplantation procedure are unacceptably high in even the most favorable circumstances. Perhaps, however, as better techniques are developed to prevent rejection and graft verus host disease and to prevent infectious complications from the transplant procedure, this treatment modality will become more reasonable.

Several other areas of research are currently in

progress to find a cure for sickle cell disease. These include the search for a drug that will inhibit the sickling phenomena by altering either the hemoglobin, the membrane, or the red cell volume. Another area of active research is in the field of molecular genetics. Examples of this research include the use of drugs to stimulate the production of fetal hemoglobin and the use of genetic engineering techniques to replace the β-S gene with a normal β-globin gene.

GENETIC COUNSELING AND SICKLE CELL SCREENING

Genetic counseling for individuals at risk for sickle cell disease and trait is an important function for the health care provider. The provider must have a thorough knowledge of the disease and the trait and an understanding of the various α- and β-thalassemic disorders and how these thalassemic conditions and other abnormal hemoglobins may interact with Hb S.

Two genes control the production of the β-chain. One β-gene resides on each of the two number 11 chromosomes within the nucleated red cells. The normal person has two normal β-globin genes. The individual with sickle cell trait has one normal β-gene and one β-S gene, which codes for β-S globin, which in turn pairs with α-globin chains to form Hb S. The individual with sickle cell anemia has two β-S globin genes. The patient with Hb SC disease has two abnormal β-globin genes, one which results in the production of β-S and the other β-C globin. The later pairs with α-globin chains to form Hb C. Depending on the type of β-thalassemic condition, the person with a trait condition for a β-thalassemic condition may have either an absent β-globin gene, a nonfunctional β-globin gene, or one that results in a reduced rate of normal β-globin synthesis.

A child inherits one β-globin gene from each parent. When both parents are normal, there is no chance that an offspring will have sickle cell trait or disease unless a spontaneous genetic mutation occurs, a very rare event. If one parent has sickle cell trait, and the other is normal, there is a 50%

chance with each pregnancy that the child will have the trait. If both parents have sickle cell trait, with each pregnancy there is a 25% chance the child will be normal, a 50% chance that the child will have the trait, and a 25% chance the child will have sickle cell anemia. If one parent has the trait and the other sickle cell anemia, with each pregnancy there is a 25% chance that the child will have the trait and a 75% chance the child will have the disease (Fig. 14-2). If both parents have sickle cell anemia, so will all offspring.

In providing counseling to a couple in whom one of the prospective parents has a sickle cell trait, it is mandatory that a β-thalassemic condition or abnormal hemoglobin be excluded in the partner. Exclusion of a β-thalassemic condition requires quantitation of hemoglobins A_2 and F, and exclusion of another abnormal hemoglobin requires a hemoglobin electrophoresis.

Counseling must contain an explanation of all family-planning options. These may include refraining from having children, adoption, artificial insemination, and abortion if the affected fetus is determined by intrauterine diagnosis to have the disease. This requires considerable sensitivity, patience, and compassion. It must always be done in a nondirected fashion with the final decision being that of the prospective parents.

With the advent of mass-screening techniques for the detection of Hb S, there has been widespread application of these procedures. When properly done and coupled with appropriate education, counseling, and follow-up, the screening can serve an important function. On the other hand, if screening is not accompanied by education, counseling, and follow-up, there is the potential for serious harm.

There are two major indications for the performance of sickle cell screening. One is the detection of the disease in the newly born child; the other is the detection of the trait in the individuals in their reproductive years so that they may make informed decisions regarding child-rearing practices.

The screening of newborns at risk for sickle cell disease has been shown by several large studies to

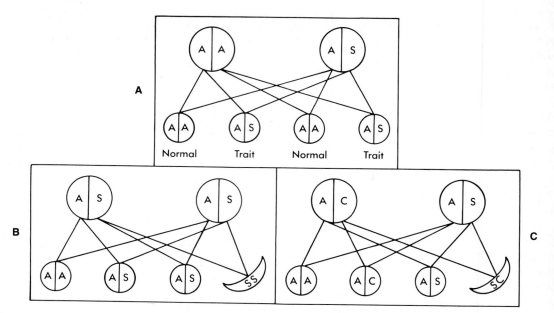

Fig. 14-2. Genetic transmission of sickle cell anemia. **A,** When one parent has normal hemoglobin (A/A) and the other parent has sickle cell trait hemoglobin (A/S), there is a 50% chance with each pregnancy that the child will have either normal hemoglobin or sickle cell trait. **B,** When both parents have sickle cell trait (A/S), there is a 25% chance that with each pregnancy the child will have sickle cell disease, a 50% chance the child will have sickle cell trait (not the disease), and a 25% chance the hemoglobin will be normal (A/A). **C,** Sickle cell combines with other hemoglobins to form variants. When one parent has hemoglobin C trait (A/C) and the other parent has sickle cell trait, there is a 25% chance with each pregnancy that the child will have either normal hemoglobin, C trait, sickle cell trait, or the disease state (Hb SC).

be an effective method to reduce infant mortality from sickle cell disease. The disease can readily be detected at birth by the combined use of cellulose acetate and agar gel hemoglobin electrophoresis. In those instances where the electrophoresis reveals an FS hemoglobin pattern, hemoglobin electrophoresis on both parents, however, is needed to classify the type of disease with certainty, since the FS pattern is found in a variety of conditions. These conditions include sickle cell anemia, sickle β-thalassemia, sickle β-8 thalassemia, and Hb S in association with the hereditary persistence of fetal hemoglobin. If both parents have the trait, the child has sickle cell anemia. If one parent has the trait and the other a β-thalassemia syndrome as determined by an increase in either the concentra-

tion of Hb A_2 and/or Hb F, then the affected child has a sickle β-thalassemia disorder. The neonate with Hb SC disease will demonstrate an FSC pattern. In this instance, studies on the parents are not required for definitive diagnosis.

For a newborn screening program to reduce infant mortality, it must be linked to an education program to teach the parents about the disease and the importance of prompt evaluation when the child is febrile or otherwise ill. The child also must have readily accessible care on a 24-hour basis. The program should also offer hemoglobin electrophoresis studies to the parents of all infants detected with sickle cell trait to determine if they are a couple at-risk for producing a child with the disease.

Screening programs for individuals in the reproductive age group should be voluntary and designed to provide them with sickle cell education and with counseling to enable them to make informed decisions regarding family planning. Educational sessions should precede screening and should stress the differences between sickle cell disease and trait. The results of screening should be presented in a confidential manner with ample opportunity for questions. Following a detailed explanation of screening results, the options of family planning should be discussed in a sensitive manner as stated previously.

NURSING CONSIDERATIONS

Sickle cell disease is a chronic disease, and as such much of the literature describing psychologic implications of chronic illness is pertinent. At the time of diagnosis, the parents are generally "shocked" by the news that their child has sickle cell disease. They often "deny" the diagnosis and think there must have been some mistake. Parents become "angry" that their child has a potentially debilitating or fatal disease. This anger can be directed toward doctors, nurses, each other, teachers, and even against their affected child or the child's siblings. Every nurse will probably recognize these symptoms as reactions to grief and loss. Parents usually shift back and forth between feelings of anger, denial, and acceptance in the course of their child's disease.

There are several frameworks to use in describing the psychologic implications of the disease. One of these is a developmental approach, which is particularly useful in reference to children's understanding of disease. A short description of some of the major issues in the developmental periods of infancy, toddlerhood, schoolage, and adolescence is presented.

Infant

When the diagnosis of sickle cell disease is made at birth or during the early infancy period, the risk of disrupting the developing parental-infant bond is possible. The "perfect child" that most parents envision may be somewhat tainted by the identification of the disease.

Although sickle cell disease is a common genetic disorder in the United States, there is considerable lack of knowledge about the disease among the general public. Sickle cell disease is often confused with types of cancer, such as leukemia, or as a nutritional disorder, such as iron deficiency anemia. Parents and grandparents frequently look for someone to put blame on for the presence of the disease. More often than not, they begin to blame each other and each other's "side of the family." Lack of knowledge and understanding perpetuates feelings of guilt and frustration in parents. The already difficult task of adjusting to a new baby is further complicated by the diagnosis. During the first few months after birth and up to the first "crisis," parents repeatedly question the accuracy of the diagnosis. The reality of the diagnosis becomes more clear with each passing crisis, and feelings of guilt surface again and again. Sometimes, guilt feelings are so intense that parents become immobilized and cannot provide necessary care for the infant or child.

Many infants progress through their infancy period with few to no problems. However, there are numerous infants who at the early age of 6 months develop repeated painful crises, sequestration crises, or severe bacterial infections.

Toddler

Toddlerhood is ordinarily an active, mobile, and energetic period of growth for the child. When painful crisis occurs, the child becomes frightened and can cope with the pain and fear in only a limited number of ways. They may cry and look to Mommy and Daddy for the help they have always provided in the past. Many times, the child is admitted to the hospital for pain management and intravenous fluids. The child is restrained, and his striving for autonomy is curtailed. Parents may feel that their role is being taken over by the nurses and doctors. Mothers may feel useless and stay home while their baby is in the hospital. Because of this the child may experience the pain of separation anxiety in addition to the pain from vaso-occlusive crisis. Every effort must be made to assist the mother and father in continuing parenting activities during the child's hospitalization and to be cognizant that parents may have other children at home. The clinician should assist the parents as needed in problem-solving during the hospitalization, since it is during these crisis periods that parents learn to trust or distrust health care providers.

Schoolage child

The schoolage child without sickle cell disease typically participates in sports activities, attends school full-time, and belongs to different groups such as scouts, church groups or others. They are beginning to look outside the family for approval. They seek recognition from peers. The child with sickle cell disease is expected to follow the same lines of psychologic-emotional development with minor modification in physical tasks.[28] Most children with sickle cell disease attend school full-time. There are times, however, when a vaso-occlusive crisis prevents the child from attending to the work assignments in school. It is highly desirable that parents contact the child's school teacher and arrange to have school work sent home for the child to do during the relative quiescent phases of the vaso-occlusive crisis. Parents must stress to the child the importance of completing assignments. This allows the child to return to the school environment without a sense of ''falling behind.'' Occasionally, it may be necessary to obtain homebound instructions, and this should be readily available to the child. Many parents and teachers become overprotective and do not allow the child to participate in normal developmental opportunities that are available to other children. Often, because the child with sickle cell disease is delayed in growth and development, teacher, parents, and peers may treat the child as being younger than their chronologic age. Classmates may tease the child because of short stature or because of other physical findings commonly observed in sickle cell disease including jaundice. Affected children may develop a poor self-image and become

isolated. If children are treated as different they begin to see themselves as different. They may also hear things that are alarming and frightening. Children need an environment that is conducive to discussing their fear with teachers or parents. In the clinic setting, health care providers can role-play with parents to help them develop communication skills with their child. Health care providers can discuss some of the issues with parents and child and assist them in problem solving.

Children with sickle cell disease are encouraged to maintain adequate hydration. This means they may have to be excused from the classroom to go to the bathroom more frequently than usual. Although children with sickle cell disease tire easily, this does not mean they should not participate in sports. They should participate up to their own level of tolerance. They can ride bikes, swim, run, and perform other physical education activities. Patients with the more severe form of sickle cell disease usually are not able to play in competitive organized sports such as basketball or football. Coaches might encourage these children to be umpires or scorekeepers. Children learn what their level of tolerance is, and this should be respected.

Children have a great deal of energy and resiliency during these schoolage years to overcome disabilities and failures and to try again. Teachers, parents, and health care providers must always concentrate on promoting the child's abilities rather than concentrating on the disabilities imposed on the child by the disease. In this way, the child will be prepared to face with confidence and competence some of the problems that lie ahead in the adolescent and adult years.

Adolescent

Some of the issues raised in the schoolage child with sickle cell disease are applicable to the teenager with sickle cell disease. The issues may potentially be magnified in teenagers. If adolescents have failed to develop a beginning sense of independence and identity separate from their sickle cell disease, they are doomed in a psychologic prison. It is during adolescence that teenagers may deny the existence of the disease and refuse to seek anticipatory or preventive medical care. This kind of behavior, this "testing" by the adolescent to see who is in control, is common in almost all teens to some degree. Health care providers must not respond to the teenager in anger for missed clinic appointments, but let him know that they are there if problems arise or for a "routine" checkup.[29]

Other issues particular to adolescents pertains to their sexual identity. Often teenagers have misguided ideas about sex. It is important to assist the teenager in obtaining appropriate and accurate information on sex and sexuality. The parents should also be included in assisting the teenager in finding acceptable resources. Genetic counseling should be included.

Setting career goals will become important to the teenager. There are certain career options that are not available to patients with sickle cell disease at this time. These are military careers or jobs requiring heavy manual labor, such as construction work.

Finally, the clinician must provide support to the parents. Many parents find it difficult to let the child grow up. Perhaps this is intensified in the parents of teenagers with a chronic illness because of the prolonged periods of dependence the teen has been required to live with. Health care providers must allow parents an opportunity to vent their frustrations about dealing with their teenager. Continuing problem solving between teen and parent will help promote healthy independence in both parents and teen.

Much of the foregoing information regarding psychologic implications of the disease is empiric and descriptive. There seems to be limitless opportunity for further research on the impact of the disease or disease complications on the individual and family.

NURSING CARE PROTOCOL FOR THE CHILD WITH SICKLE CELL DISEASE

Nursing diagnoses (problems/needs)	Goals/objectives (patient/family will:)	Interventions (nurse will:)
1. Knowledge deficit (related to diagnosis and diagnostic workup)	Describe the cause of sickle cell disease and some of the possible complications Describe how the diagnosis of sickle cell disease is made	Teach or reinforce learning regarding the cause of the disease Include written information for the patient/family Discuss with parents the hemoglobin electrophoresis and some of the genetic implications
2. Anxiety (related to diagnosis)	Decrease anxiety	Encourage family/patient to explore various support groups or other available resources Allow patient/family the opportunity to verbalize fears or misunderstandings Contact social worker or other team members as indicated for additional support

Continued.

NURSING CARE PROTOCOL FOR THE CHILD WITH SICKLE CELL DISEASE—cont'd

Nursing diagnoses (problems/needs)	Goals/objectives (patient/family will:)	Interventions (nurse will:)
3. Injury: potential for (complications of sickle cell disease)	Verbalize precautions or necessary actions to take to avoid or manage complications	Give parents phone numbers and name of persons to contact should problems arise
Dactylitis	Recognize signs and symptoms of hand-and-foot syndrome and respond appropriately	Ensure the child receives 1½ × 2 maintenance fluids (IV or PO) Strict I & O Administer analgesics as ordered Obtain vital signs q.4h. or as often as clinically indicated Apply moist heat to affected areas Provide emotional support to parents Review with parents how to administer medications and how to take a temperature
Splenic sequestration	Be able to recognize splenic sequestration in the infant and contact the appropriate persons	Review signs and symptoms of splenic sequestration including pallor, tachypnea, tachycardia, and increased spleen size Obtain vital signs as often as clinically indicated Observe for signs of hypovolemia and shock Transfuse per medical orders Ensure strict I & O Observe for signs of circulatory overload during transfusion Provide emotional support for parents/patient Review with parents/patient that this could happen again
Acute febrile illness	Recognize signs and symptoms of acute febrile illness and respond appropriately	Review with family/patient the seriousness of infections in children with sickle cell disease Monitor vital signs as often as clinically indicated Administer antipyretics and antibiotics as ordered Observe for signs of sepsis Observe for evidence of vaso-occlusive episodes Ensure strict I & O Ensure adequate hydration at 1½ × 2 maintenance

NURSING CARE PROTOCOL FOR THE CHILD WITH SICKLE CELL DISEASE—cont'd

Nursing diagnoses (problems/needs)	Goals/objectives (patient/family will:)	Interventions (nurse will:)
		Review with parents/patient how to take a temperature and how to administer medications
Aplastic crisis		Review with patient/family seriousness of aplastic crisis and the possible need for transfusion and hospitalization
		Obtain vital signs every 1-2 hr or as often as clinically indicated
		Ensure strict I & O
		Transfuse per medical orders
		Provide emotional support to patient/family
Painful crisis	Manage a painful episode at home	Review with parents/patient the signs and symptoms of painful crisis
		Ensure 1½ × 2 times maintenance fluids (IV or PO)
		Maintains phone contact with parents/patient for patients managed at home until symptoms resolve
		Administer analgesics as ordered and document effectiveness
		Review with parents how to take a temperature and how to administer medications
		Obtain vital signs q.4h. or as often as clinically indicated
		Use other comfort measures including diversion therapy and moist/dry heat to affected areas
		Encourage parents to contact child's school to obtain homework for child to do during quiescent phases of painful crisis
Priapism		Assist the patient in gentle exercise if exercise offers the patient some relief
		Assist the patient with sitz baths or hot packs
		Obtain vital signs q.4h. or as often as clinically indicated
		Maintain strict I & O
		Ensure adequate hydration at 1½ × 2 times maintenance

Continued.

NURSING CARE PROTOCOL FOR THE CHILD WITH SICKLE CELL DISEASE—cont'd

Nursing diagnoses (problems/needs)	Goals/objectives (patient/family will:)	Interventions (nurse will:)
		Administer pain medicines as ordered and document effectiveness
		Provide emotional support to the patient
Cerebrovascular accidents (acute event)	Have no neurologic damage or physical injury secondary to CVA or complications of CVA including seizures	Use seizure precautions
		Obtain vital signs q.2-4h. or as often as clinically indicated
		Transfuse per medical orders
		Contact appropriate hospital support persons
		Provide emotional support to patient/family
Cerebrovascular accidents (chronic event)	Describe the treatment for CVA to include transfusions, physical therapy, and appropriate school placement	Discuss with family/patient the rationale for transfusion therapy
		Assist family/patient in seeking appropriate resources for physical therapy and school as needed
	State the risks associated with transfusion	Explain the purpose of type and crossing of blood and potential complications of transfusion
	Develop no complications resulting from transfusion therapy	Provide appropriate nursing monitoring during transfusion
		Vital signs q.15min. for the first hour and then q.h. for the remainder of the transfusion
		Observe for signs of transfusion reactions including circulatory overload, febrile reaction, hemolytic reaction, allergic reactions
	Develop no additional CVA	Discuss signs and symptoms of CVA with parents/patient
		Discuss importance of returning to clinic at appropriate intervals for transfusion
4. Coping ineffective family: compromised	Demonstrate effective coping mechanisms necessary for optimum functioning at home, school, and community	Provide emotional support and refer to other health professionals
		Communicate with agencies and the school to facilitate optimum care at home

REFERENCES

1. Herrick, J.: Peculiar elongated and sickle-shaped red corpuscles in a case of severe anemia, Arch. Intern. Med. **6:**517, 1910.
2. Emmel, V.: A study of the erythrocytes in a case of severe anemia with elongated and sickle-shaped red blood corpuscles, Arch. Intern. Med. **20:**586, 1917.
3. Hahn, E., and Gillespie, E.: Sickle cell anemia: report of a case greatly improved by splenectomy: experimental study of sickle cell formation, Arch. Intern. Med. **39:**233, 1927.
4. Pauling, L., Itano, H., and others: Sickle cell anemia, a molecular disease, Science **110:**543, 1949.
5. Smith, C., Krwit, W., White, J.: The irreversibly sickled cell, Am. J. Pediatr. Hematol. Oncol. **4**(3):307, 1982.
6. Kim, C.: Variants of sickle cell disease. In Schwartz, E., (editor): Hemoglobinopathies in children, Littleton, Mass., 1980, PSG/Wright Publishing Co., Inc.
7. Serjeant, G.R., Serjeant, B.E., and others: Irreversibly sickled erythrocytes: a consequence of the heterogeneous distribution of hemoglobin types in sickle cell anemia, Br. J. Haematol. **17:**527, 1969.
8. Stevens, M., Padwick, M., and Serjeant, G.: Observations on the natural history of dactylitis in homozygous sickle cell disease, Clin. Pediatr. **20**(5): 311, 1981.
9. Espinosa, G.: Hand-foot roentgen findings in sickle cell anemia, JAMA **71**(2):171, 1979.
10. Sergeant, G.R., Topley, J.M., Mason, K., and others: Outbreak of aplastic crises in sickle cell anemia associated with parvovirus-like agent, Lancet **2:**595, 1981.
11. Rozzell, M., Hijazi, M., and Pack, B.: The painful episode, Nurs. Clin. North Am. **18**(1):185, 1983.
12. Cameron, B., and others: Evaluation of clinical severity in sickle cell disease, J. Nat. Med. Assoc. **75**(5):483, 1983.
13. McCaffery, M.: Nursing management of the patient with pain, ed. 2, Philadelphia, 1979, J. B. Lippincott Co.
14. Gradisek, R.: Priapism in sickle cell disease, Ann. Emerg. Med. **12**(8):510, 1983.

15. Kinney, T., and others: Priapism associated with sickle hemoglobinopathies in children, J. Pediatr. **86**(2):241, 1975.
16. Powers, D., and others: The natural history of stroke in sickle cell disease, Am. J. Med. **65:**461, 1978.
17. Sarnaik, S., and Lusher, J.: Neurological complications of sickle cell anemia, Am. J. Pediatr. Hematol. Oncol. **4**(4):386, 1982.
18. Seeler, R.: Commentary: sickle cell anemia, stroke and transfusions, J. Pediatr. **96**(2):243, 1980.
19. Wilimas, J., and others: Efficacy of transfusion therapy 1 or 2 years in patients with sickle cell disease and cerebrovascular accidents, J. Pediatr. **96:**205, 1980.
20. Russell, M., and others: Transfusion therapy for cerebrovascular abnormalities in sickle cell disease, J. Pediatr. **88:**382, 1976.
21. Kravis, E., Fleisher, G., and Ludwig, S.: Fever in children with sickle cell hemoglobinopathies, Am. J. Dis. Child. **136:**1075, 1982.
22. Landesman, S., Rao, S., and Ahonkhai, V.: Infections in children with sickle cell anemia, Am. J. Pediatr. Hematol. Oncol. **4**(4):407, 1982.
23. Barrett-Connor, E.: Bacterial infections in sickle cell anemia, Medicine **50:**97, 1971.
24. Janik, J., and Seeler, R.: Perioperative management with children with sickle hemoglobinopathies, J. Pediatr. Surg. **15:**117, 1980.
25. Fullerton, M., and others: Preoperative exchange transfusion in sickle cell anemia, J. Pediatr. Surg. **16:**297, 1981.
26. DeAngelis, C.: Pediatric primary care, ed. 2, Boston, 1979, Little, Brown & Co.
27. Schmalyer, E., Chien, S., & Brown, A.: Transfusion therapy in sickle cell disease, Am. J. Pediatr. Hematol. Oncol. **4**(4):395, 1982.
28. Chodorkoff, J., and Whitten, C.: Intellectual status of children with sickle cell anemia, J. Pediatr. **63:**29, 1963.
29. Wethers, D.: Problems and complications in the adolescent with sickle cell disease, Am. J. Pediatr. Hematol. Oncol. **4**(1):47, 1982.

CHAPTER 15

Thalassemia syndromes

MARILYN J. HOCKENBERRY and THOMAS R. KINNEY

The word *thalassemia* was first used to describe a group of individuals of Italian descent who were observed to have anemia, growth delay, and bony deformities. The Greek word for thalassemia, translated to mean "the great sea," was chosen to demonstrate the Mediterranean heritage of these patients. The thalassemia syndromes not only affect individuals of Mediterranean descent but affect individuals of other heritage including African and Asian.

HEMOGLOBIN STRUCTURE

The thalassemia syndromes are a group of hereditary disorders characterized by decreased production of one or more globin chains.[1] A hemoglobin molecule is composed of two identical pairs of globin chains with a heme moiety attached to each. Heme, an iron-containing porphyrin, is the site of oxygen binding. The globin chains are proteins that ensure reversible oxygen binding and release when the amino acid structure is normal. Four types of globins are identified and named: alpha (α,) beta (β), gamma (γ), and delta (δ).[2] The synthesis of globin chains is directed by specific genes.

Table 15-1. Composition of normal adult hemoglobin

Hemoglobin	Structure	Percentage of total hemoglobin
Hb A	$\alpha_2 \beta_2$	97
Hb A_2	$\alpha_2 \delta_2$	≤ 3.2
Hb F	$\alpha_2 \gamma_2$	≤ 1

There are four α-globin genes, two each located on the number 16 chromosome. Non-α-genes (γ, δ, β) are closely linked and reside on the number 11 chromosome.[1]

Blood from the normal older child and adult contains three types of hemoglobin. These are Hb A, Hb A_2, and Hb F. The structure and relative percentage of each hemoglobin type is summarized in Table 15-1. Hb A is composed of two α- and two β-chains. Hb A_2 is composed of two α- and two δ-chains. Hb F is composed of two α- and two γ-chains.

PATHOPHYSIOLOGY

The hallmark of the α- and β-thalassemia disorders is a reduction in Hb A synthesis as Hb A is composed of two α- and two β-chains. The severity of either α- or β-thalassemia is directly proportionate to the degree of globin chain imbalance.[1] In α-thalassemia, there is an excess of β-chains as compared with β-thalassemia where there is an excess of α-chains. The imbalance in chain synthesis may be related to one of several factors including the absence of a gene, abnormal gene structure, and transcription or translation of the genetic message.[3] Use of globin gene mapping technique or studies of globin synthesis in red cells have identified each of these types of reasons for globin chain imbalance in the thalassemia syndromes.[1]

CLASSIFICATION

Traditionally, the thalassemia syndromes have been further classified as *major, intermedia,* and *minor*.[3] These are clinical terms reflecting disease severity with major forms being the most severe. In general, major forms indicate homozygosity for the thalassemic deficit, whereas minor indicates heterogeneity. More accurate classification is provided by quantifications of gene numbers and function.[1]

Severity of disease usually correlates with the degree of globin chain synthesis imbalance.[1] Decreased synthesis of globin chains in the red cell is associated with a decrease in intracellular hemoglobin and is accompanied by microcytosis. When the imbalance is severe, ineffective erythropoiesis is observed.[2] In thalassemic red cells, there is an excess of one of the globin chains. Unable to find complementary chains with which to pair, these excess chains aggregate.[1] Unbalanced globin chains also produce oxidant stresses on the red cell membrane. Hemolysis occurs as a result of the globin chain imbalance.[2]

β-THALASSEMIAS
Thalassemia major (Cooley's anemia)

Thalassemia major, usually a homozygous condition, was first described by Thomas Cooley in 1925. Dr. Cooley evaluated a group of children who had severe anemia, massive hepatosplenomegaly, growth delay, and bony deformities (Table 15-2). His clinical description of β-thalassemia major is still valid. β-Thalassemia major occurs most commonly in the Mideast, India, Pakistan, and China.[3]

Clinical manifestation. Patients are usually identified between 6 months and two years of age when pallor and hepatosplenomegaly are noted on physical examination. Occasionally, the disease is recognized later in childhood. Affected infants may exhibit jaundice and inadequate weight gain. Bony deformities include frontal bossing, maxillary prominence, and osteoporosis. These abnormalities are typical of those associated with ineffective erythropoiesis, since they result from hypertrophy and expansion of the bone marrow in an attempt to compensate for anemia by increasing red blood cell production.[2] Expansion of the marrow cavity within the bones of the face and skull produces the characteristic thalassemia facies, which includes flattening of the nose and wide-set eyes, frontal bossing of the skull, hypertrophy of the upper maxillae, and prominent malar eminences (Fig. 15-1).[4]

Radiographic studies of the skull demonstrate dilatation of the diploic space with perpendicular bony trabeculae appearing, producing the classic "hair-on-end" appearance[4] (Fig. 15-2). The clin-

Table 15-2. The β-thalassemia syndromes

Types of β-thalassemias	Clinical features	Treatment
Thalassemia major (Cooley's anemia, homozygous thalassemia)	Severe anemia with bony deformities, hepatosplenomegaly, growth failure Develops major complications from iron overload in second decade of life	Transfusion dependent Folic acid supplementation; bone marrow transplantation is curative; splenectomy possibly needed
Thalassemia minor (high A$_2$ thalassemia trait)	Rarely symptomatic Jaundice, hepatosplenomegaly, gallstones, anemia, and reticulocytosis sometimes present Exacerbated during pregnancy, illness, or iron and folate deficiency	Folic acid supplementation
Hereditary persistence of fetal hemoglobin (HPFH)	No clinical abnormalities	None
Silent carrier thalassemia	No clinical abnormalities	None

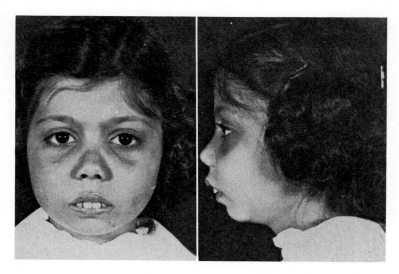

Fig. 15-1. Characteristic thalassemia facies, which includes flattening of the nose, wide-set eyes, and frontal bossing of the skull. (From Miller, D.R., Baehner, R.L., and McMillan, C.W.: Blood diseases of infancy and childhood, St. Louis, 1978, The C.V. Mosby Co.)

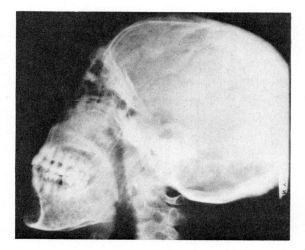

Fig. 15-2. Radiographic changes in the child with thalassemia demonstrating the classic "hair-on-end" appearance.

ical findings of the untransfused child with β-thalassemia major are summarized as follows:

General: Failure to thrive, pallor, irritability, jaundice

Head and Neck: Upper respiratory tract and ear problems; epistaxis

Chest: Frequent infections most commonly caused by pneumococci and streptococci; cardiomegaly with murmurs, arrhythmias progressing to congestive heart failure

Abdomen: Massive hepatosplenomegaly; increased risk for gallstones

Genitourinary: Impairment of renal function

Skin: Chronic leg ulceration, skin pigmentation

Skeletal: Skull—frontal bossing, flattening of the nose, dilatation of the diploic space

Maxilla—hypertrophy

Long bones—cortical thinning (Fig. 15-3); masses secondary to extramedullary hematopoiesis and accumulation of bone marrow; gout secondary to hyperuricemia

Endocrine: Endocrine dysfunction—diabetes mellitus; pituitary, thyroid, and adrenal dysfunction

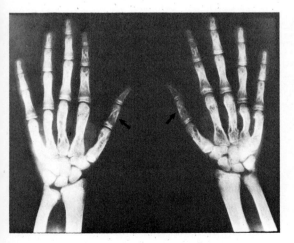

Fig. 15-3. Cortical thinning of the bones in the hand secondary to ineffective erythropoiesis caused by expansion of bone marrow.

Other: Vitamin and trace metal deficiencies, especially Vitamin E, zinc, B_{12}, folate

Laboratory features. Laboratory tools for evaluation of all thalassemic disorders are as follows:

Complete blood count
Reticulocyte count
Red blood cell indices
Evaluation of blood film
Serum iron
Total iron-binding capacity
Hemoglobin electrophoresis
Hb A and Hb F quantitations
Betke-Kleihauer Hb F stain
Bone marrow aspiration
Globin synthesis
Family studies

In thalassemia major, anemia is severe, ranging between 3 to 7 g/dl, and the mean corpuscular volume (MCV) ranges between 50 to 60 fl. Inspection of the peripheral smear shows poikilocytes, anisocytes, and severe hypochromia. Target cells and thin, folded cells containing irregular clumps of hemoglobin are seen.[5] Nucleated red blood cells are often seen. There is a neutrophilic predominance in the differential white count. Reticulocyte count ranges between 2% to 8%, inappropriately low for the degree of anemia and a reflexion of ineffective erythropoiesis.

The hemoglobin electrophoresis in untransfused patients indicates a predominance of Hb F, with levels usually in the range of 60% or greater.[4]

Treatment. Management of the child with β-thalassemia major involves supportive care. Standard therapeutic approaches endeavor to protect the child from deleterious effects of chronic anemia by a chronic red blood cell transfusion program. Folic acid supplementation at a dose of 1 mg/day is recommended.

Bone marrow transplantation is curative therapy for the child with homozygous β-thalassemia. Most affected individuals, however, do not have a compatible bone marrow donor and are not eligible for transplantation (see Chapter 22 on bone marrow transplantation).

Transfusion therapy, a major modality in the management of thalassemia major, its complications, and the role of splenectomy in these children will now be discussed.

Transfusion therapy. Transfusion therapy should be delayed in the infant until hemoglobin levels fall below 6 g/dl or signs of growth delay, progressive hepatosplenomegaly, or bony abnormalities occur. Transfusion programs are designed to maintain the hemoglobin level above 10 g/dl, which usually minimizes orthodontic and bony abnormalities. The transfused child grows normally during the first decade of life.[6] In the second decade of life, signs of hepatic, cardiac, and endocrine dysfunction usually appear, which are complications of transfusion-induced hemosiderosis.[1,7]

COMPLICATIONS OF TRANSFUSION THERAPY. Risks of chronic red blood cell transfusions include transfusion reactions, alloimmunization, transmission of infections, and iron overload.[8]

Febrile reactions may occur when frequent transfusions are administered. These reactions can be reduced with the use of packed red blood cells and the administration of antipyretics and antihistamines. Close assessment of the child receiving a blood transfusion is essential. Chapter 23 on blood products discusses appropriate nursing actions during red blood cell administration. Red cell transfusions may result in sensitization to blood group antigens. Transfusion of red cells containing antigens to which the recipient is sensitized can result in severe life-threatening reactions. Such sensitization leads to difficulty in obtaining compatible blood.

Numerous infections may be transmitted by blood transfusion. Hepatitis is the most frequently observed infection transmitted. Improvement in donor screening and use of volunteer donors have led to a reduction in the transmission of some diseases such as hepatitis B. See Chapter 23 on blood products for further detail.

Hemosiderosis, the accumulation of iron in the tissues from chronic blood transfusions, affect the cardiac, hepatic, and endocrine systems. Most patients with β-thalassemia major die of cardiac failure caused by iron overload. Pericarditis is common, with symptoms of pain, fever, and a friction rub often being auscultated initially in myocardial iron deposition.[3] Acute pericarditis is treated with bed rest, analgesics, and anti-inflammatory agents. Cardiac arrhythmias can occur, often proving fatal. Congestive heart failure may also occur, and is treated with salt restriction, diuretics, and digitalis.[2]

Hepatomegaly frequently occurs in patients over 10 years of age who have received chronic transfusions or who have chronic hemolysis of their own abnormal cells. This enlargement is primarily caused by hemosiderin deposits within the liver.[2] Accumulation of iron induces hepatic fibrosis. The degree of fibrosis and level of iron concentration can be affected by chelation therapy.[3] As discussed previously, these patients are at risk for hepatitis secondary to blood transfusions.

Endocrine disorders in children with thalassemia related to chronic iron overload are usually not manifested until the second decade of life.[2] Normal growth may occur during the first decade of life, but the adolescent's pubertal growth spurt is delayed or even absent. In females, menarche and breast development are delayed, and amenorrhea is common.[4] Males frequently lack secondary sexual characteristics, with evidence of sparse facial and body hair. Multiple endocrine abnormalities may occur secondary to iron deposition in the pancreas, adrenals, and thyroid glands.

Iron chelation therapy. Iron overload in children with thalassemia occurs both from intestinal absorption and from blood transfusions. There is approximately 1 mg iron/1 ml packed red cells. Transfusion of only 200 ml packed cells every month adds 2 g iron/year to the body.[3] It is this excessive amount of iron that is responsible for most complications of homozygous β-thalassemia in the second and third decades of life. Generalized iron loading occurs in the body's major organs. Since the development of chronic transfusion programs, emphasis has been placed on removal of iron in these overloaded patients.[9] Chelating drugs, which act to break down iron to enable excretion from the body, are now used in conjunction with chronic transfusion programs.[8]

Desferrioxamine (Desferal) is used to increase iron excretion through urine and feces. Subcutaneous infusion beginning at a dose of 20 mg/kg/day over 12 hours is the most effective method to obtain results.[9,10] A portable pump can deliver Desferal subcutaneously, most commonly used at night. Chelation therapy is expensive, with the estimated cost being over $4000/year.[5] Side effects of Desferal therapy are minimal, with minor reactions being responsive to antihistamines. Infusion sites may become indurated and should be changed daily. Administration of vitamin C is known to increase urinary excretion of iron but also has been associated with cardiac toxicity.

Splenectomy. Hypersplenism may complicate β-thalassemia major. Aggressive transfusion programs often prevent the need for splenectomy. Treatment is aimed at preventing the need for splenectomy and the associated risk for postsplenectomy sepsis. If hypersplenism develops, splenectomy is indicated to reduce the transfusion requirement, therefore slowing the rate of iron loading. Before splenectomy, these patients should be immunized with polyvalent pneumococcal vaccine because of increased susceptibility to overwhelming pneumococcal sepsis after splenectomy.[11] Prophylactic penicillin is recommended at a dose of 250 mg b.i.d.

Thalassemia intermedia

There are reported patients with homozygous β-thalassemia who have similar abnormalities as thalassemia major but suffer only a moderate degree of anemia and rarely require transfusions. This type of homozygous β-thalassemia is frequently identified as thalassemia intermedia.[12]

Problems of iron overload can occur in these patients because of the markedly accelerated erythropoiesis, which results in increased plasma iron turnover with increased GI absorption. Cardiac and endocrine complications are seen, usually 10 to 20 years later than those individuals requiring regular blood transfusions.[2]

Thalassemia minor

There are several forms of β-thalassemia minor. The most common being high A$_2$, β-thalassemia

trait. These individuals are heterozygous for a β-mutation.[13] There is a remarkable degree of heterogeneity among these patients. Most children are asymptomatic and are incidently discovered on routine examination. Life expectancy is normal.[14]

Clinical manifestations. Most individuals are asymptomatic. Mild pallor and splenomegaly are sometimes found.[15] Anemia may be exacerbated during pregnancy, concurrent illness, or with iron and folic acid deficiency.

Occasional patients are reported with high Hb A$_2$, who have unusually severe clinical symptoms including moderate anemia, splenomegaly, and bony changes.[2] Late complications of these individuals include leg ulcers and gallstones. Splenectomy may decrease the severity of these complications.[1]

Laboratory features. Diagnosis of high A$_2$ heterozygous thalassemia is established by hemoglobin electrophoresis. Hb A$_2$ is usually elevated with an average of 5.1% and Hb F mildly elevated from 2% to 5%.[2]

The hemoglobin level is frequently decreased by 1 to 3 g/dl below the normal range. The blood smear characteristically displays hypochromic (MCH less than 26 pg) and microcytic (MCV less than 75 fl) anemia. Target cells, poikilocytes, ovalocytes, and basophilic stippling are seen. Microcytosis, increased red cell count, and the presence of target cells are indicative of thalassemia trait. Iron deficiency anemia, however, must be ruled out. Family studies are extremely useful in the identification of thalassemia.

Treatment. Thalassemia minor requires no therapy. Couples at risk for having a child with homozygous β-thalassemia should receive genetic counseling.[5,8] Prenatal diagnosis of thalassemia is now available.

Other forms of β-thalassemia heterozygous states

Hb A$_2$ and F, as previously discussed, are elevated in individuals with β-thalassemia trait.[16] Variants have been described with other biochemical elevations and are discussed in the following sections.

High Hb F thalassemia trait. Individuals display a mild hypochromic, microcytic anemia with a Hb F elevated from 5% to 20%. Hb F is heterogeneously distributed in the red blood cells. The clinical features are similar to high A_2 β-thalassemia trait.[1]

Silent carrier of β-thalassemia. There are rare occasions when individuals are carriers of the β-thalassemia gene and display no hematologic evidence of the gene.[3] Normal levels of Hb A_2 and Hb F are found, yet when globin synthesis studies are performed, reduced synthesis is established. These individuals are identified when they have a child with thalassemia major.[4]

Hereditary persistence of fetal hemoglobin. Hereditary persistence of fetal hemoglobin (HPFH) is a group of uncommon disorders in which fetal hemoglobin continues to be synthesized throughout life. The Betke-Kleihauer stain is able to detect the presence of fetal hemoglobin in almost all of the red cells.[3] This disorder is not associated with any severe clinical or hematologic abnormalities in either homozygous or heterozygous conditions.

Thalassemia associated with structural hemoglobinopathies. β-thalassemia is frequently associated with other abnormal hemoglobinopathies. $β^0$-thalassemia and Hb S are common and create a severe sickling disorder clinically indistinguishable from Hb SS disease as discussed in Chapter 14. This is compared with the combination of Hb SS disease and $β^+$-thalassemia in which clinical symptoms are much less severe.

α-THALASSEMIAS

The α-thalassemias are the most difficult to classify from a clinical and genetic perspective. There are four types of thalassemias that are related to the loss of function of one to four of the α-globin chains. These include silent carrier state, thalassemia trait, Hb H disease, and hydrops fetalis as outlined in Table 15-3.

Silent carrier of α-thalassemia

This syndrome has no clinical manifestations. Red cells are usually normocytic but occasionally may be microcytic and hypochromic and demonstrate anisocytosis and poikilocytosis. The levels of Hb A_2 and F are normal. Blacks and orientals have demonstrated deletion of α-globin genes in many instances.

α-Thalassemia trait

In α-thalassemia trait, there is a significant reduction in chain synthesis. This syndrome occurs primarily in the Asian population, reaching a frequency of 20%, and seen less commonly in the African, Mediterranean, and American Black populations.[3] In orientals, the reduction of a chain syn-

Table 15-3. The α-thalassemia syndromes

α-Thalassemia syndromes	Clinical features	Hematologic features	Hb Bart's at birth (%)	Treatment
Silent carrier	None	Occasional mild microcytosis	1-2	None
α-Thalassemia trait	Occasional pallor	Red cell hypochromia, poikilocytosis, anisocytosis, and microcytosis; anemia mild or absent	5-6	None
Hb H disease	Pallor, jaundice, hepatosplenomegaly; possible gallstones	Moderately severe anemia, hypochromia microcytosis, poikilocytosis, anisocytosis, red cell inclusion bodies	20-40	Avoidance of oxidating agents; prompt treatment of infections; may require transfusions
Hydrops fetalis	Not compatible with extra-uterine life	Severe anemia, marked erythrocytes, morphology abnormalities; pronounced erythroblastemia	Predominantly Bart's	

thesis has been shown to be caused by a deletion of two α-chain globin genes.[1] In blacks both gene deletions and abnormal α-globin genes have been identified to account for this disorder.

Hb A$_2$ levels are in the low to normal range. α-Thalassemia trait is characterized by mild anemia with red cell hypochromia and microcytosis. The MCV and MCH is low, with a hemoglobin level 1 to 2 g/dl below normal for age and sex.

α-Thalassemia trait is frequently misdiagnosed as iron deficiency anemia.[4] Diagnosis of α-thalassemia trait is established in the presence of red cell abnormalities and absence of iron deficiency.[3] In the newborn period, thalassemia is readily diagnosed by the presence of Hb Bart's identified by hemoglobin electrophoresis.

Treatment is not necessary for individuals with α-thalassemia trait. Family studies and genetic counseling are important.

Hb H disease

Hb H disease is characterized by the production of H hemoglobin. Hb H is a tetramer of β-chains, which bind oxygen very tightly, and thus is useless as an oxygen-carrying protein. Hb H disease has been described most frequently in orientals and less commonly in whites and blacks. The excess of β-chains in Hb H disease is caused by a marked decreased of α-chain synthesis. This decrease of α-chain synthesis has been shown to be a result of the deletion of these α-globin genes in orientals with Hb H disease.[17]

Clinical manifestations. Children with Hb H disease exhibit a moderate degree of hemolysis and hepatosplenomegaly. The typical clinical picture is usually present by 1 year of age. Approximately 35% of these children develop facial and other bony deformities similar to that seen in β-thalassemia major.[13]

Laboratory findings. Hemoglobin ranges from 7 to 10 g/dl. Red cells are hypochromic, microcytic, and vary in size and shape.[13] Hb H is detected by hemoglobin electrophoresis. It comprises as much as 30% of the total hemoglobin. Hb A$_2$ is decreased. The bone marrow exhibits moderate erythroid hyperplasia.

Treatment. Treatment for Hb H disease includes folic acid, avoidance of oxidant agents (such as those seen in glucose 6-phosphate dehydrogenase [G6PD]), and prompt treatment of infections.[3] Transfusions may be needed occasionally, but chronic transfusion programs usually are not needed. Patients may need red cell transfusions at the time of stress such as with infections. Splenectomy may ameliorate the anemia but is not indicated unless there are significant symptoms of hypersplenism. The natural history of Hb H chain has not been well documented. Most patients appear to live into adulthood.

Hydrops fetalis

The most severe form of α-thalassemia syndrome is hydrops fetalis. It is associated with no α-chain production, and no Hb A or Hb F is produced. Because of the lack of Hb A and Hb F, extrauterine life is not possible. Affected infants are usually stillborn or survive only minutes after birth. They are grossly edematous and have massive hepatosplenomegaly. Hemoglobin electrophoresis at delivery indicates predominance of Hb Bart's. Hb Bart's is a tetramer of γ-chains and cannot function adequately as an oxygen carrier, which accounts for the fetal death.

GENETIC COUNSELING: THE THALASSEMIAS

An understanding of the mode of inheritance is essential for nurses and all professionals caring for the children and families affected by thalassemia. The chronically benign nature of most heterozygous conditions should be stressed, whereas the serious nature of the homozygous conditions should be emphasized. The risk for a couple to produce an affected offspring must be addressed after proper diagnostic studies have been performed. Mode of inheritance from heterozygous parents is diagramed in Fig. 15-4.

When one parent is normal and the other parent carries a thalassemia gene, no homozygous children will be produced, but each child will have a 50% chance of having thalassemia trait.[1] When both parents are heterozygotes for the trait, the risk

Heterozygous parent (Aa)

	A	a
A	AA Normal	Aa Trait
a	Aa Trait	aa Affected child homozygous condition

(left axis label: **Heterozygous parent (Aa)**)

Fig. 15-4. Inheritance pattern for heterozygous parents for thalassemia. *A,* Normal gene; *a,* thalassemia gene.

for producing a child with homozygous disease is 1:4 for each child born.[18]

Once a couple is determined to be at risk for having a child with a homozygous form of thalassemia, there are three options available to them regarding having children:

1. Have children regardless of the risk
2. Use artificial insemination
3. Refrain from having children

The couple must be informed about the availability of intrauterine diagnosis. The decision to terminate or continue the pregnancy must be made by the couple, but they should be allowed the opportunity to discuss their feelings of transmitting a serious chronic illness to their child.

CASE STUDY

J.W. is a 14-year-old white female of Mediterranean heritage diagnosed at 6 months of age with homozygous β-thalassemia major. She was initially noted to be severely anemic with a hemoglobin less than 5 g/dl. Her MCV was 60 with a reticulocyte count of 6%. The blood smear revealed hypochromia with anisocytosis, poikilocytosis, and nucleated red blood cells. Hemoglobin electrophoresis revealed 70% Hb F, 6% Hb A_2, and 27% Hb A.

Physical examination revealed extreme pallor with massive hepatosplenomegaly. Because of growth failure

during the first 6 months of life, a chronic transfusion program was initiated. J.W. gained weight and continued to thrive on transfusions until 10 years of age, at which time she began to show a linear decline in growth demonstrated by the height-weight percentile for age. Evaluation of her iron status revealed severe iron overload and a chelation program was initiated. Desferal was administered subcutaneously for 12 hours, 6 days a week. J.W. has since remained on a chronic transfusion chelation therapy program. She demonstrates no secondary sexual characteristics to date.

NURSING CONSIDERATIONS
β-Thalssemia major

Improved treatment has brought with it new physical and emotional problems not previously addressed. Modell summarizes major problems occurring in the patient with β-thalassemia major as being adaptation to illness, rejection of treatment, failure of puberty, infertility, difficulty in employment, isolation, and the transfer to an adult physician.[11,19]

β-thalassemia major has previously been identified as an invariably fatal disease. Young patients on chronic transfusion programs and chelation therapy now face a more hopeful future not previously encountered in their disease. These individuals should be encouraged to live every day to the fullest while looking to create a future for themselves. Their uncertain prognosis causes many patients, especially adolescents, to react with assertiveness in facing the problems of their lives.

This new found assertiveness may create problems during adolescence. Many feel a need to gain control for the first time in their life and frequently have difficulty continuing treatment. An overwhelming need to be normal may cause rebellion and lack of compliance to transfusion and chelation therapy. These patients must be given as much independence as possible, making it essential for all involved in care to allow the patient to remain an active participant.

Deleterious effects of severe β-thalassemia greatly alter the child's self-image. Failure of growth and delayed puberty cause inferiority, often substantiated by the way others treat them. The 14-

year-old who has impaired growth and development frequently is treated as a 10-year-old, causing much frustration. These individuals should be encouraged to pursue adult goals while closely monitoring their sexual development and counseling early on, since secondary impotence and amenorrhea commonly occur. Replacement therapy with hormones should be given adequately and early on.[17] Feelings of inadequacy are frequently felt by the patient with β-thalassemia major, requiring the support of sensitive caring professionals whose goals must be to provide guidance for the patient in creating a quality of life as normal as possible.

The individual with β-thalassemia major who is being treated effectively with a chronic transfusion-chelation program must strive for a quality of life that incorporates a successful socialization program, allowing the patient to attend school and eventually seek opportunities for employment.[17]

Alterations in life-style caused by an aggressive treatment program often add to the isolation the individual with β-thalassemia major feels from the disease itself. Interaction with other patients may allow for increased understanding and insight into the individual's own problems.

As patients continue to do well on aggressive therapy, patients under the supervision of pediatric care providers may need to be transferred for adult care. This changeover should be done gradually, with the patient being actively involved in the decision for transfer. A patient should never be transferred in the midst of a crisis. This transfer must be perceived as a positive move, reinforcing the patient's continued success on treatment.

The nurse plays an integral role in promoting the psychologic well-being of the patient with β-thalassemia major. Established relationships over a long period of time allow the nurse to remain actively involved in all aspects of care, giving the patient a great sense of security in the professional team.

β-Thalassemia minor

The child with β-thalassemia trait requires no specific medical treatment. Primary emphasis is placed on education of the family who must deal with its implications for inheritance. The nurse must be aware of the various disorders seen in thalassemia minor and must understand their modes of inheritance and degree of clinical severity. Knowledge of these specific thalassemias assists the family in understanding the disorder.

Family blood studies are extremely useful in identifying the specific gene abnormality in a family with thalassemia. The family must understand the rationale for testing all family members. Such an understanding enables members to undergo studies without undue frustration and fear. Prenatal testing should be presented as an option to families at risk for having severely affected offspring.

α-Thalassemias

Individuals with α-thalassemia trait, or the "silent carrier" state, frequently are not diagnosed until they have produced a child with Hb H disease or hydrops fetalis. The professional is responsible for providing or referring for genetic counseling and psychologic support. Individuals demonstrating absence of one or two of the α-genes are counseled on the risk of having an affected child when paired with another individual carrying the gene deletion. As previously discussed, families are given the options but must make their own decision whether or not to have further offspring.

Individuals with Hb H disease may require care similar to that for individuals with thalassemia major, as previously discussed. However, most children grow up to lead normal and productive lives. Transfusion therapy is rarely required, but in those who are severely affected by the deletion of three α-genes, iron overload and complications of transfusions are major nursing concerns. These individuals must be monitored closely with routine clinical visits. Avoidance of oxidative agents, as previously discussed in individuals with G6PD, should be stressed, since these agents precipitate hemolysis.

The child with hydrops fetalis cannot survive. Support of the family having a child with hydrops fetalis encompasses all aspects of the loss of a child. Guilt and blame is frequently experienced, since this is a genetic disorder. Counseling allows the parents to explore their feelings and is strongly advised.

Prenatal diagnosis is discussed when parents be-gin to think of having other children. As previously discussed, prenatal diagnosis enables families who are carriers of an affected gene to make rational intelligent decisions after discovering how severely the fetus is affected.

NURSING CARE PROTOCOL FOR THE CHILD WITH THALASSEMIA

Nursing diagnosis (patient problems)	Goals/objectives (patient/family will:)	Interventions (nurse will:)
1. Knowledge deficit (related to diagnosis)	Receive information related to diagnosis verbally and/or in printed material	Assist with and teach cause of disease; provide information related to the genetic disorder, its mode of inheritance, and clinical severity
2. Anxiety (related to diagnosis and its genetic mode of inheritance)	Demonstrate decreased level of anxiety after establishing an understanding of its mode of inheritance Share feelings and emotions with support persons	Encourage discussion of the genetic disorder and its implications Refer to other services available for counseling; provide opportunity for genetic counseling

3. Knowledge deficit (regarding care) β-Thalassemia major	Verbalize general understanding of the disorder and its implications on lifestyle
	
	Understand need for red blood cell transfusions because of severe anemia
	
	Be able to cope with demands a chronic illness places on the family
		Provide information related to the side effects of thalassemia major:
		    Delayed growth
		    Endocrine disorders
		    Bony deformities
		    Severe anemia
		Discuss need for red cell transfusions and their potential side effects (see Chapter 23 on blood products)
		Encourage discussion of concerns and assist in establishing a life-style that incorporates numerous demands placed on the family by chronic disease

NURSING CARE PROTOCOL FOR THE CHILD WITH THALASSEMIA—cont'd

Nursing diagnosis (patient problems)	Goals/objectives (patient/family will:)	Interventions (nurse will:)
	Be able to manage the child at home without added stress and frustration	Contact public health nurse to supervise care at home and support family; establish close supervision of the child by phone; develop trusting relationship with the hematology team
	Develop normal life-style that encompasses activities essential for the child's continued development	Encourage participation in activities of daily living: self care, school, interaction with peers Discuss disease with school personnel and its restrictions on the child's activities; reinforce the school's need to encourage the child to be as independent as possible
	Demonstrate ability to cope with deleterious side effects caused by severe anemia	Allow patient/family to discuss frustrations/difficulties dealing with delayed growth and sexual maturation; assist in obtaining endocrine consultation for developmental evaluation; administer appropriate hormone replacement when necessary Provide opportunities for discussion with other parents/patients who have thalassemia major Provide continuity of care to establish trust relationships Refer for additional counseling when patient/family is unable to adjust
β-Thalassemia minor	Demonstrate understanding of thalassemia trait and its mode of inheritance	Discuss mode of inheritance of thalassemia minor; review deletion or decrease in production of β-globin synthesis in terms the family can understand

Continued.

NURSING CARE PROTOCOL FOR THE CHILD WITH THALASSEMIA—cont'd

Nursing diagnosis (patient problems)	Goals/objectives (patient/family will:)	Interventions (nurse will:)
	Express concerns for the presence of thalassemia trait as a genetic disorder	Allow for expression of fears and concerns of carrying a genetic defect and producing affected offspring Review family concerns, their understanding of the disorder, and plans for follow-up Refer for genetic counseling if appropriate Discuss prenatal testing when appropriate
α-Thalassemias	Demonstrate an understanding of the genetic defect and its implications for inheritance	
α-Thalassemia trait "silent carrier" state		Discuss with patients/families affected with thalassemia trait, or "silent carrier," the absence of clinical symptoms but implications for inheritance Demonstrate mode of inheritance by diagrams
Hb H disease		Provide information to parents/families with Hb H disease regarding clinical symptoms; (may be similar to those found in thalassemia major) Reinforce that most children lead normal lives; review mode of inheritance previously discussed
Hydrops fetalis		Support families having a child die of hydrops fetalis Refer to appropriate support services: chaplain, social worker, psychologist Provide opportunity to discuss their guilt and fears for future offspring Provide for genetic counseling Discuss subsequent use of prenatal testing with future pregnancies

NURSING CARE PROTOCOL FOR THE CHILD WITH THALASSEMIA—cont'd

Nursing diagnosis (patient problems)	Goals/objectives (patient/family will:)	Interventions (nurse will:)
4. Coping, ineffective family: compromised	Demonstrate effective coping mechanisms necessary for optimum functioning at home, school, and community	Provide emotional support; refer to other health professionals as needed Introduce family to support groups if available

REFERENCES

1. Schwartz, E.: Hemoglobinopathies in children, Littleton, Mass., 1980, PSG/Wright Publishing Co., Inc.
2. Miller, D.R., Baehner, R.L., and McMillan, C.W.: Blood diseases of infancy and childhood, ed. 5, St. Louis, 1984, The C.V. Mosby Co.
3. Nathan, D.G., and Oski, F.A.: Hematology of infancy and childhood, vol. 1, Philadelphia, 1981, W.B. Saunders Co.
4. Ohene-Fremping, D., and Schwartz, E.: Clinical features of thalassemia, Pediatr. Clin. North Am. 27(2):403, 1980.
5. Bank, A.: The thalassemia syndromes, Blood 51(3):369, 1978.
6. Weiner, M., and others: Cooley's anemia: high transfusion regimen and chelation therapy, results and perspective, J. Pediatr. 92(4):653, 1978.
7. Propper, R.D., Button, L.N., and Nathan, D.G.: New approaches to the transfusion management of thalassemia, Blood 55(1):55, 1980.
8. Modell, B.: Total management of thalassemia major, Arch. Dis. Child. 52:489, 1977.
9. Piomell, S., and Graziano, J.: Reduction of iron overload in thalassemia, Birth Defects, Original Article Series 18(7):339, 1982.
10. Flynn, D.M., Hoffbrand, A.V., and Politis, D.: Subcutaneous desferrioxamine: the effect of three years treatment on liver, iron, serum, ferritin, and comments on echocardiography, Birth Defects, Original Article Series 18(7):347, 1982.
11. Modell, B.: The management of the improved prognosis in thalassemia major, Birth Defects, Original Article Series 18(7):329, 1982.
12. Reich, P.R.: Hematology, physiopathologic basis of clinical practice, Boston, 1978, Little, Brown & Co.
13. Weatherall, D.J., and Clegg, J.B.: Thalassemia syndromes, Boston, 1981, Blackwell Scientific Publications.
14. Rudolph, A.M.: Pediatrics, ed. 17, New York, 1982, Appleton Century Crofts.
15. Lanzkowsky, P.: Pediatric hematology oncology, New York, 1980, McGraw-Hill, Inc.
16. Beck, W.S.: Hematology, ed. 3, Cambridge, Mass., 1982, The MIT Press.
17. Orkin, S.H., and Nathan, D.G.: Current concepts in genetics, the thalassemias. N. Engl. J. Med. 295(13):710, 1976.
18. Waley, L.F., and Wong, D.L.: Nursing care of infants and children, St. Louis, 1979, The C.V. Mosby Co.
19. Masera, G.: The treatment of beta-thalassemia: organization, Birth Defects, Original Article Series 18(7):325, 1982.

ADDITIONAL READINGS

Alter, B.P., and others: Prenatal diagnosis of hemoglobinopathies: a review of 15 cases, N. Engl. J. Med. 295:1437, 1976.

Kan, Y., and others: Prenatal diagnosis of homozygous thalassemia, Lancet 2:790, 1975.

Modell, B.: Management of thalassemia major, Br. Med. Bull. 32:270, 1976.

Modell, C.B., and Beck, J.: Long-term desferrioxamine therapy in thalassemia, Ann. N. Y. Acad. Sci. 232:201, 1974.

Nathan, D.G.: Thalassemia: seminars in medicine, N. Engl. J. Med. 286:586, 1972.

Nienhais, A.W.: Safety of intensive chelation therapy, N. Engl. J. Med. 296:114, 1977.

Piomelli, S., others: Hypertransfusion regimen in patients with Cooley's anemia, Ann. N. Y. Acad. Sci. 232:186, 1974.

Singer, D.B.: Postsplenectomy sepsis, Perspect. Pediatr. Pathol. 1:285, 1973.

Wolman, J.J.: Transfusion therapy in Cooley's anemia: growth and health as related to long-range hemoglobin levels: a progress report, Ann. N. Y. Acad. Sci. 119:736, 1964.

CHAPTER 16

Hemophilia

MARTHA S. WARREN and CAMPBELL W. McMILLAN

Hemophilia is a sex-linked congenital bleeding disorder that primarily affects males. There are two distinct types of hemophilia: hemophilia A and hemophilia B. Hemophilia A, also known as classic hemophilia, is characterized by a deficiency or malfunction of the factor VIII clotting protein. Hemophilia B, also known as Christmas disease, is characterized by a deficiency or a malfunction of the factor IX clotting protein. Hemophilia occurs in approximately 1:10,000 newborn males. Hemophilia A is five times more prevalent than Hemophilia B. Both disorders have been noted in populations around the world. Factor VIII and IX are two of the twelve or more clotting proteins that are essential for normal blood coagulation.

A deficiency in one of the clotting proteins interferes with normal hemostasis. Hemostasis is the process by which bleeding episodes are stopped. When injury occurs to a blood vessel wall, hemostasis depends on three mechanisms: (1) vascular contraction, (2) platelet aggregation, and (3) coagulation or clot formation. The coagulation reactions involve the sequential interaction of a series of coagulation proteins with cofactors to generate thrombin, which converts fibrinogen to fibrin monomers. The fibrin monomers assemble and are cross-linked by factor XIII to form a stable clot at the site of the damaged blood vessel.[1] The clotting reactions are depicted schematically in Fig. 16-1.

HISTORY

References to hemophilia were made in the Babylonian Talmud in the fifth century AD, where it was noted that if two children died from circumcisional bleeding, the third child should not be circumcised. Otto in 1803 was the first physician to actually describe hemophilia as a sex-linked bleeding disease, observing that in "bleeding" families, only males were affected and females transmitted the disease. The "bleeding" disease was eventually named hemophilia, literally meaning "love of blood," by Hopff in 1828. Throughout the nineteenth century, various descriptions of the disease were made. Work was continued at the beginning of the twentieth century. Bulloch and Fildes in 1912 presented an extensive review of 64 pedigrees of families with bleeding disorders. All of these reports were outstanding contributions to knowledge concerning hemophilia. However, a basic understanding of the pathogenesis of hemophilia came in 1939 when Brinkhous observed that the conversion of prothrombin to thrombin is delayed in hemophilia and it could be corrected by a blood transfusion. He concluded that the basic defect in hemophilia was related to a lack of a plasma protein which he called antihemophilic factor (AHF).

It was not until 1952 that Aggeler, Biggs, and colleagues independently recognized two types of sex-linked bleeding disorders: Hemophilia A and Hemophilia B. Hemophilia B is also called Christmas disease, named after the first patient who was noted to have factor IX deficiency.[2,3] Both hemophilia A and B present identically, including the same inheritance pattern, symptomatology, and clinical manifestations. Therefore the two bleeding disorders will be discussed together throughout this chapter.

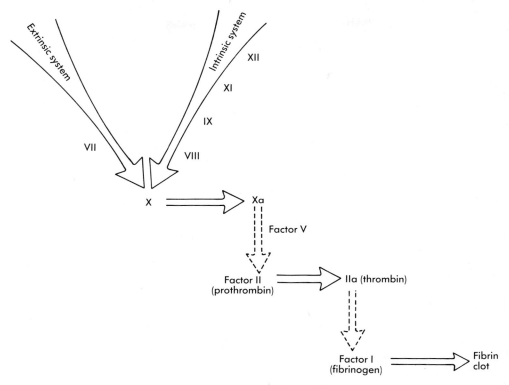

Fig. 16-1. The clotting pathway.

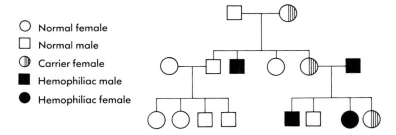

Fig. 16-2. Inheritance pattern in hemophilia.

GENETICS

Hemophilia is usually inherited as a sex-linked recessive disorder. With this sex-linked pattern, the male inherits the bleeding disorder from his mother who is a carrier of the defective gene for hemophilia. The hemophilic male then passes this gene to his daughters, but all sons of affected males will be normal. The daughters have both the gene for hemophilia and a normal gene. As a result, carriers of hemophilia will have roughly 50% levels of AHF (factor VIII) and will not experience clinical bleeding. The daughters of the hemophilic male are obligate carriers; sons of carriers have a 50% chance of having hemophilia. Daughters of carriers have a 50% chance of being carriers themselves. If the hemophilic male has only sons, the disease will not be passed on to future generations.

Rarely, a female has been diagnosed with hemophilia. If a female carrier marries a hemophilic male, female offsprings have a chance of having hemophilia.[4] Fig. 16-2 depicts a pedigree of a hemophilic family.

DIAGNOSIS

When a patient is suspected of having a bleeding disorder, a detailed history is taken before physical examination. Specific questions are designed to ascertain whether bleeding is secondary to inadequate hemostasis. For example, did the child bleed after circumcision, does the child bruise easily, does bleeding occur at the onset of injury or is bleeding delayed, and does the child take any medications? These and other similar questions can provide information needed to help make a diagnosis.

Additionally, a family history is taken and a pedigree is obtained to determine presence of bleeding in the family. If there is a history of familial bleeding, it is important to note the pattern and severity of bleeding with each family member.

Following the initial evaluation, several laboratory tests are obtained that include a prothrombin time (PT), activated partial thromboplastin time (APTT), thrombin clotting time (TCT), bleeding time (BT), and a specific factor VIII or IX assay.

The PT measures the production of thrombin and fibrin by way of the *extrinsic* clotting system (factor VII). The APTT measures the production of thrombin and fibrin by way of the *intrinsic* system (factors XII, XI, IX, and VIII). The TCT measures the conversion of fibrinogen to fibrin and is prolonged when there are low levels of fibrinogen. The factor VIII or IX assay measures the respective levels of factor VIII or IX clotting activity. In hemophilia A and B, the PTT is prolonged and the level of factor VIII or IX is low. The PT, TCT, and BT are normal.

CLASSIFICATION

Hemophilia has been divided into three main groups: severe, moderate, and mild. The severity of the disease is usually associated with the level of factor VIII or IX activity. The normal level of factor VIII or IX clotting activity in an individual ranges from 60% to 150%. The severely affected patient has less than 1% clotting activity and can bleed spontaneously, especially into joints and muscles. In moderate hemophilia, the level of factor VIII or IX is 1% to 5% of normal. Usually, there is no spontaneous hemorrhage; however, bleeding can occur with mild trauma. The mildly affected patient has factor VIII or IX levels greater than 5%. These patients rarely bleed except with trauma, surgery, or invasive dental procedures. In fact, many of these cases may go undiagnosed until such time as major trauma induces bleeding.[4]

Family members usually have the same severity of hemophilia and similar bleeding patterns. It is important to note that on occasion a person can have severe hemophilia by laboratory diagnosis, but present clinically with a milder bleeding pattern. The severity of hemophilia remains the same throughout the various generations in the family.

REPLACEMENT THERAPY

Hemostasis in the hemophiliac is achieved by infusing the deficient clotting factor. In 1840 Lane noted that by infusing the hemophiliac with whole blood, hemostasis may be obtained.[5] In 1929 Payne and Steel demonstrated that the use of plasma was more effective in raising the patient's missing clotting factor.[6] Thus the concept of using plasma products for treatment of hemophilic bleeding episodes was developed. Later, the greatest revolution for hemophiliac treatment occurred with the introduction of plasma factor concentrates in the mid-1960s.

Plasma

Fresh frozen plasma contains all the clotting factors and was the primary form of therapy used to treat hemophilia until 1964. One milliliter of fresh frozen plasma contains 1 unit of clotting factor activity. Therefore significant volumes of plasma are needed to achieve hemostasis for treatment of major bleeding episodes.

Cryoprecipitate

In 1965 Poole and Robinson demonstrated that on freezing and then thawing plasma at 4° C a precipitate forms that is rich in fibrinogen and factors VIII and XIII.[7] This precipitate, cryoprecipitate, contains approximately tenfold the amount of factor VIII found in the starting plasma. When using cryoprecipitate, sufficient levels of factor VIII may be obtained in a smaller volume, decreasing the risk of circulatory overload.

Factor VIII concentrates

Following the introduction of cryoprecipitates, the concentrates evolved. Brinkhous and his associates were among the first to develop a fractionation process used to make high-potency factor VIII concentrates. The concentrates are prepared from a further purification of the cryoprecipitates. In a typical preparation, plasma from 2,000 to 20,000 donors is pooled and fractionated, producing a freeze-dried (lyophilized) concentratrate. The freeze-dried preparation provides a longer shelf life than the other products, which makes concentrates easier for home infusion. Additionally, the concentrates are free of many extraneous proteins found is cryoprecipitate.

Factor IX concentrates

Factor IX concentrates are prepared from the plasma recovered from the supernatant from which the cryoprecipitate has been removed. Factor IX is further purified with chromatographic techniques. The factor IX concentrates contain all the vitamin K–dependent factors: II, VII, IX, and X but these are used primarily for factor IX–deficient patients.

By definition, 1 unit of clotting factor is that amount of clotting activity found in 1 ml of fresh normal pooled plasma.[8] For example, 1000 ml of plasma contains 1000 units of factor VIII or IX activity. To replace the patient's deficient clotting factor, the dosage is based on the patient's plasma volume, which is calculated on his weight. One unit of factor VIII will raise the patient's plasma level 2%. One unit of factor IX will raise the patient's plasma level 1%. A greater amount of factor IX is required, since factor IX distributes more easily into the extravascular space. The biologic half-life of factor VIII is 8 to 12 hours, and factor IX is 18 to 24 hours. Table 16-1 describes the advantages and disadvantages of products used to treat hemophilia A and B.

BLEEDING MANIFESTATIONS AND TREATMENT

Bleeding episodes can be either classified into minor or major categories (Table 16-2). The severity and anatomic location of the hemorrhage determines the classification of the bleed. Minor bleeding episodes are not life-threatening and often can be managed with treatment on an outpatient basis or with home infusion. Examples of minor bleeding include hemarthrosis, intramuscular bleeding, and mild hematuria. Major bleeding is life-threatening and requires immediate medical attention, replacement therapy raising the deficient clotting factor level 100%, and hospitalization. Major bleeds may involve the central nervous system (CNS), retropharyngeal area, retroperitoneal area, and pseudotumors. Occasionally, a minor bleed may progress into a major bleed, such as a severe intramuscular bleed compromising neurologic or vascular function.

Table 16-1. Products used for treatment of hemophilia

Product	Advantages	Disadvantages
Hemophilia A (replacement therapy)		
Fresh frozen plasma	Lower risk of hepatitis	High volume–problem circulatory overload
		Low yield of factor VIII units
		Variability of potency
		Must be stored at $-20°$ C
Cryoprecipitate	Lower risk of hepatitis	Factor VIII may vary from bag to bag
		Must be stored at $-20°$ C
		Difficult to store when using for home therapy
Concentrates		
Factorate (Armour)	High yield factor	High risk of hepatitis
Hemofil (Hyland)	VIII units, low	High risk of blood-related viruses
Humafac (Parke-Davis)	Potency stated on each bottle	
Koate (Cutter)	Reduced levels of other plasma proteins	
Profilate (Alpha)	Convenience of storage when storing	
	Long shelf life	
Hemophilia B		
Fresh frozen plasma	Lower risk of hepatitis	High volume, low yield of factor IX units
		Variability of potency
		Must be stored at $-20°$ C
Concentrates		
Konyne (Cutter)	High yield factor	High risk of hepatitis
Profilnine (Alpha)	IX units	Possible thromboembolic problems
Proplex (Hyland)		
Prothar (Armour)	Low volume	

Minor bleeds

Hemarthrosis. Hemarthrosis, or bleeding into a joint, is the hallmark of hemorrhagic problems in the hemophiliac. Joint bleeding is the most common type of hemorrhage and usually the most disabling complication associated with hemophilia. Bleeding can occur into any joint, but it most frequently occurs in the knees, elbows, ankles, hips, and shoulders (listed in order of decreasing frequency).[9] Recurrent bleeding in the joint may cause degenerative changes in the articular cartilage and inflammation of the synovium. This can ultimately lead to hemophilic arthropathy.

The pathophysiology of hemarthrosis is not entirely understood. However, two stages have been identified: an early stage and a later stage. Although

two stages have been classified, it must be noted that pathologic changes are a continual process and cannot be delineated.[9]

The early stage is characterized by synovial hypertrophy, hemosiderin deposition, breakdown of chondrocytes in the cartilage, and early fibrosis of the synovium. Release of various degradative enzymes may initiate an inflammatory response in the synovium. These pathologic changes are very similar to those found in rheumatoid arthritis.

The later stage is characterized by joint malalignment and cartilage destruction. Formation of subchrondral cysts and osteophytes on the cartilage causes a mechanical breakdown of the joint. Additionally, further fibrosis of the synovium is noted. The combination of these factors causes narrowing

Table 16-2. Signs, symptoms, and treatment of minor and major bleeds

Bleeding manifestations	Signs, symptoms	Desired level to raise factor VIII or IX
Minor		
Hemarthrosis	Early: pain, tingling sensation in joint, stiffness	30%-50%
	Later: tense, swollen, painful, joint redness, warmth	
Intramuscular	Early: muscle swelling, tightness, pain, redness, warmth	30%-50%
	Later: numbness, paresthesia, possible nerve involvement	50%-100%
Skin laceration	Oozing of blood from superficial cut	Hold cut with firm pressure
	Rapid loss of blood from deep laceration	50% before suturing
Mouth	Bleeding from gums, lips, or frenulum	50%
Gastrointestinal	Pain in abdomen, coughing up or vomiting blood, passing blood in stool, weakness, postural hypotension	50%
Hematuria	Blood in urine, urine may appear bright red to dark brown in color	
Major		
Central nervous system (Intracranial)	Headache	100% and hospitalization
	Vomiting	
	Blurred vision	
	Unequal pupils	
	Difficulty walking	
	Slurring of speech	
	Drowsiness/confusion	
	Seizures	
	Loss of consciousness	
Retropharyngeal	Tightness in throat	100% and hospitalization
	Swelling around neck	
	Difficulty swallowing and breathing	
	Possible stridor	
	Neck or throat pain	
Retroperitoneal	Pain in hip or groin	100% and hospitalization
	Difficulty with extension of leg of affected side	
	Lower abdominal pain	
Pseudotumor	Pain at site of pseudotumor	100% and hospitalization
	Partial or complete obstruction of contiguous organs	

of the joint space, a decrease in the range of motion, and the development of a flexion contracture. The previously described changes are very similar to those found in osteoarthritis. Additionally, osteoporosis may occur from disuse of the affected joint.

Hemophilic arthropathy is divided into three classes: acute, subacute, and chronic.[10]

In the *acute phase,* bleeding into the joint occurs spontaneously or as the result of minor trauma. Typically, the patient describes a tingling or bubbling sensation in the joint accompanied by stiff-

ness and pain, often called the prodrome to the hemarthrosis. When bleeding begins, the joint becomes swollen, tense, hot, tender, and very painful. The joint may be held in flexion as a result of a restricted motion and intense pain. Analgesics may be needed to alleviate pain until the bleed resolves.

The *subacute phase* is characterized by synovial hypertrophy, which usually results from several repeated bleeding episodes in the same joint. The joint becomes boggy from synovial hypertrophy and joint effusion. There is a decrease in the range of motion followed by atrophy of adjacent muscles. Joint contractures may also begin during this stage. Radiographic changes reveal early osteoporosis in the epiphyses and early changes in the joint surface.

The *chronic phase* of hemarthropathy results when degenerative changes have continued for an extended period of time. These changes are usually irreversible. Since the cartilage has been damaged, repeated bleeding is more likely to occur and a vicious cycle may ensue. Consequently, end stage arthropathy may result. Radiographic findings include irregularity in the surface of the cartilage caused by the development of osteophytes and subchrondral cysts and thinning of the cartilage.

Treatment. In the *acute phase* factor replacement therapy should be given to the patient promptly at the prodromal symptoms of bleeding. The patient's factor level should be raised 30% to 50% to achieve hemostasis.[8] Several treatments may be indicated, given every 12 hours. Adjunct therapy consists of temporarily immobilizing the joint, application of ice, and occasionally splinting.

When a major bleed occurs in a joint, arthrocentesis (joint aspiration) may be indicated during the acute phase. Sometimes, removing the large volume of blood from the joint significantly reduces the pain and decreases the possibility of blood causing destruction to the cartilage and synovium. When aspiration is required, the factor level should be raised 50% before the procedure.

In the *subacute phase,* patients are often placed on an aggressive prophylactic program to prevent further joint destruction. A typical prophylactic program consists of factor replacement therapy administered two to three times a week for several months.[11] If prophylaxis is unsuccessful, surgical intervention such as a synovectomy may be indicated. Fig. 16-3 illustrates a knee in the subacute phase.

Treatment in the *chronic phase* consists primarily in preserving the existing function of the joint, since many irreversible pathologic changes have occurred. Goals of intervention are to maintain muscle strength and range of motion. Interventions may include shoe modification for the use of an

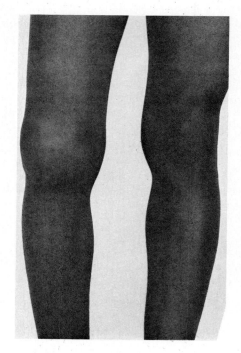

Fig. 16-3. Child's knee in the subacute phase of a bleeding episode.

assistive device during walking. Casting or traction may be required to achieve maximum extension of a flexed joint. Occasionally, surgery may be indicated for painful inflammatory joint changes. Various types of surgery include arthrodesis, osteotomy, synovectomy, or joint replacement.

Five stages of progressive hemophilic arthropathy have been described by Arnold and Hilgartner. Fig. 16-4 demonstrates a normal joint as compared with Fig. 16-5 (see pp. 260-261) which illustrates the progressive radiographic and diagrammatic changes noted in the joint. Since this current classification presents a wide clinical spectrum within the five radiographic findings, the Orthopedic Advisory Committee at the Fourteenth International Congress of the World Federation of Hemophilia recently recommended that a new radiographic classification be used. This thirteen scale classification ranges from zero (normal joint) to 13 (most

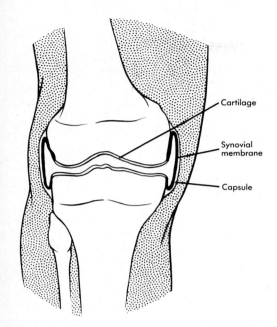

Cartilage

Synovial
membrane

Capsule

Fig. 16-4. Normal knee joint as compared with Fig. 16-5 illustrating progressive joint destruction.

extensive joint destruction).[11] However, this new classification has not been widely accepted by orthopedists.

Intramuscular hemorrhage. Hemorrhage into the muscle is another common site of bleeding in patients with hemophilia. Most frequently, this type of bleeding occurs in the calves, forearms, thighs, and iliopsoas muscle, although it may occur in any muscle.[12] Intramuscular bleeding may secondarily affect the nerves and blood vessels. Often bleeding in the muscle causes scarring and fibrosis of the connective tissue and muscle fibers. Scar tissue decreases the flexibility of the muscle and may result in contracture of the adjacent joint. For example, a hemorrhage into the calf, the gastrocnemius muscle, may result in a fixed equinus deformity. If therapy is not given promptly with this type of bleed, the scar tissue may contract and pull on the ankle, causing deformity. The patient cannot put his affected heel on the ground when in a standing position.

Another common intramuscular hemorrhage occurs in the forearm, which may result in a Volkmann's contracture. This contracture results from hemorrhage in the volar fascial compartment of the forearm. The pressure of the hematoma produces necrosis, ischemic paralysis, and atrophy of the muscle, resulting in Volkmann's contracture. The patient may experience pain, pallor, and paresthesias. To release the pressure in the forearm, surgical decompression may be indicated.

Treatment for intramuscular hemorrhage usually consists of administering factor replacement therapy to raise the patient's factor level to 50%. If numbness, tingling, or signs of neuropathy occur, additional medical intervention may be necessary.

Skin lacerations. Small superficial cuts or abrasions respond well to the application of firm pressure. Deeper lacerations may need suturing. Since suturing produces additional puncturing of the tissues, replacement therapy must be given to prevent further hemorrhage.

Mucosal bleeding. Bleeding that occurs in the mouth, gastrointestinal tract, and genitourinary tract is referred to as mucosal bleeding. Each of these areas of hemorrhage will be discussed individually.[13]

Bleeding from the mouth, gums, and lips is very common in the hemophilic child. Bleeding frequently occurs as the result of the toddler falling and tearing the frenulum or lacerating the tongue or lip. The shedding of deciduous teeth is often accompanied by gingival bleeding that may continue for days. This bleeding responds well to the use of Epsilon-amino-caproic acid (EACA), which prevents the normal lysis of the clot.

Gastrointestinal hemorrhage is another type of mucosal bleeding. It is observed most frequently in adult hemophiliacs. The occurrence of this type of bleeding may be secondary to the use of anti-inflammatory agents or aspirin-containing medications, which cause gastric irritation and interfere with platelet function. Another cause of gastrointestinal bleeding may be an organic lesion such as

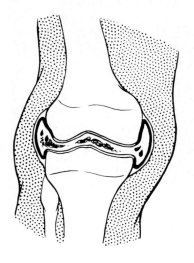
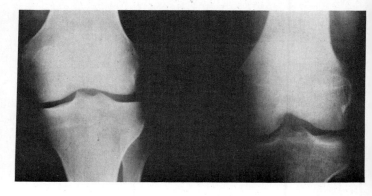

A, Stage 1

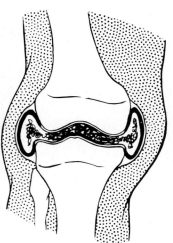
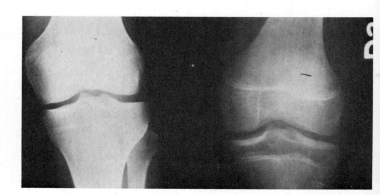

B, Stage 2

Fig. 16-5. Hemophiliac anthropathy.
A, Stage 1
Soft tissue swelling without skeletal bony abnormalities; one to two acute hemarthroses have occurred.
B, Stage 2
Characterized by early osteoporosis, epiphysial overgrowth; integrity of joint is maintained.
C, Stage 3
Disorganization of joint begins in this stage; subchondral cysts may develop in the medial and distal aspect of the bone; see bony surface irregularity; there is some preservation of joint space.
D, Stage 4
Further deterioration of stage 3; characterized by narrowing joint space.
E, Stage 5
End stage—joint is completely fused and is characterized by fibrous joint contracture; no cartilage present; loss of joint space; enlargement of epiphysis.

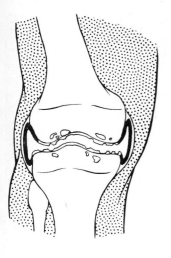
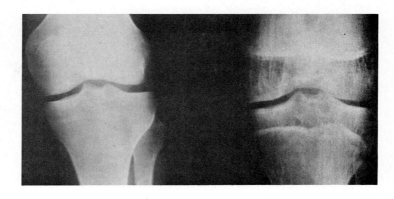

C, Stage 3

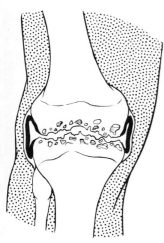
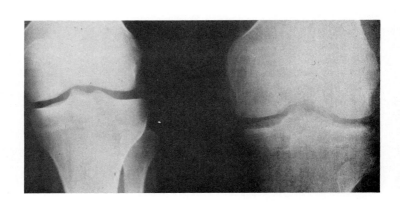

D, Stage 4

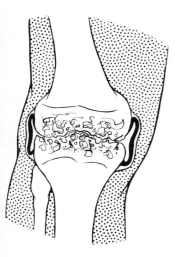
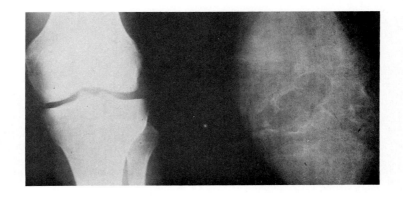

E, Stage 5

ulcer, colitis, carcinoma, or polyps. Hematemesis (or "coffee ground" emesis), abdominal pain, melena, or hematochezia may accompany hemorrhage. Occasionally, a patient may have less obvious symptoms secondary to gastrointestinal bleeding such as dizziness, dyspnea, or postural hypotension.

In patients with gastrointestinal bleeding, a diagnostic workup includes radiographic and endoscopic examination of the gastrointestinal tract. Replacement should be administered before the endoscopy, raising the patient's factor level to 100%.[8]

Hematuria Hematuria is another clinical manifestation of hemophilia. It has been observed in approximately 70% of persons with severe hemophilia and is not uncommon in young boys.[14] The amount of blood loss with hematuria is usually insignificant, although the bright red appearance of the urine gives the impression of a substantial loss of blood. Consequently, the patient or parent may be very alarmed.

The cause of hematuria is unclear, since it frequently is not related to trauma or underlying pathologic conditions. Often hematuria will abate without therapy. However, with persistent hematuria or flank pain, a urologic workup is needed to rule out infection or a pathologic process such as a benign or malignant tumor, kidney stone, glomerulonephritis, nephrosis, or structural defect. Diagnostic procedures may include intravenous pyelography (IVP), cystoscopy, or renal scan. Laboratory workup includes urinalysis, urine culture, blood urea nitrogen (BUN), and creatinine.

Treatment of gross hematuria consists of replacement therapy to raise the factor level to 50%, bed rest for several days, and liberal intake of fluids. Steroids may occasionally be used. The antifibrinolytic agent, EACA, is contraindicated, since it may promote clots that may obstruct the urinary tract.

Major bleeds

Intracranial bleeding. Intracranial hemorrhage is the most life-threatening bleed in the person who has hemophilia. The mortality has been estimated to be 34%.[15] It has been noted that children have a higher incidence of CNS bleeding than adults. CNS bleeding may be intracerebral, subarachnoid, epidural, subdural, and rarely, intraspinal. Intracerebral bleeding has the poorest prognosis. The majority of intracranial bleeding results from head trauma, although this type of bleed may occur spontaneously with no apparent underlying cause.

The most common presenting symptom of CNS bleeding is headache followed by vomiting, seizures, lethargy, irritability, confusion, obtundation, and blurred vision. Onset of these symptoms may be delayed. Occasionally, a patient may report a symptom-free period of more than 24 hours, and subsequently, may seek medical attention several days later with many of the above symptoms.[15]

Accurate diagnosis of intracranial bleeding is very important. Computed tomography (CT) scanning is the diagnostic procedure of choice, since it is noninvasive and localizes the area of bleeding. Other procedures include cerebral angiography or lumbar puncture. Skull films may be obtained to evaluate the possibility of a fracture, especially if the bleed is trauma related. CT scanning should be done on all hemophilic patients with suspected intracranial bleeding. It is not uncommon for a patient to have a severe headache with no related injury, and on CT scanning, an intracranial hemorrhage is revealed.[16]

When an intracranial bleed is diagnosed, replacement therapy is administered immediately to raise the patient's factor level to 100%. Surgery is indicated with subdural hematoma. Subarachnoid bleeding and intracranial hematomas may be medically managed with steroids to decrease cerebral edema and anticonvulsants to minimize brain injury during seizures. The patient is usually hospitalized to receive factor replacement therapy for 10 to 14 days. If treatment is given promptly, neurologic sequelae may be minimized.

Bleeding into the neck and pharynx. Bleeding into the neck, pharynx, or airway is another potential life-threatening bleed that the hemophiliac may experience. A hematoma in the neck or retropharyngeal area or on the tongue may enlarge and obstruct the airway, leading to severe respiratory difficulties. Immediate infusion of replacement therapy to raise the factor level to 100% is critical to prevent swelling that may interfere with breathing. Radiographs may be helpful in determining the presence of a mass or airway obstruction, but usually the clinical picture is diagnostic.

Occasionally, bleeding in the neck or airway may accompany a sore throat, tonsillitis, or pharyngitis. In some cases antibiotics may be required. However, if the patient has a sore throat or inflammation and complains of difficulty swallowing, replacement therapy may be necessary.

Retroperitoneal iliopsoas. Iliopsoas hemorrhage is another critical and frequent problem for the hemophiliac. The iliopsoas muscle is located in the pelvic cavity; it originates from the lumbar vertebrae and internal aspect of the ileum and inserts into the lesser trochanter of the femur. When bleeding occurs in this muscle, the hematoma may expand into adjacent fascial planes and into the retroperitoneal space. The anatomic location of this muscle makes this bleeding difficult to manage, since large volumes of blood may be lost in the retroperitoneal space. Additionally, the expansion of the hemorrhage into the retroperitoneal space may result in a femoral neuropathy caused by the pressure between the iliopsoas muscle and the inguinal ligament.[17]

The clinical expression of the iliopsoas and retroperitoneal bleed are the same. The presenting symptoms include hip flexion accompanied by pain on extension, lower abdominal pain (which may radiate to the scrotum), and iliopsoas irritation. Diagnostic procedures include CT scan of the pelvis and ultrasound examination.

Treatment consists of hospitalization, replacement therapy to raise the deficient clotting level 50% to 100% for a minimum of 5 days followed by observation until the patient is fully ambulatory.[8] Physical therapy should be instituted when the pain subsides.

Pseudotumor. The development of a pseudotumor is a rare although serious complication of hemophilia. A pseudotumor is a cystlike mass that involves muscle or bone. The mass slowly expands in size producing pressure necrosis of surrounding tissues and erosion of bony surfaces.

The cause of a pseudotumor is not certain. Several authors postulate that the bleeding may originate as a deep muscle hematoma or as a subperiosteal or intraosseous hemorrhage. Bleeding into one of these areas may not completely resolve, and an encapsulating hematoma forms. Further bleeding occurs, and the mass increases in size, causing damage to surrounding structures.[18,19]

Pseudotumors may form in any part of the body, although in children they have been noted to occur most frequently in the small bones of the hand and foot. In adults, they are commonly seen in bones adjacent to large muscles such as the femur and pelvis. The clinical picture of the pseudotumor is a painless, slowly expanding mass that often continues to grow for years before intervention is required. The wall of this mass is a tough vascular membrane. Diagnosis of the pseudotumor is confirmed by x-rays, examination, and CT scanning. Initially, the pseudotumor in children is treated with long-term prophylactic replacement therapy for 3 to 4 months. In the adult the tumor may grow so large that radiation therapy is needed. If the tumor does not respond to radiation therapy, radical surgical excision of the mass is necessary. See Table 16-2 for signs and symptoms of minor versus major bleeds and treatment.

Major surgery

All types of surgery in the hemophiliac are possible provided adequate hemostasis is maintained. In general, the only exception to this is the patient who has an inhibitor. Before surgery, a "fall off" study is completed to determine the patient's response to factor replacement therapy. If an inhibitor is detected, conventional therapy and regular surgical protocols may not be used.

Orthopedic surgery or neurosurgery generally requires replacement therapy to raise the patient's deficient clotting level 100% immediately before surgery and at least 50% for 14 days following surgery. Soft tissue surgery such as an appendectomy requires replacement therapy to raise the patient's factor level 100% before surgery and 50% replacement therapy postoperatively for 10 days.

COMPLICATIONS
Inhibitors

The development of an inhibitor is one of the most significant complications that can occur in the person with hemophilia. An inhibitor is an antibody that develops spontaneously and acts directly by inhibiting factor VIII or IX coagulant activity. It is estimated that 5% to 15% of patients with hemophilia A develop an inhibitor.[20] Persons with hemophilia B are less frequently affected. With the appearance of an inhibitor, conventional treatment becomes difficult, since both exogenous and endogenous factor VIII or IX are destroyed.

The cause of an inhibitor is not clear. In an attempt to elucidate this problem, the National Heart, Lung and Blood Institute sponsored a 13-center cooperative investigation from 1975 to 1979.[21] This investigation, the Cooperative Study of Spontaneously Occurring Factor VIII Inhibitors in Patients with Hemophilia, noted the following[21-23]:

1. An inhibitor always developed after exposure to exogenous factor VIII.
2. There was a greater tendency for the severely affected patient to develop an inhibitor.
3. There was a possible genetic predisposition; a familial tendency was observed, and brother pairs of hemophiliacs had a higher incidence in developing an inhibitor.
4. The median age for the development of an inhibitor was 16 years with the range reported as 2 to 62 years of age.

5. The black population had a greater predisposition to developing an inhibitor than other populations.
6. Bleeding frequency did not tend to increase following the development of an inhibitor.

Since the majority of patients who develop an inhibitor have hemophilia A, the following discussion will present classification and treatment of the classic hemophiliac who develops this complication. Patients with factor VIII inhibitors can be divided into three categories: the low responder, the intermediate responder, and the high responder. The low responder is defined as the patient with an inhibitor titer less than 2 Bethesda units. The intermediate responder has 2 to 10 Bethesda units. The high responder has a titer greater than 10 Bethesda units. A Bethesda unit is an arbitrary measure for quantitative activity of the antibody.

The low responding inhibitor patient usually responds well to factor VIII infusion. However, treatment must be modified by increasing the dosage of factor VIII. Occasionally, a low responder will convert to a high responder, thus making therapy more difficult.

Treatment for the high responder patient is multifaceted and must be individualized. For minor bleeding episodes, factor IX concentrate is used frequently at a dosage of 75 units/kg of body weight. Treatment for major life-threatening bleeding episodes is more complex, and there is no specific regimen that assures hemostasis. The first

Table 16-3. Therapeutic options for treatment of inhibitors to factor VIII

	Low responder	High responder
Minor bleed	Factor IX concentrate (PCC) Factor VIII concentrate (AHF)	Factor IX concentrate (PCC) Activated factor IX concentrate (APCC)
Major bleed	Factor VIII concentrate (AHF)	Titer <10 Bethesda units Factor VIII concentrate (AHF) Titer >10 Bethesda units Porcine VIII Activated factor IX concentrate (APCC) Plasmapheresis with high-dose factor VIII concentrate (AHF)

choice for a life-threatening bleeding episode is massive doses of factor VIII. This therapy can be used until the patient has an anamnestic response, at which time the body neutralizes all exogenous factor VIII, and one of the other alternative therapies must be used. Table 16-3 depicts general various therapeutic modalities that can be used to treat patients who have an inhibitor to factor VIII.

The treatment of patients with an inhibitor remains a challenge to physicians and is often controversial. The expense of treatment is extraordinary. Research continues on the various therapeutic approaches for this complex problem.

Hepatitis

Hepatitis resulting from the infusion of plasma products is another significant problem for the person with hemophilia. Frequent infusion of factor VIII or IX replacement therapy places the patient at high risk for exposure to various types of hepatitis viruses. Of the three types of hepatitis viruses—type A (infectious), B (serum), and non-A/non-B hepatitis, the latter two have been found in fractions of plasma used to make the concentrates. Since the majority of severely affected patients have been frequently transfused with the factor concentrates, the incidence of hepatitis has been high. Many of these patients do not initially have clinical symptoms; however, they do have serologic evidence of subclinical hepatitis. A recent study by White and others[24] noted that 85% of the clinically severe hemophilic patients had evidence of prior exposure to hepatitis B virus. In this same study approximately 10% of the patients were noted to have the presence of the circulating hepatitis antigen. In another study 76% of patients had at least one or more report of elevated liver enzymes SGOT (aspartate amino-transferase) or SGPT (alanine amino-transferase).[25] These figures are disturbing and must be considered in the long-term health care of the hemophiliac. However, it must be recognized that using the factor concentrates for treatment is the optimum therapy for many of these patients.

For patients who do not receive frequent exposure to plasma products, another form of therapy is available. For example, 1-deamino-8-D-arginine vasopressin (DDAVP) was approved by the FDA in 1984 for use in mild to moderate hemophilia A. DDAVP induces a transient increase in factor VIII when given intravenously. However, it has not been found to be effective in the severely affected factor VIII–deficient patient.[26]

The exact mechanism of DDAVP is not known. DDAVP may stimulate the release of factor VIII from the endothelial cells, and additionally, it may act locally on the vessel wall to increase platelet adhesiveness.[27]

Thus far, DDAVP has been especially effective in raising the patient's factor VIII level for dental extractions or oral surgery. It has been reported on occasion to be useful in other types of surgery. Studies continue on the efficacy of this drug in the treatment of various hemorrhagic problems.

Thrombosis

Thrombosis secondary to infusion of factor IX (prothrombin complex concentrates) has been noted in some patients. Typical problems are deep vein thrombosis, pulmonary embolism, and occasionally, acute disseminated intravascular coagulation. Rarely coronary thrombosis is associated with administration of these concentrates.[28]

It is not clear how the infusion of factor IX concentrate cause thrombosis, although when thromboembolic problems have occurred, patients usually have received high dosages of IX concentrates, or the concentrates have been administered more rapidly than recommended. The incidence of this type of problem is not common when recommended dosages are used. Additionally, when using the factor IX concentrate, it is also essential to know the status of the patient's liver function tests, since liver dysfunction may result in impairment in clearance of the concentrates. It has been suggested that factor IX concentrates be used with caution in patients with active liver disease, and the indications for its use should be clear and unequivocal.

Hemolysis

Hemolysis may occur as a result of the infusion of a massive dose of factor VIII concentrates. The lyophilized concentrates are made from pooled plasma containing up to 30 times the isoagglutinins (antibodies against the red cell antigens A and B) found in plasma. If a patient having blood type A, B, or AB receives a large amount of concentrate containing high titers of the isoagglutinins, acute hemolysis may occur. Patients with type O cells are not affected.[28]

Clinical symptoms that may present with hemolysis are headache and malaise, fever and chills, lower back pain, or abdominal pain. Laboratory signs associated with this type of hemolysis include a fall in the hemoglobin level, an increase in the reticulocyte count, a positive direct Coomb's test, and a decrease in the haptoglobin level. If any of these changes are noted in the patient, a hemolytic reaction should be suspected and the concentrates discontinued. An alternative therapy with type-specific or low titer concentrate may be administered.

The most serious complication secondary to this type of hemolytic reaction is acute renal failure. Occasionally, disseminated intravascular coagulation may occur.

Acquired immunodeficiency syndrome

Acquired immunodeficiency syndrome (AIDS) has recently been linked to homosexuals, drug addicts, Haitians, and hemophiliacs. Of these groups, the incidence of AIDS in the hemophilic population has been minimal. Although this incidence is low, the fear of contracting AIDS continues to be an alarming problem for persons with hemophilia.

The clinical symptoms of patients diagnosed with AIDS are general malaise, persistent fever, weight loss, diarrhea, lymphadenopathy, and chronic infection. The most characteristic laboratory studies indicate immunosuppression with a reversal of the T4/T8 (helper/suppressor cell) ratio and lymphopenia. Normal helper/suppressor cell ratio is 1.5:3.1; abnormal is 0.7 or less. Additional findings have included an abnormality in lymphocyte function and immunoglobulin synthesis. The unequivocal diagnosis of AIDS is the occurrence of an opportunistic infection in the presence of immunosuppression as manifested by an abnormal helper/suppressor ratio.[29,30]

There is considerable evidence that the cause of AIDS in the hemophilic population is related to exposure to blood products. As evidence is mounting suggesting the link of AIDS with a viral cause, it is anticipated that a vaccine will shortly be available. However, the possibility that the cause of AIDS is multifactorial still exists.

COMPREHENSIVE CARE

The concept of comprehensive care for hemophilia evolved around 1975 when federal funds were provided to support comprehensive hemophilia centers. The advantage of this system of health care delivery is to provide the patient with optimum medical care by professionals who are experienced in seeing many patients with the same illness. Members of a hemophilia multidisciplinary team include an adult and pediatric hematologist, orthopedist, dentist, psychiatrist, physical therapist, nurse coodinator, social worker, geneticist and vocational rehabilitation counselor.

Several years after the establishment of 24 federally funded hemophilia centers, a study was completed that documented highly positive results of comprehensive care. The findings of the study revealed that patients enrolled in the comprehensive centers were noted to have decreases in number of days lost from school or work, number of hospitalizations, annual cost of health care, and unemployment.[31]

Dental care

Dental care is an important component of comprehensive care. The advent of factor concentrate made dramatic changes in the delivery of dental care for the hemophilic population. However, patients with inhibitors remain difficult to manage and require very specialized care beyond the ordinary hemophilic precautions.

Before the availability of adequate replacement therapy, many dental procedures such as local anesthesia or dental extractions were impossible. Local anesthesia, such as a mandibular block predisposed the patient to the development of a dissecting hematoma. Dental extractions were life-threatening and often caused death, since postextraction hemorrhage was difficult to control. Both of these procedures are now possible with prior replacement therapy.

Another therapy used to prevent postextraction bleeding is Epsilon-amino-caproic acid (EACA). Additionally, EACA has been effective in controlling bleeding associated with tongue laceration, gingival bleeding, and other dental-related bleeding. The mechanism of action of EACA is to prevent the activation of plasminogen to plasmin, which indirectly inhibits the lysis of a clot. Plasmin is a nonspecific proteolytic enzyme found in tissues and saliva. It is activated secondary to tissue injury such as a dental extraction. Amicar is the trade name for EACA. When used with dental work or bleeding in the mouth, the recommended dosage of Amicar is 50 mg/kg of body weight administered by mouth every 6 hours for 8 to 10 days.

Psychosocial issues

The diagnosis of hemophilia often brings about many emotions within the parent. Common feelings include disbelief, anger, fear of the unknown, anxiety, and guilt. Because the mother carries the defective gene and passes it on to her son, many mothers experience feelings of guilt. Those who do not overcome these feelings can have difficulty with issues of overprotection and a need to try to compensate for their son. Other relationships within the family may also be affected. An abnormally close relationship between mother and son may develop and lead to exclusion of the father. Some siblings resent the attention the hemophilic child receives and the disruption bleeding episodes cause to the family's normal life-style.

In the toddler stage, parents need to accept the fact that they cannot prevent bleeding by limiting their son's activities, although the usual safety measures for children of this age should be stressed. One of the toddler's major developmental needs is for exploration and movement. It is a learning process to know when to seek medical treatment, and it can be anxiety-provoking to deal with hospital procedures. Blood drawing and venipuncture necessitates the child to be still and confined, often causing much crying at this age. Parents who

deal with their situation calmly can decrease anxiety in the child, since children take cues from parents.

Preschool years are important for learning to play with other children and for preparing the child for school entry. Ideally, by this time the family is comfortable in leaving the child with others. School personnel need to be taught the basic facts about hemophilia so that they will not be afraid of the child and deal with him inappropriately. Most hemophilic children attend regular school and classroom. Physical education teachers must be instructed regarding which activities may predispose the child to bleeding. Physical activities are individualized depending on the child's physical limitations resulting from joint damage and frequency of bleeding.

Often parents need help from a nurse or social worker knowledgeable about hemophilia in working with the school. Many hemophilic boys may have hospitalizations that require long school absences. In this case, continuing school classwork by tutoring or hospital classroom is essential.

Although some hemophilic boys have a smooth adolescence, others engage in excessive risk-taking. Adolescents can be very moody and have difficulty communicating; therefore it is important to try encouraging them to express their needs and concerns. All adolescents are sensitive to body image, and hemophilic boys with noticeable body changes such as joint contractures may be especially sensitive. At this age, being a part of the peer group is important. However, many hemophilic boys may not be able to keep up with the group because of physical limitations. Additionally, it is recommended that they not play contact sports such as football and soccer. All attempts should be made to encourage the development of other interests and hobbies.

Ideally, by the time a boy reaches adolescence, he has been instructed in home infusion or he is interested in learning this skill. Home infusion can provide the boy with a sense of control, independence, and decision-making in the management of his illness.

The importance of school and preparation for the

competitive job market is another area that should be considered. Often the child may not be able to follow other family members' footsteps in jobs requiring physical labor. Many employers know nothing about hemophilia, and because of misconceptions about the illness, they will not consider the hemophiliac for a job. Vocational rehabilitation can provide assistance with career counseling, training, and job placement.

Financial concerns are a major concern to the family with a hemophilic child. The expense of hemophilia has been reported to range from $8000 to $22,000 a year.[31] Often, the social worker refers the family to various agencies for assistance with financial problems relating to their illness. Other referral sources may include referrals to vocational rehabilitation, mental health agencies, and school counselors. The role of the health professional is multifaceted in helping the child and family with various hemophilia-related issues.

Home therapy

In Texas in 1961 home therapy was first introduced by Dr. Richard Halden, who used plasma.

Subsequently, Dr. Frederick Rabiner and Dr. Margaret Telfer at the Michael Reese Hospital in Chicago used cryoprecipitate for home infusion.[32] When the factor concentrates became available in the late 1960s the concept of home therapy became a viable option in treatment since the concentrates could be stored, reconstituted, and administered more easily than the other plasma products. However, it was not until 1975, when comprehensive hemophilia centers were established, that the majority of patients were instructed in home therapy. At that time nurse coordinators designed specific protocols for the management of patients instructed in home infusion.

Home therapy is a program in which the patient and/or family members are taught how to administrate the deficient clotting factor intravenously. The rationale of home therapy is to provide the patient with prompt adequate replacement therapy. Before home therapy was introduced, many patients had to wait hours in an emergency room or clinic to receive therapy. Home therapy greatly changed the lives of many patients. Fig. 16-6 illustrates a mother infusing her child at home.

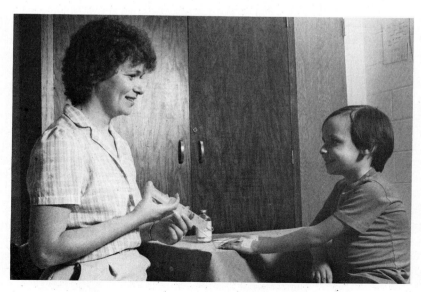

Fig. 16-6. Home infusion of factor by the child's mother.

The advantages of home therapy are numerous; by receiving early treatment, the patient has less damage to the area of bleeding, less pain, and less disruption of his normal life-style. Additionally, home therapy offers the patient a dimension of control and independence and a sense of well-being.

CONCLUSION

Medical care for the patient with hemophilia has changed dramatically over the past few decades because of the introduction of factor concentrates and advent of home therapy. Early, adequate treatment has provided the hemophiliac with a much better life-style, both physically and socioeconomically. Additionally, the life span for the hemophiliac has been significantly increased as a result of the availability of modern treatment. However, patients continue to have problems such as hepatitis with concomitant liver diseases related to the infusion of blood products. More recently, the possibility of contracting AIDS has become a major concern for many in this patient population.

Basic and clinical research continues at a rapid pace. There is hope in the near future for developing a synthetic specific blood clotting factor concentrate using recombinant DNA techniques. The development of such products lend hope to patients in terms of eliminating blood-related complications.

NURSING CONSIDERATIONS

The hemophilia nurse has a role with many diverse duties. The wide-ranging responsibilities of this role include patient education, instruction of home therapy, triage and treatment of bleeding episodes, and coordination of the hemophilia center. Since hemophilia is a chronic illness that has multidimensional effects on the patient and entire family, the nurse must have an in-depth understanding of the medical and psychosocial implications of this disease.

There is a strong focus on preventive education with the family. With the diagnosis of hemophilia, the nurse begins the educational process by providing the family with a basic understanding of hemophilia and guidelines of what to expect with the long-term effects of this bleeding disorder. As the child gets older and has more bleeding episodes, the nurse gives more specific information about sites and severity of bleeding. Often the parent is very anxious with the anticipation of the first bleed. However, with the experience of the child's bleeding and the knowledge gained through further educational sessions, the anxiety is usually reduced.

During the toddler and preschool years, the parents seek medical treatment for the child at the local physician's office or emergency room. However, when the child is around 4 to 6 years of age, the parents frequently express an interest in learning home therapy. The instruction of home therapy is individualized and is best accomplished on a one-to-one basis with a family member or the patient. The home therapy session is comprehensive and is designed to teach venipuncture technique, reconstitution of the factor concentrates, aseptic technique, indications for treatment, and the correct dosages to use for various bleeding episodes. Possible complications such as allergic transfusion reactions or hepatitis and the method of documentation of treatment are also included. Additional information that is discussed during the sessions are general guidelines that the parent should know such as the fact that all aspirin-containing medications should be avoided, since aspirin may prolong bleeding. Intramuscular injections should not be given because of potential hematoma formation. However, immunizations may be given intramuscularly, if a small-gauge needle is used and pressure is held at the injection site for at least five minutes.

Triage and treatment of bleeding episodes is another important function of the nurse. Because of the complex nature of hemophilia, the patient forms a close relationship with the hemophilia center staff and often uses the center as the primary facility for medical treatment. Frequently, the patient is treated by the nurse in the center for acute, non–life-threatening bleeding episodes. Additionally, the nurse triages many medical problems by phone recommending appropriate intervention and therapy for specific bleeding episodes.

There is a strong emphasis on comprehensive care in hemophilia. The nurse is an integral member of the multidisciplinary team and often is the person who coordinates continuity of care for the patient with the various team members. Following evaluation of the patient in the clinic, the nurse collaborates with the team and subsequently communicates any pertinent medical information to the patient's school, personnel employer, or family member. The nurse assumes the role of the patient's advocate when school systems, employers, or other health care givers have misconceptions or biases regarding hemophilia. Education is an ongoing process with the patient and family.

NURSING CARE PROTOCOL FOR THE CHILD WITH HEMOPHILIA

Nursing diagnoses (problems/needs)	Goals/objectives (patient/family will:)	Interventions (nurse will:)
1. Diagnostic workup and cause of hemophilia	Understand purpose of diagnostic workup (purpose of blood tests, physical examination)	Provide parents with verbal information regarding blood tests and other related tests
	Understand cause of hemophilia (inheritance transmission, gene mutation)	Explain the genetic pattern of hemophilia; provide example of a pedigree diagram
2. Knowledge deficit (related to clinical manifestations of hemophilia)	Understand basic knowledge of hemophilia and hemostasis; define what causes the bleeding to continue longer	Provide verbal and written information on hemophilia (pamphlets, booklets)
	Understand when to seek medical treatment; identify signs and symptoms related to bleeding (see Table 16-2)	Teach what to expect with initial bleeding episodes, signs and symptoms to observe (for instance with hemarthrosis limitation in movement of a joint, pain or tingling sensation in a joint) (see Table 16-20)
		Instruct treatment of minor versus major life-threatening bleeding; stress importance of contacting the hemophilia center with major bleeds
		Explain what are typical bleeding problems during the following: Infancy—bruising Toddler age—bleeding in mouth, tongue, frenulum, usually secondary to child falling; occasional hemarthrosis Preschool to schoolage—hemarthrosis intramuscular, occasional hematuria

NURSING CARE PROTOCOL FOR THE CHILD WITH HEMOPHILIA—cont'd

Nursing diagnoses (problems/needs)	Goals/objectives (patient/family will:)	Interventions (nurse will:)
		Adolescent—all types of bleeding episodes Stress not to panic with visible bleeding, since hemorrhaging in hemophilia is not faster but longer
3. Anxiety (related to diagnosis and implications of a chronic illness; fear of the unknown)	Decreased anxiety by education	Encourage family to verbalize fears and concerns related to diagnosis; stress that emotional support is often needed for families who have a child with a chronic illness. Provide education to allay anxiety Introduce family to other hemophilic families Provide information regarding resources such as the National Hemophilia Foundation and local hemophilia chapter Encourage parent to contact the hemophilia center as problems arise Provide family with guidelines such as the child should be encouraged to participate in most activities except contact sports; encourage parents not to be overprotective; encourage general safety precautions that are used with toddler and young children Provide financial counseling if needed; explore agencies that may assist families (Crippled Children's, Medicaid, special plans with private insurance companies)
4. Coping, ineffective family: compromised	Demonstrate effective coping mechanisms necessary for optimum functioning at home, school, and community	Provide emotional support; refer to other health professionals as needed Introduce family to support groups if available

REFERENCES

1. Moake, J.L., and Funicella, T.: Common bleeding problems, Clin. Symp. **35**(3):2, 1983.
2. Brinkhous, K.: A short history of hemophilia with some comments on the word "hemophilia." In Brinkhous, K., and Hemker, H.C., editors: Handbook of hemophilia, Amsterdam, 1975, Excerpta Medica.
3. Hougie, C.: Hemophilia and related conditions—congenital deficiencies of prothrombin (factor II), factor V, and factors VII to XII. In Williams, W.J., and others, editors: Hematology, New York, 1983, McGraw-Hill, Inc.
4. Miller, C.: Genetics of hemophilia and von Willebrand's disease. In Hilgartner, M.W., editor: Hemophilia in the child and adult, New York, 1982, Masson Publishing USA, Inc.
5. Lane, S.: Haemorrhagic diathesis: Successful transfusion of blood, Lancet **1**:185, 1840.
6. Payne, W.W., and Steen, R.E.: Haemostatic therapy in hemophilia, Br. Med. J. **1**:1150, 1929.
7. Pool, J.G., and Robinson, J.: Observation of plasma banking and transfusion procedures for haemophilic patients using a quantitative assay for antihaemophilic globulin (AHG), Br. J. Haematol. **5**:24, 1959.
8. Hilgartner, M.W.: Factor replacement therapy. In Hilgartner, M.W., editor: Hemophilia in the child and adult, New York, 1982, Masson Publishing USA, Inc.
9. Arnold, W.D., and Hilgartner, M.W.: Hemophilic arthropathy, J. Bone Joint Surg. **59-A**(3):287, 1977.
10. Greene, W.B., and Raney, R.B.: Musculoskeletal complications of hemophilia. In Wilson, F., editor: The musculoskeletal system basic processes and disorders, Philadelphia, 1983, J.B. Lippincott Co.
11. Greene, W.B., and Wilson, F.C.: The management of musculoskeletal problems in hemophilia: Part III. In Evarts, C.M., editor: Instructional course lectures of the American Academy of Orthopaedic Surgeons, vol. XXXII, St. Louis, 1983, The C.V. Mosby Co.
12. Greene, W.B., and Wilson, F.C.: Pathophysiologic and roentgenographic changes in hemophilic arthropathy: Part II. In Evarts, C.M., editor: Instructional course lectures of the American Academy at Orthopaedic Surgeons, vol. XXXII, St. Louis, 1983, The C.V. Mosby Co.
13. Hilgartner, M.W., and McMillan, C.W.: Coagulation disorders. In Miller, D.R., and others, editors: Smith's blood diseases of infancy and childhood, St. Louis, 1978, The C.V. Mosby Co.
14. Lazerson, J., and Gomperts, E.: Renal disease in hemophilia. In Hilgartner, M.W., editor: Hemophilia in the child and adult, New York, 1982, Masson Publishing USA, Inc.
15. Eyster, M.E., and others: Central nervous system bleeding in hemophiliacs, Blood **51**:1179, 1978.
16. Gilchrist, G.S., Piepgras, D.G., and Roskos, R.: Neurologic complications in hemophilia. In Hilgartner, M.W., editor: Hemophilia in the child and adult, New York, 1982, Masson Publishing USA, Inc.
17. Dietrich, S.L., Luck, J.V., and Martinson, A.M.: Musculoskeletal problems. In Hilgartner, M.W., editor: Hemophilia in the child and adult, New York, 1982, Masson Publishing USA, Inc.
18. Forbes, C.D.: Clinical aspects of the hemophilias and their treatment. In Ratnoff, O.D., and Forbes, C.D., editors: Disorders of hemostasis, New York, 1984, Grune & Stratton, Inc.
19. Gilbert, M.S., Kreel, I., and Hermann, G.: The hemophilic pseudotumor. In Hilgartner, M.W., editor: Hemophilia in the child and adult, New York, 1982, Masson Publishing USA, Inc.
20. Shapiro, S.S.: Genetic predisposition to inhibitor formation. In Hoyer, L.W., editor: Factor VIII inhibitors, New York, 1984, Alan R. Liss, Inc.
21. Gill, F.M.: The natural history of factor VIII inhibitors in patients with hemophilia A. In Hoyer, L.W., editor: Factor VIII inhibitors, New York, 1984, Alan R. Liss, Inc.
22. McMillan, C.W.: Clinical patterns of hemophilic patients who develop inhibitors. In Hoyer, L.W., editor: Factor VIII inhibitors, New York, 1984, Alan R. Liss, Inc.
23. Roberts, H.R., and Cromartie, R.: Overview of inhibitors to factor VIII and IX. In Hoyer, L.W., editor: Factor VIII inhibitors, New York, 1984, Alan R. Liss, Inc.
24. White, G., and others: Chronic hepatitis in patients with hemophilia A: histologic studies in patients with intermittently abnormal liver function tests, Blood **60**:6, 1982.
25. Cederbaum, A.I., Blatt, P.M., Levine, P.H.: Abnormal serum transaminase levels in patients with hemophilia A, Arch. Intern. Med. **142**:481, 1982.
26. Mannucci, P.M., and others: A new pharmacologic approach to the management of hemophilia and von Willebrand's disease, Lancet **1**:869, 1977.
27. Barnhart, M.I., Chen, S., and Lusher, J.M.: DDAVP: does the drug have a direct effect on the vessel wall? Throm. Res. **31**:239, 1983.
28. Forbes, C.D.: Clinical aspects of the hemophiliacs and their treatment. In Ratnoff, O., editor: Disorders of Hemostasis, New York, 1984, Grune & Stratton, Inc.
29. Apuzzo-Berger, D.: A.I.D.S.: could you be at risk? RN **46**:2, 1984.
30. White, G.C., and Lesesne, H.R.: Hemophilia, hepatitis, and the acquired immunodeficiency syndrome, Ann. Intern. Med. **98**(1):403, 1983.
31. Aledort, L.M.: Lessons from hemophilia, N. Engl. J. Med. **306**:10, 1982.
32. Eyster, E.E.: Home therapy programs. In Hilgartner, M.W., editor: Hemophilia and the adult, New York, 1982, Masson Publishing USA, Inc.

CHAPTER 17

Polycythemia in children

DAVID BECTON

Polycythemia, or erythrocytosis, is an uncommon condition in children in which there is an unusually high number of red blood cells. In adults, polycythemia can be defined as a hemoglobin concentration above 18 g/dl or a red cell count greater than 6 million/mm^3.[1] The definition is not so simple in children, however, since the normal values for hemoglobin concentration and red cell count vary considerably with age. Table 17-1 lists the normal range of these values at various ages throughout childhood.

Another important concept in the understanding and description of polycythemia is the red cell mass, which is a reflection of the total number of red cells in the circulation at a given time.[2] The red cell mass is a measure of the volume of red cells/unit of body weight, usually expressed in terms of ml/kg. It is not affected by increases or decreases in the plasma volume as are the hemoglobin concentration and red cell count, both of which are described in terms of units of volume (g/dl or cells/mm^3).

The red cell mass can be measured by injecting a sample of radiolabeled red cells into the patient and calculating the amount of dilution of the radiolabel over a 10-minute period.[3] Table 17-2 demonstrates that when red cell mass is increased, there is a compensatory increase in total blood volume, which is the sum of the red cell mass and the plasma volume.

When a patient has excessive fluid losses because of dehydration, burns, or adrenal dysfunction, the resulting elevation of hemoglobin concentration and red cell count suggests polycythe-

mia. This is termed relative polycythemia because in fact there is not an actual increase in red cell mass but only a relative increase in red cell concentration because of the decreased plasma volume.[4] On the other hand, absolute polycythemia exists when there is an increase in red cell mass because of increased production of red cells, leading to an elevation of hemoglobin concentration and red cell count. Therefore an important first step in understanding polycythemia is the distinction between relative (caused by loss of plasma volume) and absolute (caused by increased red cell mass) polycythemia. Only the latter will be discussed subsequently in this chapter.

Table 17-1. Normal values for hemoglobin concentration and red cell count at various ages

Age	Mean hemoglobin (g/dl)	Red cell count ($\times 10^6$ cells/ mm^3)
Birth	16.5	4.7
3-6 months	11.5	3.8
2 years	12.5	4.6
6 years	13.5	4.6
15 years		
male	14.5	4.9
female	14.0	4.6
>20 years		
male	15.5	5.2
female	14.0	4.6

Modified from Rudolph, A., editor: Pediatrics, ed. 16, New York, 1977, Appleton-Century-Crofts, Inc.

Table 17-2. Relationship between blood volume, red cell mass, and plasma volume in normal and polycythemic patients

	Normal		Absolute polycythemia		Relative polycythemia	
	Male	Female	Male	Female	Male	Female
Total blood volume	70 ± 5	65 ± 5	>75	>70	<65	<60
Red cells mass	30 ± 3	25 ± 3	>36	>32	30 ± 3	25 ± 3
Plasma volume	40 ± 2	40 ± 2	>40	>40	<35	<35

All units ml/kg.

NORMAL ERYTHROPOIESIS

Red cells are made in the bone marrow as the end product of an orderly process of proliferation and differentiation.[5] This gradual process involves several identifiable stages of maturation through which each cell must pass. The last step includes the extrusion of the nucleus from the cell just before the cell is released into the circulation and occurs after the cell has manufactured its full complement of hemoglobin. Newly released cells contain small amounts of RNA and can be identified and quantitated by special staining as reticulocytes. Once in the circulation, the normal life span of the red cell is about 100 to 120 days. Senescent red cells are destroyed and removed by the spleen. Thus there is a need for replacing approximately 1% of the red cell mass each day, and the normal reticulocyte count is 0.5% to 1.5%. When erythrocyte production is increased, the reticulocyte count is usually greater than 2%.

The marrow has a remarkable capacity for enhancing erythropoiesis when necessary. Shortened red cell survival (hemolytic anemia), acute or chronic blood loss, and tissue hypoxia lead to increased red cell production, sometimes to six or eight times normal. The best defined mechanism of regulation of erythropoiesis is that involving the hormone erythropoietin. Erythropoietin has a direct stimulatory effect on red cell precursors, so that increased serum erythropoietin levels lead to increased red cell proliferation and an eventual increase in the release of mature red cells from the marrow.[6] Erythropoietin is made in the kidney, and its rate of manufacture is a reflection of the oxygenation of the tissues in which it is made. Conditions leading to relative tissue hypoxia such as severe pulmonary or cardiac disease, high altitudes, abnormal hemoglobins that do not release or carry oxygen normally, severe anemia, or compromised renal blood flow can lead to increased erythropoietin production, increased plasma erythropoietin, and therefore increased stimulation and proliferation of marrow erythroid precursors. However, many patients with hemolytic anemia and increased marrow production, as reflected by an increased reticulocyte count, have normal erythropoietin levels. The "feedback" mechanism responsible for the increased erythropoiesis in these patients is uncertain.

CLINICAL FEATURES

The age at which children with polycythemia are diagnosed varies depending on the etiologic factors. A hemoglobin concentration obtained during a "routine" examination may disclose an abnormally high value in an asymptomatic patient. When symptoms are present, they result from increased whole blood viscosity, leading to impaired circulation. Common presenting complaints include ruddy complexion, headache, fatigability, and dyspnea. Less commonly, bleeding, night sweats, pruritis, and weight loss are present. The presence and severity of these symptoms are related to the underlying disorder and to the severity of the polycythemia. Common physical findings include plethora, conjunctival engorgement, purpura, hypertension, and rarely in children, organomegaly. Other physical findings present are those of the underlying disorder such as cyanotic heart disease, severe pulmonary disease, renal disease, or neoplastic disease.

Other than the obvious increase in hemoglobin concentration and red cell counts, screening laboratory findings are nonspecific and unhelpful except in polycythemia vera (to be discussed).

SPECIFIC CAUSES OF ABSOLUTE POLYCYTHEMIA

As stated previously, absolute, or true, polycythemia is the presence of an increased red cell mass. Absolute polycythemia can be associated with increased (secondary) or normal (primary) erythropoietin levels.

Increased erythropoietin levels (secondary polycythemia)

Tissue hypoxia leads to an increase in the production of erythropoietin, which subsequently increases the red cell mass.[7] The most common causes of tissue hypoxia in childhood are congenital cyanotic heart disease and severe parenchymal pulmonary disease such as cystic fibrosis. The elevated erythropoietin level seen in such cases is considered appropriate, since it is in response to hypoxia.[8,9] Usually, the hematocrit does not exceed 60%. Since the increased hemoglobin concentration enhances oxygen-carrying capacity, treatment to reduce the hematocrit might be detrimental. As the hematocrit approaches 70%, circulatory sludging may occur and lead to exercise intolerance. Some patients require regular phlebotomy to avoid this complication. If the underlying disease can be treated effectively, the red cell mass will return to normal.

Patients whose hemoglobin has an unusually high oxygen affinity have well-oxygenated blood, but since the hemoglobin does not appropriately release oxygen, the tissues are poorly oxygenated. The abnormal hemoglobins Hb Chesapeake and Hb Bethesda are two examples of high oxygen affinity variants; affected patients are polycythemic because of the elevation in erythropoietin production secondary to tissue hypoxia.[10] Phlebotomy is rarely necessary because the hematocrit usually does not exceed 60%. The diagnosis can be made by hemoglobin electrophoresis.

Some patients with severely compromised renal blood flow may have local tissue hypoxia and a subsequent increase in erythropoietin production. The level of polycythemia in such patients rarely warrants phlebotomy; in any case, the compromised renal blood flow will usually be corrected following its identification, leading to recovery from the polycythemia.

Occasionally, neoplastic tissues produce excessive quantities of erythropoietin in the absence of known hypoxia.[11] This is considered inappropriate erythropoietin, since there is no tissue hypoxia. In childhood the most common tumor associated with increased erythropoietin levels are cerebellar hemangioblastoma, hepatocellular carcinoma, and adrenal adenoma. Again, once the primary disorder is identified and corrected, polycythemia ceases to be a problem.

Low to absent erythropoietin levels (primary polycythemia)

Patients with primary polycythemia have no systemic or local tissue hypoxia and do not have elevated erythropoietin levels. Therefore the bone marrow is autonomously producing red cells at a faster rate than is necessary to replace normal red cell loss. There are two main types of primary polycythemia: polycythemia vera and benign familial polycythemia.

Polycythemia vera is considered a myeloproliferative disorder, since there is abnormal uncontrolled proliferation in the bone marrow of erythroid cells.[12] The overall incidence of polycythemia vera is approximately 1/100,000 but is much less common in children. The peak age is the early 60s. The cause is uncertain; the pathogenesis involves uncontrolled erythropoiesis. Erythropoietin levels are usually quite low unless the patient is being phlebotomized, but erythroid proliferation is markedly increased.

The diagnosis of polycythemia vera is based on the presence of strict diagnostic criteria such as an increased red cell mass, a normal arterial oxygen saturation (>92%), and splenomegaly. Leukocytosis (white blood count >12,000 cells/mm³), thrombocytosis (platelet count >400,000 cells/mm³), elevated leukocyte alkaline phosphatase scores, and elevated vitamin B_{12} levels are frequently seen in polycythemia vera. Erythroid cells from affected patients can be cultured in vitro without the addition of exogenous erythropoietin, unlike normal erythroid cells.

Treatment may include regular phlebotomy cytotoxic chemotherapy (usually chlorambucil) or radiotherapy with intravenous ³²P. Children are managed initially with repeated phlebotomies if possible; chemotherapy or radiotherapy is reserved for those with aggressive disease or malignant transformation. Adults with polycythemia vera are at greatly increased risk for developing acute myelogenous leukemia; it is uncertain whether the rare affected child will share this fate.

Benign familial polycythemia is similar to polycythemia vera in that the red cell mass is strikingly increased without elevated levels of erythropoietin.[13] Affected patients are, however, otherwise completely normal, and the prognosis is much more favorable. As the name would suggest, this appears to be an inherited disorder although spontaneous cases are not at all uncommon. The pathogenesis is uncertain. Erythroid cell cultures from patients with benign polycythemia require an exogenous supply of erythropoietin, indicating a basic difference in the pathogenic mechanism from that of polycythemia vera.

Other than the signs and symptoms associated with polycythemia in general, there are no specific clinical features. The white cell and platelet counts are normal, and organomegaly is absent. Asymptomatic patients require no therapy. Patients whose hematocrits are >60% may have exercise intolerance, dyspnea, bleeding tendencies, or other symptoms. These patients can be managed with intermittent phlebotomies, which will reduce the hematocrit so that the patient becomes asymptomatic. Any patient requiring frequent phlebotomies will eventually become iron deficient, causing a reduction in mean cell volume (MCV) of the red cells which will further ameliorate the hyperviscosity. There is no evidence that patients with benign familial polycythemia are prone to developing myelogenous leukemia or other myeloproliferative disorders. Most patients continue to have elevated hematocrits, often requiring phlebotomies, into adulthood.

DIAGNOSTIC APPROACH TO POLYCYTHEMIA

If there are no clinical findings suggesting excessive water or plasma losses (relative polycythemia), a diagnostic plan should be formulated to determine if the patient has primary or secondary polycythemia. If erythropoietin assays were simple and available in many clinical laboratories, this distinction could be made easily. Since these assays are not in widespread use, a search is made for discovering common causes of secondary polycythemia. Arterial oxygen saturation and the P_{50} O_2 for hemoglobin can be easily measured. If the oxygen saturation is greater than 92%, then significant cardiac or pulmonary disease can be ruled out as the cause of polycythemia.

The presence of a normal P_{50} O_2 for hemoglobin indicates a normal oxygen affinity, thereby ruling out the presence of an unusual hemoglobin variant with a high oxygen affinity. If these tests are normal, a search for renal pathologic findings, specifically compromised arterial blood flow, is indicated using intravenous pyelography and perhaps renal arteriography. Computed tomography of the posterior fossa should be considered to look for a cerebellar hemangioblastoma.

If all of these tests—the history, family history, and the physical examination fail to indicate a secondary cause, then primary polycythemia is more probable, and urine or serum erythropoietin assays should be obtained. If erythropoietin is elevated, a further search for a cause of secondary polycythemia should be made. If erythropoietin is low or absent, primary polycythemia has been confirmed, and the main differential is between polycythemia vera and benign familial polycythemia. The latter disorder is much more common in children, and in the absence of other suggestive features of polycythemia vera, such as leukocytosis, thrombocytosis, or organomegaly, should be considered the correct diagnosis. Culture of erythroid stem cells in the absence and presence of erythropoietin is sometimes helpful in distinguishing these two disorders.

CASE STUDY

A 13-year-old white male was having a camp physical examination performed when a hemoglobin value of 21 g/dl was obtained. The boy was referred to his pediatrician for further evaluation. He was found to be asymptomatic; exercise tolerance was excellent. There had been no previous hospitalizations or serious illnesses. A review of his medical records revealed a hemoglobin of 13 g/dl at 2 months of age and 14.5 g/dl at 6 years of age. Family history revealed that there were no known blood disorders, but that his father was well-known for his hearty complexion. Physical examination revealed a plethoric but healthy appearing adolescent in no distress; vital signs were normal. Conjunctival engorgement was noted. There was no organomegaly and no evidence of bruising or petechiae.

Laboratory evaluation revealed a hemoglobin of 19.8 g/dl; white blood count and platelet counts were normal. Leukocyte alkaline phosphatase and the vitamin B_{12} level were normal. Arterial blood gases revealed an oxygen saturation of 96% and a P_{50} O_2 hemoglobin of 27 mm Hg (normal). Hemoglobin electrophoresis, serum electrolytes, serum creatinine, and liver functions were all normal. Red cell mass was measured using ^{51}Cr-labeled erythrocytes and was found to be markedly elevated (38 ml/kg).

Chest x-ray examination and electrocardiogram were normal. Serum and urine assays for erythropoietin were obtained and revealed values at the very low end of the normal range. A diagnosis of benign familial polycythemia was made. No therapy was begun, but blood counts were recommended every 3 months.

NURSING CONSIDERATIONS

There are no specific nursing considerations in caring for the child who has polycythemia. Signs and symptoms related to an increased red cell mass may or not be observed. A careful history may reveal headaches, easy fatigability, and dyspnea. Careful assessment should include a thorough history and observation and documentation of specific signs and symptoms.

NURSING CARE PROTOCOL FOR THE CHILD WITH POLYCYTHEMIA

Nursing diagnoses (patient problems)	Goals/objectives (patient/family will:)	Interventions (nurse will:)
1. Knowledge deficit related to diagnosis	Understand the diagnosis and major concerns for the child with polycythemia	Discuss disease process and its specific pathogenesis Review common symptoms the disease may cause: headache, fatigue dyspnea
Related to management of the disorder	Be able to state the common therapeutic modalities in managing polycythemia.	Evaluate level of understanding regarding management Review method for phlebotomy in children and its rationale

Continued.

NURSING CARE PROTOCOL FOR THE CHILD WITH POLYCYTHEMIA—cont'd

Nursing diagnoses (patient problems)	Goals/objectives (patient/family will:)	Interventions (nurse will:)
2. Anxiety (emotional distress related to the disorder)	Have decreased anxiety Express feelings regarding diagnosis	Encourage verbalization of fears and concerns Contact other health professions as necessary.
3. Injury: potential for (tissue hypoxia)	Detect signs and symptoms related to increased red cell mass	Review history for presence of headaches, easy fatigability, dyspnea Assess for symptoms including ruddy complexion, plethora, conjunctival engorgement, purpura, hypertension, and rarely in children, organomegaly.
4. Coping, ineffective family: compromised	Develop adequate coping mechanisms Display basic understanding of the child's disorder	Provide support as needed by involving appropriate health care personnel

REFERENCES

1. Castle, W.B.: In Beck, W.S., editor: Hematology, ed. 2, Cambridge, Mass, 1977, The MIT Press.
2. Bentley, S.A., and Lewis, S.M.: The relationship between total red cell volume, plasma volume, and venous hematocrit, Br. J. Haematol. **33:**301, 1976.
3. Hillman, R.S., and Finch, C.A.: Red cell manual, ed. 4, Philadelphia, 1974, F.A. Davis Co.
4. Berlin, N.I.: Diagnosis and classification of the polycythemias, Semin. Hematol. **12:**339, 1975.
5. Nathan, D.G., Housman, D.E., and Clake, B.J.: The anatomy and physiology of hematopoiesis. In Nathan, D.G., and Oski, F.A., editors: Hematology of infancy and childhood, ed. 2, Philadelphia, 1981, W.B. Saunders Co.
6. Krantz, S.B., and Jacobson, L.O.; Erythropoietin and the regulation of erythropoiesis, Chicago, 1970, The University of Chicago Press.
7. Balcerzak, S.P., and Bromberg, P.A.; Secondary polycythemias, Semin. Hematol. **12:**353, 1975.
8. Bing, B.J., and others: Physiological studies in congenital heart disease. VI. Adaptations to anoxia in congenital heart disease with cyanosis, Bull. Johns Hopkins Hosp. **83:**439, 1948.
9. Gallo, R.C., and others: Erythropoietic response in chronic pulmonary disease, Arch. Intern. Med. **113:**559, 1964.
10. Erslev, A.J.: Hemoglobinopathies producing erythrocytosis. In Williams, W.J., editor: Hematology, ed. 3, New York, 1983, McGraw-Hill, Inc.
11. Thorling, E.B.: Paraneoplastic erythrocytosis and inappropriate erythropoietin production, a review, Scand. J. Haematol. Suppl. **17:**1, 1972.
12. Murphy, S.: Polycythemia vera. In Williams, W.J., editor: Hematology, ed. 3, New York, 1983, McGraw-Hill, Inc.
13. Adamson, J.W.: Familial polycythemia, Semin. Hematol. **12:**383, 1975.

CHAPTER 18

Childhood neutropenia

DAVID BECTON

Polymorphonuclear leukocytes, or neutrophils, are an important component of the body's defense mechanism. When there are insufficient numbers of circulating neutrophils, the host is predisposed to infection by pyogenic bacteria and fungi. The normal absolute neutrophil count (total white blood count × the percentage of neutrophils) ranges between 3500 and 4000 cells/mm³ after infancy in white children and between 3000 and 3500 cells/mm³ in black children. Although neutropenia is defined as the presence of fewer than 1500 neutrophils/mm³, significant infections rarely occur unless the neutrophil count drops below 500 cells/mm³.[1-3]

Neutropenia can be caused by two mechanisms: decreased production by the bone marrow or increased destruction in the circulation. An understanding of the normal development and life span of neutrophils is necessary to properly assess the importance of these mechanisms.[4,5] The normal maturation of neutrophils is outlined in Fig. 18-1. The myeloblast is the earliest recognizable neutrophil precursor in the bone marrow and usually comprises about 1% of all nucleated marrow cells. Within 24 hours, each myeloblast undergoes differentiation and mitotic division to produce the promyelocyte. Over the next 24 hours, further differentiation and division result in the production of the myelocyte.

Myeloblasts, promyelocytes, and myelocytes comprise the mitotic pool in the granulocytic series. They undergo an average total of five mitotic divisions so that one myeloblast eventually gives rise to 32 metamyelocytes. The later cells—metamyelocytes and band forms— continue to differentiate gradually into mature neutrophils but no longer divide. These cells form the maturation and storage pool. The average time period from myeloblast to mature neutrophil is about 10 days. Outside the marrow, about half of the body's neutrophils are in the bloodstream, or circulating pool. The remainder are adherent to vessel walls and comprise the marginal pool. There is probably continual interchange between the circulating and marginal pools. The average circulating half-life of the mature neutrophil is only about 6 hours. Therefore the need is great for continual replenishment by the bone marrow to maintain adequate numbers of circulating neutrophils.

The regulatory mechanisms controlling the production of neutrophils have not been fully defined.[6,7] Regulation of the production of red cells and platelets appears to involve a circulating hormone, which has a direct effect on the development of immature cells within each line in the bone marrow. No similar hormone has been identified for the granulocytic line. The number of circulating neutrophils can be increased in three ways. The marginal pool, consisting of neutrophils adherent to vessel walls, can quickly be recruited to the circulating pool in response to stress such as infection or trauma. Demargination follows endogenous epinephrine released in response to the stressful event.[8] Demargination can be mimicked, for diagnostic purposes, by pharmacologic epinephrine. Second, the bone marrow can allow early release of "storage" neutrophils and more immature forms such as bands and metamyelocytes

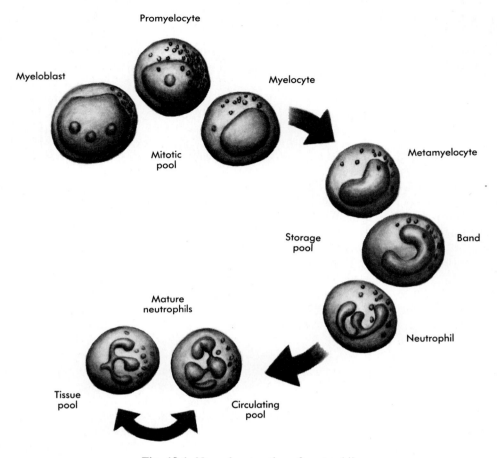

Fig. 18-1. Normal maturation of neutrophils.

in response to stressful stimuli. Corticosteroid administration leads to a similar release of storage neutrophils. Finally, increased commitment of uncommitted stem cells to the neutrophil cell line leads to an increased number of cells progressing through neutrophil maturation and an eventual increase in circulating neutrophils. This level of regulation is probably more affected by the number of peripheral neutrophils, through an unidentified feedback mechanism, than it is by acute events such as stress or infection.

These levels of regulation can be evaluated with varying degrees of precision by specific laboratory investigations. As mentioned previously, administration of pharmacologic epinephrine or corticosteroids normally leads to release of neutrophils from the marginal or storage pools, respectively. Failure to respond to these signals with an appropriate increase in the neutrophil count offers insight into the location of the defect causing neutropenia. An examination of a stained bone marrow aspirate or biopsy permits an approximate quantitation of the neutrophil precursors in various stages of maturation, allowing a diagnosis to be made when marrow failure is the cause of neutropenia.

CAUSES OF NEUTROPENIA IN CHILDREN

The common causes of childhood neutropenia are as follows:

Disorders associated with decreased marrow production
    Benign familial neutropenia
    Severe congenital neutropenia (Kostmann's syndrome)
    Neutropenia associated with other congenital anomalies
        Pancreatic exocrine insufficiency (Shwachmann-Diamond syndrome)
        Constitutional aplastic anemia (Fanconi's anemia)
        Reticular dysgenesis
    Cyclic neutropenia
    Toxin exposure
    Nutritional deficiencies
    Marrow infiltration
    Infection
Disorders associated with decreased neutrophil survival
    Infection
    Immunologic
        Autoimmune
        Isoimmune
        Drug-related

It is helpful to group these disorders on the basis of their general pathophysiologic mechanism, either as a failure of marrow production or an increased peripheral destruction of neutrophils.

Disorders associated with decreased marrow production

Benign familial neutropenia. Benign familial neutropenia is, as the name suggests, a mild form of inherited neutropenia caused by decreased production of neutrophils by the bone marrow.[1] The inheritance may be autosomal dominant or recessive, and isolated cases with no family history are not uncommon. Clinical manifestations are mild and include superficial skin or gingival infections. The neutrophil count rarely falls below 300 cells/mm[3]. Examination of bone marrow morphology reveals adequate numbers of early myeloid precursors but a relative decrease at the band or mature neutrophil level. This implies a "maturational arrest" in myeloid differentiation, the exact cause of which is uncertain. Since the clinical manifestations are minimal and the prognosis is excellent, no specific therapy is indicated other than normal supportive and antibiotic therapy for infections. Most affected children "outgrow" this illness during the preschool years.

Severe congenital neutropenia. Severe congenital neutropenia (Kostmann's syndrome) is a disorder characterized by autosomal recessive inheritance and chronic neutropenia.[9] The neutrophil count is usually less than 200 cells/mm[3]. Affected infants usually succumb in the first months of life to severe respiratory or skin infections by pyogenic bacteria. The marrow is depleted of early and late myeloid precursors. Corticosteroids and splenectomy have been unsuccessful in increasing the neutrophil count and improving survival. Antibiotic therapy and supportive measures are usually inadequate in controlling infection in affected infants. Bone marrow transplantation has been used with encouraging early results.[10]

Neutropenia associated with other anomalies. Several inheritable disorders with striking phenotypic abnormalities are associated with neutropenia. Shwachman-Diamond syndrome is characterized by small stature, pancreatic exocrine insufficiency, metaphyseal chondrodysplasia, and neutropenia.[11,12] The onset is usually in the first 2 years of life and is similar to that of cystic fibrosis, with malabsorption, failure to thrive, and recurrent respiratory tract infections. Pancreatic insufficiency can be improved by the administration of replacement enzymes, but there is no therapy for the neutropenia. Many patients die of infection in early childhood.

Constitutional aplastic anemia, or Fanconi's anemia, is frequently associated with anomalies of several organ systems and the gradual onset of bone marrow failure, including neutropenia.[13] This disorder has been reviewed elsewhere (Chapter 13).

Reticular dysgenesis is a syndrome in which there is severe deficiency of myeloid and lymphoid development.[14] Affected patients have neutropenia, lymphopenia, and absence of lymphoid tissue. Erythroid and platelet development is normal. Most infants with reticular dysgenesis die of severe infections early in life.

Cyclic neutropenia. Cyclic neutropenia is a unique disorder characterized by recurrent episodes of neutropenia.[15,16] These episodes occur at intervals of approximately 21 days. Bone marrow examination several days before the onset of neutropenia demonstrates reduced numbers of granulocytic precursors. A marrow examination at the time of neutropenia will usually reveal recovery of early precursors, indicating the impending improvement in the neutrophil count. In most instances the period of neutropenia is only a few days. Symptoms occur only during neutropenic periods and primarily consist of superficial skin and mucous membrane infections, adenitis, and malaise. These infections are rarely serious and occur usually in younger children, since the disorder tends to improve with age. Therapy is usually directed at the specific infectious complications, although occasionally corticosteroids have been successfully employed to increase the neutrophil count. The diagnosis of cyclic neutropenia is made when biweekly neutrophil counts obtained over a 6- to 8-week period demonstrate the cyclic nature of the neutropenia.

Toxin exposure. Toxic chemicals and drugs can cause neutropenia by suppressing normal marrow function.[17] Organic chemicals and heavy metals have a direct toxic effect on marrow progenitors, as do cytotoxic chemotherapeutic drugs and radiation. Common pharmacologic agents such as phenothiazines, sulfonamides, and anticonvulsants, particularly when used chronically, may also interfere with marrow proliferation of neutrophil precursors. Complete blood counts of patients taking these drugs should be obtained at regular intervals. Marrow suppression by toxic agents is usually dose-related and reversible, although occasional instances of irreversible complete marrow aplasia have been reported.

Nutritional causes. Specific nutritional deficiencies can lead to neutropenia and other hematologic disorders. Folic acid and vitamin B_{12} are necessary for the normal production of granulocytes. Folate deficiency is more common in children and in most cases is seen in infants fed a goat's milk diet. Deficiency states of folate and vitamin B_{12} are usually diagnosed following the onset of the associated megaloblastic anemia, but neutropenia is not an uncommon finding. The response to appropriate therapy is usually brisk, and the prognosis is excellent. Copper deficiency is unusual in the normal population, but it can occur in infants maintained on parenteral nutrition that does not contain copper supplementation. The hematologic manifestations of copper deficiency include microcytic anemia and neutropenia.[18] Supplemental copper usually provides a complete hematologic recovery.

Marrow infiltration. Replacement of marrow space by malignant cells crowds out normal marrow elements and prevents their normal proliferation and differentiation, leading to neutropenia, thrombocytopenia, and anemia. Leukemia, lymphoma, and neuroblastoma are the neoplastic processes that most commonly infiltrate the marrow in children.[19] Storage diseases, osteopetrosis, and myelofibrosis cause neutropenia by a similar pathologic mechanism.[20] The diagnosis of these disorders is suggested by history and physical examination findings and can be confirmed by a marrow examination. If treatment is successful in removing the malignant cells from the bone marrow, normal cells will return, and the blood counts will become normal.

Infection. Infections, particularly those caused by viruses, can cause transient marrow suppression leading to neutropenia. The exact mechanism is not known, but immune mediation may be important.[21] Although usually mild, neutropenia caused by viral infection is quite common; many cases are probably not diagnosed because of the transient nature and mildness of the neutropenia. The onset is usually within 1 to 2 weeks following the viral syndrome, and the duration is in most cases a few days to a few weeks. The absolute neutrophil count rarely falls below 500 cells/mm³. Since it is a self-limited disorder, specific therapy is not necessary, although antibiotics may be required for febrile episodes until the neutrophil count returns to normal.

Overwhelming bacterial infection can also lead to marrow suppression, particularly in infants. When the infection is adequately treated, marrow function returns to normal, and eventually the neutrophil count recovers.

Disorders associated with decreased neutrophil survival

Infection. Severe infections, particularly bacterial sepsis, are sometimes associated with shortened neutrophil life span, presumably secondary to increased use, immune phenomena, or both. Decreased neutrophil survival, especially if accompanied by marrow suppression as discussed previously, may impair the host's ability to successfully fight the infection. The mediators of this shortened survival are unknown, but bacterial endotoxin may play a role.[22] Neutrophil survival returns to normal following appropriate treatment of the infection, and in fact an improving neutrophil count is an early sign that the treatment is effective.

Immune disorders. Autoimmune neutropenia, although less common, is analogous to autoimmune hemolytic anemia and autoimmune thrombocytopenia (ITP). Affected patients possess an antibody directed against their own blood cells, in this case, their neutrophils.[23] Antibody-coated neutrophils are destroyed by the reticuloendothelial cells in the spleen so that neutrophil survival is shortened. If the increased destruction is not fully compensated by increased production by the marrow, neutropenia will result. Clinical manifestations are usually mild and consist of upper respiratory, mucosal, and superficial skin infections. Frequently, a viral syndrome will precede the onset of autoimmune neutropenia. As is the case with autoimmune hemolytic anemia and ITP, many patients will benefit from corticosteroid therapy. Autoimmune neutropenia is more likely than the other autoimmune hematocytopenias to accompany or precede a systemic autoimmune disorder such as systemic lupus erythematosus or rheumatoid arthritis. Therefore these diagnoses should be considered in a patient with autoimmune neutropenia even in the absence of other features of collagen-vascular disease.[24]

Neonatal immune neutropenia is a result of the transplacental transfer of antibodies directed against infant neutrophils. The maternal antibodies may be directed against specific antigens present on the infant's neutrophils (inherited from the father) that are not present in the mother's neutrophils, a situation analogous to the Rh-related hemolytic disease of the newborn.[25] Alternatively, the mother may have antibodies to her own neutrophils (autoimmune neutropenia) because of a collagen-vascular disease. These antibodies can be passively transferred to her infant and cause neonatal neutropenia. In either type, infants can be severely affected with serious pyogenic infections including sepsis, pneumonia, meningitis, omphalitis, and cellulitis. Vigorous supportive therapy is necessary until the level of maternal antibodies falls to a level to allow a normal neutrophil count, a process that may require 2 to 3 months. Transfusion of maternal neutrophils may be beneficial to infants with severe infections if the maternal antibodies are directed against infant-specific antigens but are not helpful if the mother has autoimmune neutropenia.

Occasionally, drugs will cause neutropenia on an immune basis.[26] Such instances may be accompanied by systemic symptoms of an allergic reaction or anaphylaxis, but frequently neutropenia is the only manifestation of drug sensitivity. Since many of the same drugs that cause marrow suppression such as sulfonamides, anticonvulsants, and penicillins also cause immune-related neutrophil destruction, the exact mechanism of neutropenia in patients receiving these medications may be obscure unless systemic symptoms are present indicating drug sensitivity. In either case, neutropenia associated with a common offending agent should lead to the discontinuation of the medicine, which usually results in a steady increase in the neutrophil count, regardless of the mechanism of neutropenia.

EVALUATION OF THE CHILD WITH NEUTROPENIA

An orderly and systematic approach leads to a more efficient diagnostic evaluation of the child with neutropenia (Table 18-1).[10] A thorough history discovers the onset, duration, and severity of the symptoms related to neutropenia. The relationship to viral syndromes or other symptomatic illnesses, medications or other possible toxic exposures, and heritable conditions will also be beneficial. Pertinent physical findings include the presence of anomalies suggestive of one of the syndromes associated with neutropenia and the extent of acute infectious lesions related to the neutropenia itself. A complete blood count including examination of the peripheral blood film is the single most important initial laboratory observation, providing quantitative and qualitative information regarding white cells, red cells, and platelets.

Once the diagnosis of neutropenia has been confirmed, in the absence of a readily identifiable associated syndrome or toxic exposure, a diagnostic plan should be formulated. Since in most cases the child will not be desperately ill, time is a very important diagnostic ally. A period of observation of 6- to 8-weeks can be beneficial for two reasons: (1) neutropenia caused by viral infection or drug exposure is usually self-limited and will improve during that period; (2) the customary 21-day cycle of cyclic neutropenia can be detected by twice-weekly neutrophil counts during the observation period. Many hematologists prefer to perform a marrow examination before this time of observation; the decision to do so is based on clinical suspicion of the presence of a serious marrow pathologic condition at the time of presentation.

If after 6 to 8 weeks there is no improvement in the neutrophil count, more specific diagnostic tests are justified. Serum folate, cobalamin (vitamin B_{12}), and copper levels document the presence of deficiencies of these nutrients. Erythrocyte sedimentation rate, rheumatoid factor, LE prep, FANA, complement components, and immunoglobulins can all be measured to investigate the diagnosis of a collagen-vascular disorder. A stool trypsin level can be measured if Shwachman-Diamond syndrome is suspected, and a karyotype will demonstrate chromosomal breaks if Fanconi's anemia is present. Neutrophil antibodies can be measured in a few laboratories; their presence indicates autoimmune neutropenia, which is usually secondary to a viral infection or a collagen-vascular disease such as systemic lupus erythematosus or juvenile rheumatoid arthritis.[27]

Investigation of neutrophil kinetics can be accomplished by two specific laboratory maneuvers. The epinephrine stimulation tests involve a subcutaneous injection of 0.01 cc/kg of 1:1000 epi-

Table 18-1. Diagnostic evaluation of neutropenia in children

Observation	Diagnostic information
History	Age, sex, diet, developmental history, family history, drug or toxin exposure, onset of infections or related symptoms
Physical examination	Nature of infectious lesions, growth and development, presence of anomalies
Laboratory evaluation	
Complete blood count, blood smear	Involvement of other cell lines
Biweekly white cell count and differential × 6-8 weeks	Chronicity, possible cyclic nature of neutropenia
Bone marrow aspirate and biopsy	Quantitations and qualitative evaluation of marrow production of neutrophils and other cell lines
Epinephrine stimulation	Estimation of marginal pool
Corticosteroid stimulation	Estimation of marrow storage pool
Neutrophil antibodies	Role of immune mediated destruction
Karyotype	Possible chromosome disorders
ESR, LE prep, FANA, immunoglobulins, complement	Possible collagen-vascular disease
Stool trypsin	Possible Shwachman-Diamond syndrome

nephrine followed by measurements of the neutrophil count at 15-minute intervals for 1 hour. This test allows an approximation of the marginal pool of neutrophils, since epinephrine causes demargination. The neutrophil count should increase by 50% to 100% during the observation period if the marginal pool is intact. Corticosteroid administration (200 mg hydrocortisone succinate intravenously) followed by neutrophil counts at regular intervals for 6 to 12 hours allows an estimation of the size and availability of the bone marrow storage pool. Neutrophils are recruited from this pool into the bloodstream following the dose of corticosteroids; an increase of fewer than 3000 cells/mm^3 in the neutrophil count suggests an inadequate marrow storage pool.

THERAPY

Therapeutic recommendations can usually be made in a straight-forward manner once a diagnosis is established. The most common causes of childhood neutropenia can be "treated" effectively by removal of the offending agent (drug or viral infection) and time (weeks to months). Benign familial neutropenia usually causes no significant infections, and again, time (months to years) usually resolves the problem. Cyclic neutropenia itself cannot be treated effectively, but oral antibiotics usually control the infections that occur during neutropenic periods. Neutropenia caused by marrow infiltration resolves if the primary disease causing the invasion of marrow can be treated effectively. The treatment of idiopathic aplastic anemia and Fanconi's anemia is discussed in Chapter 13. The exocrine pancreatic insufficiency of Shwachman-Diamond syndrome is ameliorated with oral pancreatic enzyme therapy, but the associated neutropenia is unresponsive. Vigorous supportive care is necessary to avoid fatal pyogenic infections. Bone marrow transplantation offers the only hope at present for patients with severe congenital neutropenia (Kostmann's syndrome) and reticular dysgenesis who will otherwise usually die in early infancy. Nutritional deficiencies causing neutropenia can be easily treated with appropriate replacement; recovery is usually brisk and complete.

Autoimmune neutropenia is usually responsive to corticosteroid therapy. If, as is often the case, an underlying disorder such as systemic lupus erythematosus or rheumatoid arthritis is discovered, specific therapy directed at that disorder may lead to a resolution of the neutropenia. Conversely, relapses of the systemic illness may be accompanied by the recurrence of neutropenia. If neonatal neutropenia is caused by a maternal antibody directed against a paternal-inherited antigen on the infant's neutrophils, transfusion of maternal neutrophils, against which the antibody would have no effect, can be temporarily beneficial. This maneuver should be reserved for times of extreme clinical suspicion of infection, since there may be a limit to the number of donations the mother can make. If the passively acquired antibody is diverted against maternal neutrophils (autoimmune neutropenia), the transfusion of maternal neutrophils to the infant will be of no benefit. In these cases, corticosteroid therapy or removal of antibody by exchange transfusion may be beneficial and is indicated if infectious complications are present. The titer of passively transferred antibodies is usually low enough by 2 to 3 months of age to allow a normal neutrophil count. Until that time, and especially in the first few days of life, vigorous supportive care may be necessary to prevent and treat pyogenic infections.

NURSING CONSIDERATIONS

The febrile child with neutropenia poses a special problem, regardless of the cause of the neutropenia.[28] If the neutrophil count is less than 500 cells/mm^3, persistent fever over 38.3° C (101° F) should be considered to be of bacterial origin until proven otherwise. Admission to the hospital is therefore usually necessary. Following appropriate cultures (blood, throat, urine), parenteral antibiotic therapy is started. Antibiotics should be used in a combination that will effectively treat bacteria derived from the skin (such as *staphylococcus aureus*) and the gastrointestinal tract (Gram-negative coliforms). Usually a semi-synthetic penicillin or a cephalosporin is combined with an aminoglycoside.

If a specific bacterial pathogen is isolated, specific antibiotic therapy is designed for a complete treatment course of at least 10 to 14 days. Longer therapy may be necessary for certain organisms or if neutropenia persists. Even if no organism is identified, broad-spectrum antibiotic coverage should be continued until the child is afebrile or neutropenia has resolved. Many regional blood centers can by leukopheresis obtain granulocyte concentrates for transfusion. Until there is more information regarding their effectiveness and until they are more readily available, granulocyte transfusions are restricted to specific patient indications:

1. Proven systemic bacterial or fungal infections
2. Persistent fever despite broad-spectrum antibiotic therapy
3. Absolute neutrophil count less than 500 cells/mm^3, without expectation for improvement in the near future

When the neutropenic child is hospitalized, several special precautions should be observed. Although protective isolation is not necessary, strict hand washing is essential for all health care workers and visitors with potential patient contact. Staff members, visitors, and other patients with apparent contagious illnesses should be restricted from the child's room. All skin punctures for phlebotomy or intravenous access should be preceded by careful washing of the skin with a providine-containing solution. Skin wounds and intravenous catheter sites should be observed frequently.

It should be remembered that in neutropenic patients, the usual signs of inflammation that accompany soft tissue infection may be less impressive than in the normal person; the index of suspicion should be great. Manipulation of the skin, oral mucosa, perineum and rectum should be minimal; rectal temperatures and enemas are forbidden while neutropenia persists. If the child is not hospitalized, similar precautionary measures should be taken. Family members and friends with possible contagious illnesses should be kept away. The child should not go to day-care centers, school, church nurseries, or other areas where there are likely to be large groups of people such as shopping malls or amusement parks until the neutropenia has resolved. In most cases, once the neutrophil count is greater than 500 cells/mm^3, no restrictions are necessary.

NURSING CARE PROTOCOL FOR THE CHILD WITH NEUTROPENIA

Nursing diagnoses (patient problems)	Goals/objectives (patient/family will:)	Interventions (nurse will:)
1. Knowledge deficit (related to diagnosis)	Receive information regarding the diagnosis; demonstrate understanding of its meaning Gain knowledge of side effects and requirements for home care	Assist in discussing the diagnosis, its cause, and complications Discuss in detail the risk of infection and precautions necessary to prevent complications from neutropenia
2. Anxiety (emotional distress related to possible complications of neutropenia)	Demonstrate decreased anxiety; share feelings and concerns with others	Provide opportunities to discuss parents'/child's concerns regarding the diagnosis; assist in identifying other support persons to the family

NURSING CARE PROTOCOL FOR THE CHILD WITH NEUTROPENIA—cont'd

Nursing diagnoses (patient problems)	Goals/objectives (patient/family will:)	Interventions (nurse will:)

3. Injury: potential for (infection)	Exhibit awareness of risk of infection because of neutropenia Demonstrate knowledge of precautions necessary to prevent complications of neutropenia	Discuss in detail major concerns for the child with neutropenia
		
		The child is at risk for development of an overwhelming infection
		Fever over 38.3° C (101° F) in a child with an absolute granulocyte count less than 500 mm^3 requires *immediate* assessment and initiation of intravenous antibiotics. (Signs of infection [i.e., erythema, edema, warmth] may not be present due to neutropenia even when an infection exists.) (Localized infections will heal more slowly [i.e., cuts or lesions on extremities, mouth ulcers])
		Give out any written material on infection
		Review precautions essential for prevention of infection in the child with neutropenia:
		  Never allow the child to go barefoot, which increases the risk for cuts or lesions that will not heal readily
		  Enforce stringent oral hygiene with close assessment for mouth ulcerations
		  Prevent undue exposure to individuals who are ill
		  Practice good hand washing at all times
		  Prevent any rectal manipulation (i.e., rectal temperature, enemas) that will increase the child's risk for infection
		  Maintain good nutrition, enforcing well-balanced meals
		  Should development of infection occur, see nursing care protocol for the child with neutropenia and fever in Chapter 24

4. Coping, ineffective family: compromised	Demonstrate effective coping mechanisms necessary for optimum functioning at home, school, and the community	Provide emotional support and refer to other health professionals as needed Communicate with other agencies and the school to facilitate optimum care at home Stress importance of re-establishing a normal life-style

NURSING CARE PROTOCOL FOR THE CHILD WITH NEUTROPENIA AND FEVER

Nursing diagnoses (patient problems)	Goals/objectives (patient/family will:)	Interventions (nurse will:)
1. Injury: potential for (risk for overwhelming infection with granulocyte count <1000)	Early detection of signs of sepsis	Monitor vital signs closely for changes in the following: Pulse becoming weak and rapid *Normal pulse ranges* 1-6 yr 90-110 beats/min 6-12 80-95 beats/min 12-16 75-80 beats/min Shallow rapid respirations *Normal respirations* 1-6 yr 20-30 breaths/min 6-12 15-25 breaths/min 12-16 15-20 breaths/min Drop in blood pressure *Normal systolic mean pressure* 1-6 yr 90 mm Hg 6-12 100 mm Hg 12-16 113 mm Hg Drop in temperature Change in level of consciousness Assess skin for diaphoresis, ashen color, poor capillary filling Check urine output hourly (Urine output should not fall below 0.5 cc/kg/hr.) Notify physician immediately for any of the above
	Receive appropriate antibiotic therapy	Administer antibiotics after blood cultures are obtained according to physician orders Check dosage to ensure adequate coverage Observe for reaction to antibiotic during infusion: check vital signs Observe for rash Assess any complaints
2. Comfort, alteration in: pain (malaise, discomfort, irritability because of fever)	Be able to rest comfortably	Take temperature at least every 4 hr For temperature >38.3° C, notify physician if blood cultures and acetaminophen are not routinely ordered (If ordered draw blood cultures before administering acetaminophen.) For temperature >39° C, give patient tepid sponge bath or tub bath; use light clothing and bedding If chills occur, discontinue measures to cool patient

NURSING CARE PROTOCOL FOR THE CHILD WITH NEUTROPENIA AND FEVER—cont'd

Nursing diagnoses (patient problems)	Goals/objectives (patient/family will:)	Interventions (nurse will:)

3. Fluid volume deficit, potential	Be adequately hydrated	Maintain strict I & O
		Continue to assess for signs of dehydration
		Signs of dehydration
		  Loss of skin turgor
		  Dry mucous membranes
		  Acute weight loss
		  Decreased tearing
		  Soft, sunken, eyeballs
		  Sunken anterior fontanel
		  Oliguria and concentrated urine (specific gravity daily normal 1.010-1.025)
		Ensure patent IV with appropriate rate
		Force fluids every 1 hr while awake

4. Injury: potential for (seizures in infants and young children)	Demonstrate no seizure activity	Assess closely for undue irritability, sudden screaming, hallucinations, staring, tremors; report any of these signs immediately Notify physician immediately of rapid rise in temperature that is not reduced by sponging or other measures previously stated
5. Injury: potential for (invasion of organisms producing secondary infections)	Demonstrate no site of infection	Daily check mouth for ulcerations and redness, skin punctures for edema or redness, anal region for fissures or breakdown Remove adhesive bandages daily Auscultate lungs every shift Ambulate when afebrile Follow cultures daily

REFERENCES

1. Pincus S.H., and others: Chronic neutropenia in childhood, Am. J. Med. **61:**849, 1976.
2. Karayalcin, G., and others: Pseudoneutropenia in American Negroes, Lancet **1:**387, 1972.
3. Rudolph, A.M., editors: Pediatrics, ed. 16, New York, 1977, Appleton-Century-Crofts, Inc.
4. Nathan, D.G., Housman, D.E., and Clarke, B.J.: The anatomy and physiology of hematopoiesis. In Nathan, D.G., and Oski, E.A., editors: Hematology of infancy and childhood, Philadelphia, 1981, W.B. Saunders Co.
5. Quesenberry, P., and Levitt, L.: Hematopoietic stem cells, N. Engl. J. Med. **301:**755, 1979.
6. Lichtman, M.A., and others: The regulation of the release of granulocytes from normal marrow. In Greenwelt, T.J., and Jamieson, G.A., (editors): The granulocyte: function and clinical utilization, New York, 1977, Alan R. Liss, Inc.
7. Moore, M.A.S.: Humoral regulation of granulopoiesis, Clin Haematol. **8:**287, 1979.
8. Mishler, J.M., and Sharp, A.A.: Adrenaline: further discussion of its role in the mobilization of neutrophils, Scand. J. Haematol. **17:**78, 1976.
9. Kostmann, R.: Infantile genetic agranulocytosis: a review with presentation of ten new cases, Acta. Paediatr. Scand. **64:**362, 1975.
10. Baehner, R.L., and Boxer, L.A.: Disorders of granulopoiesis and granulocyte function. In Nathan, D.G., and Oski, F.A., editors: Hematology of infancy and childhood, Philadelphia, 1981, W.B. Saunders Co.
11. Shwachman, H., and others: The syndrome of pancreatic insufficiency and bone marrow dysfunction, J. Pediatr. **65:**645, 1964.
12. Shmerling, D.H., and others: The syndrome of exocrine pancreatic insufficiency, neutropenia, metaphyseal dysostosis and dwarfism, Helv. Paediatr. Acta. **24:**547, 1969.
13. Fanconi, G.: Familial constitutional panmyelopathy, Fanconi's anemia. I. Clinical aspects, Semin. Hematol. **4:**233, 1967.
14. DeVall, D.M., and Seynhaeve, V.: Reticular dysgenesis, Lancet **2:**1123, 1959.
15. Guery, D. IV, and others: Periodic hematopoiesis in human cyclic neutropenia, J. Clin. Invest. **52:**3220, 1973.
16. Morley, A.A., and others: Familial cyclic neutropenia, Br. J. Haematol. **13:**719, 1967.
17. Pisciotta, A.V.: Immune and toxic mechanisms in drug-induced agranulocytosis, Semin. Hematol. **10:**279, 1973.
18. Al-Rashid, R.A., and Spangler, J.: Neonatal copper deficiency, N. Engl. J. Med. **285:**841, 1971.
19. Bernard, C.W., and others: Current concepts of leukemia and lymphoma: etiology, pathogenesis and therapy, Ann. Intern. Med. **91:**758, 1979.
20. Boxer, L.A., and others: Myelofibrosis myeloid metaplasia in childhood, Pediatrics **55:**861, 1975
21. Habib, M.A., and others: Profound granulocytopenia associated with infectious mononucleosis, Am. J. Med. Sci. **265:**339, 1973.
22. Berthrong, M., and Cluff, L.E.: Studies of the effect of bacterial endotoxins on rabbit leukocytes. I. Effect of intravenous ingestion of the substances with and without induction of the local Schwartzman reaction, J. Exp. Med. **98:**331, 1953.
23. Lalezari, P., and Rahel, E.: Neutrophil-specific antigens: immunology and clinical significance, Semin. Hematol. **11:**281, 1974
24. Storkebaum, G., and others: Autoimmune neutropenia in systemic lupus erythematosus, Clin. Res. **26:**155A, 1978.
25. Boxer, L.A., and others: Isoimmune neonatal neutropenia, J. Pediatr. **80:**783, 1972.
26. Weitzman, S.A., and Stossel, T.P.: Drug-induced immunological neutropenia, Lancet **1:**1068, 1978.
27. Boxer, L.A., and Stossel T.P.: Effects of anti-neutrophil antibodies in vitro: quantitative studies, J. Clin. Invest. **53:**1534, 1974.
28. Pizzo, A.P.: Infectious complications in the young patient with cancer: etiology, pathogenesis, diagnosis, management and prevention. In Levine, A.S., editor: Cancer in the young, New York, 1982, Masson Publishing USA, Inc.

CHAPTER 19

Platelet disorders of childhood

MARILYN J. HOCKENBERRY and THOMAS R. KINNEY

Platelets are essential for a variety of functions including hemostasis, phagocytosis, inflammatory responses, and endothelial support.[1] The most essential role of the platelet, or thrombocyte, is to promote hemostasis. Disorders of platelets are caused by numerous diseases that present with thrombocytopenia as a secondary complication. Bone marrow dysfunction related to replacement diseases (i.e., leukemia, lymphoma) or marrow failure (i.e., aplastic anemias, chronic disease) have been discussed earlier in previous chapters. This chapter will review common causes of platelet disorders not previously discussed.

THE PLATELET

The normal platelet is a small round disc without a nucleus that measures 1 to 2 mm in diameter and is one fourth the size of a normal red blood cell. The normal platelet count ranges from 150,000 to 450,000 cells/mm[3] and has a mean circulating span of 8 to 10 days. Two thirds of the body's platelets circulate, while one third remains in the spleen.

The platelet normally flows freely through the body's vascular system. However, when vascular injury occurs, platelets begin adherence to the exposed collagen and other vascular components. Collagen stimulates platelet adherence more than any other substance in the vessel wall.[1] Platelet aggregation following their interaction with collagen is mediated through the release of adenosine diphosphate (ADP).[2] Platelets then begin to aggregate, changing their shape to form sticky, spiny spheres that bond to each other and surrounding substances. This aggregation of platelets, along with exposed collagen, promotes activation of plasma coagulation factors that trigger thrombin clot generation[3] (see Chapter 16 on hemophilia).

PLATELET DISORDERS

Platelet disorders occurring in childhood are caused primarily by impairment in production, increase in destruction, or by platelet dysfunction as shown in Fig. 19-1. These disorders can be acquired or inherited.

Thrombocytopenia caused by increased destruction may occur through both immune and non-immune mediated responses. These states are characterized by adequate megakaryocytes in the bone marrow, decreased platelet survival time, and the presence of large platelets on the peripheral smear. Thrombocytopenia secondary to decrease in the platelet production is characterized by reduced numbers of megakaryocytes in the bone marrow.

Disorders causing hypersplenism, where platelets are sequestered in the spleen, may cause a drastic decrease in circulating platelets. Thrombocytopenia is caused by inadequate platelet distribution and increased platelet destruction occurring in the spleen.[2]

APPROACH TO THE CHILD WITH A BLEEDING PROBLEM

Evaluation of a child with bleeding involves a detailed history and physical examination. A thorough initial assessment can help to establish a cause and often distinguish between a platelet disorder or coagulation protein abnormality.

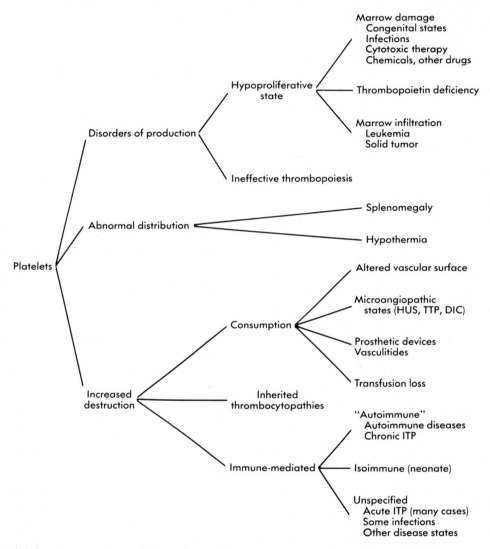

Fig. 19-1 Physiologic classification of thrombocytopenia in childhood is depicted. *HUS*, hemolytic uremic syndrome; *TTP*, thrombotic thrombocytopenic purpura: *DIC*, disseminated intravascular coagulation; *ITP*, idiopathic thrombocytopenic purpura. (Adapted from Lightsey, A.L., Jr.: Pediatr. Clin. North Am. **27**(2):293, 1980.)

History

A detailed history must include family history of bleeding. Pattern of inheritance frequently points to a specific diagnosis as seen in individuals who have factor VIII and IX deficiencies, which are sex-linked recessive disorders. Hereditary disorders usually are manifested soon after birth, whereas acquired disorders may occur at any time.

Coagulation protein abnormalities, when severe, produce joint and muscle bleeding, whereas platelet abnormalities are more commonly associated with skin and mucous membrane bleeding. Prolonged bleeding occurring immediately after trauma and not alleviated by pressure reveals impaired hemostasis.

Dietary history is essential in determining deficiencies that may cause increased bleeding. Deficiency of vitamin C, essential for normal collagen formation, will cause a vascular defect causing hemorrhage in the skin and mucous membranes. Hematuria, melena, and orbital or subdural hemorrhage may also occur.[1] Coagulation factors II, VII, IX, and X are dependent on vitamin K, essential for prothrombin formation. When vitamin K is depleted, it may cause prolonged bleeding and oozing of minor wounds to generalized ecchymoses and life-threatening surface hemorrhage.[1]

A careful drug history is essential. Ingestion of aspirin-containing compounds may produce prolonged bleeding by interference of platelet function.[1] Numerous drugs are known to cause platelet dysfunction and should be evaluated as a possible etiologic factor.

Careful evaluation of onset of bleeding, its location, relation to trauma, and surgery must be considered. It is helpful to evaluate the presence of prolonged, uncontrollable bleeding following dental extraction that continues for hours after extraction.[2]

Physical examination

Symptomatic children with platelet disorders usually have low platelet counts; however, the severity of hemorrhage does not always correlate with the platelet count. Frequently, children display no overt bleeding unless the platelet count falls below 20,000 mm[3]. Petechiae and ecchymoses may or may not be present in children with platelet counts of 50,000 mm[3].[1] There are some disorders that will be discussed later in this chapter that cause bleeding in the presence of a normal platelet count. Classic signs and symptoms of thrombocytopenia include spontaneous bleeding in the skin and mucous membranes, forming small pinpoint hemorrhages called petechiae or larger bruises called purpura. Less commonly, epistaxis, oozing from gums, hematuria, melena, or hemorrhagia may develop. Rarely, children with thrombocytopenia present with gastrointestinal or central nervous system bleeding.[4]

Laboratory evaluation

Initial laboratory evaluation of the child with petechiae and ecchymosis should include a complete blood count, platelet count, and examination of the peripheral blood smear. An accurate assessment of the platelet count can be obtained from the standard blood film. The blood count may suggest an underlying cause for the decreased platelets, thus all cellular elements should be examined closely. Size of the platelets may assist in further establishing the diagnosis. Young platelets appear larger, and their presence suggests active thrombopoiesis in the bone marrow and increased turnover of platelets.[4]

Bone marrow examination is usually warranted in the presence of thrombocytopenia. Presence of megakaryocytes in the bone marrow assists in differentiating thrombocytopenia caused from destruction or abnormal distribution as compared with bone marrow failure or infiltration[4] (Fig. 19-2).

Tools to assist in determining whether or not a clotting disorder exists are discussed in Chapter 16 on hemophilia. Diagnostic evaluation of associated illnesses determined by the physical examination and history are essential to help determine an underlying cause for bleeding.

ACQUIRED PLATELET DISORDERS
Idiopathic thrombocytopenic purpura

Idiopathic thrombocytopenic purpura (ITP) is an acquired hemorrhagic disorder resulting in excess

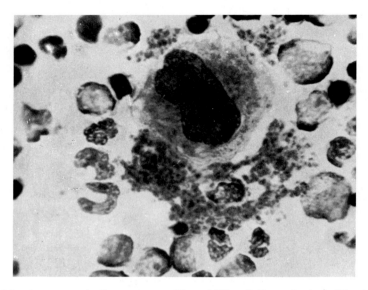

Fig. 19-2. Megakaryocytes in bone marrow. (From Miller, D.R., and others: Blood diseases of infancy and childhood, St. Louis, 1984, The C.V. Mosby Co.)

destruction of circulating platelets. It is the most common type of thrombocytopenic disease in childhood.[2] Over one half of the cases occur before 15 years of age. At this age the disease is usually a benign, self-limiting condition with spontaneous recovery within a matter of weeks to months.[5] This form of ITP, entitled acute ITP, has an acute onset with a peak age of onset between 2 to 6 years with equal sex distribution.[6]

Over 50% of children with ITP will recover within 1 to 3 months of onset, and 80% to 90% will demonstrate normal platelet counts by 4 months after diagnosis.[2] Thrombocytopenia remaining in approximately 10% of the patients beyond 6 to 12 months duration is classified as chronic ITP. At onset of ITP, it is difficult to differentiate the acute from chronic type. Table 19-1 demonstrates differing features among the two types of ITP.

Acute ITP is associated with a prior illness, most frequently viral in nature. Common childhood exanthems and live virus immunizations, particularly rubella, have also anteceded onset of ITP.[2] A majority of these cases occur in the winter and spring, at the time of greatest incidence of viral infections. Thrombocytopenia usually occurs 10 to 14 days following onset of infection, illness, or immunization.

Etiology. Specific pathogenesis of ITP remains unclear although it appears that the platelet membrane is altered by a virus or viral antigen-antibody complex that has an affinity for sites on the platelet surface. These immune complexes interact with the platelet by means of an Fc receptor site on the platelet. This immune mediated response, resulting in antiplatelet antibody formation, causes increased destruction of platelets by the reticuloendothelial system of the spleen.[2] Association of virus and thrombocytopenia is well established, with the more common viruses being varicella, rubella, rubeola, mononucleosis, and those frequently seen with pharyngitis.[2]

Clinical manifestations. In the majority of children, onset is acute, with a benign history of a child who has suddenly developed easy bruisabil-

Table 19-1. Classifying features of acute versus chronic childhood ITP

Finding	Acute ITP	Chronic ITP
Age	Less than 10 years	Greater than 10 years
Onset	Preceding viral infection, childhood exanthem, immunization	Unknown cause
Sex	Equal sex distribution	More common in females
Platelet count	Less than 20,000 per mm^3	20,000-75,000 per mm^3
Immunoglobulins	Normal IgA	Decreased IgA
Platelet associated antibody IgG	Markedly elevated	Moderately elevated
Eosinophilia and lymphocytosis	Common	Rare
Duration	2-6 weeks	Months to years
Prognosis	Spontaneous remission in 80% of patients	Chronic in nature

ity. Careful history should include evaluation of recent infections, childhood exanthems, or immunizations. Bleeding under the skin is the major sign of ITP, with petechiae and purpura being present on every child at diagnosis. Epistaxis occurs in 25% of these children. Hematuria and oral and gastrointestinal bleeding are rare, seen only in 5% to 10% of children at diagnosis.[5] Extent of purpura and petechiae varies from mild to severe.

Other findings of the physical examination include minimum splenomegaly, which is a common finding among normal children. Shotty lymphadenopathy may be present.[7]

Laboratory findings. Thrombocytopenia may be severe, with platelet counts in the range of 1,000 to 20,000 mm^3. Few platelets are seen on the peripheral smear and, when seen, are large and abnormally shaped. Children with chronic ITP frequently express higher platelet counts initially, with a range between 20,000 to 75,000 mm^3. Acute ITP may present with a lymphocytosis reflecting a recent viral infection. A mild eosinophilia is seen in approximately 25% of children with ITP. Platelet antibody tests may be used to evaluate the extent of antibody formation. Direct platelet antibody results indicate antibody mediated response within the cytoplasm as compared with indirect results, which measure circulating antibodies within the plasma.

Bone marrow examination reveals an increased number of megakaryocytes. Eosinophilia may also be seen in the bone marrow.

Diagnosis of ITP in a child should demonstrate the following findings[8]:

1. Physical examination reveals petechiae and ecchymoses in an otherwise normal appearing child. Minimum splenomegaly and lymphadenopathy are found.
2. Peripheral blood smear reveals thrombocytopenia only.
3. Bone marrow aspiration shows normal to increased numbers of megakaryocytes with normal erythroid and myeloid constituents.
4. Underlying etiologic factors as a cause for thrombocytopenia are absent.

Treatment

Acute ITP. A primary goal of management of the child with acute ITP is prevention of complications secondary to thrombocytopenia. Restriction of a child's activities to prevent bleeding is a major goal of supportive care until the platelet count has recovered. Contact sports should be avoided. Young children should be fitted with a protective helmet during play to prevent head trauma. Extra measures to prevent falling should be pursued such as preventing the young child from crawling up stairs and padding the child's crib. Avoidance of drugs that interfere with platelet function such as aspirin and many antihistaminic preparations should be stressed. Intramuscular or arterial punctures, rectal temperatures, enemas, nasogastric intubation, and suctioning should be avoided.

Controversy remains in the use of corticosteroids in acute ITP. It is felt that administration of corticosteroids induces an earlier rise in platelet counts in many children. This earlier rise reduces the child's risk for developing major bleeding, thus decreasing anxiety in parents.

Corticosteroids are used in a dosage of prednisone 2 mg/kg/day orally in divided doses for 2 to 4 weeks.[8] Short courses of steroids are associated with few or no side effects.[8] Steroids prove to do a number of functions in ITP: inhibit phagocytosis of antibody-coated platelets in the spleen and prolong platelet survival; improve capillary resistance; and inhibit platelet antibody production.[7] On termination of steroid treatment the child will demonstrate one of three responses: the platelet count returns to normal and will remain so for life; thrombocytopenia recurs once prednisone is discontinued; thrombocytopenia persists with little or no improvement seen with steroid therapy.[2] Further corticosteroid therapy is discouraged once an initial trial is attempted unless the child demonstrates increased bleeding problems after steroids have been discontinued and has had some benefit with the initial course of steroids. The lowest possible dose should be used on an every-other-day schedule.

Platelet transfusions are of no benefit in the child with ITP because of rapid destruction of platelets in the spleen and increased antibody formation with transfusion of platelets. When life-threatening bleeding occurs, an emergency splenectomy must be performed to stop platelet destruction.

When a child with ITP continues with intermittent or consistent clinical symptoms beyond 6 months, the disorder becomes chronic, and new therapeutic considerations are pursued.

Chronic ITP. The major focus of treatment continues with supportive care to prevent complications from major bleeding episodes. Children who maintain a stable platelet count ranging from 30,000 to 50,000 mm³ can be watched indefinitely with relatively few restrictions. This observance period is critical for the child under 10 years of age who has a good chance for spontaneous recovery. Children over 10 years of age rarely demonstrate recovery after 1 year of onset of ITP.

Splenectomy may be considered when a child continues with thrombocytopenia and persistent hemorrhagic symptoms that are difficult to control.[2] Elective splenectomy should be delayed until a child is over 4 years of age because of increased risk of overwhelming sepsis. Benefits of splenectomy demonstrate a remission of ITP in 70% of children who have refractory ITP.[1] This is attributed to the removal of the major site for destruction of platelets and production of platelet antibodies.

Risks of splenectomy must be seriously considered. The family and the child must know these risks and participate in the decision for the surgery. Decisions for splenectomy should not be made in a hurry, except in children with life-threatening hemorrhage. Pneumococcal vaccination should be administered before surgery to protect against pneumococcal infection. The child should begin a prophylactic regimen of penicillin twice daily for life because of the increased risk of overwhelming sepsis following splenectomy. Children undergoing splenectomy for ITP should be supported during surgery with steroids, if they were used previously, to prevent adrenal insufficiency caused by stress of surgery. Thrombocytosis is frequently observed following splenectomy with counts sometimes rising over 1 million. Thrombotic complications secondary to increased platelets are rarely, if ever, observed in these patients.

Recent trends are being considered in the treatment of chronic ITP that are hoped to delay or even exclude the need for splenectomy. Use of intravenous immunoglobulin is now being investigated as an alternative to splenectomy. Its mode of action is unclear although it is thought to interfere with fixation or absorption of immunoglobulin on the platelets or with uptake of immunoglobulin by the platelets.[9]

Immunologic suppression has been used in

children with ITP not responding to prednisone and splenectomy. Azathioprine, 6-mercaptopurine, cyclophosphamide, and the vinca alkaloids have been used to promote platelet stimulation.[10] Children with chronic ITP manifesting life-threatening bleeding may require plasma exchange to rapidly remove antibodies interfering with platelet function and promoting platelet destruction. Treatment with fresh frozen plasma has been used to control bleeding in a small number of children but was of short duration.[10]

Thrombocytopenia associated with autoimmune disorders

Thrombocytopenia is associated with a number of diseases that are autoimmune in nature. Immunologically induced thrombocytopenia can occur with disorders such as systemic lupus erythematosus, Evan's syndrome, rheumatoid arthritis, nephritis, Hashimoto's thyroiditis, Graves' disease, myasthenia gravis, immunodeficiency syndromes, and atrophic gastritis.[2,11]

Clinical expression of thrombocytopenia in children with one of these autoimmune disorders is similar to chronic ITP. Thrombocytopenia is caused by the development of platelet-specific antibodies.[1] Management places primary emphasis in controlling the underlying autoimmune disorder, while following the guidelines previously discussed under treatment of the child with chronic ITP.

Drug-induced platelet disorders

Ingestion of specific drugs may create a decrease in the platelet count by causing marrow depression or decreasing platelet destruction. Many of these drugs are associated with aplastic anemia and have been discussed in Chapter 13 on childhood anemias. Other drugs may cause platelet dysfunction, creating a tendency for prolonged bleeding episodes.

Numerous antibiotics have an adverse effect on platelet function. Carbenicillin is the most extensively studied antibiotic known to cause platelet dysfunction.[12] The majority of individuals exposed to carbenicillin in dosages used to treat Gram-negative sepsis will have a prolonged bleeding time, usually occurring within 24 hours after initiation of the drug and persisting for days.[13] Penicillin has also been known to inhibit platelet function. Ampicillin and cephalothin have been associated with increased stool blood loss in patients who were already thrombocytopenic.[14]

Aspirin inhibits platelet aggregation and prolongs the bleeding time by several minutes in most individuals who have no underlying illness.[15] These defects can be detected after a single dose of aspirin and can last for several days. Among other drugs that may produce platelet dysfunction are the tricyclic antidepressants, antihistamines, ethyl alcohol, nitrofurantoin, dextran, pyrizadine compounds, phenothiazines, and numerous anesthetics.[16,17]

Clinical manifestations. Acute hemorrhagic findings involving the mucous membranes may develop within 1 to 12 hours after administration of a drug in a previously sensitized patient. Systemic manifestations may develop readily with the presence of chills, fever, and later arthralgias.

More commonly, clinical manifestations resemble those found in acute ITP. These findings are self-limited, disappearing once the drug has been discontinued. Careful history is essential, giving detail to the dosage and duration of each drug ingested. Once the cause is established, the drug should be avoided.

Treatment. Duration of platelet dysfunction induced by drugs is usually short, lasting less than 2 weeks. Supportive care to prevent complications of bleeding should be pursued. The drug should be discontinued. Further discussion of drug-induced marrow suppression is reviewed in the Chapter 13.

Microangiopathic destructive thrombocytopenia

Destructive thrombocytopenia associated with nonimmunologic microangiopathic disorders has been discussed previously in Chapter 13 on childhood anemias. Hemolytic anemia and thrombocytopenia occur. Common syndromes include hemolytic uremic syndrome and thrombotic thrombocytopenic purpura although similar platelet and red blood cell changes are observed in a variety of disorders. Disseminated diseases, surgical cardiac repair, and disseminated intravascular coagulation may produce thrombocytopenia secondary to a microangiopathic process.[10,18]

Hemolytic uremic syndrome

Hemolytic uremic syndrome (HUS) is an acquired disorder seen in the infant and toddler 6 months to 2 years of age. HUS is preceded by onset of bloody diarrhea, vomiting, and abdominal pain.[19] Anemia occurs a few days after onset of initial symptoms and is followed by complications of renal insufficiency, which include hematuria, oliguria, hypertension, edema, and seizures. Microangiopathic hemolytic anemia and thrombocytopenia are caused by damage to the red cells and platelets as they travel through the injured glomerular capillaries and renal arterioles.[20]

Primary treatment is aimed toward treatment of renal failure. Administration of platelets is rarely necessary and should be avoided unless severe hemorrhage occurs.

Thrombotic thrombocytopenic purpura

Thrombotic thrombocytopenic purpura (TTP) is an acquired disorder seen primarily in adolescents and adults. This disorder is characterized by microangiopathic hemolytic anemia, thrombocytopenia, and neurologic symptoms. Paresthesias, seizures, altered state of consciousness, and personality changes are seen in patients with this disorder.

Renal impairment including the onset of hematuria, proteinuria, and azotemia may develop. Fever is a common finding.

This disorder is caused by proliferative microvascular injury with resultant onset of platelet fibrin formation. This results in the formation of thrombin in the capillaries and arterioles, which causes fragmentation of red blood cells and increased use of platelets.[2]

Significant mortality is associated with TTP. Supportive care is of major importance, placing emphasis on those organs most severely affected.

Aggressive corticosteroid therapy with splenectomy is thought to be of some benefit in TTP.[21] Plasma exchange transfusions and repeated plasma infusions have been used in some patients with encouraging results.[22,23]

Thrombocytopenia caused by transfusions

Thrombocytopenia has been observed in individuals receiving massive amounts of blood in the form of transfusions with compatible blood. This is observed in trauma victims or patients requiring extensive surgery such as for scoliosis. A decrease in platelet count is thought to be from a dilution of the patient's platelet pool by large quantities of blood, deficiency of platelets in the donated blood, and inability of the patient's megakaryocytes to compensate for the rapid depletion of platelets in the peripheral circulation.

Significant clinical complications are rare. Treatment consists of replacing platelets in circulation by administering platelet transfusions or the use of fresh whole blood.

Thrombocytopenia with infections

Onset of infection in a child frequently causes bone marrow suppression as discussed early in Chapter 13 on childhood anemias. Thrombocytopenia is associated with bacterial, fungal, rickettsial, viral, and protozoal infections.

Platelet counts less than $150,000/mm^3$ occur in 60% to 80% of children with Gram-positive or Gram-negative sepsis.[24] There are several mechanisms for thrombocytopenia in children with septicemia. Bacteria may cause endothelial damage, leading to platelet aggregation. Bacterial products may bind directly to platelets causing destruction. There is speculation that decreased platelets in septicemia is also mediated by immune mechanisms.[25]

Thrombocytopenia associated with giant hemangioma

Numerous individuals with giant cavernous hemangiomas, or Kasabach-Merritt syndrome, are known to have thrombocytopenia associated with it.[2] These hemangiomas are congenital, thus bleeding manifestations usually are seen within the first few weeks of life. The size of the hemangioma has no impact on the degree of thrombocytopenia. Occurrence of cavernous hemangiomas occurs in 1% to 8% of children less than 1 year of age.[2] Most lesions spontaneously regress by 5 years of age.

Clinical manifestations. The hemangiomas may be superficial and located separately from other structures or they may involve bone or other viscera including the tongue, thorax, liver, and spleen.[26] Typically, development of hemorrhagic complications are preceded by changes in the hemangioma. There may be increase in its size, consistency, or color. This is followed by more characteristic findings associated with thrombocytopenia such as ecchymosis and petechiae.

Treatment. Careful observance of the hemangioma and periodic platelet counts are appropriate methods for management. Corticosteroids may be used in an attempt to decrease the size of the lesion and increase the platelet count. Hemangiomas located in areas that are at risk to compromise vital organs require more aggressive therapy and may warrant surgical removal or radiation. Major complications result from hemorrhage, airway obstruction, and infection. When these symptoms occur, aggressive treatment must be pursued.

INHERITED PLATELET DISORDERS
Wiskott-Aldrich syndrome

Wiskott-Aldrich syndrome is a rare X-linked recessive disorder, characterized by eczema, thrombocytopenia, and increased susceptibility to infections.[2] Thrombocytopenia is thought to be caused by increased destruction of abnormally functioning platelets.

Clinical manifestations. Clinical evidence usually becomes obvious with the first 6 months of life. Physical examination reveals petechiae, purpura, generalized eczema, hepatosplenomegaly, and evidence of infection. Recurrent chronic otitis media is a common finding.

Significant thrombocytopenia is present, with the platelet count being below 50,000 mm³. Small, infrequent platelets are seen on the smear and are

a key finding in this disorder. Bone marrow aspiration reveals adequate numbers of megakaryocytes, which may be abnormal in appearance.[2]

Treatment. Treatment is limited to supportive care and management of recurrent infections. Prognosis of Wiskott-Aldrich syndrome is poor. Affected males rarely survive to adulthood and usually develop complications of infection or bleeding. There is an increased incidence of malignancy, specifically lymphomas, which may increase the complications of this disorder.[1] Topical corticosteroids may be used to control eczema. Systemic corticosteroids are not effective in the treatment of thrombocytopenia and may aggravate the existing immunodeficiency.[1] Platelet transfusions may be used to control severe bleeding. Bone marrow transplantation after total body irradiation is now being pursued as a new mode of treatment.[27]

Giant platelet disorders

Bernard-Soulier syndrome. Bernard-Soulier disease is a rare inherited disorder with hemorrhagic symptoms beginning in infancy.[28] Striking abnormalities in platelet morphology with a varying degree of clinical severity of bleeding are seen. There is a prolongation of the bleeding time, abnormal prothrombin consumption, and varying platelet count in the presence of usually large platelets.

Bleeding may be severe and even fatal. The type of bleeding is similar to that seen in other platelet disorders. The bleeding disorder is not benefited by corticosteroid therapy or splenectomy.[29] Management is controlled by administration of platelet transfusions when bleeding occurs.

May-Hegglin anomaly. May-Hegglin anomaly is a rare autosomal dominant trait characterized by the presence of giant platelets. One third of these individuals have thrombocytopenia. Peripheral smear reveals large platelets that vary in size and shape. Leukocytes may contain basophilic patches called Döhle bodies, which are RNA material.[2] The platelet defect in this disorder has not been fully established. The majority of these patients have no bleeding manifestations, and the anomaly is found as an incidental finding.[30]

Thrombocytopenia absent radii syndrome. Thrombocytopenia absent radii is a congenital disorder characterized by deficiency of megakaryocytes in association with skeletal abnormalities.[2] The finding of thrombocytopenia purpura with bilateral absence of the radii in infancy establishes the diagnosis. Bone marrow examination reveals decreased and defective megakaryocytes with normal or increased numbers of other cells.

In some infants affected with this syndrome, there is increased gastrointestinal bleeding with exposure to cow's milk. Elimination of cow's milk in these infants decreases the amount of bleeding.[2]

Prognosis is favorable if the infant survives the first year of life. Corticosteroid therapy and splenectomy are of no benefit in these infants.[1] Red blood cell and platelet transfusions should be used as supportive therapy. Cow's milk should be excluded from the diet of children showing gastrointestinal symptomatology.

Glanzmann's thrombasthenia. Glanzmann's thrombasthenia is a rare, autosomal recessive disorder that presents with nonthrombocytopenic purpura, prolonged bleeding time, and a deficient or absent clot retraction. Platelets do not aggregate with ADP in about 80% of these patients.[29]

These patients present with similar symptoms seen in chronic ITP. Purpura begins in early infancy, with hemorrhagic symptoms usually being non–life-threatening.[2] The platelet count is normal with the absence of normal platelet clumping seen on peripheral smear. Coagulation tests, prothrombin time (PT), and partial thromboplastin time (PTT) are normal. Platelet function tests are abnormal with an Ivy bleeding time commonly being greater than 10 minutes. Platelet aggregation studies are abnormal.

Treatment involves supportive care with blood products. Splenectomy and corticosteroids are of no benefit.

ADP storage pool disease

Storage pool disease is a rare autosomal dominant disorder characterized by mild nonthrombocytopenic purpura and abnormal second phase aggregation of platelets caused by a lack of storage of ADP and a failure of the ADP release mechanism of normal stores.[31] Storage pool is frequently associated with other systemic diseases. Clinical manifestations vary according to the underlying abnormality. There are no clinical symptoms that distinguish this disorder from other thrombocytopathies.

Diagnosis of storage pool disease is established by demonstration of decrease or absence of ADP stores. Isotopic techniques are used along with electron microscopy.

There is no specific treatment, since the bleeding tendency is mild and life-threatening hemorrhage is rare. The use of aspirin should be avoided. Supportive blood products should be used when increased bleeding may occur (such as in surgery).

VASCULAR DISORDERS
Henoch-Schönlein purpura

Henoch-Schönlein purpura is an acquired disorder seen in children who initially have a nonthrombocytopenic purpura with joint and visceral abnormalities.[1] It occurs most frequently in children between the ages of 2 to 7 years, with males more commonly being affected. There is a high incidence of prior upper respiratory tract infection occurring 1 to 3 weeks before the onset of purpura.

Clinical manifestations. The child presents with purpura involving the buttocks and lower extremities. A maculopapular erythematous rash is common with the presence of urticaria. Petechial lesions may be present as seen in Fig. 19-3. Presence of purpura is symmetric and ranges in color from dark red to purple and brown as old lesions fade and new appear. Joint involvement is common with children presenting with nonmigratory polyarthralgias in the ankles and knees.[2] Edema is a frequent finding and occurs on the dorsum of the hands and feet, scalp, lip, ears, and periorbital area.[1]

Gastrointestinal manifestations may include midabdominal pain with nausea and vomiting and bloody mucous stools. Intussusception may occur.

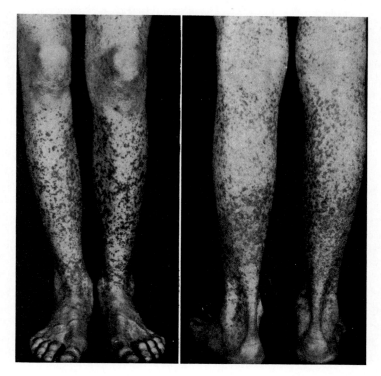

Fig. 19-3. Ecchymoses and petechiae caused by spontaneous bleeding in child with Henoch-Schönlein purpura. (From Miller, D.R., and others: Blood diseases of infancy and childhood, St. Louis, 1984, The C.V. Mosby Co.)

Renal involvement is present in as many as 50% of children and is the most serious long-term complication of this disorder.[1] Renal symptoms include hematuria and proteinuria. Central nervous system complications are rare but have been described.

Laboratory findings. Diagnosis of Henoch-Schönlein purpura is established by clinical examination. It is, however, crucial to monitor function of all organs and to determine the extent of renal involvement. Laboratory evaluation should attempt to identify any preceding illnesses associated with the onset of Henoch-Schönlein purpura.

Treatment. Supportive care is crucial for management of the child with Henoch-Schönlein purpura. Underlying infections must be treated appropriately. Arthralgias should be controlled by analgesics and sedation. Acetaminophen should be prescribed instead of aspirin.

Prednisone therapy is used in children with abdominal manifestations in an attempt to reduce edema of the bowel. Its use may also provide pain relief from polyarthralgias. Prednisone will not alter the extent of renal impairment.

Approximately 50% of these children will recover within a month of the onset of purpura. During this month, frequent recurrences of skin lesions and abdominal pain are seen. Prognosis and ultimate recovery is excellent, with long-term renal complications occurring in less than 15% of children who had initial renal involvement.[5]

CASE STUDY

J.L. is a 5-year-old white female who was seen by her pediatrician because of increased bruising of the lower extremities and frequent nosebleeds occurring in the past 2 days. Until this visit, J.L. had been in excellent health. Past history is unremarkable. She had recovered from a viral illness 2 weeks previously consisting of high fever and upper respiratory congestion. This viral illness lasted for 3 days and was treated symptomatically. Physical examination revealed multiple areas of petechiae and ecchymoses located on all extremities. Pinpoint hemorrhagic areas were noted on the buccal mucosa bilaterally. The spleen was palpable 2 cm below the left costal border. Laboratory studies indicated hemoglobin 10.8 g/dl, white blood cell count 5 mm³, and a platelet count of 4,000 mm³. A bone marrow aspiration was performed revealing normal numbers of megakaryocytes, with normal erythroid and myeloid constituents. Direct platelet antibody studies were markedly elevated. J.L. was diagnosed with idiopathic thrombocytopenic purpura and was begun on prednisone 2 mg/kg/day in three divided doses for 14 days. On day 14 J.L. demonstrated a platelet count of 88,000 mm³ and was placed on a steroid taper.

NURSING CONSIDERATIONS

A major goal of nursing care is directed toward prevention of bleeding episodes. Initial discussion of the cause for bleeding must include establishment of the family's understanding of the disorder and assessment of their ability to care for the child at home. Precautions to decrease the risk of bleeding must be emphasized and is no easy task. Infants and toddlers with platelet disorders are at increased risk for falls, bruises, and minor cuts because of their primitive motor development. Their environment should be made as safe as possible by padding the crib; using cushions or upholstered chairs instead of hard metal or wood frames in the play area; purchasing toys that have no hard, sharp edges; and dressing the child in long sleeves and long-legged pants with padding at the elbow and knees to protect for falls. A helmet is frequently used to prevent head injury. Close supervision of play should exist at all times. The child in school should refrain from contact sports that could cause trauma and subsequent bleeding. Activities such as diving and motorcycle riding should be restricted, since they increase the chances of head injury. The school must be notified of these restrictions and asked to keep close supervision of the child while at school.

Local measures used to control bleeding should be taught to the child and parents. Bleeding from a wound or close to the skin should be managed with pressure to the area for at least 10 to 15 minutes to allow clot formation and then application of cold compresses to promote vasoconstriction.[32] Appropriate teaching can prevent excessive blood loss when trauma occurs.

Mucous membranes are common sites of bleeding when the platelet count falls below 20,000 mm³. Dental care remains essential, and the use of a water pik or sponge-tipped disposable toothpick should be recommended. Adolescents should be asked to refrain from using razors because of the difficulty they create in causing minor cuts. In addition, intramuscular injections, arterial punctures, enemas, rectal temperatures, nasogastric intubation, and suctioning should be avoided if possible.

One complication in children with a platelet disorder is cerebral hemorrhage. Parents should be instructed to take the child to the hospital immediately should head trauma occur. Children with a platelet disorder who experience headaches, blurred vision, diplopia, nausea and vomiting, or a decreased sensorium should be seen immediately by a physician. Cerebral hemorrhage is a life-threatening condition and should be pursued as such.

The child who is at increased risk for bleeding presents the nurse with a difficult dilemma. Pursuance of tasks essential for growth and development are essential and yet may produce increased risks for the child. The nurse must continue to be creative in identifying activities and providing guidance to the child and family in the day-to-day management of the disorder.

NURSING CARE PROTOCOL FOR THE CHILD WITH A PLATELET DISORDER

Nursing diagnosis (problems/needs)	Goal/objectives (patient/family will:)	Interventions (nurse will:)
1. Knowledge deficit (related to cause of bleeding)	Receive information related to underlying cause.	Provide information related to the cause of bleeding
	Verbally explain reason for increased risk of bleeding	Assist with explaining underlying etiology Give available information on the disorder.
2. Anxiety (emotional distress related to the disorder and its diagnostic evaluation)	Demonstrate decreased level of anxiety Share feelings with support persons	Encourage verbalization of fears and concerns Discuss specific tests and their importance in determining the cause of bleeding Refer to other services (chaplain, social worker)
3. Home maintenance management, impaired	Make environment as safe as possible	Assist the parents in making the environment as safe as possible: *Infant and toddler:* Pads on the crib, soft toys without edges, long-sleeved shirts and pants with pads in the knees and elbows: use of a helmet during play; close supervision during play; removal of furniture with hard, sharp edges; use of soft foods *Schoolage:* Restriction of contact sports; refrain from activities that would increase chance of cerebral hemorrhage (i.e., diving, motorcycle riding, ice skating or roller skating, horseback riding); pursuance of normal life-style in relation to these restrictions; use of toothettes and soft toothbrushes for oral care *Adolescent:* Continuation of restrictions for schoolage child with adolescent making individual decisions regarding activities and restrictions (allow for independence)
	Discuss appropriate limit-setting patterns to control behavior	Discuss with school verbally and in writing restrictions essential for the child Suggest use of Medic Alert identification in case of emergency

Continued.

NURSING CARE PROTOCOL FOR THE CHILD WITH A PLATELET DISORDER—cont'd

Nursing diagnosis (problems/needs)	Goal/objectives (patient/family will:)	Interventions (nurse will:)

4. Knowledge deficit (measures for local control of bleeding)	Implement measures at home to stop bleeding once it occurs	Review procedure for local control of bleeding:
		  Apply pressure to areas for 10-15 min
		  Immobilize area if possible
		  Apply cold compresses
		  When nose bleeding occurs, have patient sit up and lean forward while applying pressure to the nose for 10-15 min
		Instruct family to notify physician that bleeding has occurred

5. Injury potential for (bleeding)	Demonstrate awareness of severity of the disorder Be able to state appropriate situations where the child needs immediate medical attention Awareness of need for platelets to control bleeding	Teach importance of notifying health care team immediately when head trauma has occurred or change in sensorium, increased complaints of headaches, dizziness, or altered vision develops; gastrointestinal bleeding develops (tarry stools, hematemesis); local bleeding is not controlled by pressure or ice Administer platelets as ordered by physician (see Chapter 23 on blood products for nursing considerations in the administration of platelets)
6. Coping, ineffective family: compromised	Be able to cope with adjustments necessary for maximum functioning at home and at school Maintain positive self-concept	Provide emotional support; refer to other health care professionals as needed Encourage independence in spite of restrictions

REFERENCES

1. Miller, D.R., and others: Smith's blood diseases of infancy and childhood, St. Louis, 1978, The C.V. Mosby Co.
2. Nathan, D.G., and Oski, F.A.: Hematology of infancy and childhood, Philadelphia, 1981, W.B. Saunders Co.
3. Weiss, H.J.: Platelet physiology and abnormalties of platelet function, N. Engl. J. Med. **293**(11):531, 1975.
4. Lightsey, A.L.: Thrombocytopenia in children, Pediatr. Clin. North Am. **27**(2):293, 1980.
5. Lusher, J.M., and others: Idiopathic thrombocytopenic purpura in children, Am. J. Pediatr. Hematol. Oncol. **6**(2):149, 1984.
6. Dunn, N.L., and Maurer, H.M.: Prednisone treatment of acute idiopathic thrombocytopenic purpura of childhood, Am. J. Pediatr. Hematol. Oncol. **6**(2):159, 1984.
7. Lanzkowsky, P.: Pediatric hematology-oncology, New York, 1980, McGraw-Hill, Inc.
8. Sartornis, B.A.: Steroid treatment of idiopathic thrombocytopenic purpura in children, Am. J. Pediatr. Hematol. Oncol. **6**(2):165, 1984.
9. Imbach, P., and others: Intravenous immunoglobulin for idiopathic thrombocytopenic purpura (ITP) in childhood, Am. J. Pediatr. Hematol. Oncol. **6**(2):171, 1984.
10. Russell, E.C., and Maurer, H.M.: Alternatives to splenectomy in the management of chronic idiopathic thrombocytopenic purpura in childhood, Am. J. Pediatr. Hematol. Oncol. **6**(2):175, 1984.
11. Karpatkin, S., and Lackner, H.L.: Association of antiplatelet antibody with functional platelet disorders, Am. J. Med. **59**(5):599, 1975.
12. Brown, C.H., and others: The hemostatic defect produced by carbenicillin, N. Engl. J. Med. **291**(6):265, 1974.
13. Malpass, T.W., and Harker, L.A.: Acquired disorders of platelet function, Semin. Hematol. **17**(4):242, 1980.
14. Schichter, S.J., and Harker, L.A.: Thrombocytopenia: mechanisms and management of defects in platelet production, Clin. Haematol. **7**:523, 1978.
15. Stuart, M.J., and others: Platelet function in recipients of platelets from donors ingesting aspirin, N. Engl. J. Med. **287**(22):1105, 1972.
16. Weiss, H.J.: Platelet physiology and abnormalities of platelet function, N. Engl. J. Med. **293**(12):580, 1975.
17. Meischer, P.A.: Drug-induced thrombocytopenia, Semin. Hematol. **10**:311, 1973.
18. Harker, L.A., and Slighter, S.J.: Studies of platelet and fibrinogen kinetics in patients with prosthetic heart valves, N. Engl. J. Med. **283**(24):1302, 1970.
19. Brain, M.C.: The haemolytic-uremic syndrome, Semin. Hematol. **6**:162, 1969.
20. Aster, R.H.: Thrombocytopenia due to enhanced platelet destruction. In Williams, W.J., and others, editors: Hematology, New York, 1977, McGraw-Hill, Inc.
21. Schwartz, J.P., Rosenburg, A., and Cooperberg, A.A.: Thrombotic thrombocytopenic purpura: successful treatment of two cases, Can. Med. Assoc. J. **106**:1200, 1972.
22. Lian, E.C.-Y., and others: Presence of a platelet aggregating factor in the plasma of patients with thrombotic thrombocytopenic purpura and its inhibition by normal plasma, Blood **53**:33, 1979.
23. Ryan, P.F.J., Cooper, J.A., and Firkin, B.G.: Plasmapheresis in the treatment of thrombotic thrombocytopenic purpura, Med. J. Aust. **1**:69, 1979.
24. Corrigan, J.J.: Thrombocytopenia: a laboratory sign of septicemia in infants and children, J. Pediatr. **85**:219, 1974.
25. Kelton, J.G., and others: Elevated platelet-associated IgG in the thrombocytopenia of septicemia, N. Engl. J. Med. **300**(14):760, 1979.
26. Shim, W.K.T.: Hemangiomas of infancy complicated by thrombocytopenia, Am. J. Surg. **116**:896, 1968.
27. Parkman, R., and others: Complete correction of the Wiskott-Aldrich syndrome by allogenic bone marrow transplantation, N. Engl. J. Med. **298**:921, 1978.
28. George, J.N., and others: Bernard-Soulier disease: a study of four patients and their parents, Br. J. Haematol. **48**:459, 1975.
29. Stuart, M.: Inherited defects of platelet function, Semin. Hematol. **12**(3):233, 1975.
30. Lusher, J.M., and Barnhart, M.I.: Congenital disorders affecting platelets, Semin. Thromb. Hemost. **4**:123, 1977.
31. Baldini, M.G., and Myers, T.J.: One more variety of storage pool disease, JAMA **244**(2):173, 1980.
32. Whaley, L.F., and Wong, D.L.: Nursing care of infants and children, St. Louis, 1979, The C.V. Mosby Co.

PART III

TREATMENT MODALITIES

CHAPTER 20

Chemotherapy

NANCY FERGUSON NOYES

Research in cancer chemotherapy has brought forth complex and effective treatment protocols requiring highly skilled nursing intervention. The nurse must have an understanding of the actions and toxicities of chemotherapeutic agents to effectively manage the patient and restore optimum levels of function. This chapter focuses on the development, actions, toxicities, and administration of chemotherapeutic agents. Additionally, the role of the health professional in educating children and families about chemotherapy is discussed.

DEVELOPMENT OF CHEMOTHERAPEUTIC AGENTS

From available documentation, Hippocrates (460 to 375 BC) was the first to classify neoplastic diseases. Leonides of Alexandria (AD 180) was the first to develop the idea of surgically removing tumors.[1] Very little advancement in cancer therapy was seen until 1865, when Lissaeur first demonstrated the effect of potassium arsenite on leukemia and various malignancies.[2]

The modern age of cancer chemotherapy began during the 1940s when Huggins and Hodges reported that patients with prostatic cancer benefited from the administration of estrogens.[3] During the same decade, scientists at Yale University observed that nitrogen mustard gases used in chemical warfare during World War II caused severe myelosuppression and selectively damaged the lymphatic system and bone marrow.[4] Researchers then began to study nitrogen mustard's effect on malignancies and found that it drastically reduced tumor cell growth. By the 1950s, numerous other effective chemotherapeutic agents were discovered, including actinomycin D, cyclophosphamide, 5-fluorouracil, and the vinca alkaloids. Tumor and pharmacology research continued during the 1960s and 1970s, leading to the development of many more beneficial therapies. The principal historic developments in cancer chemotherapy are summarized in Table 20-1.[5,6]

CONCEPTS OF PROTOCOL DEVELOPMENT

Advances in cancer chemotherapy research led to clinical trials to test drug effectiveness. A clinical trial is an experiment designed to answer precise questions about a certain agent within a patient population.[7] Most clinical trials involve randomization of patients into different treatment modalities in an effort to prevent conscious or unconscious bias on the part of the investigator. Patients are stratified according to prognostic factors and then are randomized into treatment groups. This ensures an adequate balance of important prognostic variables among the treatment arms being compared. Thus no single agent or therapy is weighed toward a good or poor prognostic factor.

Chemotherapeutic agents are classified into three phases in clinical trials. Phase I involves the first administration of a new drug to humans.[1] The goals of this phase are to develop a maximum tolerated dose (MTD) on a given schedule and route of administration; to establish toxicity patterns and determine if they are reversible, tolerable, and predictable; and to determine the drug's effectiveness on specific tumors. Phase II involves an evaluation of the antitumor effects of specific drug therapy. The MTD is used to test the drug's effectiveness.

Table 20-1. Principle historic developments of cancer chemotherapy

Approximate date	Agent	Disease treated
1865	Potassium arsenite	Leukemia, various malignancies
1893	Cooley's toxins	Various malignancies
1941	Estrogens	Carcinoma of the prostate
	Androgens	Carcinoma of the breast
1945	Nitrogen mustard	Lymphoma and solid tumor
1948-1950	Adrenocorticosteroids and antifolates	Leukemia, lymphoma, multimyeloma, acute leukemia, and choriocarcinoma
1950-1955	6-Mercaptopurine	Acute leukemia
	Actinomycin D	Wilms' tumor, choriocarcinoma, testicular tumor
	Busulfan	Chronic granulocytic leukemia
1955-1960	Cyclophosphamide	Lymphoma and solid tumors
	Vinca alkaloids	Lymphoma, acute leukemia, reticuloendothelial malignancy of childhood and choriocarcinoma
	5-Fluorouracil	Carcinoma of the breast and GI tract
	Progestins	Endometrial carcinoma
	Mitotane	Adrenal carcinoma
1960-1965	Hydroxyurea	Chronic granulocytic leukemia
	Procarbazine	Hodgkin's disease
	Cytosine arabinoside	Acute leukemia
	Nitrosoureas	Lymphoma, brain tumor and solid tumors
	Daunorubicin	Acute leukemia
1965-1970	L-asparaginase	Acute leukemia
	cis-Platinum	Testicular and ovarian tumors
	DTIC	Melanoma
1970-Present	Doxorubicin	Sarcomas and a wide spectrum of other tumors
	Bleomycin	Lymphoma, head and neck cancer

From Haskell, C.M.: Cancer treatment, Philadelphia, 1980, W.B. Saunders Co.

Effectiveness is a measurable and reproducible decrease in tumor size over a certain time period. Phase III involves giving a drug to larger patient populations to confirm the effectiveness shown in phase II trials and to investigate unexpected toxicities and possible benefits in other malignancies.[7]

The use of treatment protocols has led to further treatment successes in the childhood cancers. Protocols are carefully designed modes of therapy for each specific type of tumor and are constructed by medical oncology experts. Each protocol is evaluated for safety and effectiveness in achieving long-term remissions or cures. National cooperative studies involving many institutions have led to substantial breakthroughs in treatment development and evaluation. In 1968 the limited success

of antineoplastic agents in the treatment of Wilms' tumor led to the formation of the National Wilms' Tumor Study. This cooperative study has resulted in increased knowledge and more effective treatment of Wilms' tumor. Since that time, many other national study groups have evolved, including Southwest Oncology Group (SWOG), Children's Cancer Study Group (CCSG), and the Pediatric Oncology Group (POG).

SINGLE AGENT VERSUS COMBINATION CHEMOTHERAPY

Historically, the potential for resistance to one form of chemotherapy has led to the development of drug combinations. Drug resistance develops as a result of altered metabolism of drugs, impermeability of the cell to active compounds, altered specificity to an inhibited enzyme, increased production of a target molecule, increased repair of cytotoxic lesions, and, in some cases, bypass of inhibited reactions by alternative biochemical pathways.[8] By administering multiple agents, many pathways in cellular biosynthesis are attacked, leading to more effective tumor inhibition and arrest.[7] Another aspect of combination chemotherapy is the sensitivity of a given tumor to certain agents. Specific agents that are individually active against a tumor are often combined to enhance effectiveness.[7] When many choices of agents exist within a class, selection is based on the type of dose-limiting toxicity likely to be produced by other agents employed in the combination.

The final aspect of chemotherapy development has involved the use of intermittent drug schedules to enable greater intensity in treatment. One theoretic advantage is that the drug combination exerts a selective killing effect on the tumor, and an interval between courses allows bone marrow and immunologic recovery.[9]

There are several criteria used in the selection of combination chemotherapy. Only those drugs shown to be effective as single agents against the tumor in question are included in a combination. Certain drugs that are ineffective against the tumor yet minimize dangerous toxicities to normal tissues are also included in combination therapies. These drugs are called ''rescue'' agents. Drugs included in the combination should have different modes of action to minimize the potential for drug resistance and should have different clinical toxicities.[8,10,11]

GENERAL OBJECTIVES OF CHEMOTHERAPY

The objective of chemotherapy can be cure or palliation. Cure is complete eradication of tumor, residual tumor, and metastatic disease. Palliation is partial eradication or temporary control of tumor with prolongation of life and symptomatic relief.[12]

Response to chemotherapy is measured in different ways. Bakowski classifies response of solid tumors to treatment as complete, partial, no re-

Table 20-2. Commonly used criteria for objective response and disease progression in solid tumors

Complete response	Complete disappearance of all demonstrable disease
Partial response	>50% reduction in the sum of the products of the longest perpendicular diameter of discrete measurable disease with no demonstrable disease progression elsewhere
No response	No change in the size of any measurable lesion or <50% reduction of measurable disease as shown above
Progression	>50% increase in the sum of the products of the largest perpendicular diameter of any measurable lesions

From Chemotherapy of cancer, by H. Bakowski. Copyright © 1977, Wiley Publishing Co. Reprinted by permission of John Wiley and Sons, Inc.

Table 20-3. Karnofsky's performance scale

Rating	Status
100	Normal activity
90	Minor symptoms with normal activity
80	Activity with some effort
70	Unable to do heavy work; does self-care
60	Requires assistance; can do self-care
50	Needs much assistance
40	Disabled; home care
30	Severely disabled; hospital care
20	Very ill
10	Moribund
0	Dead

From See-Lasley, K., and Ignoff, R.J.: Manual of oncology therapeutics, St. Louis, 1981, The C.V. Mosby Co.

sponse, and progression of disease as seen in Table 20-2.

The response of leukemia to treatment is often measured by the percentage of leukemic cells in the bone marrow and peripheral circulation. Karnofsky rates functional response according to the patient's ability to continue in activities of daily living as seen in Table 20-3.

Three factors that affect the response of malignancies to chemotherapy are the physiologic state of the patient, the cellular and biochemical characteristics of the tumor, and the pharmacokinetics of the chemotherapeutic agent.[13]

Physiologic state includes nutritional status, immunologic status, metabolic and excretory capabilities, presence or absence of infection or additional illness, and age. Infants are more susceptible to drug toxicities because of immaturity of body systems.[14] Chemotherapy doses are often reduced by one half to one fourth and gradually increased to tolerance. However, older children can often tolerate higher doses of drugs than adults.

The histopathology of the tumor and the extent of disease at diagnosis also affect the response to chemotherapy. Highly malignant, disseminated disease is more difficult to eradicate on the basis of tumor bulk alone. Certain tumors such as acute lymphocytic leukemia are very sensitive to chemotherapy, whereas others such as brainstem glioma and acute myelocytic leukemia are not. If a tumor is localized, often excision and/or radiation may be sufficient to eradicate the disease.[14]

Pharmacokinetics of chemotherapeutic agents involve how a drug is absorbed, metabolized, and biotransformed.[15-17] Because drug absorption varies at different sites, a variety of routes to administer cancer chemotherapy are used to optimize drug availability.[13] Oral, intramuscular, subcutaneous, intravenous, intrathecal, intra-arterial, and regional routes are currently used. The route selected delivers maximum concentrations of the drug over desired time intervals. Guidelines and precautions regarding each route are discussed later in this chapter. Many chemotherapeutic agents are inert until they are activated by the host's normal tissues or by tumor cells.[8] This process is called biotransformation. An example of biotransformation is cyclophosphamide, which becomes active against tumor cells after it is metabolized by the liver.[8]

DOSAGE AND SCHEDULING

The dosage and frequency of drug cycles depend on the patient's response to the therapy and the toxicities that occur. The optimum dosage is that which achieves a maximum cytotoxic effect with minimum toxic effects on normal cells.

The use of body surface area in place of body weight alone as the basis of dosage calculation of chemotherapy has been suggested.[18,19] However, in childhood cancers, both body surface area and body weight are used for various drugs. Fig. 20-1 demonstrates calculation of body surface area by use of the (M^2) nomogram.[20]

CLASSIFICATION AND ACTIONS OF CHEMOTHERAPY
Cell growth and differentiation

The life cycle of a proliferating cell from one mitosis to the next is divided into four phases: the mitotic phase (M), gap 1 (G_1), the DNA synthetic phase (S), and gap 2 (G_2) as shown in Fig. 20-2.[13] During the S phase, the cell grows by synthesizing proteins. During the M phase, the cell divides to make two cells. G_1 and G_2 are considered to be resting states of the cell. The main difference between normal cells and cancer cells is that tumor cells have fewer restraints on their growth.[13]

Anticancer drugs interfere with cellular growth in a variety of ways.[13,21,22] They can inhibit nucleic acid biosynthesis or alter the nucleic acid structure. They can inhibit protein synthesis or mitosis and can alter the general hormonal environment of the body. Several agents exert their influence during the S phase of the cell cycle. These are called "S-phase specific" drugs, and include cytosine arabinoside and hydroxyurea. Other agents such as 6-mercaptopurine, methotrexate, and 5-fluorouracil also inhibit DNA synthesis during the S phase. However, they may concurrently inhibit RNA and protein synthesis, thereby preventing the cells from entering the more sensitive S phase. These agents are termed "self-limited S-phase specific" agents. "Cycle nonspecific" drugs produce a direct effect on DNA; hence, their activities are not enhanced by administration during the S phase. "Cycle nonspecific" drugs include the alkylating agents, nitrosoureas, and most of the antibiotics. Fig. 20-3 demonstrates the mechanisms of action of the var-

Nomogram for determination of body surface area from height and weight:

A straightedge placed from the patient's height (left column) to his
weight (right column) will give his body surface area (middle column).†

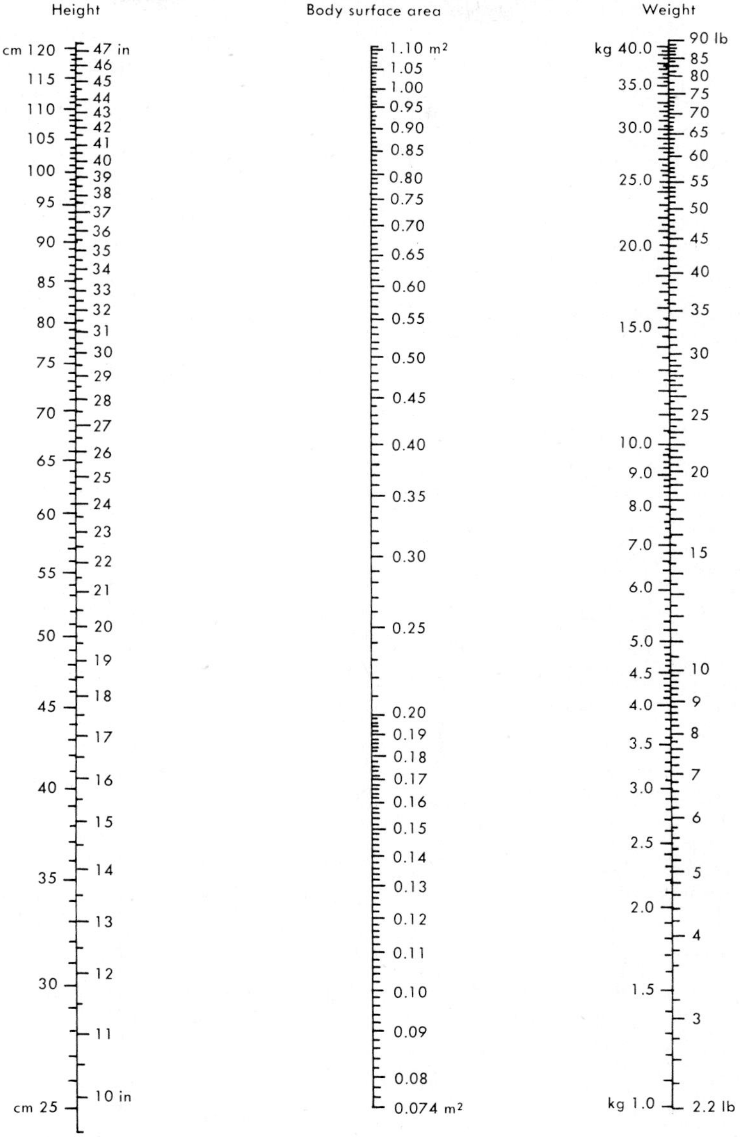

Height	Body surface area	Weight
cm 120 — 47 in	1.10 m²	kg 40.0 — 90 lb
46	1.05	85
115 — 45	1.00	35.0 — 80
44		75
110 — 43	0.95	70
42	0.90	30.0 — 65
105 — 41	0.85	60
40		
100 — 39	0.80	25.0 — 55
38	0.75	50
95 — 37	0.70	
36		45
90 — 35	0.65	20.0
34	0.60	40
85 — 33		
32	0.55	35
80 — 31		15.0
30	0.50	30
75 — 29		
28	0.45	
70 — 27		25
26	0.40	10.0
65 — 25		9.0 — 20
24	0.35	8.0
60 — 23		7.0 — 15
22	0.30	6.0
55 — 21		
50 — 20	0.25	5.0
19		4.5 — 10
45 — 18		4.0 — 9
17	0.20	3.5 — 8
	0.19	
	0.18	3.0 — 7
40 — 16	0.17	
	0.16	6
15	0.15	2.5
	0.14	
35 — 14	0.13	5
13	0.12	2.0
	0.11	4
30 — 12	0.10	1.5
11	0.09	3
	0.08	
cm 25 — 10 in	0.074 m²	kg 1.0 — 2.2 lb

*From Documenta Geigy scientific tables, ed. 7, courtesy CIBA-Geigy Limited, Basle, Switzerland.
†From the formula of Du Bois and Du Bois, Arch. Intern. Med. 17:863, 1916. $S = W^{0.425} \times H^{0.725} \times 71.84$, or log S = log $W \times 0.425$ + log $H \times 0.725$ + 1.8564 (S = body surface in cm², W = weight in kg, H = height in cm)

Fig. 20-1. Body surface area of children. (From See-Lasley, K., and Ignoffo, R.J.: Manual of oncology therapeutics, St. Louis, 1980, The C.V. Mosby Co.)

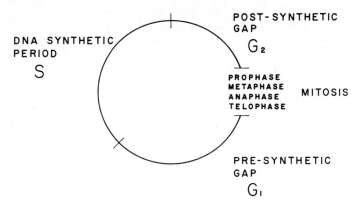

Fig. 20-2. The cell cycle. (From Sutow, W.W., Fernbach, D., and Vietti, T.: Clinical pediatric oncology, St. Louis, 1984, The C.V. Mosby Co.)

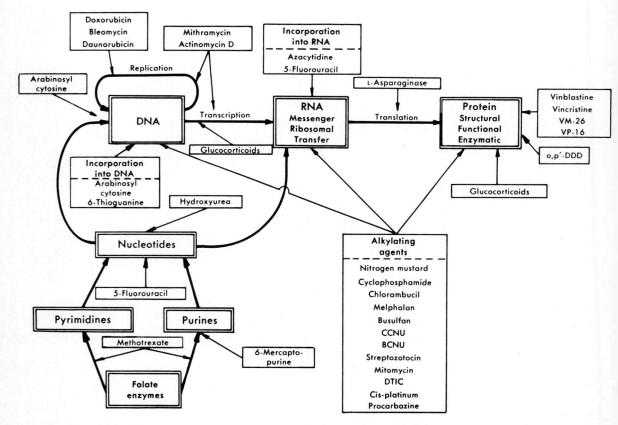

Fig. 20-3. Sites of action of antineoplastic agents. (From Sutow, W.W., Fernbach, D., and Vietti, T.: Clinical pediatric oncology, St. Louis, 1984, The C.V. Mosby Co.)

ious drugs. Table 20-4 (pp. 316-319) lists specific information (strength, storage, route of administration, major uses, and special considerations) for each antineoplastic agent.

Classification of agents

Alkylating agents cause breaks in the DNA molecule and the cross-linking of its twin strands, thus interfering with DNA replication and transcription of RNA. Subsequent protein synthesis is disrupted, resulting in death of the cell.[13] As a class, alkylating agents are considered cell cycle phase nonspecific.[23,24] Alkylating agents include nitrogen mustard derivatives, cyclophosphamide, chlorambucil, melphalan, busulfan, dacarbazine, and nitrosoureas.

Antibiotics are natural products of the soil fungus *Streptomyces*. They bind with the DNA molecule and block RNA production.[25,26] They are cell cycle phase nonspecific.[23] Agents in this class include actinomycin D, doxorubicin, daunomycin, bleomycin sulfate, mithramycin, and mitomycin C.[8]

Antimetabolites are structurally similar to normal metabolites of the cell and act as substrates for the enzyme of the metabolites they resemble. They bind to the enzyme, decrease its activity, and undergo conversion to products that become nonfunctioning macromolecules.[8] Antimetabolites are subdivided into nucleoside analogues (cytarabine, Cytosar, arabinosylcytosine), purine analogues (thioguanine, 6-mercaptopurine), and folic acid antagonists (methotrexate).[8] Except for 5-fluorouracil, these drugs are cell cycle specific.[23]

Corticosteroids enter the cell passively and bind to macromolecules in the cytoplasm. After entering the molecules, the steroids bind with DNA and modify the transcription process.[13] Drugs in this class include prednisone, hydrocortisone, prednisolone, and dexamethasone.[13] If a corticosteroid is given to a patient for more than 14 days, it must be tapered slowly. Oral corticosteroids suppress endogenous adrenal steroid production. If exogenous steroids are withdrawn too quickly, the adrenals do not have enough time to produce adequate quantities of corticosteroids on their own. Thus the slightest insult to a body (i.e., illness, injury) can lead to profound shock.

Vinca alkaloids bind to microtubular proteins within cells, causing mitotic arrest.[27] In large concentrations, these drugs can also eradicate nonproliferating cells and exert complex effects on RNA and protein synthesis.[28] They are cell cycle phase specific.[8,23,27] Drugs in this class include vincristine (Oncovin) and vinblastine (Velban).[23]

Miscellaneous drugs include procarbazine (Matulane), hydroxyurea, mitotane, L-asparaginase, and platinum complexes.[8] A classification of the various chemotherapeutic agents is as follows*:

Alkylating agents
Busulfan	Melphalan
Chlorambucil	Uracil mustard
Cyclophosphamide	Thio-TEPA
Mechlorethamine	Hexamethylmelamine
	Triethylenemelamine

Antimetabolites
Cytosine arabinoside	6-Mercaptopurine
5-Fluorouracil	Methotrexate
5-Fluoro-2'-deoxyuridine	6-Thioguanine

Antibiotics
Adriamycin	Daunorubicin
Bleomycin	Mithramycin
Actinomycin D	Mitomycin C

Steroid hormones
Androgens	Progestational steroids
Estrogens	Adrenal steroids
Antiestrogens	

Metaphase inhibitors
Vinblastine	VM-26
Vincristine	VP-16

Miscellaneous
L-Asparaginase	Nitrosoureas (BCNU, CCNU, methyl-CCNU)
o,p'DDD (mitotane)	Procarbazine
Hydroxyurea	*cis*-Platinum diamine dichloride
	DTIC

*From Horton, J., and Hill, G.: Clinical oncology, Philadelphia, 1977, W.B. Saunders Co.

Table 20-4. Antineoplastic agents

Agent	Strength and storage	Stability	Route of administration	Major uses	Special considerations
Actinomycin D (Dactinomycin, Cosmegen)	0.5-mg vials; room temperature	Discard unused portion; light sensitive	IV; avoid extravasation	Ewing's sarcoma; osteogenic sarcoma; testicular cancer (CA); rhabdomyosarcoma; Wilms' tumor	Impaired excretion with hepatic damage; do not use diluent preservative
Arabinosylcytosine (cytosine arabinoside, Ara-C, Cytosar, cytarabine)	100- and 500-mg vials; refrigerate	Stable 12 hr	IV; IM; SQ; IC; IT	Acute granulocytic and lymphocytic leukemia	Infuse slowly to avoid nausea and vomiting
Asparaginase (Elspar)	10,000-U vial; refrigerate	Stable 48 hr at 4° C	IV; IM	Acute lymphocytic leukemia (ALL)	Anaphylaxis may be very abrupt; be prepared to handle
5-Azacytidine (5-Aza-C)	100-mg vial; refrigerate	Stable 8 hr	IV	Acute granulocytic leukemia	Do not reconstitute in 5% G/W; infuse slowly
BCNU (bis-chloroethyl-nitrosourea); (carmustine)	100-mg vial-refrigerate	Discard unused portion	IV; avoid extravasation	Brain tumor; colorectal CA; gastric adenocarcinoma; hepatoma; Hodgkin's disease; non-Hodgkin's lymphoma (NHL)	Infuse slowly to prevent hypotension; delayed and sustained myelosuppression
Bleomycin (Blenoxane)	15-U vial; room temperature	Stable 28 days at 4° C	IV; IM; SQ; IC	Hodgkin's disease; NHL; testicular carcinoma	Observe for hypotension; may cause pulmonary fibrosis, pyrexia
Busulfan (Myleran)	2-mg tablet; room temperature	Stable	Oral	Chronic granulocytic leukemia	May cause pulmonary fibrosis
CCNU (chloroethylmethyloy-clohexyl-nitrosourea) (lomustine)	10-, 40-, 100-mg capsules; refrigerate; avoid moisture	Stable	Oral on empty stomach	Brain tumor; colorectal CA; Hodgkin's disease	Delayed and sustained myelosuppression
Chlorambucil (Leukeran)	2-mg tablets; room temperature	Stable	Oral	Chronic lymphocytic leukemia; Hodgkin's disease; non-Hodgkin's	Cumulative myelosuppression

amine dichloride)	powder; refrigerate	used portion; light sensitive	travasation	lar CA	mulative renal impairment
Cyclophosphamide (Cytoxan, Endoxan)	100-, 200-, and 500-mg vials; room temperature	Stable 24 hr at 4°C	IV; oral	ALL; NHL; ovarian CA; rhabdomyosarcoma; chronic lymphocytic leukemia; Ewing's sarcoma; Hodgkin's disease; neuroblastoma	Keep patient well hydrated for 12-24 hr after administration
Daunorubicin (Daunomycin, Rubidomycin)	20-mg vials; orange crystals; room temperature	Avoid extravasation; light sensitive	IV	ALL; acute granulocytic leukemia; neuroblastoma	Cumulative cardiomyopathy Do not exceed 550 mg/m^2 total dose, less with cardiac irradiation; impaired excretion with hepatic damage
Dimethyl-triazenoimidazolecarboxamide (DTIC, DIC, dacarbazine)	100- and 200-mg vials; white powder; refrigerate	Stable 72 hr at 4°C; light sensitive	IV; avoid extravasation	Hodgkins disease; neuroblastoma; general sarcoma	
Doxorubicin (Adriamycin, Adria)	10- and 50-mg vials; red-orange crystals; room temperature	Stable 48 hr at 4°C; light sensitive	IV; avoid extravasation	Wilms' tumor; acute granulocytic leukemia; osteogenic sarcoma; rhabdomyosarcoma; general sarcoma; thyroid, testicular CA; Ewing's sarcoma; hepatoma; Hodgkin's disease; NHL; neuroblastoma	Cumulative cardiomyopathy; do not exceed 550 mg/m^2 total dose, less with cardiac irradiation; impaired excretion with hepatic damage
5-Fluorouracil (fluorouracil, 5-FU)	500 mg/10 ml ampule; clear liquid; room temperature; protect from light	Discard unused portion	IV; IC; oral; avoid extravasation	Breast CA; colorectal CA	Impaired excretion with hepatic damage
Hydroxyurea (Hydrea)	500-mg capsules; 2-gm vial; white powder; room temperature	Stable 48 hr at 4°C	Oral; IV	Chronic granulocytic leukemia	Impaired excretion with renal damage

Adapted from Sutow, W.W., Fernbach, D., and Vietti, T.: Clinical pediatric oncology, St. Louis, 1984, The C.V. Mosby Co.

Continued.

Table 20-4. Antineoplastic agents—cont'd

Agent	Strength and storage	Stability	Route of administration	Major uses	Special considerations
Melphalan (L-phenylalanine mustard; L-PAM, Alkeran; L-sarcolysin)	2-mg tablets; 100-mg vials; white powder; room temperature	Stable 1 hr at 4° C	Oral; IV; avoid extravasation	Ovarian CA; testicular CA; seminoma	Myelosuppression
6-Mercaptopurine (Purinethol, 6-MP)	50-mg tablets; 500-mg vial; white powder; room temperature	Discard unused portion	Oral; IV	Acute granulocytic leukemia; ALL; chronic granulocytic leukemia	Reduce dose to one fourth if patient receiving allopurinol
Methotrexate (amethopterin, MTX)	2.5-mg tablets; 5-, 50-, 500-mg and 10-m vial; yellow powder or liquid; room temperature	Stable; light sensitive	Oral; IV; IM; IT; IC	ALL; medulloblastoma, osteogenic sarcoma; rhabdomyosarcoma; testicular CA	Impaired excretion with renal damage; with huge doses, hydrate and alkalinize urine
Methyl CCNU (Semustine)	2.5-mg vial; yellow powder	Stable at 4° C; use immediately	IV; avoid extravasation	Brain tumor; colorectal CA; gastric adeno CA; pancreatic adeno CA	
Mithramycin (Mithracin)	10-, 50-, and 100-mg vials	Stable at 4° C; avoid moisture	Oral on empty stomach	Testicular CA	Prolonged and sustained myelosuppression
Mitomycin C (Mutamycin)	5-mg vial; gray-purple powder; room temperature	Stable 14 days at 4° C	IV; avoid extravasation	Colorectal adeno CA; gastric adeno CA; pancreatic adeno CA	
Nitrogen mustard (Mustargen; HN2; mechloro-	10-mg vial; white powder; room temperature	Use immediately	IV; IC; avoid extravasation	Hodgkin's disease; non-Hodgkin's lymphoma	Avoid contact with skin and eyes

Drug	Supply/Storage	Stability	Administration	Uses	Special considerations
(o,p'-DDD): (Mitotane, Lysodren)	room temperature				trauma; caution with liver disease
Procarbazine (Matulane)	50-mg capsules; room temperature	Stable	Oral	Brain tumor; NHL; lymphoma; Hodgkin's disease	Do not use with phenytoin (Dilantin) or MAO inhibitors
Streptozotocin	20-m vial; white powder; room temperature	Stable	IV	Hodgkin's disease; islet cell CA; malignant carcinoid	Caution with renal disease
6-Thioguanine (6-TG)	50-mg tablets; 75-mg vial; white powder; room temperature	Discard after 24 hr	Oral; IV	ALL; acute granulocytic leukemia	
Vinblastine (Velban, VBL)	10-mg vial; white powder; refrigerate	Stable 30 days at 4°C	IV; avoid extravasation	Hodgkin's disease; nonHodgkin's lymphoma; testicular CA	Neuropathies
Vincristine (Oncovin, VCR)	1- and 5-mg vials; white powder; refrigerate	Stable 14 days at 4°C	IV; avoid extravasation	ALL; Ewing's sarcoma; Hodgkin's disease; neuroblastoma; NHL; rhabdomyosarcoma; Wilms' tumor	Neuropathies
VM-26 (4'-1 demethyl-epidopophyllotoxin B-D-thenylidene glucoside)	100-mg vial		IV infusion over 45 min; avoid extravasation	Brain tumor; NHL; Hodgkin's disease	Caution with liver disease
VP-16 (4'demethyl-epidopophyllotoxin-B-D-thylidene glucoside)	10-mg vial		IV infusion over 15-60 min; unstable in dextrose	Acute granulocytic leukemia	

PRINCIPLES AND GUIDELINES FOR USE OF CHEMOTHERAPY

The decision to use chemotherapy as a treatment modality is based on many factors. First, chemotherapy is used only after a diagnosis of malignancy has been well established histologically. In some cases such as brainstem tumors, histologic diagnosis may be impossible to obtain, and diagnosis is based on clinical findings and computed tomography scans. Second, chemotherapy should be used only if there are adequate facilities to monitor the potential toxicities of the agent. Third, objective evidence of the tumor must be followed to assess its response to the drug.

After an appropriate need for chemotherapy is established, it is important to follow specific guidelines for the administration of such therapy. Intravenous infusion sites should be chosen carefully. Generally, the forearm is the preferred site of chemotherapy administration, yet conflicting views do exist. The dorsum of the hand is preferred over the wrist, and both are preferred over the antecubital fossa. The forearm and wrist are painful and technically difficult sites. Many clinicians prefer the dorsum of the hand because of easy and early visualization of possible infiltration. The antecubital fossa is a very difficult site to determine infiltration and is used only if other sites cannot be found. A butterfly needle or angiocath is used for giving chemotherapy. *cis*-Platinum breaks down aluminum, and angiocaths should be used in giving this agent. After insertion, the needle is taped down distally to allow visualization of the infusion site. Normal saline (5 cc) is injected into the vein to determine its patency before the drug is given. A small amount of blood can be withdrawn to check for the vein's integrity and flow. The IV tubing is flushed with 3 to 5 cc of normal saline between drugs if more than one agent is given. If extravasation with normal saline occurs, another site on a different extremity or proximal to the extravasated site is selected. Infusing in a distal point on the same vein can cause serious extravasation downstream. Blood is aspirated after every 1 to 2 ml of solution administered to ensure adequate needle

position in the vein. The injection site is checked for redness, pain, and swelling. The drug injection is followed with 0.5 to 1 ml of normal saline to flush the tubing and needle of all the drug.

When multiple drugs are given, the nonvesicant agents are usually injected first. If all the drugs are vesicants, the one with the least amount of diluent is injected first. Although many clinicians feel that injecting the nonvesicant drug first is best in the event of an immediate infiltration, others feel that it is best to administer the vesicant therapy before the vein's integrity is compromised. With multiple subcutaneous or intramuscular injections, alternate injection sites are used. A combination of cold compresses followed by heat is recommended to enhance drug absorption.

Precautions in preparation and handling of chemotherapeutic agents

Much concern has arisen over the potential hazard to the health professionals chronically exposed to chemotherapeutic agents. Because of this concern, research is being conducted to look at long-

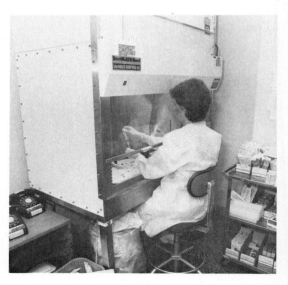

Fig. 20-4. Proper use of a vertical laminar flow hood for mixing chemotherapy.

term risk from chronic exposure to chemotherapy. Protective eyewear, masks, gloves, and gowns may or may not be helpful for preventing exposure while mixing chemotherapeutic agents.[29] A vertical laminar air flow hood is used when available as seen in Fig. 20-4. When a hood is not available, an area isolated from people and food is recommended.

Disposal of materials

Proper disposal of syringes, vials, needles, IV bags, tubing, and other materials used for chemotherapy is essential. Vials and ampules should be disposed of in specifically designated waste cans for chemotherapeutic agents. Needles used to mix and administer therapy should be dispensed in special needle containers. IV bags, tubing, and empty vials or ampules of chemotherapeutic agents should not be discarded into regular waste containers. Remaining agents not used should be sent to the pharmacy for proper disposal. When drawing up drug dosages into syringes, any excess drug should be eliminated into properly labeled waste areas and not into the sink or waste can.

Precautions with vesicant therapy

Many vesicant agents, including vincristine (Oncovin), nitrogen mustard, and doxorubicin (Adriamycin), pose significant clinical problems with extravasation into subcutaneous tissue. Extravasation leads to pain and induration at the IV site, swelling of the affected extremity, tissue necrosis, functional impairment, full thickness skin loss, and damage to underlying tendons and neurovascular structures as seen in Fig. 20-5.[30-34] Prevention is ideal, yet even under the best of circumstances, tissue extravasation can occur. Unfortunately, most labels that accompany commercially available chemotherapeutic agents warn of the damages of extravasation but fail to recommend management. Research is currently being done to determine the best technique for management of extravasation, since there is a lack of agreement in the literature regarding optimum management. Cohen[35] reports that, empirically, intravenous hydrocortisone or local ice applications have been used to treat extrav-

asations. There is no evidence, however, that either treatment is particularly beneficial.[35]

Basic guidelines should be followed when administering vesicant agents. Joints with underlying tendons and areas of extensive soft tissue and neurovascular bundles should be avoided.[34,36,37] The vein should be large enough to handle IV fluid administration, and the medication should be injected "piggyback" through a Y-site injection over 2 to 5 minutes.[30,31,34,37] The longer an agent takes to infuse, the greater the chances of extravasation. This is especially true in a highly anxious and combative child who must be restrained for administration of chemotherapy. Close supervision should be provided during the drug administration to recognize infiltrations promptly. If extravasation oc-

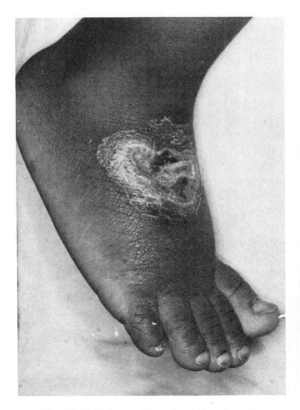

Fig. 20-5. Extravasation of a vesicant agent.

curs, the IV should be discontinued immediately, and the appropriate physician should be notified. Depending on institution policy, hydrocortisone may be administered intravenously before discontinuing the IV, and ice may be applied for 24 hours after the extravasation occurs. The area is observed for increased pain, swelling, and redness, and the patient is observed for fever. The extravasation site is cleaned daily with soap, water, and hydrogen peroxide. In many institutions, a surgeon is commited to evaluate an infiltration site. Op-site dressing may be applied to the area to prevent infection and tendon injury. Erythematous streaking along the route of the vein can occur during doxorubicin injections and does not necessarily indicate drug infiltration. However, if in doubt, the IV should be discontinued and restarted at another site.

Indwelling catheters

Many pediatric patients are on prolonged treatment protocols that require repeated venipunctures for drug therapy, administration of blood products and fluids, periodic blood studies, nutritional support, or antibiotics. Several methods of long-term venous access are available, including the Hickman, Broviac, Medicina, Evermed, and Infusaid indwelling catheters, as well as arteriovenous (AV) fistulaes[38-44] (Fig. 20-6). The large-bore Hickman catheter has been shown to be well suited for venous access and is superior to AV fistulaes as a means of repeated entry into the vascular system.[39] Insertion of indwelling catheters and AV fistulaes is usually done under general anesthesia in the operating room. In certain situations, insertion of a Broviac catheter may be done under local anesthesia in older children.[39] (See Fig. 20-7 for proper placement of a Broviac catheter.)

Complications of indwelling catheters include infection, bleeding, thrombus formation, and damage to the catheter itself. Standard guidelines to determine when removal of the catheter is necessary include[43,45,46] (1) phlebitis which does not improve with warm soaks within 48 hours, (2) catheter occlusion, (3) documented bacteremia not re-

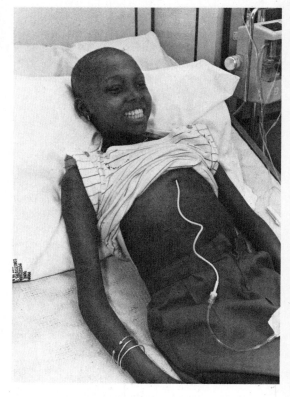

Fig. 20-6. Broviac catheter used as a means for long-term venous access.

sponding to antibiotic therapy in 72 hours, (4) documented fungemia, and (5) persistent fever of unidentified cause in neutropenic patients after an empiric trial of antibiotic therapy. The success of catheter use is dependent on careful and consistent care of the catheter after insertion.

Regional chemotherapy

Regional chemotherapy has been used in localized carcinomas and sarcomas. Regional chemotherapy is the infusion, perfusion, or injection of chemotherapeutic agents into a limited anatomic area to obtain higher drug concentrations and thus a greater biologic effect.[28] Improved response rates

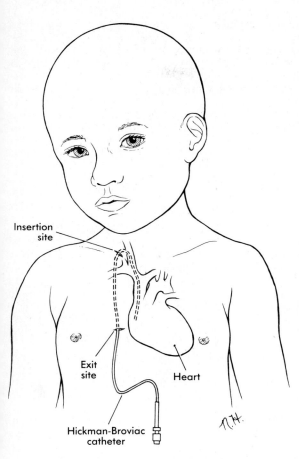

Insertion site

Exit site

Heart

Hickman-Broviac catheter

Fig. 20-7. Hickman/Broviac catheter placement.

can occur with direct infusion of the agent into the appropriate artery such as with intra-arterial chemotherapy for osteosarcoma.[47] However, these responses are not dramatic and have limited application to pediatric tumor management.

MANAGEMENT OF SIDE EFFECTS

Cells differ greatly in their growth rates and susceptibility to environmental changes. They also differ in their susceptibility to chemotherapy. In general, the most rapidly growing cells are most susceptible to the effects of chemotherapy. Normal bone marrow, hair follicles, and intestinal epithe-lium, which multiply rapidly, are the cells most sensitive to growth inhibition by chemotherapeutic agents. Tumors have different rates of growth, and their reponsiveness often correlates with growth rate. To obtain a therapeutic response, the physician must often prescribe doses of chemotherapy that produce systemic toxicity. It is hoped that the damaged tumor cells recover more slowly than the affected normal tissue. Specific nursing management of toxicities caused by chemotherapeutic agents is shown in Table 20-5.

Nausea and vomiting

Nausea and vomiting occur as frequently when drugs are given intravenously as when they are given orally. Thus these effects occur as a result of the chemotherapeutic agent's effect on particular areas of the brain. See Table 20-6 for the emetic potential of various chemotherapeutic agents.

There are several antiemetics currently used for the control of nausea and vomiting, with the most widely used group being the phenothiazines as shown in Table 20-7. Phenothiazines are psychotropic drugs that have sedative and antiemetic effects. Common adverse reactions include extreme drowsiness and extrapyramidal effects closely resembling parkinsonism. Acute extrapyramidal reactions can be treated with intravenous Benadryl. To ensure constant therapeutic blood levels of an antiemetic, doses should be started before the nausea begins and repeated at intervals according to specific drug instructions.

Psychogenic vomiting can occur when a child is anxious about therapy and begins to vomit or gag when he thinks about, sees, or smells the drug. It is important to identify the child's anxieties and use stress reduction techniques to help the child adapt to such treatments.

A patient with severe nausea and vomiting is observed for signs of dehydration, including sunken eyes, decreased skin turgor, and dryness of the mouth. Fluids are replaced intravenously if necessary, and antiemetics are continued to decrease vomiting.

Table 20-5. Nursing management of antineoplastic drug toxicities

Actinomycin	Nausea and vomiting may occur, requiring an emetic on a regular basis. Good oral hygiene is necessary. Mouth ulcers are common. Monitor enzymes and hematologic changes. Avoid extravasation.
Arabinosylcytosine	Be careful to not confuse this drug with Cytoxan. May need to premedicate with an antiemetic. Good oral hygiene is necessary. Monitor hematologic changes.
Asparaginase	With initial dose, may give 1 to 2 units intradermally as a test dose for potential anaphylaxis. Epinephrine and hydrocortisone should be at the bedside with each injection, along with an airway. Alternate sites for IM injection on a regular basis. Check serum amylase and prothrombin time/partial thromboplastin time (PT/PTT), and repeat through course. Check for symptoms of pancreatitis.
5-Azacytidine	Infuse slowly. Monitor hematologic changes.
BCNU	Infuse slowly in proper diluent over 1 hour to minimize the pain of injection. Apply ice to infusion site if necessary. May need to premedicate with an antiemetic. Monitor hematologic changes.
Bleomycin sulfate	With initial dose, give 1 to 2 units subcutaneously to test for potential anaphylaxis. Have airway, epinephrine, and hydrocortisone at bedside for initial does. *Document cumulative dosage.* Antipyretic and antihistamine help to decrease fever and chills. Do not exceed *top dose of agent.* Perform pulmonary function studies before and during treatment.
Busulfan	Instruct patient not to chew tablets. Carefully note for any cough, shortness of breath, or tachycardia before administering. Monitor hematologic changes.
CCNU	May need an antiemetic with therapy. Continue if nausea and vomiting persist. Monitor hematologic effects.
Chlorambucil	Instruct patient not to chew tablets. Monitor hematologic effects.
cis-Platinum	Before administration, check all renal studies for normalcy. Prehydrate the patient as per protocol. Strict I & O. Premedicate with an antiemetic and continue on a routine basis. Check for signs of ototoxicity such as ringing in the ears or dizziness. Monitor hematologic changes. May need to administer Lasix and/or mannitol for decreased urine output.
Cyclophosphamide	Instruct patient not to chew tablets. Strict I & O should be monitored with decreased urine output. IV fluids may be necessary. With high doses, hydrate patient before and 12 to 24 hours after administration of drug as per protocol. Report any hematuria and pain. Monitor hematologic changes.
Daunorubicin	Before initiation of therapy, do a baseline electrocardiogram (ECG) and echocardiogram. Monitor serum chemistries and hematologic studies. Monitor liver enzymes regularly. Maintain good oral hygiene. Administer an antiemetic as necessary. Do not exceed top dose of medication. Avoid extravasation.
DTIC	Premedicate with antiemetic and continue if necessary on a regular basis. Infuse according to protocol. Monitor hematologic changes.
Doxorubicin	Avoid extravasation of drug. Premedicate patient with antiemetic and continue on a regular basis if necessary. Instruct patient that urine may turn red with drug excretion. Do not exceed *cumulative dosage.* Do a baseline ECG and echocardiogram before each administration of the drug. Good oral hygine is necessary. Monitor hematologic and serum chemistries regularly, especially liver enzymes.
5-Fluorouracil	Instruct patient that veins may become discolored with injection. Maintain good oral hygiene. Monitor hematologic changes.

Table 20-5. Nursing management of antineoplastic drug toxicities—cont'd

Hydroxyurea	Monitor hematologic changes.
Melphalan	Instruct patient not to chew tables. Monitor hematologic changes.
6-MP	Reduce dosage if patient is also receiving allopurinol. Monitor for hematologic changes.
Methotrexate	Monitor renal function, serum chemistries, and hematologic studies before administration of each treatment. Good oral hygiene should be maintained. With increased dosages of methotrexate, it is essential to give Leucovorin factor on time as ordered by the protocol of treatment. Strict I & O. With decreased urine output, hydrate and alkalinize the patient before and after treatment according to treatment protocol. Administer an antiemetic as needed.
Methyl CCNU	Do not mistake this drug for CCNU. Give antiemetics before therapy and continue if necessary. Monitor hematologic changes.
Mithramycin	Premedicate with antiemetics and give regularly if needed. Monitor hematologic changes. Avoid extravasation.
Mitomycin C	Premedicate with antiemetics and give regularly if needed. Monitor hematologic changes. Maintain good oral hygiene. Avoid extravasation.
Nitrogen mustard	Warn patient that vein discoloration may occur. Monitor hematologic changes and serum chemistries before administration. Premedicate with an antiemetic and continue on a regular basis. Emesis soon after administration is often seen.
Ortho, para-DDD	Monitor liver enzymes before administration of drug. Monitor for hematologic changes. In the event of severe shock or trauma, steroids may be needed. Because of CNS problems, warn patient against doing tasks that require mental alertness. Monitor behavior and neurologic status.
Procarbazine	Monitor hematologic changes. Instruct patient to swallow capsule whole. Instruct patient to avoid the following foods and drink: alcohol, ripe cheese, bananas, and yeast products. Avoid using concurrently with tricyclic antidepressants and sympathomimetic drugs. Use with caution with barbiturates, narcotics, and antihistamines. Give antiemetics as needed.
Streptozotocin	Premedicate with an antiemetic and continue as needed. Monitor renal functioning and hematologic changes. Monitor blood urea nitrogen (BUN), and weekly creatinine.
6-TG	Maintain good oral hygiene. Monitor liver enzymes carefully.
Vinblastine	Avoid extravasation. Instruct patient to report numbness, tingling, and pain in extremities. Give stool softeners with chronic constipation.
Vincristine	Avoid extravasation. Instruct patient to report numbness, tingling, and pain in extremities. May need to give stool softeners with chronic constipation.
VM-26	Monitor hematologic changes. Give antiemetics as needed. Monitor for allergic reaction and hypotension.
VP-16	Monitor hematologic changes. Give antiemetics as needed. Monitor for allergic reaction and hypotension.

Table 20-6. Emetic potential of antineoplastic drugs

Severe >75% chance for nausea and vomiting	Moderate 25%-75% chance for nausea and vomiting	Mild to none <25% chance for nausea and vomiting
Azacytidine (rapid injection)	Azacytidine (slow infusion)	Bleomycin
Carmustine	Cytarabine	Busulfan
Cyclophosphamide	Etopside	Chlorambucil
(high dose parenteral)	Hexamethylmelamine	Fluorouracil
Dacarbazine	Mitotane	Hydroxyurea
Dactinomycin	Procarbazine	L-Asparaginase
Daunorubicin	Razoxane	Melphalan
Doxorubicin	Teniposide	Mercaptopurine
Lomustine	Thiotepa	Methotrexate
Mechlorethamine	Vinblastine	Mitomycin C
Mithramycin		Thioguanine
Semustine		Vincristine
Streptozotocin		

From See-Lasley, K., and Ignoffo, R.J.: Manual of onocology therapeutics, St. Louis, 1981, The C.V. Mosby Co.

Essential nursing considerations for appropriate use of antiemetic therapy involve the following:

1. It is more effective to use antiemetics to prevent nausea and vomiting than to treat it after it has begun.
2. Patterns of sickness should be determined. Onset and duration of nausea and vomiting should be documented. Most cancer chemotherapy agents do not produce sickness longer than 48 hours.
3. Antiemetic therapy should be started before the anticipated nausea and vomiting at a time interval in which the clinician is certain a therapeutic blood level of the antiemetic will be present when vomiting is anticipated. The best time of administration may not be immediately before the injection of chemotherapy agents or other forms of therapy.
4. To ensure constant therapeutic blood levels of an antiemetic in patients, dosage times of administration should be written on a sheet of paper or patient medication calendar to encourage patient compliance.
5. Antiemetic therapy should be given throughout the entire anticipated duration of nausea and vomiting, then discontinued.
6. Antiemetics given on a p.r.n. basis should be avoided.

Anorexia and weight loss

The ability of patients to maintain adequate caloric intake while receiving chemotherapy is compromised by food aversions, changes in taste acuity, emetic-inducing properties of chemotherapy agents, and the psychologic and metabolic effects of the disease. Children can develop aversions to familiar and preferred foods when receiving gastrointestinal toxic therapy. The tumor itself can generate anorexia, although the mechanism is not well understood. Depression may also be a factor in the development of anorexia and weight loss. Malnutrition can result from anorexia, nausea, and vomiting.

At diagnosis, the child should undergo a full nutritional assessment, including weight, height, anthropometric measurements, and complete dietary history. Weight should be monitored closely during chemotherapy treatments. Oral caloric supplements can be offered if the patient is unable to eat solid foods. The dietician may offer suggestions of more palatable foods and smaller, more nutritious meals. Progressive weight loss may neces-

Table 20-7. Commonly used antiemetics for nausea and vomiting

Name	Dosage	Route	How Supplied	Precautions
Phenergan (Promethazine)	0.5mg-1mg/kg	PO,PR, or IV q.4-6h.	10-mg, 25-mg tablets; 12.5-mg,25-mg suppositories; 25-mg ampules	Occasional autonomic reactions such as dryness of mouth, blurred vision, or dizziness; mild hypotension possible with IV infusion
Thorazine (Chlorpromazine)	0.5mg-1mg/kg	PO, PR, or IV q.4-6h.	10-mg, 25-mg tablets; 25-mg suppositories; 25-mg ampules	Extrapyramidal symptoms (EPS) possible; autonomic reactions common as above; hypotension when give IV; give slowly; use Benadryl if EPS occur
Compazine (Prochlorperazine)	2.5 mg for children under 20 kg, 5 mg over 20 kg	PO,PR, or IV q.6-12h.	5-mg, 10-mg tablets; 2.5-mg, 5-mg suppositories; 10-mg ampules	Not frequently used intravenously due to hypertension; EPS possible; autonomic reactions common; Benadryl may be used
Torecan (Thiethylperazine)	10 mg q.6h. (dosage not established in small children)	PO,PR (rarely IM) q.6h.	10-mg tablets; 10-mg suppositories; 10-mg ampules	EPS possible; Benadryl may be used; autonomic reactions common; severe hypotension with intravenous infusion
Metaclopramide (Reglan)	1-2 mg IV slowly over 5 min; 30 min before infusion; 2, 4, and 6 hours after infusion; give with dexamethasone 20 mg IV and Benadryl 25-50 mg IV	IV, PO	5-mg/ml vials; 2-mg tablets	Extrapyramidal effects; always use Benadryl and steroid; may cause diarrhea
Lorazepam	0.05 mg/kg not to exceed 4 mg IV 1 hr before infusion & q 4 hr after	IV	2-mg/ml and 4-mg/ml tubexes	Effective with *cis*-platinum therapy; causes extreme sedation, mild hypertension, and amnesia

sitate the initiation of nasogastric feedings or intravenous hyperalimentation. See Chapter 26 for more details.

Constipation

Vincristine may cause severe constipation, colicky abdominal pain and paralytic ileus. On physical examination, the rectum may be found to be empty; however, a flat plate x-ray examination may show an upper colon impaction. Enemas and suppositories are avoided in the immunocompromised patient yet are sometimes necessary in children with painful impactions. A prophylactic regimen against constipation is recommended for patients receiving vincristine.[1] Such a regimen may include stool softeners, a diet rich in bulk, and generous fluid intake.

Diarrhea

Diarrhea can be caused by cytarabine, daunorubicin, 5-fluorouracil, hydroxyurea, nitrogen mustard, and methotrexate. Metaclopramide, an antiemetic, may also cause diarrhea. Monitoring of intake and output is necessary in patients with severe diarrhea. The frequency and consistency of stools should be recorded. If dehydration occurs, intravenous rehydration may be necessary. The dietician can offer foods that may be tolerable. If excoriation of the buttocks occurs, sitz baths may offer relief.

Bone marrow suppression

There is a progressive fall in the number of leukocytes and platelets in the peripheral blood following administration of chemotherapy. The onset of leukopenia and thrombocytopenia usually occurs within 7 to 10 days after giving the drug, and the nadir (lowest blood counts) occurs at approximately 14 days after giving the drug. The bone marrow usually recovers within 21 to 28 days.

Careful monitoring of blood counts is important, especially during the nadir period. Patients with neutropenia are susceptible to infection and are encouraged to avoid large crowds of people and to maintain meticulous body hygiene. Staff members with infections or illnesses should avoid patients with neutropenia. Reverse isolation has been used for these patients yet has not proven to be effective in reducing the incidence of infection. In addition, reverse isolation can cause the child to feel abandoned by staff and family.[1] Intravenous sites, skin breakdown, and oral lesions must be monitored for infection, and IV tubing should be changed daily. When temperature elevations occur, antipyretics may be used after appropriate cultures have been obtained. Acetaminophen is preferred over aspirin, since aspirin interferes with blood clotting. Antibiotics ordered by the physician should be started immediately in the patient with neutropenia and fever. See Chapter 24 on management of infections. Rectal temperatures, which could lead to infection or bleeding, are avoided.

Children with thrombocytopenia are prone to bleeding. Nosebleeds are common and are frightening to children and parents. If epistaxis occurs, the patient should sit upright and apply pressure by squeezing the nose for up to 15 minutes.[1] Uncontrolled bleeding secondary to thrombocytopenia is treated by intravenous platelet infusions. Bleeding of the oral mucosa can occur secondary to thrombocytopenia, especially with platelet counts below 20,000. It usually presents as intermittent oozing and can be quite disturbing for the patient. A clean oral cavity can decrease the incidence of oral complications. However, using toothbrushes is not recommended for patients with platelet counts of less than 20,000. Toothettes are helpful in cleaning the oral cavity without undue trauma.

Anemia can also result from chemotherapy yet is not as life-threatening as neutropenia and thrombocytopenia. Since the life span of a red blood cell is much longer than that of a platelet or white blood cell, the production rate in the bone marrow is much slower. Chemotherapy does less damage to cells such as red blood cells that are produced more slowly, yet repeated doses can eventually lead to a decreased red blood cell count. Washed and packed red blood cell infusions may be necessary to alleviate symptoms of anemia.

Hyperuricemia

Hyperuricemia develops from an increase in uric acid from the tumor burden or from increased lysis of tumor cells after chemotherapy. The kidney is unable to excrete such large amounts of uric acid. Symptoms of hyperuricemia include lethargy, nausea and vomiting, hematuria, renal colic, oliguria, and anuria. If untreated, renal failure and death can follow. Specific treatment protocols discuss particular management of hyperuricemia. One such protocol recommends premedicating the patient 48 hours before treatment with allopurinol (Zyloprim, Lopurin), hydrating adequately during treatment, and alkalinizing the urine with oral acetazolamide (Diamox). Allopurinol reduces both the serum and urinary uric acid levels by inhibiting the formation of uric acid. It inhibits conversion of xanthine to uric acid.

Renal complications

Intravenous *cis*-platinum and methotrexate can cause renal failure secondary to acute tubular necrosis. The patient's renal status must be evaluated before each dose of these drugs. This evaluation usually involves a 24-hour urine collection for creatinine clearance, a serum creatinine, uric acid, and BUN. Poorly functioning kidneys are unable to clear creatinine well, and the resulting creatinine clearance level is low. Patients often take home a urine collection container between hospital admissions to collect urine the day before admission for their next course of chemotherapy. They should be instructed on the proper technique for obtaining a urine collection. During the actual infusion of *cis*-platinum or methotrexate, the patient is monitored closely for decreased urine output and hypertension. Adequate hydration is essential during and after the drug infusion to flush the drug out of the kidneys.

Liver complications

Cytarabine, 6-mercaptopurine, and methotrexate can cause liver dysfunctions, which are detected by abnormal liver function tests (transaminase, SGOT, SGPT). Liver function tests are done frequently in children taking these agents, and if found to be abnormal, their dosage is decreased, or they are discontinued altogether.

Stomatitis

Symptoms of oral mucositis and inflammation often occur as early as 2 to 3 days after adminis-

tration of certain chemotherapeutic agents, including methotrexate, 6-mercaptopurine, doxorubicin, and actinomycin D.[48] Stomatitis is seen either locally or generally on the lips, tongue, buccal mucosa, palate, gingiva, and floor of the mouth as seen in Fig. 20-8. Careful observation of the oral mucosa and good oral hygiene are the keys to prevention. The patient with mild mucositis should brush teeth with a soft nylon toothbrush or toothette, using a salt and soda water rinse consisting of 1 teaspoon salt, 1 teaspoon soda in a glass of tepid water every 4 hours while awake.[48] Flossing is not recommended. The patient with severe mucositis should clean the oral cavity with gauze dipped in a solution of 5 ml sodium bicarbonate in 500 ml saline solution twice a day with equal rinses of two while awake.[48] A "magic mouthwash" preparation consisting of hydrocortisone, nystatin, and Benadryl may be used in severe mucositis. A nystatin preparation of 100,000 ml should be used when oral thrush is present. Commercial preparations should be avoided because of their alcohol and phenol content. Lemon glycerine substances are contraindicated in severe mucositis, since they are ineffective in cleaning plaque and debris from teeth and the acidity of the swab decalcifies teeth.[48] Lemon glycerine is also painful to denuded epithelium.[49] Mechanical and bacterial trauma can dis-

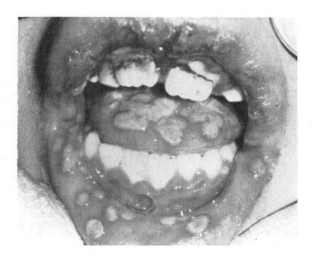

Fig. 20-8. Severe stomatitis following a course of methotrexate therapy.

rupt the integrity of oral mucosa, leading to an entry site for infection.[48] Ulcerations can be treated by allowing the patient to swish with unflavored xylocaine before meals, bedtime, and oral care.[48]

Irritated and ulcerated oral tissues are highly sensitive to temperature changes and pressure.[50] There may be decreased taste acuity and difficulty in talking, chewing, or swallowing.[49] To ensure adequate nutrition, a modified, bland, semisoft diet is recommended.

Alopecia

The most bothersome side effect of chemotherapy for many children is loss of their hair. It is important to inform them that alopecia is a temporary phenomenon and that the hair will return when chemotherapy is completed. If an older child chooses to wear a wig, it is important to obtain one before the hair begins to fall out. Younger children tend to dislike wigs because of the discomfort and may prefer to wear caps, scarves, or nothing at all. Children in warm climates should be instructed to wear protection or sunscreen when outside, since the head may become sunburned with sun exposure.

Neurologic problems

Vincristine and vinblastine can cause paresthesias, peripheral neuropathies, decreased tendon reflexes, and motor weakness. These symptoms may disappear with discontinuation of therapy yet can persist.[1] 5-Fluorouracil can cause cerebellar ataxia within 8 to 12 months following treatment, especially if it is given concurrently with hydroxyurea. *cis*-Platinum can cause VIII cranial nerve toxicity and subsequent high-frequency hearing loss. Hearing tests should be done before the administration of each course of the drug.[14]

Pulmonary problems

Busulfan can lead to pulmonary fibrosis after prolonged use, and bleomycin can lead to pneumonitis and/or fibrosis as its maximum cumulative dose is reached. Pulmonary problems are exacerbated in patients with prior lung irradiation of pulmonary disease. Pulmonary function studies and chest x-ray examinations that indicate pulmonary fibrosis may lead to discontinuation of treatment.

Reproductive problems

Many chemotherapeutic agents can affect the growth and differentiation of developing embryos. Patients and families need education about potential changes in ovarian and testicular functioning with chemotherapeutic agents. Contraceptive devices should be recommended to sexually active adolescents to avoid mutagenesis and teratogenesis in fetal development. Menses may become irregular or stop while on certain drugs. Sterility may develop in boys after taking some chemotherapeutic agents.[1] Adolescent boys who are beginning treatments may choose to have sperm frozen so that they have the option of artificial insemination later in life if treatment causes sterility.

Miscellaneous toxicities

L-Asparaginase, which is produced by *Escherichia coli* bacteria, can cause hypersensitivity reactions, including urticaria, fever, chills, and anaphylaxis.[14] These reactions vary in degree and can be treated with epinephrine and hydrocortisone. If hypersensitivity reactions do occur, it is recommended to change to Erwinia Asparaginase, which is produced by bacteria other than *Escherichia coli* and is less likely to cause reactions.

Doxorubicin (Adriamycin) can cause cardiotoxicity in a cumulative dose exceeding 550 mg/m^2 of body surface area. Many pediatric references recommend giving no more than 450 mg/m^2, and before each dose, a chest x-ray examination and echocardiogram are done to evaluate cardiac status.

Cyclophosphamide (Cytoxan) crystallizes in the bladder and can cause hemorrhagic cystitis in the patient who is not well hydrated before and during therapy.[14] Hemorrhagic cystitis can be life-threatening and can occur immediately or days after cyclophosphamide is given.

Several chemotherapeutic agents such as methotrexate, 6-mercaptopurine, and procarbazine can cause skin rashes, which usually disappear when the drug is stopped.

Patients often take other medications concurrent with chemotherapy. The potential interactions between those medications and chemotherapeutic agents must be recognized to avoid potential hazards and to maximize the clinical effectiveness of the drug therapy. Drug interactions to be aware of are listed in Table 20-8.

EDUCATING THE CHILD AND FAMILY ABOUT CHEMOTHERAPY

One of the most important functions of the pediatric oncology nurse is patient and family teaching about the diagnosis and management of the treatment. Well-informed families understand their child's therapy and are better able to anticipate and manage side effects. It is important that children and parents have written information about specific chemotherapeutic agents so that the side effects and toxicities can be reviewed. The treatment schema is also a helpful tool for the family to plan ahead for future therapies.

Many other community professionals, including the local physician, school nurse, and teachers, are involved in the care of the child with cancer and require proper information about diagnosis and treatment. The local physician often plays a vital role in the administration of chemotherapy and management of drug toxicities. See Fig. 20-9 for an example of instructions for preparation and administration of chemotherapy. The school nurse assesses and interacts with the child on an ongoing basis, and can refer problems to appropriate professionals. The school teacher plays an integral and vital role in the child's life, and is able to alleviate fears, educate other children in the classroom, and maximize the child's capacity to function normally in the school setting. (See Chapter 30 and Fig. 20-10 for an example of a letter to the school.)

Table 20-8. Drug interactions

Name	Drug interaction
BCNU and Tagamet	Tagamet enhances leukopenia and thrombocytopenia caused by the BCNU.[51]
Methotrexate and antibiotics	Antibiotics alter the gastrointestinal flora, leading to altered absorption of oral methotrexate.[52] Some antibiotics can cause prolonged excretion of methotrexate.
Cyclophosphamide (Cytoxan) and Chloramphenical	Chloramphenical prolongs the half-life of Cytoxan possibly by inhibiting hepatic metabolism.[53]
6-Mercaptopurine and allopurinol	Allopurinol inhibits xanthine oxidase, which inactivates 6-mercaptopurine. This leads to an enhancement of 6-mercaptopurine toxicity. Patients receiving both drugs may require a 25% reduction of the original 6-mercaptopurine dose.[54-56]
Methotrexate and folic acid	A decreased response to methotrexate occurs when combined with vitamins containing high levels of folic acid. Folic acid is needed for cell growth and longevity, and methotrexate is a folic acid antagonist.[57]
Methotrexate and probenecid	Probenecid enhances serum methotrexate concentration. A reduction of methotrexate may be necessary when probenecid is taken.[58,59]
Methotrexate and salicylates	Salicylates cause a reduction of methotrexate clearance by 35% reduction in plasma protein binding by 30%.[60]
Methotrexate and L-asparaginase	There may be an inhibition of methotrexate across the cell membrane by L-asparaginase.[61]
Methotrexate and vincristine	Vincristine enhances methotrexate uptake.[61]
Alkylating agents and succinyl-choline	Alkylating agents can suppress acetocholinesterase and prolong apnea if succinylcholine is used with general anesthesia.[62]
Procarbazine and Tyramine	Tyramine, which is found in wine, beer, and certain cheeses, may potentiate the nausea and vomiting from procarbazine.[1]

NAME _____ DATE_____

Instructions for Preparation and Administration of Chemotherapy

DRUG _____

DOSE _____

Preparation

1) Reconstitute ( ) _____mg vials with_____ cc sterile _____.
                  ( ) _____mg vials with_____ cc sterile _____.
                  ( ) _____mg vials with_____ cc sterile _____.

2) Withdraw _____cc of the mixture in the _____ mg vial.
             _____cc of the mixture in the _____ mg vial.
             _____cc of the mixture in the _____ mg vial.

   This equals a total dose of _____ mg of the drug.

Administration

   Administer: ☐ Sub Q; ☐ IV Push; ☐ IV Drip w/fluids; ☐ IM;

                 ☐ Other _____ On _____

Precautions

☐ Myelosuppression   The WBC and platelet count may be lowered with this drug. Please check the CBC before administering the drug. If the absolute neutrophil count is < 1000* or the platelet count is ≤ 100,000, please consult us prior to drug administration.

☐ Potential extravasation necrosis   Assure good venous access. We inject sterile saline to check for extravasation before and after drug administration. When infusing the drug, we check for blood return every 1-3 ml of drug. We recommend local SQ injection of hydrocortisone at any site of infiltration, followed by application of ice packs to area. However, these maneuvers do not have proven efficacy.

☐ Potential anaphylaxis   As a precautionary measure, we have benadryl and epinephrine (1:1,000) readily available to reverse an allergic reaction. We also observe the child in the clinic for 20 minutes after the chemotherapy injection to check for delayed reactions.

☐ Nausea and Vomiting   Premedication with an antiemetic is often helpful. Antiemetics can be utilized every 4-6 hours after administration of drug.

☐ Other. See attached drug sheet. _____

_____

*Absolute neutrophil count = WBC x (% polys + % bands + % metas)

Fig. 20-9. Example of instructions for preparation and administration of chemotherapy.

I. Introduction

Your student_____, is currently
being treated at _____ for acute
lymphocytic leukemia. This disease, a form of cancer, is the
principle type of leukemia affecting children and is
characterized by an abnormal invasion of blood-forming organs
with abnormal blood cells. This invasion interferes with the
normal production of white blood cells necessary for blood clotting.
The child is, therefore, at risk for infection and bleeding upon
diagnosis and prompt medical treatment is necessary.

The child immediately begins treatment with the goal of
obtaining a full remission (free of leukemic cells). In recent
years, the chances of going into remission, for long periods of
time, has significantly improved and potential "cures" are
possible.

We feel the school plays a major part in every child's life
and children with cancer gain special benefits and satisfaction
from being normal, productive learners and achievers.

II. Current Status of Your Student

A. Medications your student is on:

B. Length on therapy:

C. Anticipated date to go off therapy:

D. Anticipated number of days the child will miss school:

   1. For treatment:

   2. For hospitalization:

   3. For clinic visits:

III. Treatment Schedule

A. Generalized treatment:

B. Drugs and potential side effects:

C. Supportive care for side effects from medications.
There are a variety of side effects that you, as the
teacher, can recognize and possibly help alleviate with
parental permission.

   1. Nausea - if severe, allow child to lie down and rest.
   Do not force the child to eat lunch, but possibly try
   a carbonated beverage or saltine crackers to settle
   the stomach.

Continued.

Fig. 20-10. Example of nurse's letter to teacher of child receiving chemotherapy.

2. <u>Vomiting</u> - if the child vomits infrequently, follow above instructions. If the child is vomiting frequently, call the parents and send the child home. If the child should vomit any blood, immediately call the parents and they will call the medical treatment team.

3. <u>Mouth</u> <u>Sores</u> - most of the treatment for mouth sores will be at home but it is important for the teacher to recognize that these may cause for lack of appetite at school.

4. <u>"Pot Belly"</u> - one of the medications, Prednisone, will cause weight gain, a pot belly and some possible swelling. These will subside as the child goes off the medication and is not to be mistaken for severe weight gain.

5. <u>Clumsiness</u> <u>or</u> <u>weakness</u> <u>in</u> <u>extremities</u> - possibly one of the drugs may cause the child to trip and fall unusually or he may complain of weakness in extremities. Please inform the parents of any such changes so that they can inform us and we subsequently may alter the medications.

6. <u>Precautions</u> <u>with</u> <u>radiation</u> <u>therapy</u> - it is recommended by most radiotherapists that the child refrain from being in the direct sunlight while undergoing radiation therapy. After the therapy is complete, there are no such restrictions. The child will most likely lose his hair during this phase of treatment, but it will grow back with time.

7. <u>Fatigue</u> - fatigue may be common during the initial phase of the child's treatment. This is usually when he receives his most intensive therapy. It will subside and you may notice only some occasional instances of fatigue because his blood counts are low. The child is the best judge of his limitations at that time.

8. <u>Headache</u> - headaches should be treated, with parental permission only, with medication. <u>Tylenol</u> <u>should</u> <u>be</u> <u>given</u> <u>instead</u> <u>of</u> <u>aspirin</u> <u>because</u> <u>aspirin</u> <u>can</u> <u>affect</u> <u>blood</u> <u>clotting</u>.

IV. <u>Medical</u> <u>Concerns</u> <u>and</u> <u>Discipline</u> <u>Management</u>

It is important to treat the child as normal as possible while he/she is in school. There are times, however, when you have other health related concerns about your student.

A. As a general rule, young children with cancer should be allowed to participate in any age-suited activities. Most children know their own limitations and do not need to be cautioned against over-exertion. If you are unsure of a particular activity, however, feel free to contact either the parents or medical treatment team concerning specific limitations.

B. In general, there are not special precautions with most infections except for shingles (herpes zoster), chicken-pox, and regular measles. If there is an actual or expected exposure to any of these infections, it is essential to report this to the parents and/or the medical treatment team immediately. Young people who are on chemotherapy have a much lower resistance to infection and are especially susceptible to these diseases.

Fig. 20-10 cont'd.

C. Children with cancer should have routine vision and hearing tests. These children are subject to the same problems and illnesses as any young child. Children on chemotherapy, however, should refrain from getting vaccinations because their immune system differs from other children.

D. Cancer is not dangerous or contagious to others. This is often a misunderstood concept and needs to be clarified to other students at school.

E. It is often difficult to distinguish how best to not over-protect the child, and yet establish an appropriate concern for potential limitations the child with cancer might have. It is important to report unusual behaviors such as excessive physical complaints (such as headaches, etc.), etc. to the parents and medical treatment team for clarification.

V. Emotional Impact of the Disease

The child with cancer is most happy when he/she is allowed to continue as normal a life as possible. If they are treated differently, they often become fearful and feel isolated from their other peers.

The child who experiences physical changes from treatment and/or their disease is particularly conscious of such changes. Teasing by class peers is usually an indication of their fears and lack of understanding about the child's illness. It is important, with parental permission, to explain changes that may be anticipated in the sick child to the class before the child returns to school to aid in their understanding of the illness. When discussing the child's disease to the class, it is important to answer all questions openly and honestly and to foster a positive attitude about the child's illness.

It is important to have open communication between the child and his peers so that the child feels he is part of the classroom and is not isolated or rejected by others.

VI. The Child in School

An important link in the child's attitude and participation in school is the parent-teacher conferences. Conferences should be held periodically to assess not only physical adjustment, but psychological adjustment to the classroom setting. You, as a teacher, are an important part of the child's total care. We are truly interested in any information you may have re: copies of parent-teacher conferences, the child's health and psychosocial development, etc.

Please feel free to contact me at any time.

Thank you,

Fig. 20-10 cont'd.

THE FUTURE OF CHEMOTHERAPY

Because of long-term remission rates and potentially curable forms of childhood cancer, the field of pediatric oncology holds many exciting challenges for the future. Many clinical trials are currently being done to test experimental drug effectiveness. Clinicians are now researching the long-term effects of cancer therapy and ways to alleviate such effects (see Late Effects, Chapter 32). Such information will be helpful in creating more effective and less toxic chemotherapeutic agents.

REFERENCES

1. Kurtz-Bouchard, R., and Owens-Speese, N.: Nursing care of the cancer patient, ed. 4, St. Louis, 1981, The C.V. Mosby Co.
2. Lissauer: Zwei falle von leucaemie, Berliner Klinische Wochenschift 2:403, 1865.
3. Huggin, C., and Hodges, C.V.: The effect of castration, of estrogen and other androgens injected on serum phosphatases in metastatic carcinoma of the prostate, Cancer Res. 1:293, 1941.
4. Morra, M., and Potts, E.: Choices: realistic alternatives in cancer treatment, New York, 1980, Avon Books.
5. Burchenal, J.H.: The historical development of cancer chemotherapy, Semin. Oncol. 4:135, 1977.
6. Cline, M.J., and Haskell, C.M.: Cancer chemotherapy, ed. 3, Philadelphia, 1979, W.B. Saunders Co.
7. Carter, B., Curt, M., and Curt, H.: Cancer chemotherapy, New York, 1977, John Wiley & Sons, Inc.
8. Haskell, C.M.: Cancer treatment, Philadelphia, 1980, W.B. Saunders Co.
9. Hersh, E.M., Carbone, P.P., and Freireich, E.J.: Recovery of immune responsiveness after drug suppression in man, J. Lab. Clin. Med. 67:566, 1966.
10. Capizzi, R.L., and others: Combination chemotherapy: theory and practice, Semin. Oncol. 4:227, 1977.
11. Frei, E., and others: New approaches to cancer chemotherapy with methotrexate, N. Engl. J. Med. 292(2):846, 1975.
12. Sutow, W.W.: Chemotherapy in childhood cancer and appraisal, Cancer 18(1):1585, 1965.
13. Koch-Weser, J.: Bioavailability of drugs, N. Engl. J. Med. 291(1):233, 1974.
14. Sutow, W.W., Vietti, T.J., and Fernbach, D.J.: Clinical pediatric oncology, ed. 4, St. Louis, 1984, The C.V. Mosby Co.
15. Chabner, B.A., and others: Clinical pharmacology of anticancer drugs, Semin. Oncol. 4:165, 1977.
16. Bischoff, K.B.: Some fundamental considerations of the applications of pharmacokinetics for cancer chemotherapy, Cancer Chemotherapy, 59(4):777, 1975.
17. Apple, M.A.: New anticancer drug design: past and future strategies. In Beck, F.F., editor: Cancer, a comprehensive treatise, vol. 5, New York, 1977, Plenum Publishing Corp.
18. Crawford, J.D., Terry, M.E., and Rourke, G.M.: Simplification of drug dose calculation by application of surface area principle, Pediatrics 5:783, 1950.
19. Pinkel, D.: The use of body surface area as a criterion of drug usage in cancer chemotherapy, Cancer Res. 18(2):853, 1958.
20. Shirkey, H.C.: Drug dosage in infants and children, JAMA 193(6):443, 1965.
21. Wheeler, G.B., and others: Comparison of the effects of several inhibitions of the synthesis of nucleic acids upon the viability and progression through the cell cycle of cultured H Ep. no. 2 cells, Cancer Res. 32(2):2661, 1972.
22. Van Putten, C.M.: Cell kinetic data relevant for the design of tumor chemotherapy schedules, Cell Tissue Kinet. 7:493, 1974.
23. Hill, B.T., and Basergar, R.: The cell cycle and its significance for cancer treatment, Cancer Treat. Rev. 2:159, 1975.
24. Proceedings of the symposium on cell kinetics and cancer chemotherapy, Cancer Treat. Rep. 60(2):1679, 1976.
25. Umezawa, H.: Principles of antitumor antibiotic therapy. In Holland, J.F., and Frei, E., editors: Cancer medicine, Philadelphia, 1973, Lea & Febiger.
26. Waring, M.: Variation of the supercoils in closed circular DNA by binding of antibiotics and drugs: evidence for molecular models involving intercalation, J. Mol. Biol. 54:247, 1970.
27. Proceedings of the 16th annual meeting of the society for economic botany, Cancer Treat. Rep. 60(2):973, 1976.
28. Goodman, L.E., and Seligman, A.M.: Regional chemotherapy. In Holland, J.F., and Frei, E., editors: Cancer Medicine, Philadelphia, 1973, Lea & Febiger.
29. Wilson, J.P., and Solimando, D.: Antineoplastics: a safety hazard, Am. J. Hosp. Pharm. 38(1):624, 1981.
30. Benjamin, R.S.: A practical approach to adriamycin toxicology, Part 3, Cancer Chemother. Rep. 6(2):191, 1975.
31. Bowers, D.G., and Lynch, J.B.: Adriamycin extravasation, Plast. Reconstr. Surg. 61(1):86, 1978.
32. Chait, L.A., and Dinner, M.I.: Ulceration caused by cytotoxic drugs, S. Afr. Med. J. 49(4):1935, 1975.
33. Drugan, L.H., and Braine, H.G.: Necrosis of the hand after daunorubicin infusion distal to AV fistula, Ann. Intern. Med. 9(1):58, 1979.
34. Reilly, J.J., Neifeld, J.B., and Rosenberg, S.A.: A clinical course and management of accidental adria extravasation, CA 40(3):2053, 1977.
35. Cohen, M.: Amelioration of adriamycin skin necrosis: an experimental study, Cancer Treat. Rep. 63(6):1003, 1979.
36. Bowles, D.G., and Lynch, J.B.: Adriamycin extravasation, Plast. Reconstr. Surg. 61(1):86, 1972.

37. Rudolph, R., Stein, R.S., and Palitto, R.A.: Skin ulcers due to adriamycin, Cancer **38**(1):1087, 1976.
38. Hickman, P.D., and others: A modified right atrial catheter for access to the venous system in marrow transplant recipients, Surg. Gynecol. Obstet. **148**(2):871, 1979.
39. Wade, J.C., Newman, K.A., and Schimpff, S.S.C.: Two methods for improved venous access in acute leukemia patients, JAMA **246**(1):140, 1981.
40. Abraham, J., Mullen, J.L., and Jacobsen, N.: Continuous central venous access in patients with acute leukemia, Cancer Treat. Rep. **63**(1):209, 1979.
41. Blacklock, H.A., and others: Use of a modified subcutaneous right-atrial catheter for venous access in leukemic patients, Lancet **1**(2):993, 1980.
42. Blume, K.G., and others: The use of the right atrial catheter in bone marrow transplanatation for acute leukemia, Exp. Hematol. **6**:636, 1978.
43. Thomas, J.H., and others: Hickman-Broviac catheters, indications and results, Am J. Surg. **140**:791, 1980.
44. Thomas, M.: The use of Hickman catheters in the management of patients with leukemia and other malignancies, Br. J. Surg. **66**:673, 1979.
45. Reed, W.P., and others: Prolonged venous access for chemotherapy by means of the Hickman catheter, CA **52**(1):189, 1983.
46. Buttino, J., and others: Long-term intravenous therapy with peripherally inserted silicone Elastomer central venous catheters in patients with malignant diseases, CA **43**(2):1937, 1979.
47. Sullivan, R.D., Norcross, J.N., and Watkins, E.: Chemotherapy of metastatic liver cancer by prolonged hepatic artery infusion, N. Engl. J. Med. **270**:321, 1964.
48. DeBiase, C.B., and Komues, B.K.: An oral care protocol for leukemia patients with chemotherapy-induced oral complications, Spec. Care Dent. **3**(5):208, 1983.
49. Dalffler, R.: Oral hygiene measures for patients with cancer, Cancer Nurs. **3**:347, 1980.
50. Toth, B.B., and Hoor, R.E.: Oral dental care for the pediatric oncology patient, Cancer Bull **34**(2):69, 1982.
51. Selker, R.G., Moore, P., and LoDolce, D.: Bone marrow depression with cimetidine and lomustine, N. Engl. J. Med. **299**(2):834, 1978.
52. See-Lasley, K., and Ignoffo, R.J.: Manual of oncology therapeutics, St. Louis, 1981, The C.V. Mosby Co.
53. Faber, O.K., and Mourid, S.H.T.: Cyclophosphamide activation and corticosteroids, N. Engl. J. Med. **291**(1):211, 1974.
54. Coffey, J.J., and others: Effect of allopurinol on the pharmacokinetics of 6 MP in cancer patients, Cancer Res. **32**(1):1283, 1972.
55. Calabro, J.J., and Castleman, B.: Case records of the Massachusetts General Hospital, N. Engl. J. Med. **286**(1):205, 1972.
56. Berns, A., and others: Hazards of combining allopurinol with thiopurine, N. Engl. J. Med. **286**(1):730, 1972.
57. Methotrexate product information, Reuce River, New York, 1979, Lederle Labs.
58. Aherne, G.W., and others: Prolongation and enhancement of serum methotrexate concentration by probenecid, Br. Med. J. **1**:1097, 1978.
59. Ramer, A., and others: Probenecid inhibition of methotrexate excretion from CSF in dogs, J. Pharmacokinet. Biopharm. **6**:389, 1977.
60. Leigler, D.G., and others: The effect of organic acids on renal clearance of methotrexate in man, Clin. Pharmacol. Ther. **10**:849, 1969.
61. Chabree, B.: Pharmacologic principles of cancer treatment, Philadelphia, 1982, W.B. Saunders Co.
62. Gurman, G.M.: Prolonged apnea after succinylcholine in a case treated with cytostatics for cancer, Anesth. Anal. **51**(5):761, 1972.

ADDITIONAL REFERENCES

Dodd, M., and Mood, D.: Chemotherapy: helping patients to know the drugs they are receiving and their possible side effects, Cancer Nurs. **4**(4):811, 1981.
Greene, P.E., and Fergusson, J.H.: Nursing care in childhood cancer: late effects of therapy, Am J. Nurs. **82**(3):443, 1982.
Trester, K.: Nursing management of patients receiving cancer chemotherapy, Cancer Nurs. **5**(3):201, 1982.
Operstemy-Berry, D., and Heusinkveld, K.B.: Prophylactic antiemetics for chemotherapy associated nausea and vomiting, Cancer Nurs. **6**(2):117, 1983.
Gawley, E., and Kramer, R.: Improving cancer patients adjustment to infusion chemotherapy: evaluation of a patient education program, Cancer Nurs. **6**(5):373, 1983.
Waskerwitz, M.J.: Special nursing care for children receiving chemotherapy, J. Assoc. Pediatr. Oncol. Nurs. **1**(1):16, 1984.
Williams, L.T., Peterson, D.E., and Overholser, C.D.: Acute periodontal infection in myelosuppressed oncology patients: evaluation and nursing care, Cancer Nurs. **5**(6):465, 1982.
Gross, J., Johnson, B.L., and Bertino, J.R.: Possible hazards of working with cytotoxic agents, Oncol. Nurs. Forum **8**(4):10, 1981.

CHAPTER 21

Radiation therapy

EDWARD C. HALPERIN

Radiation therapy plays a major role in the treatment of childhood malignancies. Nurses involved in the care of children with cancer should have a basic understanding of the principles and practice of modern radiation oncology. This chapter reviews the essential concepts of this discipline.

WHAT IS RADIATION?

The term *radiation* is derived from the Latin word *radiatus*. It is defined as the action or process of emitting radiant energy in the form of waves or particles.[1] We encounter many examples of radiation in our daily lives: light waves, heat waves, radio waves, ultraviolet waves. In radiation therapy, we make use of x-ray, gamma rays, and heavy particle rays. Although it is often useful to think of radiation as waves, we may also conceive of it as small packets of energy traveling through space. These "packets" or "particles" have different names depending on the type of radiation. The packet of energy of the x-ray and the gamma ray is called a photon. Radiation therapy also uses radiation waves of various atomic particles: electrons, neutrons, and protons. Each of the various radiation waves has its own unique physical properties and therefore its own unique uses in clinical practice.

The unit of radiation dose is called the rad or the centiGray (abbreviated as cGy). One rad equals 1 centiGray. Since the accepted international unit of radiation is the *cGy*, it will be the term used throughout this chapter. Many medical centers, however, still use the term *rad*. One cGy is defined as the amount of radiation that results in the absorption of 100 ergs of energy in 1 g of material. One hundred cGy equals 1 Gray (abbreviated as Gy) (i.e., 100 cGy = 1 Gy).

HOW IS THERAPEUTIC RADIATION GENERATED?

External beams of therapeutic radiation can be generated by cobalt 60 (Co^{60}) units, cesium 137 (Cs^{137}) units, Van de Graaff generators, linear accelerators, betatrons, and cyclotrons. Radiation for implant radiotherapy can be generated by radium or by radium substitute isotopes.

Co^{60} external beam machine

Radioactive Co^{60} emits gamma rays with energies of 1.17 and 1.33 million electron volts. The Co^{60} may be housed in a shielded box (Fig. 21-1). A piston drives the Co^{60} into the "on" or exposed position. At the conclusion of the treatment session, the piston pulls the Co^{60} back into the "off" position.

Linear accelerators

Linear accelerators may be used to produce either x-rays or electrons. Because of the sharp beam definition and the ability to generate many different electron and photon energies, linear accelerators have become the principal radiotherapy machine in many departments. Within the machine, electrons are fired from an electron gun into an accelerator tube. The electrons are swept down the tube by intense electrical fields. The electrons may be used to strike a target and produce x-rays or they

□ The author thanks S.F. Halperin, C. Belvin, L. Harris, and C. Schmidt for reviewing the manuscript. Ms. Jody Hobbs typed the manuscript.

can be directly emitted from the machine (Fig. 21-2). Electrons are used for therapy in situations where it is desirable to administer relatively superficial irradiation. X-rays are used for therapy directed more deeply into the body.

Implant radiotherapy

Direct implantation of sealed sources of radioactive material into or adjacent to a tumor is a technique for cancer treatment. This technique is occasionally used in the pediatric patient. Radioactive needles or small radioactive seeds may be placed directly into tissue. Alternatively, sealed sources may be placed in a body cavity or on a body surface immediately adjacent to the malignant area. Several types of radioactive material are commercially available for these purposes. The most commonly used are radium 226, cesium 137, radon 222, gold 198, iodine 125, and iridium 192. There is a general trend away from the use of radium and radon because of shielding and storage problems. Therefore cesium, iodine, and iridium have become more popular.

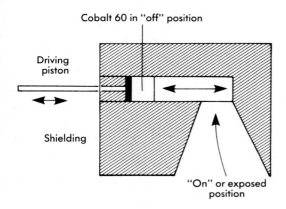

Fig. 21-1. The cobalt 60 machine.

ANCILLARY RADIOTHERAPY EQUIPMENT
Simulator

There must be a mechanism of converting the concept of irradiating a certain amount of tissue into a practical plan. The specific number of radiation beams (also called radiation ports), their size, and their angles of entry into the body must be determined. The simulator is a machine that assists in the development of an actual treatment approach.

The simulator reproduces, or "simulates," the radiotherapy treatment machine (i.e., Co^{60} or linear

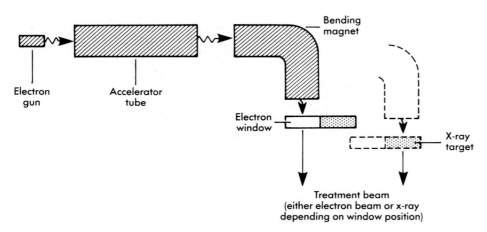

Fig. 21-2. The linear accelerator.

accelerator). The simulator contains, however, a diagnostic x-ray tube instead of a high-energy radiation source. The physician may plot the angles of the radiation beams and determine the beam size required and document each proposed "port" with a diagnostic x-ray. This diagnostic film is used to show the tumor volume and the location of any appropriate lead blocks. In this way a high energy treatment plan can be developed without exposing the patient unnecessarily to radiation from cobalt or the linear accelerator.

Immobilization devices

Precision irradiation of childhood tumors, with protection of vital normal body structures, requires detailed treatment planning. Even the most careful planning of field size and field angles will, however, be of no avail if there is significant patient movement during therapy. An immobilization device is frequently necessary to eliminate motion. The device is intended to hold the area to be treated in a comfortable but rigid position during irradiation. There are many different commercially available and "homemade" devices. These include plaster body and limb casts, plastic head holders, plastic body "cradles" that self-mold around part of the body, and wooden arm or leg boards (Figs. 21-3 and 21-4). The child must be introduced to the immobilization device and be allowed to examine it, touch it, and determine that it will cause

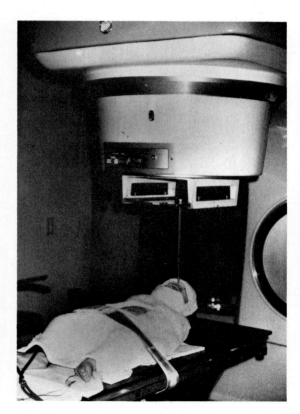

Fig. 21-3. Retinoblastoma treatment: the anesthetized child in a stabilization device for therapy.

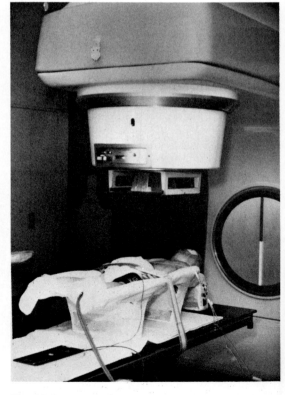

Fig. 21-4. Medulloblastoma treatment: stable prone position.

neither pain nor harm. After a few sessions with the device, most children over the age of 3 years will put themselves into it without complaint.

Anesthesia

Children over 3 years of age rarely require anesthesia for radiotherapy. Children 2 to 3 years of age may require some sedation. In general, the requirement for a stable position during irradiation necessitates anesthesia for those children less than two. Anesthesia may be given by the rectal, intramuscular, or intravenous route. Intravenous or intramuscular ketamine generally provides excellent results. Anesthesia is given under the direct supervision of an anesthesiologist. Misguided efforts to be "kind" to the child by avoiding anesthesia may compromise the possibility of tumor control and increase the risk of radiation side effects because of patient motion.

BIOLOGIC EFFECTS OF IONIZING RADIATION

When radiation interacts with living tissue, the possibility exists of direct action of the radiation on critical sites in cells. These critical sites might include, but not be limited to, the cell's chromosomes, membrane, or intracellular organelles. The radiation might raise the target to an excited state (ionized) and set off a chain of reactions that would lead to a biologic change. The effect of radiation directly on critical cellular sites is called the *direct action*.

Alternatively, when radiation interacts with living tissue the possibility exists of an indirect action of radiation on critical sites in cells. The radiation may raise various substances in the cells to an ionized state. These excited substances may, in turn, interact with critical targets and set off the chain of reactions leading to a biologic change. Since the majority of living tissue consists of water, the most obvious candidate for the intermediate substance is the water molecule. The action of radiation on critical cellular targets by way of intermediate substances is called the *indirect action*. The indirect action accounts for most of radiation's biologic effects.[2]

When radiation interacts with a water molecule, the photon or electron may raise the water to an excited (ionized) state.

$$H_2O + Radiation \rightarrow H_2O^+ + Electron^-$$

H_2O^+ is a positively charged ion. An *ion* is defined as an atom or group of atoms having a charge of positive or negative electricity. The H_2O^+ ion is extremely short lived and can decay by interacting with another water molecule.

$$H_2O^+ + H_2O \rightarrow H_3O^+ + OH°$$

$OH°$ is a free radical. A *free radical* is an extremely reactive group of atoms with a very short half-life (0.0001 seconds or less) that carries an unpaired electron on its outer shell. The highly reactive $OH°$ free radical can chemically interact with, for example, DNA. The reaction of $OH°$ with DNA occurs principally at the level of the pyrimidine bases.

By virtue of its reaction with DNA, the $OH°$ free radical can produce biologic changes. These biologic changes include single strand chromosome breaks, double strand chromosome breaks, and damage to the pyrimidine bases of the DNA. These events may result in cell death. In radiobiology, the terms *cell death, survival,* or *killing* are used in the sense that is standard in microbiology. These terms refer to the ability of an individual cell to multiply into a macroscopic colony. *Death* therefore is equivalent to the inability to reproduce.[3]

The biologic effects of ionizing radiation are briefly summarized: radiation most commonly acts indirectly on the critical DNA target through its action on water. Radiation produces highly reactive free radicals that damage the DNA double helix. This damage may manifest itself as cellular loss of reproductive capability.

Effects of radiation on normal tissue

The concept of a "tolerable" dose. The dose of radiation tolerable by an organ cannot be characterized as an absolute number. Rather, a dose of radiation to the entire substance of an organ may be associated with a certain probability of a radiation-induced complication. This concept is referred to as the minimal tissue tolerance dose (TTD).[4]

The $TTD_{5/5}$ is usually used in clinical practice and is defined as that dose of radiation associated with a 5% rate of complications occurring within 5 years of treatment. The use of the $TTD_{5/5}$ concept is frought with pitfalls. In general, $TTD_{5/5}$ refers to "whole organ" doses of which the clinician must be aware. For example, the $TTD_{5/5}$ is usually higher if less than 100% of an organ is irradiated. The $TTD_{5/5}$ when the entire heart is irradiated is 4500 cGy. When, however, only 20% of the heart is irradiated, the $TTD_{5/5}$ is 6000 cGy. Before invoking a $TTD_{5/5}$ in practice, one must be aware of how much of an organ was treated. In addition, $TTD_{5/5}$ is usually used in the context of 180 to 200 cGy/fraction. That is to say that the $TTD_{5/5}$ of the heart is approximately 180 cGy/fraction for 25 fractions or 200 cGy/fraction for 22 fractions. As the dose/fraction increases, the $TTD_{5/5}$ decreases.

Effects of total body irradiation

Data in this field are derived from total body irradiation (TBI) exposures for bone marrow transplantation, animal experimentation, radiation accidents, and the Atomic Bomb Casualty Commission. Three toxic syndromes resulting in death following TBI have been described.[5] Within 1 to 2 months following 200 to 800 cGy of TBI, bone marrow aplasia will result in death from pancytopenia. Obviously, the success or failure of bone marrow transplant is dependent on successful engraftment to obviate the *bone marrow syndrome*. Within 3 to 10 days following a single TBI exposure of about 1000 cGy, death may result from diarrhea, vomiting, malabsorption, and dehydration—a *gastrointestinal syndrome*. Finally, single exposures of 10,000 cGy will result in death within a few hours from central nervous system decompensation. This irreversible situation is called the *CNS syndrome*.

Effects of radiation on specific organs

Central nervous system

Eyes. The human eye contains several structures that are, to varying degrees, sensitive to irradiation. The lens is a highly sensitive structure and rela-tively low-radiation doses can produce partial or total lens opacification (i.e., cataract formation). The minimum dose to produce cataracts may be as low as 200 cGy. The $TTD_{5/5}$ is approximately 500 cGy.[6]

Radiation damage to the cornea can produce severe pain and corneal necrosis. The $TTD_{5/5}$ for the cornea is 5000 cGy.

High doses of radiation are given to the retina during the treatment of retinoblastoma.[7] Retinal hemorrhage and vascular occlusion may occur as late effects of irradiation. The retinal $TTD_{5/5}$ of 5500, however, rarely needs to be exceeded in clinical practice.

Brain. The effects of radiation on the brain may be divided into acute and late changes. The acute changes following irradiation may include headache, nausea, and vomiting. Within a few weeks following cranial irradiation, children may go through a period of fatigue and slowed mentation (somnolence syndrome).

The tolerance of the child's brain to radiotherapy is among the most important topics in clinical pediatric radiation oncology.[8] Children irradiated to the brain, when less than 2 years of age, run a substantial risk of moderate to severe mental retardation as a late effect. Children irradiated to the brain have a risk of late complications, which are a function of the child's age, time of treatment, dose of irradiation administered, volume of the brain encompassed in the radiation field(s), chemotherapy administered intravenously and/or intrathecally, and disease being treated. Children treated when older than 2 years have a risk of late damage, which decreases with age. Minimization of the treated volume would be expected to reduce complications. The concurrent or sequential use of cranial radiotherapy and intrathecal methotrexate may increase the risk of late complications over that seen with either modality alone (see Chapter 31 on late effects of treatment). Finally, the insult to functioning brain of an intracranial malignancy may decrease the resistance of normal tissue to radiation-induced damage.

Subtle changes in neurologic function are, in

some individuals, seen following whole brain doses in excess of 2000 Gy. Frank histologic radiation damage is not seen until much higher doses. The $TTD_{5/5}$ for the brain is between 5000 and 6000 cGy. Radiation injury to the optic nerves or chiasm is rare if the total dose to the chiasm is 4500 cGy and the dose/fraction is less than or equal to 200 cGy.

Spinal cord. Radiation effects on the spinal cord are separable into acute and late effects. Acute transient radiation myelopathy occurs 2 to 4 months following spinal irradiation. The clinical syndrome is characterized by an electrical shock–like sensation following neck flexion (Lhermitte's sign). The syndrome is usually self-limiting.

Late radiation damage to the spinal cord usually occurs 12 to 24 months following irradiation. The late syndrome is a radiation transection with paraplegia or quadraplegia. It is generally irreversible. The $TTD_{5/5}$ for the spinal cord is 4500 cGy.[4]

Digestive tract

Salivary glands. The salivary glands may be irradiated during the treatment of rhabdomyosarcoma of the head and neck, lymphoepithelioma of the nasopharynx, and other childhood malignancies. The parotid glands may, after the first one or two fractions of radiotherapy, swell and become painful. This "radiation parotiditis" is usually self-limited and is adequately treated with aspirin. Parotid irradiation may be accompanied by an elevation in serum amylase.[9]

Radiation damage to salivary function will result in an increase in the viscosity of the saliva and a decrease in its volume. The patient may complain of a dry mouth. An increase in oral fluids should be prescribed. In severe cases, artificial saliva may be indicated. Since the saliva constitutes part of the natural defense against tooth decay, meticulous attention to oral hygiene is necessary to reduce the development of caries.[10]

Oral mucosa. The intraoral mucosa will, after approximately 2000 cGy of irradiation, become erythematous. At doses greater than 4000 cGy, epithelial desquamation may occur. Regeneration of the epithelium after irradiation generally takes 14

to 21 days. Telangiectasia and fibrosis of the oral mucosa may be seen as a delayed effect of high-dose radiotherapy.

Esophagus. Carcinoma of the esophagus during childhood is extremely unusual. The esophagus may, however, be irradiated during the treatment of mediastinal lymphoma, neuroblastoma, and during pulmonary irradiation. In a manner similar to the oral cavity, the esophageal mucosa will be affected by radiotherapy. Dysphagia and odynophagia will occur at doses of 2000 cGy. An anesthetic gargle such as viscous lidocaine or aspirin chewing gum may relieve symptoms. Symptoms usually abate 14 to 21 days following cessation of irradiation.

Stomach. Acute postirradiation nausea may occur following treatment of the stomach. Antiemetics, administered before and after therapy, usually attend to the problem. Radiation ulceration of the stomach may occur after a dose of 4500 cGy.[11] This is, however, an unusual complication of pediatric radiotherapy.

Liver. The administration of moderate- to high-dose radiotherapy to the liver may produce hepatic enlargement, tenderness, and elevation in serum liver function tests. Radiation hepatitis is a potentially fatal complication characterized, in its late stages, by fibrosis. The $TTD_{5/5}$ for the radiation of the entire substance of the liver is 2500 cGy.

The radiosensitivity of the liver is increased by several chemotherapeutic agents. Children with right-sided Wilms' tumor who receive chemotherapy and right hemiabdomen irradiation are susceptible to radiation hepatopathy if a large portion of the organ is treated.[12]

Small intestine. The intestinal mucosa is susceptible to radiation damage. Postirradiation nausea and vomiting may follow irradiation of the abdominal contents. Diarrhea and cramping occur following 2000 to 3000 cGy of treatment. Delayed complications of radiotherapy include small bowel obstruction, malabsorption, and fistula formation. The $TTD_{5/5}$ for small bowel is 4500 cGy.[13]

Large intestine. Radiation damage to the large bowel generally presents as frequent diarrheal bowel movements and/or tenesmus. It is generally seen after 2500 to 5000 cGy of treatment. The problem may be addressed by prescribing diphenoxylate, tincture of paregoric, or tincture of opium. Diarrhea usually resolves 7 to 14 days following completion of radiotherapy. Persistent proctitis, rectal ulceration, or stenosis is usually not seen at doses less than 6000 cGy.[14] Fortunately, in childhood malignancy, a pelvic dose of this size is usually not required.

Lung. Radiation effects on the lung are a function of the total dose of radiation administered and of the volume treated. Doses in excess of 2000 cGy to both lungs may produce radiation pneumonitis. This disorder is characterized by dyspnea, dry cough, tachypnea, tachycardia, and radiographic pulmonary infiltrates.[15] It may be fatal. The $TTD_{5/5}$ for whole lung irradiation is 2000 cGy. However, several chemotherapeutic agents are known to increase lung sensitivity to radiation. Therefore the dose for whole lung irradiation when chemotherapy is also given, should be restricted to 1200 to 1800 cGy.[16]

Limited volumes of the lung may be irradiated to higher doses (4000 to 6500 cGy). Such doses will produce permanent localized pulmonary fibrosis within the radiation portal, which will be visible on chest x-ray examination.

Heart. Radiation-induced heart disease can be either acute or late. Acute pericarditis occurs within 1 year of therapy and is characterized by fever, pleuritic chest pain, and a pericardial friction rub. Since, in my experience, radiation pericarditis is clincally indistinguishable from other causes of pericarditis, the diagnosis is made by inference and exclusion. The late effects of cardiac irradiation include constrictive pericarditis and, in some cases, myocardial fibrosis. The $TTD_{5/5}$ for the heart is 4500 cGy.[17] This dose may be approached in the treatment of lymphoma. A special left ventricle lead block is often used to reduce the risk of complications.[18]

Urinary tract

Kidney. Large field irradiation of the abdomen during the therapy of rhabdomyosarcoma, neuro-

blastoma, Wilms' tumor, germ cell tumors, and lymphomas may require inclusion of one or both kidneys in the portal. Late radiation nephropathy from radiotherapy may be characterized by shrunken kidneys, anemia, proteinuria, hypertension, and/or uremia. The damage is irreversible. Because the $TTD_{5/5}$ for the kidneys is 2000 cGy,[19,20] careful attention must be paid to renal shielding.

Bladder. Acute radiation cystitis is frequent during pelvic irradiation. The syndrome is characterized by urinary frequency and pain on urination. Such symptoms are usually self-limited. If a dose greater than 6000 cGy is given, urinary abnormalities may be permanent. Because hemorrhagic cystitis is a well-known potential complication of cyclophosphamide therapy, radiation to the bladder should not be given concurrently with cyclophosphamide unless absolutely necessary.

Reproductive organs. The testes are directly irradiated in children for the treatment of testicular involvement by acute lymphoblastic leukemia.[21] Doses used in this clinical situation (18 to 24 Gy) produce permanent sterilization. The function of the testosterone-producing Leydig cells may not be significantly affected.

Pelvic irradiation may encompass the ovaries. Doses in excess of 1500 to 2500 cGy may produce sterilization. The ovaries may be moved, during a staging laparotomy for Hodgkin's disease, to avoid their being irradiated. This procedure is called an oophoropexy.[22] In some adolescents, menstruation may cease during and following radiotherapy but will resume later.

When any area of the body is irradiated, there will be some scattered irradiation of the gonads. The extent and duration of the effect on reproduction function of this scattered radiation will be determined by the dose to the gonads.

Hematopoietic. Circulating lymphocytes are acutely sensitive to the lethal effects of ionizing radiation. Even if little or no bone marrow is included in the radiotherapy field, the peripheral lymphocyte count will fall because of destruction of cells "in-transit" through the field. Peripheral red blood cells, white blood cells other than lymphocytes, and platelets are relatively insensitive to radiotherapy; the bone marrow precursors of these cells are, however, quite sensitive. Therefore irradiation of a large area of bone marrow will produce a diminution in peripheral counts as a function of the half-lives ($T_{1/2}$) of the circulating elements: red blood cells ($T_{1/2}$ = 120 days), polymorphonuclear leukocytes ($T_{1/2}$ = 6 to 7 hr), platelets ($T_{1/2}$ = 8 to 10 days). A dose of 2000 cGy to an area of bone marrow will permanently obliterate hematopoietic function at that site.[23,24]

Bones. The growth of a child's bones, at the epiphyseal plate, will be slowed by a dose in excess of 600 cGy to the plate. A dose in excess of 2000 cGy will arrest growth.[25] If only part of the growth plate is irradiated, asymmetric growth will result. The reduction in a child's potential for growth, by radiation, will depend on the child's age at the time of treatment, the number and location of bones irradiated, and the effects of other therapies. For example, symmetric irradiation of the spinal column of a young child will significantly reduce the ultimate sitting height. If the legs are spared, the standing height will be affected to a lesser extent.

Irradiation of the buds of the permanent teeth, to a dose greater than 1000 cGy, will cause failure of eruption of the teeth.[26] Irradiation of the globe for retinoblastoma will often produce subsequent failure of eruption of the upper second molar.

Integument. Fractionated radiotherapy to the skin will produce erythema with doses in excess of 2000 cGy. Dry desquamation is seen at approximately 4000 cGy and moist desquamation of 5000 to 6000 cGy. These reactions resolve substantially within a few weeks following irradiation. Topical application of lotions other than bland emollients should be avoided during radiotherapy. Topical agents should always be applied after, rather than before, the daily irradiation treatment. One should avoid irradiating "through" the topical agent and jeopardizing the skin. Corn starch may be useful in moist intertriginous areas. Topical cortisone is often used following a course of radiotherapy to reduce superficial inflammation.

Epilation will occur after doses of 500 to 1000 cGy. If the total dose to the hair follicle exceeds 4500 cGy, hair loss may be permanent. The area of hair loss will correspond to the radiation portal.

Endocrine glands. Irradiation of the thyroid gland during head and neck radiotherapy (i.e. Hodgkin's disease, rhabdomyosarcoma) can result in hypothyroidism—even occurring several years later.[27] The incidence of late hypopituitarism following pituitary irradiation is unknown. When it occurs, it primarily manifests itself as a growth hormone deficiency.[28]

CONCLUSION

Irradiation is a powerful tool for the treatment of malignant disease in children. Therapeutic irradiation may be generated by a cobalt 60 machine, a linear accelerator, or by a sealed source of radioactive material. A simulator is often used to design treatment portals. Patient immobilization is required for reproducible daily treatments.

Radiation, acting indirectly on DNA via water, produces cellular loss of reproductive capability. Careful attention must be paid to the radiation tolerance of normal tissues during the design and conduct of a course of treatment.

REFERENCES

1. Woolf, H.W., editor: Webster's new collegiate dictionary, Springfield, 1979, G. & C. Merriam Co.
2. Hall, E.J.: Radiobiology for the radiologist, Hagerstown, 1978, Harper & Row, Publishers, Inc.
3. Puck, T.T., Marcus, P.I.: Action of x-rays on mammalian cells, J. Exp. Med. **103**:653, 1956.
4. Rubin, P., Casareh, G.W.: A direction for clinical radiation pathology: the tolerance dose. In Vaeth, J.M., editor: Frontiers of radiation therapy and oncology, vol. 6, Baltimore, 1972, University Park Press.
5. Hemplemann, L.H., Lisca, H., and Hoffman, J.G.: The acute radiation syndrome: a study of nine cases and a review of the problem, Ann. Intern. Med. **36**:279, 1952.
6. Merriam, G.R.: Radiation dose to the lens in treatment of tumors of the eye and adjacent structures: possibilities of cataract formation, Radiology **71**:357, 1958.
7. Abramson, D.H., Jereb, B., Ellsworth, R.M.: External beam radiation for retinoblastoma, Bull. N. Y. Acad. Med. **57**:787, 1981.
8. Eiser, C.: Intellectual abilities among survivors of childhood leukemia as a function of CNS irradiation, Arch, Dis. Child. **53**:391, 1978.

9. van den Brenk, H.A.S., and others: Serum amylase as a measure of salivary gland radiation damage, Br. J. Radiol. **42:**688, 1969.

10. Fromm, M., and others: Treatment of soft tissue sarcomas of the head and neck, Int. J. Radiat. Oncol. Biol. Phys. **10**(Suppl. 2):87, 1984.

11. Hamilton, E.E.: Gastric ulcer following radiation, Arch. Surg. **55:**394, 1947.

12. Tefft, M., Mitus, A., and Jaffe, N.: Irradiation of the liver in children: acute effects enhanced by concomitant chemotherapeutic administration, Am. J. Roentgenol. **111:**165, 1971.

13. Friedman, M.: Calculated risks of radiation injury of normal tissue in the treatment of cancer of the testis. Proceedings of the second national cancer congress. vol. I, 390, 1952.

14. Montana, G.S., and others: Analysis of results of radiation therapy for state III carcinoma of the cervix, Int. J. Radiat. Oncol. Biol. Phys. **10**(Suppl. 2):138, 1984.

15. Gross, N.J.: Pulmonary effects of radiation therapy, Ann. Int. Med. **86:**81, 1977.

16. D'Angio, G.J., chairman: National Wilms' Tumor Study—3, Philadelphia, 1979, National Wilm's Tumor Study.

17. Stewart, J.R., and Fajardo, L.F.: Radiation-induced heart disease: clinical and experimental aspects, Radiol. Clin. North Am **9:**511, 1971.

18. Glatstein, E., and Kaplan, H.S.: Determination of tumor extent and tumor localization of Hodgkin's disease and non-Hodgkin's lymphomas. In Levitt, S.H., and Tapley, N.: Technological basis of radiation therapy: practical clinical applications, Philadelphia, 1984, Lea & Febiger.

19. Luxton, R.W., and Kunkler, P.B.: Radiation nephritis, Acta Radiol. **2:**169, 1964.

20. Kunkler, PB., Farr, R.F., and Luxton, R.W.: The limit of renal tolerance to x-rays, Br. J. Radiol. **25:**190, 1952.

21. Saiontz, H.I., and others: Testicular relapse in childhood leukemia, Mayo Clin. Prac. **53:**212, 1978.

22. Kaplan, H.S.: Hodgkin's disease, ed 2, Cambridge, Mass., 1980, Harvard University Press.

23. Rubin, P., editor: Radiation biology and pathology syllabus, Chicago, 1975, American College of Radiology.

24. Haas, G.S., and others: Differential recovery of circulating T cell subsets after nodal irradiation for Hodgkin's disease, J. Immunol. **132:**1026, 1984.

25. Probert, J.C., Parker, B.R., and Kaplan, H.S.: Growth retardation in children after megavoltage irradiation of the spine, Cancer, **32:**634, 1973.

26. Moss, W.T., Brand, W.N., and Bahiforo, H.: Radiation oncology: rationale, technique, results, St. Louis, 1979, The C.V. Mosby Co.

27. Markson, J.L., and Flatman, G.E.: Myxedema after deep x-ray therapy to the neck, Br. Med. J. **1:**1228, 1965.

28. Sheline, G.E., and Tyrrell, B.: Pituitary adenomas. In Phillips, T.L., and Pistenmaa D.A., editors: Radiation oncology annual 1983, New York, 1984, Raven Press.

CHAPTER 22

Bone marrow transplantation

JOLEEN KELLEHER

Marrow transplantation offers a therapeutic option for children with hematologic and oncologic disorders involving the bone marrow, when these diseases are refractory to conventional therapy. The bone marrow as an organ essential to life, is responsible for production of red blood cells, platelets, and granulocytes. As an immunologic competent organ, it is rich in lymphocytes and offers both humoral and cell-mediated immunity. Replacing diseased or deficient marrow with healthy marrow reconstitutes these hematologic and immunologic functions.

Research advances in tissue typing, supportive care during marrow aplasia, and prevention and treatment of post-transplant complications have improved the success of marrow transplantation for leukemia, immunologic deficiencies, and congenital or acquired regenerative anemia. Table 22-1 summarizes the diseases currently treated with marrow transplantation.

Theoretically, marrow transplantation could be of benefit for any malignant disorder that demonstrates a steep dose response curve to therapy of which marrow toxicity is the dose-limiting factor.[1] Research studies continue to evaluate the efficacy of this treatment modality for refractory Hodgkin's disease and selected solid tumors such as neuroblastoma.

DONOR SELECTION

As with other organ transplants, a major impediment to successful grafting is the immunologic reaction of donor and recipient tissue. Tissue typing is essential to provide identification of histocompatibility between donor and recipients. Compatibility is largely determined by two tests: human leukocyte antigen (HLA) typing and mixed lymphocyte culture (MLC) reaction. The HLA complex is easily identified and tested in the white blood cells.[2]

HLA antigens are located on chromosome 6, containing four separate loci (HLA-A,B,C,D) on two different haplotypes. Each individual inherits one HLA-A, B, C, D gene (haplotype) from the mother and one from the father. Theoretically, non-twin siblings have a 1 in 4 chance (25%) of being HLA identical. In families with more than one sibling, there is a 35% to 40% chance of having an HLA-matched donor.[3] To extend the availability of compatible donors, the use of nonsibling (unrelated) individuals who are HLA-identical with the child is being investigated. With computerization of HLA-A, -B, -C, -D typing, it is technically feasible to have a large volunteer unrelated donor pool. The chance of finding an unrelated HLA-matched donor is approximately 1:5,000.

After HLA compatibility is determined, the lymphocytes of the donor and recipient are combined in culture media to determine MLC reactivity. This test further establishes HLA-D compatibility. Reactivity indicates potential for graft versus host disease, and a nonreactive MLC signals compatibility.

Red cell incompatibility is no longer a barrier to marrow transplantation. By using plasma exchange or immunoabsorbent columns, A or B antibodies can be removed from the recipient before transplant.

Table 22-1. Common diseases transplanted, conventional therapy, and recommended time to transplant

Diseases transplanted	Conventional therapy	Recommended time to transplant
Acute lymphoblastic leukemia	Chemotherapy	After first relapse
Acute nonlymphoblastic leukemia	Chemotherapy	First remission
Chronic granulocytic leukemia	Chemotherapy	Chronic accelerated phase or blast crisis
Lymphoma	Chemotherapy and/or radiotherapy	After first relapse
Severe aplastic anemia	Androgens, glucocorticoids Blood transfusions Antithymocyte globulin	At time of diagnosis
Thalassemia	Blood transfusions Chelation therapy	Within first few years of life
Wiskott-Aldrich syndrome	Passive immunity therapy Platelet transfusions Antibiotics	Anytime
Severe combined immunodeficiency (SCID)	None	At time of diagnosis

TYPES OF TRANSPLANTS

There are three basic types of transplants: autologous, syngeneic, and allogeneic.

Autologous grafting involves the aspirations of the child's own marrow, cryopreservation of that marrow, and reinfusion after chemoradiotherapy administration treats the underlying disease.

Syngeneic grafting occurs between identical twins. The donor and recipient are genetically mirror images of each other, and engraftment is assured with minimum complications.

Allogeneic transplants are usually those between HLA-matched siblings (or nonsiblings). However, recent studies are underway using HLA-mismatched related donors and recipients. Marrow is treated with either lectin or monoclonal antibiotics before infusion. Each technique removes harmful mature T lymphocytes from donor marrow.[4]

RECIPIENT'S ENVIRONMENT

Depending on availability and institutional protocol, marrow transplants can be successfully done in either a private nonsterile room or a laminar airflow sterile unit. Studies indicate that patients in the laminar airflow units have less major local infection and less septicemias in the early post-transplant phase.[5] However on discharge from the hospital, there is no difference in acquisition of late transplant infections between patients placed in a laminar airflow unit and those transplanted in a private room.

Private rooms must have sinks for hand washing on entering and leaving the room. Masks may or may not be worn as indicated by protocol. Contact with other than family members should be minimized, and no live plants or fresh fruits are allowed in the patient area.

Children considered at high risk should be placed in the sterile environment. Those at risk include any child with an immune deficiency disorder, congenital or acquired anemias, established infection before transplant, mismatched donor, and children in leukemic relapse.

The laminar airflow room is designed for single patient occupancy, consisting of a sterile patient zone, marked off by a plastic curtain wall, and an anteroom where families can visit the child without disturbing the sterile environment. High-efficiency filters and continuous sterile horizontal airflow in the patient zone assist in maintaining the sterile zone. Decontamination of the child's skin and gastrointestinal tract prohibit growth of endogenous pathogens. Microbial suppression of the alimentary tract with oral nonabsorbable antibiotics includes a combination of vancomycin hydrochloride liquid, tobramycin sulfate liquid, polymyxin B sulfate, and nystatin oral suspension. This solution is swished and swallowed three times daily. Skin decontamination involves bathing with an antimicrobial soap (chlorhexidine gluconate) before entry into the laminar airflow room and daily thereafter paying special attention to the axilla and groin. Persistent skin organisms are diminished with topical application of antibacterial and antifungal powders and ointments. A triple antibiotic ointment and nystatin ointment are applied four times daily to the ears, the nares, the umbilicus, and the rectal area. Triple antibiotic powder and antifungal nystatin powder are applied four times daily to the axilla and groin. A solution of vancomycin, hydrochloride, polymyxin B sulfate, and neomycin sulfate is sprayed through a nebulizer into each nostril three times daily, eradicating organisms of the nose and pharynx.[6]

Weekly surveillance cultures of the nose, mouth, vagina, and rectum monitor the degree of microbial suppression and alert the physician to acquisition of new or resistant micro-organisms.

Each room is provided with necessary sterile equipment and supplies. Equipment that cannot be steam or gas sterilized is soaked in a Betadine bath or disinfectant. Sterile zone including walls are cleaned daily. An indication that cleaning techniques are providing a germ-free environment results from negative room cultures.

Sterile or low bacteria diets should be provided by the dietary department to further reduce the incidence of micro-organism acquisition.

Nursing care can be performed by indirect contact from the anteroom. All intravenous solutions and blood products can be infused through extension tubing that passes into the sterile room from the anteroom. Direct nursing care requires putting on a mask, hat, sterile booties, sterile gown and sterile gloves. Once in the patient zone, normal nursing functions can be performed like bed changes, bath, physical assessment, and certain nursing treatments.

Psychologically, this extreme form of isolation can have adverse effects, with some children becoming withdrawn, depressed, developmentally regressed, and having difficulty sleeping. An attempt should be made to create an environment that has items familiar to the child like a favorite book, picture, blanket, or dolls and provides space and equipment for play and expression such as crayons and paper. Family members should be encouraged to "grow-up" and enter the patient zone for direct daily interaction with the child.

TRANSPLANTATION PROCESS

Marrow transplant requires a family commitment, a short hospitalization for the donor, several months hospitalization for the ill child, and long-term readjustment to a new level of wellness. The complications of treatment can be life-threatening. It is impossible to predict the severity and outcome of complications. Early assessment, detection, and intervention can decrease the mortality and morbidity of the child undergoing transplant.

Pretransplant preparation

Careful medical and psychosocial preparation of the marrow donor and recipient is important. Preparation can be done in an outpatient setting before admission to the transplant unit. Medically, both donor and recipient receive an extensive history and physical examination. Additional procedures for the recipient include pulmonary function tests, bone marrow aspiration to determine current disease status, electrocardiogram, liver enzyme and electrolyte tests, and screening for hepatitis and cytomegalovirus (CMV).

A conference involving medical and nursing staff, a social worker, and the family is held to outline treatment plans, discuss various protocols and randomizations, and to answer questions the family and/or child may have regarding the course of treatment. Donors may have concerns about inhibition of marrow function or of acquiring leukemia with marrow donation. The family and donor need reassurance that normal marrow function resumes after donation. Encouraging family members to participate in all aspects of caring for the ill child may help them feel a part of the success of transplant.[7]

Venous access. A right atrial catheter (RAC) is usually inserted before transplant. The Hickman right atrial catheter is the most frequently used. Major catheter advantages are easy accessibility to the child's circulatory system and minimum restriction of the child's daily activity. Blood samples except coagulation screens and arterial blood gases are drawn from the catheter, eliminating the discomfort of repeated venipunctures. The large bore (1.6 mm) allows administration of blood products, parenteral nutrition, and intravenous medications without risk of occlusion or infiltration. Depending on vein size, availability, age of child and surgeon's recommendation, a single or double lumen right atrial catheter is inserted.

Before catheter insertion, play therapy can be initiated, enabling the child to better cope with the impending procedure.

Placement of a catheter is carried out under local or general anesthesia. Decision for anesthesia should be made jointly by parents and medical staff based on their perception of child's ability to cooperate during the procedure.[8]

When handling the inserted catheter, aseptic technique must be used. After blood samples are drawn from the catheter, the line is irrigated with heparinized saline to reduce the risk of coagulation within the catheter internal lumen.

No more than 5 cc/kg/day of blood should be removed from the catheter. This safety measure prevents hemodynamic problems. A blood draw flow sheet is helpful in maintaining accurate records of blood loss from sampling.

Nursing responsibilities involve daily catheter exit site examination and cleaning. Any change such as redness, purulent drainage, or induration with tenderness should be noted; the area should be cultured and physician notified. Securing the Hickman dressing and line can be difficult with an active child. The use of a Ray Marshall shield stockinette and clamping the catheter to the inside of child's clothing with clamps can safely secure the line.

Conditioning (immunosuppressive) regimen. All children except infants with severe immunologic deficiency disease are immunologically competent and capable of rejecting marrow grafting, unless they are prepared with some form of immunosuppressive therapy (conditioning regimen). This regimen achieves three goals: reduces graft rejection by destroying immune system, eliminates any malignant cells, and prepares marrow cavity for donor engraftment.

High-dose chemotherapy, usually cyclophosphamide is used to prepare patients with nonmalignant diseases. Some clinical settings do use total body irradiation (TBI) to further reduce the incidence of graft rejections, especially if the patient has had multiple blood transfusions.[9]

A combination of high-dose chemotherapy (usually cyclophosphamide) and TBI is the conditioning regimen for children with malignancies. Children with leukemia also receive a series of intrathecal injections of methotrexate as prophylaxis against central nervous system relapse.

Cyclophosphamide affects rapidly proliferating cells and is a powerful marrow depressant. Doses range from 40 to 60 mg/kg/day for 2 to 4 consecutive days, depending on disease and protocol. It is administered over 30 to 60 minutes. Nursing care following cyclophosphamide infusion involves minimizing the side effects of treatment. Adverse effects include nausea, vomiting, alopecia, cardiomyopathy, inappropriate antidiuretic hormone (IADH) syndrome, skin rash, and hemorrhagic cystitis. Peak time for nausea and vomiting is 12 hours after administration. An antiemetic regimen should be initiated ½ to 1 hour before the dose of cyclophosphamide and continued on a regular schedule until 24 hours after last dose of chemotherapy. Combinations of antiemetics such as droperidol and metaclopramide are effective agents. Extrapyramidal symptoms are peculiar to this combination and easily controlled with addition of diphenhydramine.

Electrocardiogram taken before each dose of cyclophosphamide and examined for reduced voltage or nonspecific S-T segment changes will indicate cardiac toxicity. Severe cardiomyopathy may indicate a need to discontinue cyclophosphamide and replace with another cytotoxic agent. Assessment for fluid overload and edema is essential. If congestive heart failure occurs, indicated treatment is fluid and sodium restriction, digoxin, and diuretics. However, cyclophosphamide-induced failure is usually resistant to treatment.[10]

Hemorrhagic cystitis results from cyclophosphamide metabolites, excreted in the urine, reacting with the bladder epithelium. Prevention involves intravenous hydration at twice maintenance for children greater than 20 kg and 1½ times maintenance for children less than 20 kg. Voiding every 2 hours to eliminate toxic metabolites from the bladder is necessary. Some children may need a Foley catheter inserted to ensure adequate emptying of the bladder. Urine is tested every void for blood. If hematuria develops and persists, hydration may need to be prolonged.

Inappropriate antidiuretic hormone secretion causes fluid retention and is treated with intravenous furosemide if urine output drops below 3 to 4 cc/kg/hr. Before diuretic administration, an IV fluid challenge of 10 cc/kg should be given to spare kidneys a hypovolemic episode. Intake and output is recorded hourly, urine specific gravity checked hourly, and weights taken to monitor fluid status twice daily.

Total body irradiation adds further immunosuppression and aids in destruction of tumor cells, penetrating privileged chemoresistant sites like the central nervous system and testes.[11] The length of time needed to administer TBI (one-time dose or fractionated) and the age of the child may necessitate sedation to ensure that the child remains in a safe, comfortable position. For those children receiving TBI, nursing care focuses on controlling adverse reactions to treatment such as nausea, vomiting, diarrhea, fever, and parotiditis. The severity varies and appears to be reduced with the administration of fractionated doses. Antiemetic regimens can be initiated before TBI and continued throughout treatment. Diarrhea is variable and treated symptomatically. Adequate hydration and accurate intake and output are essential in preventing hypovolemia during this period.

Bilateral parotiditis may appear 4 to 24 hours following irradiation and usually resolves in 72 hours. It can be painful and is treated with ice packs and acetaminophen.[12] Fever following treatment is usually a result of acute tissue destruction, although infection must be ruled out and appropriate cultures (blood, urine, throat, and stool) should be obtained. Fever usually dissipates in 4 to 6 hours.

Sterility and cataracts are long-term complications of TBI. Young males should have the option of sperm banking before treatment is initiated. Corrective lenses or lens implants may be necessary for treatment of cataracts after transplantation.

Day of transplant

The day of transplant begins with aspiration of marrow from the donor. Risk of marrow donation is relatively minimal (e.g., pain, stiffness, and possible infection at aspiration site). The greatest risks are those of general anesthesia. Donor marrow replenishes itself within a few days. Under sterile conditions, in an operating room, donor marrow is aspirated from the anterior and posterior iliac crests. Multiple aspirations are necessary to obtain appropriate marrow volume (10 to 15 cc/kg). This volume is dependent on donor and recipient physical size. After aspiration, the marrow is placed in a beaker and mixed with tissue culture media and heparin (without preservative) to prevent coagulation. The marrow is then filtered twice, once through a course screen and once through a fine screen, to remove bone and fat particles. Before transferring marrow to a transfusion bag, a cell count and culture are taken. A corrected nucleated cell count above 3×10^8/kg for aplastic anemia and 1.0×10^8 for leukemia is considered an adequate sample.

The marrow is administered like a blood transfusion through the Hickman catheter over approximately 4 hours. Unlike a blood transfusion, the marrow is *unirradiated* and unfiltered. Marrow stem cells enter the general circulation and migrate through the blood to marrow cavities where they proliferate and undergo a normal maturation process.

Children receiving autologous marrow undergo a similar process for donor donation. After aspiration, marrow is preserved in 10% DMSO and frozen at -180° C. On the day of transplant, marrow is rapidly thawed in a 37° C water bath with subsequent rapid infusion of unirradiated, unfiltered marrow. The day of marrow infusion is considered as day *0*.

During marrow infusion, nursing assessment includes monitoring for fluid overload, pulmonary emboli, reaction to white cells in marrow, and rarely, bacterial contamination of the marrow. Changes in vital signs, complaints of dyspnea, chest pain, chills, hives, and fever may indicate problems. Infusion should be slowed, the physician notified and reactions treated symptomatically. Diuretics or phlebotomy may be necessary if cardiac failure occurs. A fever less than 38.5° C needs complete culturing (blood, urine, throat, and stool). Initiation of broad-spectrum antibiotics may be necessary if infection is suspected. Marrow infusion should continue despite complications. Slowing the infusion may diminish symptoms.

POST-TRANSPLANTATION COMPLICATIONS

Profound marrow aplasia exists for 2 to 4 weeks after marrow infusion. This is the most critical time for the child, since it is impossible to predict the outcome and severity of complications. Nursing care can do much to alleviate the child's distress and discomfort. Providing continuity and consistency of nursing care using the primary nursing model is essential for early intervention of subtle changes that may indicate impending complications or improvements. Until marrow stem cells can migrate and proliferate in the marrow cavity, supportive care is essential for survival. The nurse is involved in maximizing nutritional support, maintaining fluid and electrolyte balance, protecting the child from exogenous and endogenous sources of infection, controlling pain, and assessing and preventing hemorrhagic complications. In addition, complications such as renal failure, venocclusive disease, and acute graft versus host disease can create severe multi-organ failure.

Nutrition

Nutritional complications result from the conditioning regimen and post-transplant complications. They include nausea, vomiting, diarrhea, fever, infection, mucositis, changes in taste sensation and salivary flow, and failure to thrive. These problems often occur together and prevent the child from maintaining adequate oral caloric intake, increasing the potential of morbidity and mortality. Total parenteral nutrition is initiated after the last dose of chemotherapy and continued until the child is able to consume adequate calories orally. The goal of parenteral therapy is to prevent negative nitrogen balance, loss of lean body mass without creating excessive fluid and caloric overload.

The availability of various percents of amino acid solution, dextrose solution, and lipid emulsions enables varied parenteral nutrient regimens as clinical condition indicates.[13] To allow physiologic adjustment to hypertonic dextrose infusions, parenteral nutrition can be initiated with a 10% dextrose, amino acid combination. As the body equilibrates and serum glucoses are less than 200 mg/ml and urine glucose is negative, dextrose concentrations can be increased to 25% to 35%, depending on caloric needs. Regular insulin may be added to dextrose solutions to control glucose intolerance. Serum and urine glucoses should be monitored daily during parenteral therapy.

Lipid emulsions of 10% and 20% are concomitantly infused with dextrose solutions to prevent essential fatty acid deficiency and to add calories for children with glucose intolerance. Lipid clearance tests should be performed weekly to verify metabolism of the fat emulsion.

As the child resumes oral nutritional intake, emphasis is placed on caloric and fluid content of diet to prevent weight loss and dehydration. Discerning the cause of anorexia and working within the constraints of the etiology is a challenge whether it be GVHD or psychologically induced. For the child and the parent, nutritional teaching should focus on a gradual return to normalcy, not immediate emphasis on a balanced diet. Eating is not enjoyable after transplant because of the dramatic taste changes and reduction of salivary flow. Parents should be instructed to have food available but to avoid making eating an issue. Supplementary vitamins are necessary during this transition time.

Fluid and electrolyte balance

Homeostasis (body's ability to maintain fluid balance) is difficult to maintain because of complications of high-dose chemoradiotherapy, massive IV infusions, frequent blood transfusions, and sepsis. The osmotic gradient across the body fluid compartments is constantly shifting to compensate for these changes. Daily fluid and electrolyte monitoring is essential to identify problems. Maintenance fluid needs can be calculated for children not experiencing major fluid excess or deficits. Replacement fluids or fluid restriction may be necessary as clinical condition of the child changes. Common fluid and electrolyte problems are summarized in Table 22-2.

Replacement of fluid and electrolyte losses is

Table 22-2. Common transplant fluid and electrolyte problems, possible causes and interventions

Problem	Possible causes	Interventions
Extracellular fluid (ECF)		
Excess	Renal dysfunction caused by Nephrotoxic drugs Decreased renal blood flow (venocclusive disease [VOD], treatment of shock, steroid therapy, rapid infusion of saline solution)	Diuretics Sodium and fluid restriction Concentration of total parenteral nutrition (TPN), IV medication solutions
Deficit	Acute gastrointestinal graft versus host disease (GVHD) Fever Vomiting Nasogastric drainage Excessive diuretic use	Fluid replacement with similar fluid composition Frequent, accurate assessment of fluid status
Intracellular fluid (ICF)		
Excess (total body excess)	Excessive oral water intake Inappropriate ADH-like syndrome caused by cyclophosphamide	Free water restriction Avoidance of rapid IV infusions
Deficit (total body deficit)	Fever Severe skin GVHD Diabetes insipidus Prolonged artificial respiration Decreased water intake (not a frequent problem)	D_5W or oral water replacement

Continued.

Table 22-2. Common transplant fluid and electrolyte problems, possible causes and interventions—cont'd

Problem	Possible causes	Interventions
Sodium imbalances		
Hypernatremia	Water loss Rapid saline infusion	D_5W or oral water replacement Sodium and fluid restriction: oral, parenteral nutrition (PN), IV solutions, sodium-containing antibiotics Free water restriction
Hyponatremia	Saline loss: Sweating Gastrointestinal losses Severe skin GVHD Excessive free water intake	
Potassium imbalance		
Hyperkalemia	Acute renal failure Spironolactone	Immediate removal of IV and PN potassium Rapid IV administration of hypertonic glucose with insulin Hemodialysis NOTE: Kayexalate enemas or oral solutions are not recommended because of questionable gastrointestinal absorption
Hypokalemia	Amphotericin B Thiazide diuretics Gastrointestinal losses (GVHD, infectious enteritis, emesis) Corticosteroids Anabolism	Increase PN potassium (allows continuous coverage) Potassium piggyback NOTE: Oral replacement generally ineffective because of poor absorption and intolerance
Hypomagnesemia	Renal wasting caused by cyclosporine, amphotericin B, tobramycin, and gentamicin Excessive gastrointestinal losses Anabolism	Increase magnesium in PN IV magnesium bolus
Hypermagnesemia	Diuretics Hypokalemia and hypomagnesemia Respiratory alkalosis Anabolism Hyperkalemia	Phosphate piggybacks
Hypocalcemia	Hypoalbuminemia Excessive phosphate administration	Calcium decreases 0.8 mg by each 0.1 g drop in serum albumin Delete calcium from PN
Hypercalcemia	Tumor lysis Renal failure	Saline hydration/diuretics Steroids Mithramycin Calcitonin

Table 22-3. Major fluid losses after transplant and appropriate replacement

Fluid loss	Recommended replacement
Vomiting	cc/cc with D$_5$ ¼ – ½ NS + electrolytes
Excessive GVHD diarrhea	cc/cc with D$_5$ ¼ – ½ NS + electrolytes
Bright red bloody stools (as in severe gastrointestinal GVHD)	cc/cc of packed red blood cells or whole blood as clinically indicated
Fever/mucositis	Replace only if patient is symptomatic for hypovolemia with D$_5$ ½ NS + electrolytes
Ascites associated with venocclusive disease (VOD)	Replace with albumin, packed red cells

based on the amount lost and clinical symptoms. Whatever the fluid losses, replacement should be made with those of similar composition (Table 22-3).

Nursing assessment of the child's hydration status should include daily weights; vital sign monitoring; examination of skin turgor; daily serum potassium, sodium, glucose, blood urea nitrogen (BUN) and creatinine levels; monitoring of urine specific gravity and gastrointestinal losses; and examination of peripheral pulses for adequate perfusion. Vital sign changes may occur late in the case of hypovolemia, since children can quickly vasoconstrict peripherally in the presence of hypovolemia to maintain adequate blood pressure and preserve blood flow to vital organs. On examination, the higher the coolness of the lower extremity, the more critical the hypovolemia.

Stomatitis

Deterioration of oral mucosa results from the conditioning regimen and can be mild to severe. Strict attention to good oral hygiene is important in minimizing oral colonization of bacteria and fun-

gus. Frequent saline mouth rinses, use of a soft toothbrush, and oral suctioning keeps the mouth clean of mucous and debris and reduces the risk of disseminated infection. Special attention should be given to young children and infants, since they are not capable of independently performing a mouth care regimen. Oral assessments are done every shift to check for dryness, redness, ulcerations, white plaque, and changes in salivation.

Mouth pain resulting from mucosal deterioration can be controlled by topical anesthetics (e.g., dyclone) in the early stages of mucositis. Progressive deterioration and pain may require parenteral narcotics. A morphine drip starting with 0.05 mg/kg is an excellent pain medication. Titrating the medication to severity of pain and vital signs can maintain the child in a relatively pain-free and alert state. At all times, an oral airway should remain at the child's bed in case of obstructions due to mucositis and pharyngeal swelling. Healing of the mucosal lining does not occur until engraftment occurs and granulocytes are seen in peripheral blood smears.

Hemorrhage

Hemorrhagic incidences during marrow aplasia and thrombocytopenia are increased with infection, fever, and graft-versus-host disease. Children should be checked for signs of petechiae, ecchymoses, epistaxis, bleeding gums, hematuria, uncontrolled menses, guaiac positive stools and neurological changes. Daily monitoring of blood counts are important. To prevent and control hemorrhage, platelet counts are maintained above 20,000/mm^3 with the support of random, community and family donors, until child's own megakaryocytes are proliferating. Megakaryocytes do not proliferate until about 1-2 weeks after evidence of engraftment. Packed red blood cell transfusions are needed to maintain a hematocrit between 25-30 percent. Usually 10 cc/kg per transfusion is adequate unless the child is profusely bleeding and then infusions are titrated to vital signs. Treatment of hemorrhage is dependent on the site of bleeding and child's response to platelets. Nasal bleeds can be controlled with packing, pressure and instruction not to blow the nose forcibly. Gastrointestinal bleeding can be minimized with the use of antacids. Provera is administered to control menses. Topical cocaine or thrombin can be applied to gum bleeds. Avoidance of rectal temperatures, intramuscular injections and use of soft toothettes for mouth care help to minimize traumatic bleeding.

Venocclusive disease

Venocclusive disease (VOD) is a clinical syndrome of the liver occurring early after transplant. Children with a history of liver disease before transplant who received high-dose chemoradiotherapy as a conditioning regimen and/or are undergoing a second transplant are at risk for developing VOD after bone marrow transplant. This syndrome involves the fibrous obliteration of the terminal hepatic venules and sublobular veins. This results in inappropriate shunting of blood away from the liver. Fluid containing sodium and albumin is shifted from the intravascular to the extracellular, extravascular space. This results in intravascular volume depletion and subsequent decrease of the renal blood flow. Renal compensatory mechanisms attempt to counteract the intravascular volume loss, creating significant fluid retention with subsequent dramatic weight gain, oliguria, and sodium retention. A vicious cycle develops with the continuance of the abnormal fluid shifts. Clinical manifestations are sudden weight gain, right upper quadrant pain, hepatomegaly, ascites, jaundice, elevated bilirubin, normal or mildly elevated SGOT and alkaline phosphatase, and encephalopathy. Treatment is nonspecific. The therapeutic goal is to facilitate a reversal of intravascular volume depletion. Supporting recommendations are restricting fluid and sodium, maintaining osmotic pressure with colloids, performing infusions (i.e., PRBC, albumin), and using an aldosterone antagonist diuretic (i.e., aldactone). By administering aldactone, renal sodium and water excretion is increased which theoretically helps prevent extravascular accumulation.

Early detection is important in preventing progressive fatal VOD. If the child survives, recovery is gradual following engraftment. Nursing assessments include daily weights, daily abdominal girth measurements, strict intake and output, and central venous pressure monitoring.

Infection

Infections are the major cause of morbidity and mortality after transplant. Malnutrition, lengthy marrow aplasia, long-term hospitalization, break in the cutaneous barrier with marrow aspirations, insertion of right atrial catheters, and radiation predisposes the child to infection. Avoidance of rectal temperatures and medication and urinary catheterizations, early initiation of aggressive pulmonary toilet, consistent mouth care, daily bath with antimicrobial soap, and maintaining isolation are necessary prophylactic infection measures.

Despite prophylactic attempts, infections do occur and are difficult to detect. Children may not produce pus or an inflammatory response as a result of lack of granulocytes.[14] Routine admission surveillance cultures should be done to provide baseline infectious information. Children are usually infected by resident flora, either endogenous (normal flora) or acquired exogenous (from hospital environment), that become a part of the child's normal flora after admission. Culturing should include nose, throat, rectum, and urine.

Consistent monitoring of signs and symptoms of infection should include changes in vital signs, temperature higher than 38.5° C, shaking chills, redness or pain at a site not previously affected, malaise, decreased alertness, cough, increased respiration rate, white plaques in the mouth, and urinary frequency or burning. Skin, mouth, throat, perirectal area, and right atrial catheter site should be checked for redness, swelling, tenderness, and/or drainage. Lungs should be auscultated and respiratory rate monitored. Weekly laminar airflow patient cultures should be taken and monitored for colonization. Any infection left untreated during marrow recovery can lead to dissemination and death.

Broad-spectrum antibiotics are initiated when the granulocyte count drops below 500/mm³ and the child is febrile (38.5° C or higher) despite no causative organisms cultured. With any temperature spike above 38.5° C, a chest x-ray examination is ordered; blood, urine, and throat cultures obtained; and acetaminophen given to reduce fever. More specific antibiotics are prescribed when the causative agent is identified.

Antibiotic therapy should be continued until the child is afebrile and the granulocyte count remains above 500/mm^3 for several days. Antifungal therapy (amphotericin B) can be initiated if the child does not become afebrile after 72 hours of empiric antibiotic therapy or immediately if there has been one or more surveillance sites positive for fungus.[15] Antifungal treatment is continued according to the antibiotic therapy regimen. Persistent fever, blistering of lips, or blisterlike lesions in the mouth may be indicative of herpes simplex viral infection (HSV). Appropriate cultures should be taken and acyclovir treatment ordered. Although acyclovir does not eliminate the virus, it does shorten virus excretion and accelerates crusting and healing of lesions. This infection can spread rapidly causing severe painful mucocutaneous lesions (Fig. 22-1) and if untreated, can progress to gastric infection or HSV pneumonia. The virus can spread to the eyes in young children who place their hands in their mouth and then rub their eyes. Eighty percent of children with seropositive HSV before transplant will develop a HSV infection. The first outbreak will generally occur in the first 2 weeks after transplant, which is usually the height of stomatitis. Once treatment is discontinued, HSV reactivation can occur. Studies are being conducted regarding the usefulness of prophylactic acyclovir in children with seropositive HSV before transplant.

Interstitial pneumonia occurs as a late infectious complication and warrants close pulmonary and vital sign assessment. Initial signs and symptoms are often subtle, including increasing nonproductive, dry cough, slow increase of respiratory rate, fever, tachypnea, and finally radiologic abnormalities.

A diagnosis of interstitial pneumonia is difficult, and most often open lung biopsy is the only definitive diagnostic procedure. Biopsies are performed

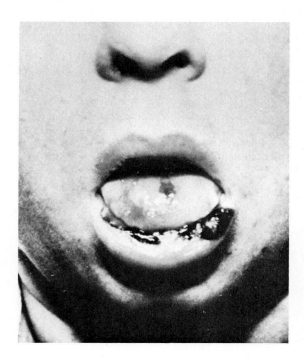

Fig. 22-1. A boy 18 days after transplantation with herpes simplex stomatitis.

within 24 hours of clinically suspected interstitial pneumonia if the child's platelets can be maintained above 50,000/mm^3. The cytomegalovirus (CMV) is the most common type of interstitial pneumonia and has the highest fatality rate. Nearly 90% of those diagnosed with CMV pneumonia die, since there is no adequate treatment.

Idiopathic pneumonia occurring in about one third of patients with interstitial pneumonia is a syndrome where no infectious agent can be identified. This may be a direct toxicity of the intensive chemoradiotherapy and not an infectious process. Signs and symptoms are similar to other interstitial pneumonias. Treatment may require the use of anti-inflammatory agents and supportive mechanical ventilation if the child is unable to support respiratory effort.

Pneumocystis carinii pneumonia has essentially been eliminated since the initiation of post engraftment prophylaxis with trimethoprim-sulfamethoxazole.[16]

Varicella zoster virus infections can occur within the first year after transplant and are treated with acyclovir at the first sign of cutaneous dissemination or visceral involvement. Any suspected lesion should be cultured and the child placed in direct isolation away from other transplantation patients.

Graft versus host disease

The capacity of the body to recognize materials as foreign to themselves and to neutralize, eliminate, or metabolize them with or without injury to the host tissue is the physiologic mechanism known as immunity. This can be either a cell-mediated response (T lymphocytes) or humoral response (B lymphocytes). It is the cell-mediated immune response (antigen sensitive T lymphocyte) that is responsible for the graft versus host disease reaction and threatens 30% to 50% of children with allogeneic grafts.

The donor marrow produces lymphocytes that proliferate, recognize the immunologic incompetent recipient as foreign, and mount an attack at the cellular level against the recipient. Damage results from an accumulation of lymphocytes and macrophages.[17] Immunosuppresive children receiving nonirradiated blood products can have the same physiologic response of graft versus host disease. For this reason, all blood products except marrow are irradiated with 1500 rad before infusion. This adequately inhibits proliferation of lymphocytes without damage to platelets, granulocytes, or red cell function.[18]

Prophylactically, attempts to prevent graft versus host disease include selection of a histocompatible donor, irradiation of all blood products, protective environment, and use of cyclosporine and methotrexate as prophylaxis medications.[18] These medications are intended to reduce and/or delay the reactivation of lymphocytes and antigens by slowing the rate of engraftment.

Methotrexate and cyclosporine as prophylactic agents are given in combination or alone, depending on the institutional protocol. Methotrexate in

low dose is given IV push on specific days after transplant. Cyclosporine is given before transplant and then twice daily either IV or PO for 6 months after transplant. Because of the potential of renal toxicity, cyclosporine levels, BUN, and creatinine are monitored daily and dose adjustments made when creatinine doubles.

Despite prophylaxis, graft versus host disease still occurs. Target organs are the skin, liver, and gastrointestinal tract. One or more of these organs can be involved. Symptoms can be transient and self-limiting or severe and life-threatening. The onset of graft versus host disease can occur as early as 1 to 3 weeks after transplant and is directly associated with engraftment. Diagnosis of acute graft versus host disease is difficult. Often symptoms can be confused with other causes (e.g., drug reactions, viral or fungal infections, irradiation, venocclusive disease or hepatitis.) Assessment of consistent, characteristic lesions and conditions help to determine diagnosis.

Early clinical evidence of acute graft versus host disease can be in the skin. Involvement ranges from mild maculopapular rash to general erythroderma with desquamation reminiscent of second-degree burns. Diagnosis is made by skin biopsy. Liver involvement includes a mild to severe rise in liver function tests associated with right upper quadrant the gastrointestinal tract results from a degeneration of mucosa and mucosa glands and ranges from production of green, watery guaiac positive stools to bright red, bloody stools with evidence of mucosal sloughing. Nausea, vomiting, abdominal pain, and ascites may develop as well. Treatment is directed at reducing the number of donor lymphocytes and alleviating discomfort by managing symptoms of the acute graft versus host disease reaction. Table 22-4 summarizes current medications, doses, and side effects. These drugs are used singularly or in combination with each other, depending on the child's response and the institutional protocol.

Supportive care involves applying creams such as hydrocortisone to the skin to reduce the discomfort of itching. If there is evidence of blistering and

Table 22.4. Current graft versus host disease treatment, dosage, and side effects

Medication	Dosage	Side effects
Cyclosporine	IV: 1.5 mg/kg q.12h. PO: 6.25 mg/kg q.12h.	Rise in bilirubin Doubling of creatinine Renal tubular damage Hypomagnesium Hypertension Tremors, anorexia, nausea, depression, increased hair growth—all reversible by lowering the dose
Antithymocyte globulin (ATG)	15 mg/kg/day (divided into two doses) given every other day × 6 doses	Fevers, chills, tremors Rise in bilirubin Arthralgia Myalgia Serum sickness
Steroids	2 mg/kg divided in four doses q.6h. IV, 1-14 days 1 mg/kg q.6h. 14-21 days, then taper according to clinical response	Glucose intolerance Hypertension Fluid retention Impaired phagocyte function Catabolism
Monoclonal	Variable × 7 days	Serum sickness Arthralgia Effusions B cell proliferation

skin sloughing, application of silver sulfadiazene (silvadene) and use of a burn sheet provide protection against infection.

Fluid losses from gut graft versus host disease can be in excess of several liters per day. Intravenous fluid replacement is given to replace losses. Composition of the solution should be similar to what is being excreted. Monitoring the child's weight, urine ouput, urine specific gravity, vital signs, skin turgor, and stool loss will clinically indicate the degree of hypovolemia created by the loss of fluid. Avoidance of antidiarrheal agents is recommended. They do not decrease the secretory loss of volume in the gut but only decrease the motility of the gut, creating pooling of fluid in the gastrointestinal tract and a false sense of decreased fluid losses from mucosal lining. Morphine sulfate or meperidine may relieve pain and cramping aggravated by oral intake. Depending on the severity of the gastrointestinal involvement, a child may need to be N.P.O. to rest the bowel and diminish nausea and vomiting. Advancing to a normal diet is possible by using a graft versus host disease diet plan (Table 22-5).

As yet, no cure for graft versus host disease has been demonstrated. The family and child need support in dealing with body image changes, frustration, depression, and uncertainty of survival.

Psychosocial impact

Choosing marrow transplantation as an alternative treatment is a family crisis. Although hope and potential gains are great, so too is the emotional cost. Understanding by the transplant team of the factors influencing emotional balance is critical to supporting the family and child. Identification of previous hospitalization and coping styles, degree of geographic dislocation and disruption, and hidden stressors (e.g., marital conflicts, financial problems, recent losses) may help in maximizing the family's coping strategies and minimizing the emotional cost of treatment. It is important that staff not expect to solve all emotional conflicts within families.

Table 22-5. Gastrointestinal graft versus host disease diet recommendation based on clinical symptoms

Phase	Clinical symptoms	Diet	Clinical symptoms of diet intolerance
1 NPO	Gastrointestinal cramping Large volumes of watery diarrhea Gastrointestinal protein losses Depressed serum albumin Severely reduced transit time Small bowel obstruction or diminished bowel sounds Nausea and vomiting	Oral: NPO	
2 Introduction of oral feeding	Minimum gastrointestinal cramping Diarrhea less than 500 ml/day Guaiac negative stools Improved transit time (minimum 1½ hours) Infrequent nausea and vomiting	Oral: Isosmotic, low-residue beverages initially	Increased stool volume or diarrhea Increased emesis Increased abdominal cramping
3 Introduction of solids	Minimum or no gastrointestinal cramping Formed stool	Oral: Allow introduction of solid foods: Minimum lactose Low fiber Low fat Low total acidity Without gastric irritants	As in phase 2
4 Expansion of diet	Minimum or no gastrointestinal cramping Formed stool	Oral: Minimum lactose Low fiber Low total acidity No gastric irritants If stools indicate fat malabsorption: low fat	As in phase 2
5 Resumption of regular diet	No gastrointestinal cramping Normal stool Normal transit time Normal albumin	Oral: Progress to regular diet by introducing restricted food slowly: Acid foods with meals Fiber-containing foods Lactose-containing foods	As in phase 2

Unlike adults, children are in various growth and developmental periods. Despite illness and treatment, growth and development continue. There should be an initial assessment of the child's developmental stage, and adjustments of daily schedule should be made to allow for activities that facilitate development appropriate for the child's age and degree of illness.

Young children need an established routine and designated time for rest and play periods. Parents should be interviewed regarding methods of discipline, so staff and parents can be consistent with their approach and expectation of the child. The nonverbal communication from drawings may assist the nurse in understanding the child's anxieties and perception of treatment.

Adolescents developmentally are caught between the past and future and are attempting to work through independent-dependent conflicts with parents. Both parents and adolescents need help in being open about their feelings without being judgmental. Frustration for the adolescent results from temporarily having to depend on others, often expressing moodiness, secretiveness, resentfulness, and rage. Parents may see themselves needing to be more involved with decision making, monitoring the teenager's activities, and giving advice, especially if the adolescent becomes critically ill.

Parents should be encouraged to divide their energies carefully by alternating with each other in spending time with the sick child and other siblings. Siblings can be resentful or feel left out as attention is focused on the ill child and parents become unavailable.

Particular emotional tones characterize each stage of the transplant. The early pretransplant phase focuses on hope of the possibility of cure from a fatal disease. During the actual transplant period, fear intensifies and particular concern is focused on the potential complications. During the posttransplant period, there is vacillation between fear of losing the child and hope of cure as there is fluctuation in the child's medical condition. At discharge from the hospital, families express ambivalence. They are grateful for being able to leave but concerned and fearful of assuming the major responsibility for daily care of the child. Isolation is increased as the family leaves the supportive network of the transplant staff and other families.

DISCHARGE HOME

Depending on patient proximity to the transplant center, discharge to home could be immediately on discharge from the hospital or as long as 100 days after transplant. The family and child are taught how to care for the central line catheter if still in place, how to give medications at home, what symptoms to observe that may indicate recurrence of graft versus host disease, infection, and bleeding.

Medical follow-up is provided by a local physician, including monitoring of blood counts and maintaining protocol treatments. Protective measures such as avoiding large crowds and not returning to school for 6 to 9 months after the transplant are emphasized. The family and child need reinforcement that return to pretransplant stamina level will be slow and progressive, taking up to 12 months for full energy recovery.

LATE COMPLICATIONS

The majority of long-term complications are secondary to chronic graft versus host disease. This disease may range from mild to severe and may develop as an extension of acute graft versus host disease or after a period of well-being. The manifestations include hyperpigmentation, scleroderma with joint contractures, alopecia, ocular and oral sicca, vaginal and esophageal strictures and webbing, restrictive pulmonary disease, chronic liver disease and generalized wasting. Histologically, chronic graft versus host disease resembles the systemic collagen vascular diseases, especially lupus erythematosus profundus. Children with this disease have a higher incidence of psychosocial problems such as lower self-esteem, poor body image, clinical depression, and emotional instability secondary to immunosuppressive therapy. Psychologic intervention may be indicated if problems are severe and disabling. To prevent late complications, research continues to examine less toxic conditioning regimens, more successful prevention and treatment of graft versus host disease, and faster recovery of immunocompetence in marrow recipients. This will contribute to improving disability-free survival of children treated with marrow transplant.

CONCLUSION

Theoretically, the actual marrow transplant is simple. It is the preparatory treatment and post-transplant complications that create a complex and multifactorial challenge. As active members of the transplant team, nurses require skill and knowledge in pediatrics, oncology, critical care, clinical research, and psychosocial issues of crisis and loss. As optimum care is provided, overall survival and quality of life can improve for those children undergoing marrow transplantation.

REFERENCES

1. Thomas, E.: Bone marrow transplantation: present status and future expectations. In Isselbacher, K., Adams, R., and Braunwald, E., editors: Harrison's principles of internal medicine, New York, 1982, McGraw-Hill, Inc.
2. Parker, N., and Cohen, T.: Acute graft-versus-host disease in allogeneic marrow transplantation, Nurs. Clin. North Am., **18**(3):569, 1983.
3. Nuscher, R., and others: Bone marrow transplantation, Am. J. Nurs. **84**(6):764, 1984.
4. Thomas, E.: Marrow transplantation for malignant diseases, J. Clin. Oncol. **1**(9):517, 1983.
5. Buckner, C., and others: The role of a protective environment and prophylactic granulocyte transfusions in marrow transplantation, Transplant. Proc. **10**(1):255, 1978.
6. Lindgren, P.: The laminar air flow room, Nurs. Clin. North Am. **18**(3):553, 1983.
7. Hutchison, M., and Itoh, K.: Nursing care of patient undergoing bone marrow transplantation for acute leukemia, Nurs. Clin. North Am. **17**(4):697, 1982.
8. Doran, L.: Care of the Hickman catheter in children, Nurs. Clin. North Am. **18**(3):579, 1983.
9. Camitta, B., Storb, R., and Thomas, E.: Aplastic anemia: pathogenesis, diagnosis, treatment and prognosis, N. Engl. J. Med. **306**(12):712, 1982.
10. Caspi, A., and McArtor, R.: Cyclophosphamide-induced cardiomyopathy, Hosp. Formulary **17**:115, 1982.
11. Thomas, E.: Marrow transplantation for marrow failure or leukemia, Compr. Ther. **6**(7):69, 1980.
12. Stream, P., Harrington, E., and Clark, M.: Bone marrow transplantation: an option for children with acute leukemia, Cancer Nurs. **3**(3): 195, 1980.
13. Cunningham, B., and others: Nutritional considerations during marrow transplantation, Nurs. Clin. North Am. **18**(3):585, 1983.
14. Potter, S.: Critical infections in the pediatric oncologic patient, Nurs. Clin. North Am. **16**(4):699, 1981.
15. Meyers, J., Flournoy, N., and Thomas, E.: Nonbacterial pneumonia after marrow transplantation: a review of ten years' experience, Rev. Infect. Dis. **4**(6):1119, 1982.
16. Neiman, P., and others: Interstitial pneumonia following marrow transplantation for leukemia and aplastic anemia. In Gale, R., and Fox, C., editors: Biology of bone marrow transplantation, New York, 1980, Academic Press.
17. Bellanti, J.: Immunology, Philadelphia, 1971, W.B. Saunders Co.
18. Weiden, P., and others: Fatal graft-versus-host disease in a patient with lymphoblastic leukemia following normal granulocyte transfusion, Blood **57**(2):328, 1981.

ADDITIONAL READINGS

Anderson, M., Aker, S., and Hickman, R.O.: The double lumen Hickman catheter, Am. J. Nurs. **82**:272, 1982.

Besinger, W.I., and others: Immunoabsorption for removal of A and B blood group antibodies, N. Engl. J. Med. **304**:160, 1981.

Brown, M., and Kiss, M.: Standards of care for the patient with "graft-versus-host disease" post marrow transplant, Cancer Nurs. **4**:191, 1981.

Buckner, C.D., and others: High-dose cyclophosphamide therapy for malignant disease: toxicity, tumor response and the effects of stored autologous marrow, Cancer **29**:357, 1972.

Cliff R., and others: Allogeneic marrow transplantation for acute lymphoblastic leukemia in remission using fractionated total body irradiation, Leuk. Res. **6**:409, 1982.

Dunlop, J.: Critical problems facing young adults with cancer, Oncol. Nurs. Forum **9**:33, 1982.

Ford, R., McClain, K., and Cunningham, B.: Veno-occlusive disease following marrow transplant, Nurs. Clin. North Am. **18**:563, 1983.

Gardner, G., August, C., Githers, J.: Psychological issues in bone marrow transplantation, Pediatrics **60**:625, 1977.

Johnson, F.L., and others: A comparison of marrow transplantation with chemotherapy for children with acute lymphoblastic leukemia in second or subsequent remission, N. Engl. J. Med. **305**:846, 1981.

Layton, P.B., Gallucci, B.B., and Aker, S.N.: Nutritional assessment of allogeneic bone marrow recipients, Cancer Nurs. **4**:127, 1981.

McKusick, V.A.: Immunogenetics. In Harvey, A.M., editor: The principles and practice of medicine, ed. 12, New York, 1980, Appleton-Century-Crofts.

Meyers, J.D., and others: Prevention of cytomegalovirus infection by cytomegalovirus immune globulin after marrow transplantation, Ann. Intern. Med. **98:**442, 1983.

Patenaude, A.F., Szymanski, L., and Rappeport, J.: Psychological costs of bone marrow transplantation in children, Am. J. Orthopsychiatry **49:**409, 1979.

Sanders, J.E., Thomas, E.D., and the Seattle Marrow Transplant Group: Marrow transplantation for children with non-lymphoblastic leukemia in first remission, Med. Pediatr. Oncol. **9:**423, 1981.

Shulman, H., and others: An analysis of hepatic venocclusive disease and centrilobular hepatic degeneration following bone marrow transplantation, Gastroenterology **79:**1178, 1980.

Stroot, V.: Fluid and electrolytes: a practical approach, ed. 2, Philadelphia, 1977, F.A. Davis Co.

Sullivan, K.M., and others: Late complications after marrow transplantation, Semin, Hematol. **21:**53, 1984.

Tesler, A.S.: High dose total body irradiation prior to bone marrow transplantation, UCLA Cancer Center Bulletin p. 5, 1978.

Thomas, E.D.: Bone marrow failure and bone marrow transplantation. In Petersdorf, R.G., Adams, R.D., and Braunwald, E., editors: Harrison's principles of internal medicine, ed. 10, New York, 1983, McGraw-Hill, Inc.

Weiden, P.L., and others: Antileukemic effect of graft-versus-host disease in human recipients of allogeneic marrow graft, N. Engl. J. Med. **300:**1068, 1979.

Weiden, P. L., and the Seattle Marrow Transplant Team: Graft vs host disease in allogeneic marrow transplantation, In Gale, R.P., and Fox, C.F., editors: Biology of bone marrow transplantation, New York, 1980, Academic Press.

Weiden, P.L., and others: Antileukemic effect of chronic graft versus host disease: contribution to improve survival after allogeneic marrow transplantation, N. Engl. J. Med. **304:**1529, 1981.

Witherspoon, R.P., and others: Recovery of antibody production in human allogeneic marrow graft recipients: influence of time posttransplantation, the presence or absence of chronic graft-versus-host disease and antithymocyte globulin treatment, Blood **58:**360, 1981.

Yusko, J.: Care of patient receiving radiation therapy, Nurs. Clin. North Am. **17:**631, 1982.

CHAPTER 23

Blood products

ROSALIND BRYANT and JOHN KOEPKE

Professionals involved in pediatric hematology and oncology must know what blood products are available, their properties, methods of preparation, actions, efficacy, storage, mode of administration and possible complications. Risks of transfusion range from transmission of infectious diseases to isoimmunization and incompatibility. The physician must weigh the potential danger against expected benefit when ordering a transfusion. From another perspective the nurse must administer many different blood components, each requiring special handling techniques. This chapter will provide those involved in hemotherapy with useful information of blood products, compatibility testing, typing and grouping, expected results of infusion, storage requirements, administration techniques, and complications associated with blood transfusions.

BASICS IN IMMUNOHEMATOLOGY

Basavanthappa defined a blood transfusion described in ancient Egyptian writings as the transference of blood from a healthy individual to one suffering from a grave degree of anemia caused by either hemorrhage or disease.[1] Much later, blood transfusions became an effective means of treatment with the discovery of ABO blood groups by Landsteimer in 1902. This was followed some years later with the discovery of the Rh or Rhesus factor by Wiener. Basic information related to blood grouping is found in Table 23-1. As noted in the table, a person with a particular ABO red cell antigen possesses a corresponding serum antibody, or isoagglutinin. AB is the universal recipient because it possesses no isoagglutinins. Group O is the universal donor, since these red cells possess neither A or B red cell antigens. For example, if the supply of A red cells is exhausted, a type A patient can be safely transfused with type O red cells, since the recipient does not have isoagglutinins directed against the transfused O cells.[2]

Wiener, the discoverer of the Rh factor, noted approximately 85% of all individuals possess the Rh (D) antigen or agglutinogen on the surface of their red cells. The remaining 15% of human beings do not possess the Rh (D) antigen. If an Rh-negative individual receives Rh-positive cells, he would almost always form antibodies to the foreign Rh (D) antigen and become immunized. For this reason, blood is also tested for Rh-negative agglutinin in addition to A and B antigens.

Other contributions that aided the use of blood transfusions included the development of a method for preventing blood clotting for long periods after collection by adding an anticoagulant. Sodium citrate prevents coagulation by chelating calcium ion, a necessary component for clotting. Lautit and Mallison followed with the development of a solution to maintain red cell viability for longer periods than with citrated blood by using acid-citrate dextrose (ACD).[1]

Along with determining compatibility and preservation of blood, fairly strict guidelines for donor centers have been established to aid in the selection of suitable donors. Each prospective donor is assessed for physical fitness and given a brief clinical examination with a determination of the hemoglobin level. Individuals with a history of recent in-

Table 23-1. ABO system antigens and antibodies

Group	Subgroups	Erythrocyte antigens	Serum antibodies (isoagglutinins)	Incidence	
				Whites	Blacks
O	None	None	Anti-A Anti-A$_1$ Anti-B	45%	49%
A	A$_1$	A,A$_1$	Anti-B	40%	27%
	A$_2$	A			
B	None	B	Anti-A Anti-A$_1$	11%	20%
AB	A$_1$B	A,A$_1$,B	None	4%	4%
	A$_2$B	A,B			

fections, severe allergies, malignant diseases, or use of certain medications are not taken as donors. Once the donor is selected, the blood is collected. The blood is tested for hepatitis, AIDS, and blood cell antibodies in addition to ABO and Rh testing. Screening for antibodies is performed by using the antiglobulin test also known as a Coombs' test. This allows for the discovery of antibodies either in serum (the indirect antiglobulin test) or attached to the surface of red cells (the direct antiglobulin test).

Crossmatching with the recipient's blood is performed by testing the serum of the recipient against red cells of the donor to determine the presence or absence of any agglutination and to determine compatibility between donor and recipient. The crossmatch procedure may take 45 minutes to 1 hour. Since many times blood that is ordered is not transfused, a more efficient, yet safe method called type and screen (T and S) procedure has been developed. The blood sample from the patient is tested by a sensitive indirect antiglobulin technique and ABO typing. If no antibodies are found, ABO units can be issued on a moment's notice without the lengthy Coombs' crossmatch procedure.[3]

BLOOD CELL PRODUCTS

In the next several sections, various products available for transfusion will be discussed. Formerly, only whole blood was available for trans-

fusion. With a number of technical breakthroughs, in particular development of the plastic blood collection bags, whole blood is now most often fractionated into its several components, which are transfused separately depending on the individual patient's needs.

Whole blood

In the past, whole blood containing red cells, plasma, and buffy coat had been recognized as the most appropriate treatment for acute hypovolemia. Supplies of blood and its components made possible dramatic advances in surgery and treatment of trauma. Whole blood was greatly overused in the past, often resulting in shortages. Increased concentrations of plasma and potassium and ammonia, increased antigenic load of plasma antigens, and possible infusion of donor antibodies were problems resulting from whole blood transfusions. With the advent of newer separation techniques, use of whole blood has greatly decreased with its various components being used for more specialized purposes.

Today, availability of plastic containers has made it possible to separate freshly donated units of blood into red cells, platelet concentrates, fresh frozen plasma, and antihemophilic cryoprecipitate in a closed system without the hazard of bacterial contamination. Fortunately, the densities of red cells, platelets, white cells, and plasma differ suf-

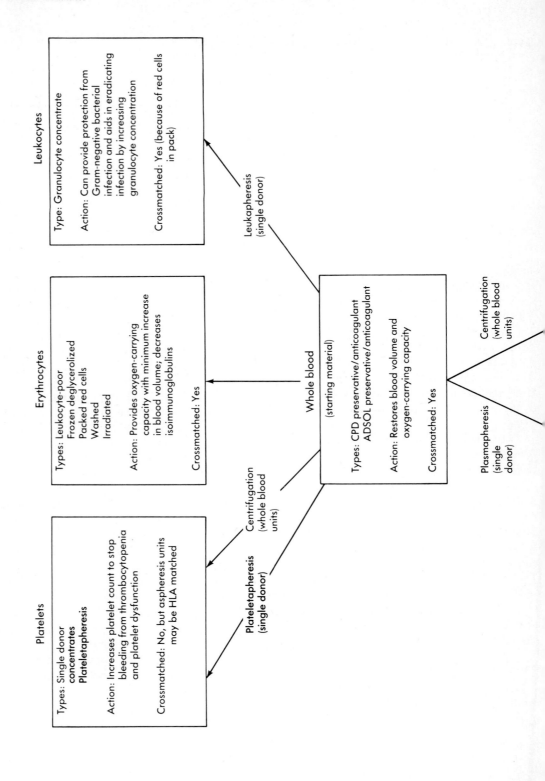

Leukocytes

Type: Granulocyte concentrate

Action: Can provide protection from
Gram-negative bacterial
infection and aids in eradicating
infection by increasing
granulocyte concentration

Crossmatched: Yes (because of red cells
in pack)

Erythrocytes

Types: Leukocyte-poor
Frozen deglycerolized
Packed red cells
Washed
Irradiated

Action: Provides oxygen-carrying
capacity with minimum increase
in blood volume; decreases
isoimmunoglobulins

Crossmatched: Yes

Platelets

Types: Single donor
concentrates
Plateletapheresis

Action: Increases platelet count to stop
bleeding from thrombocytopenia
and platelet dysfunction

Crossmatched: No, but aspheresis units
may be HLA matched

Whole blood

(starting material)

Types: CPD preservative/anticoagulant
ADSOL preservative/anticoagulant

Action: Restores blood volume and
oxygen-carrying capacity

Crossmatched: Yes

Leukapheresis
(single donor)

Centrifugation
(whole blood
units)

Plateletapheresis
(single donor)

Centrifugation
(whole blood
units)

Plasmapheresis
(single
donor)

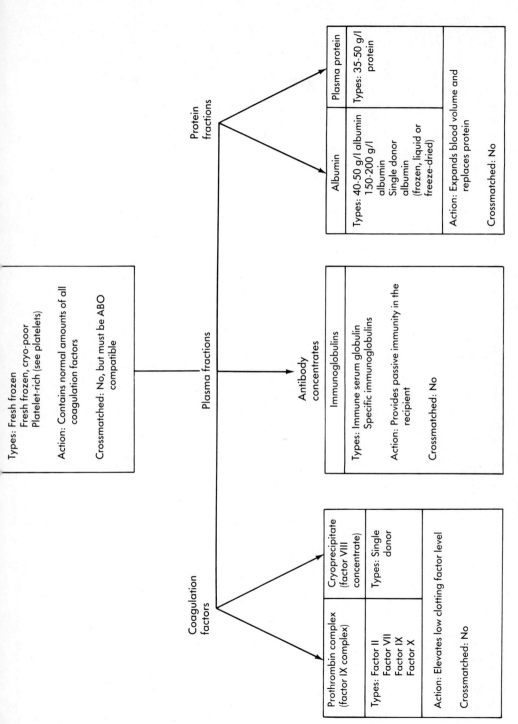

Fig. 23-1. Flow diagram of blood component production.

ficiently to make separation by centrifugation feasible.[4] In treating massive hemorrhage, whole blood may be used or combinations of packed red blood cells (PRBC's), fresh frozen plasma (FFP) and platelet concentrates. There is no longer any need for fresh whole blood; the patient's needs can be met with products available in the blood bank.

Blood is stored at $4° \pm 2°$ C for 35 days in the blood bank refrigerator, having been collected in anticoagulant preservative (CPD-A1 = citrate-phosphate-dextrose adenine solution). This solution has 15% to 20% less citrate ion than A.C.D. solution previously employed. CPD-A1 also maintains a higher diphosphoglycerate (DPG) level in red cells, which has an increased affinity of hemoglobin for oxygen. Banked blood is relatively deficient in platelets, factors V and VIII. Other components must be used if the patient has thrombocytopenia or is factor V or factor VIII deficient. Although whole blood may be transfused during acute hemorrhage, hypovolemic shock, or exchange transfusion, it may be contraindicated in these situations of adequate blood volume and availability of specific components.

Administration must include use of a filter or microaggregate filter recipient set (to be discussed later) to remove microaggregates of platelets, leukocytes, and fibrin found in whole blood. The blood warmer was developed to avoid profound hypothermia that may occur with transfusion of large volumes of blood at $4°$ C. Clinicians working with patients with renal failure who are receiving blood should observe the patient for signs of cardiac arrhythmias caused by an increase in serum potassium level. The usual time for a transfusion is no more than 4 hours through a 20- to 18-gauge needle. In the young child, volumes may be less, but blood should also be infused over 3 to 4 hours using a 22-gauge needle.

Red blood cells (packed cells)

The most commonly used blood product is red blood cells, which are given to raise hematocrit and hemoglobin levels. Red cells carry less risk of volume overloading and are indicated in any anemic patient with (1) heart failure—to prevent circulatory overload; (2) renal failure because of added K^+ and H^+ in whole blood; (3) bone marrow failure; (4) debilitated, elderly, or young patients.

The advantages of using red blood cells are several and include the following:

1. Decreased volume load
2. Decreased citrate load
3. Decreased waste products load (K^+, ammonia, Na^+, organic acid)
4. Decreased risk of reactions to plasma antigens
5. Risk of transmitting serum hepatitis may be reduced (this is controversial)

The disadvantages of red blood cells are as follows:

1. Slow flow rate caused by increased viscosity (Packed cells may be diluted with normal saline to increase flow rate.)
2. Inadequate volume replacement in acute blood loss
3. Deficiency of coagulation factors
4. Deficiency of plasma proteins

Red blood cells are available in several forms, as listed in Fig. 23-1. Red blood cells are prepared, by sedimentation or centrifugation, from a single unit of whole blood. A unit of packed cells contains less plasma and smaller amounts of plasma constituents because it is the component remaining after removal of most of the plasma. Extensive use of red cell transfusions allows the community blood bank to prepare many units of platelets, cryoprecipitate, fresh frozen plasma, albumin, plasma protein fraction, and gamma globulin. This makes possible the use of various components from 1 unit of blood for several patients.

In a child, 5 cc/kg of packed red cells should raise the hemoglobin 1 g. For example, a 20-kg child with a hemoglobin of 7 g/dl should be transfused 300 cc of packed red cells to raise the hemoglobin to 10 g/dl. Most children can safely receive 15 ml/kg of packed cells as a constant infusion at a rate of 5 ml/kg/hr.

Children requiring more than 15 ml/kg to obtain an acceptable hemoglobin level may be transfused over 2 days at 10 to 15 ml/kg/day. When more must be transfused in 1 day, packed cells may be

given with several hours between the two transfusions.

When red blood cells are prepared from a single
plastic container, they have a shelf life of 24 hours
from the time of preparation. However, if red cells
are prepared in the closed multibag system, the red
cells have the same dating period as the original
container of whole blood. The storage and administration is essentially the same as for whole blood.

Frozen red cells

Frozen red blood cells are separated by centrifugation. Plasma is removed and the cells diluted
with approximately 100 cc of sterile glycerol cryo-
protective solution. The glycerolized cells are frozen and can be stored at a temperature of $-80°$ C
($-112°$ F) or colder for years. The freezing process allows blood to be frozen and stored for autologous transfusion or for stock piling of rare cell
types. Once thawed, they must be used within 24
hours. Thawed red cells are sequentially washed
with electrolyte solutions containing decreasing
amounts of glycerol.

Although frozen red cells have numerous advantages over conventionally stored blood, a major
disadvantage is the greater expense of processing.
Extensive washing used to remove glycerol blood
group antibodies, microaggregation plasma proteins, plasma electrolytes and other potentially toxic products is expensive.

Leukocyte-poor red cells

Another type of red cell preparation is the leukocyte-poor red cell pack. The leukocyte-poor red
cell concentrate contains at least 80% of the original red cells in the donor unit but less than 25%
of the leukocytes from the original unit. The preparation of leukocyte-poor blood can be performed
by centrifugation, filtration, freezing, and washing
or by washing techniques alone.

IRRADIATION OF BLOOD CELL PRODUCTS

Irradiation of red cell concentrates or other blood
components is done for any case in which the recipient may be immunoincompetent. This includes
intrauterine transfusion (IUT), exchange transfusion following IUT, and platelet and granulocyte
transfusions in leukemia or other patients with a
malignancy who may be receiving chemotherapy.
Irradiation of blood products is the method of
choice for preventing graft versus host disease in
transplant recipients and also can be used for the
immunosuppressed host.[5] Irradiation with 1500 to
5000 cGy (centiGrays or rads) is effective in destroying the replicating ability of the transfused
lymphocyte. Reducing the number of viable lymphocytes can also be accomplished by use of frozen
deglycerolized red blood cells, red blood cells prepared by inverted centrifugation, by automated
washing techniques or cotton wool filtration.[5] Both
leukocyte-poor red cell concentrates and irradiated
red cell concentrates are similar to red blood cells
in their dosage, administration, and hazards.

PLATELETS, RANDOM DONOR UNIT

Platelets are megakaryocyte cytoplasmic fragments necessary for normal blood coagulation.
They are decreased in a variety of conditions. Platelets can be separated from a unit of whole blood,
separated from platelet-rich plasma, or separated
by plateletapheresis and concentrated for more efficient transfusion.

The platelet concentrate consists of platelets separated from whole blood collected from a single
donor. Whole blood must be maintained at 20° to
24° C and concentrate must be separated within 6
hours. The expiration date is 72 hours after collection from whole blood.

A single donor unit of platelets contains not less
than 5.5×10^{10} platelets suspended in 40 to 50 ml
of plasma. It is stored under constant agitation (on
a rotator) at 20° to 24° C. The usual dose in a
pediatric patient with bleeding and a platelet count
below 25×10^9/liter is 0.2 units/kg of platelets.
The half-life of platelets is 3 or 4 days, so transfusions must be repeated every 2 to 4 days.[6]

PLATELETS, APHERESIS UNITS

Platelets prepared by apheresis are similar to single donor unit platelets. However, apheresis units
generally contain more than 3.3×10^{11} platelets.[7]

Apheresis means the separation of cells from plasma and returning plasma back to the donor.[8]

Plateletapheresis platelet concentration is prepared by centrifugal separation of platelets from whole blood with a continuous or intermittent return of platelet-poor whole blood to the donor. Consequently, numerous platelets are collected from a single donor. Each plateletapheresis platelet concentrate contains approximately 3.5×10^{11} platelets in an average volume of 300 cc.

Platelets, either pooled single donor units or apheresis units, are indicated for the treatment of bleeding resulting from thrombocytopenia or abnormality of platelet function. They also may be useful prophylactically in thrombocytopenia secondary to chemotherapy to maintain adequate levels of circulating platelets and to prevent bleeding.

As with other blood products, filters should be used when platelets are transfused. A nonwettable clot filter is preferred, since microaggregate filters tend to retain platelets. Platelets should be administered as rapidly as possible using a rate of approximately 10 min/unit. When there is a possibility of fluid overload, the infusion can be slowed to infuse over 1 to 2 hours but no longer than 4 hours. A platelet count may be ordered 1 to 2 hours after transfusion to confirm effectiveness of the transfusion.

Chills and fever reactions are common in patients receiving platelet transfusions and are often caused by immunization of platelet and leukocyte antigens from previous transfusions. It is now recognized that refractory patients can be successfully transfused with platelets from HLA-compatible siblings or from unrelated donors matched as closely as possible for similar HLA phenotypes. Ideally, in the future, compatible platelets can be supplied to isoimmunized thrombocytopenic patients, decreasing patient reactions to platelet infusions.

GRANULOCYTES

A granulocyte pack is a concentrate of separated leukocytes. Such a preparation may also contain a large number of platelets and red blood cells, depending on the method of preparation. Granulocytes can be prepared by centrifugation and/or sedimentation with chemical agents from single units of fresh whole blood. The most common method of preparation is granulocyte apheresis. In granulocyte apheresis, blood is drawn from a donor, and granulocytes are removed by centrifugation or filtration in a manner analogous to plateletapheresis.

Granulocyte concentrates are used as supportive therapy in neutropenic (granulocytes $<0.5 \times 10^9$/ liter) patients with Gram-negative bacterial infections that are not responsive to antibiotics (see Chapter 24 on management of infections). Granulocyte transfusions have been used successfully in septic leukopenic patients and in patients undergoing aggressive chemotherapy with refractory neutropenia.

A significant disadvantage of granulocyte concentrates is that they take a number of hours to collect and must be infused within 24 hours of collection. Granulocytes are kept at 20° to 24° C until used for transfusion. Granulocytes are infused using a standard filter, since the microaggregate filters will also filter out granulocytes. They are given at a rate of 1 unit over 4 hours.

Efficacy of the pheresis procedure (cell separator) is measured by the number of circulating granulocytes harvested and ranges from 5 to 30 $\times$ 10^9. The number of granulocytes may also be increased by premedicating the donor with corticosteroids. In studies reported to date, the most striking beneficial effect has been achieved in patients transfused daily for at least 3 or 4 days who have had lysis of fever and in some cases cures.[4] Most common side effects exhibited during granulocyte treatment are chills, fever, and sometimes severe hypotension. These side effects have been minimized by administering the transfusion at no more than 10^{10} cells/hr and premedication before the transfusion[4] (see Chapter 24 on management of infections).

PLASMA COAGULATION FACTORS

The recognized plasma coagulation factors most frequently encountered, cryoprecipitate and factor

IX complex (factors II, VII, IX, and X), will be discussed in this section (see Fig. 23-1).

Cryoprecipitate is a preparation that concentrates factor VIII and fibrinogen obtained either from plasma or plasmapheresis units. The process involves freezing and thawing plasma and subsequent collection of insoluble precipitate. It is used as a source of factors VIII and XIII and fibrinogen.

Single donor factor VIII cryoprecipitate is the mainstay of therapy for classic (antihemophilic factor deficient) hemophilia. It is available frozen and as a lyophilized superconcentrate in powder form, which must be kept refrigerated. Both products may be kept for at least a year.

This component is not only used for treatment of classic hemophilia but also von Willebrand's disease. It is also useful for replacing fibrinogen or factor XIII. ABO compatible cryoprecipitate is preferred but not required. When large volumes of ABO incompatible cryoprecipitate are given, the recipient may develop a positive direct Coombs' test and even mild hemolysis.

Each unit contains an average of 80 units of factor VIII and 200 mg of fibrinogen in 5 to 15 ml of plasma. It must be thawed at 37° C before transfusion and must be given intravenously through a microfilter within 6 hours after thawing. It should be stored at room temperature after thawing.

When cryoprecipitate is transfused as a source of fibrinogen, it may be expected that half the activity will be lost in the first half hour. The remainder will survive with a half-life of 36 to 90 hours.

Normal dosage is considered 4 bags cryoprecipitate/10 kg of body weight repeated at intervals to maintain fibrinogen levels above 100 mg/dl. These patients should be monitored by periodic partial thromboplastin time (PTT). The PTT is the most readily available screening test for coagulation factor deficiencies. It is designed to detect all clinically significant coagulation factor deficiencies, except factor VII and factor XIII.[5]

FACTOR IX COMPLEX

Factor IX complex is a stable, dried, purified, plasma fraction consisting of coagulation factors II (prothrombin), IX (Christmas factor), and X (Stuart-Prower factor). Each container has approximately 500 units of factor IX and roughly the same levels of factors II, VII, and X as in fresh normal plasma.

It is intended for use in treatment of patients with deficiency of factor IX or infants with significant hemorrhage as a result of factor II, VII, IX, and X deficiency. Children and adults with proven factor II, VII, IX, and X deficiency caused by acquired hepatic insufficiency who are bleeding or being considered for surgery are treated with factor IX complex. The prothrombin time (PT) is used to monitor levels of factors II, V, VII, and X.[5]

The coagulation concentrates carry the same high risk of hepatitis and AIDS as other concentrates prepared from plasma pools of large numbers of donors. There is also a fair amount of evidence that coagulation concentrates have some tendency to induce thromboses in the recipient.[4] For these reasons, it may be wise to use plasma transfusion therapy for milder episodes of bleeding. For more detailed discussion on disorders related to reduced levels of plasma coagulation factors, see Chapter 16 on hemophilia.

PLASMA AND PLASMA FRACTIONS
Fresh frozen plasma

Single donor fresh frozen plasma (FFP) is plasma separated from a freshly donated single unit of blood and frozen within 6 hours after collection. Freezing is done in a mechanical freezer at or below −40° C or with a combination of solid carbon dioxide and an organic solvent such as alcohol.[8] When continuously maintained at temperatures of −18° C or colder (preferably below −30° C), FFP has an expiration date 1 year after collection. When thawed immediately before use, it is a source of all plasma coagulation factors.

Single donor FFP is used in treatment of patients with deficiencies of clotting factor V, XI, and XIII and when specific concentrates for factor VIII, or II, VII, IX, or X are not available. It is also useful for treatment of multiple deficiencies caused by liver disease, defibrination syndrome, or disseminated intravascular coagulopathy. However, FFP should not be used when the coagulopathy can be corrected with a more specific therapy (e.g., vitamin K or cryoprecipitate).

FFP cryoprecipitate-poor, is prepared by thawing FFP at 4° C and then removing the cold precipitated AHF (antihemophilic factor). The plasma liquid contains only small amounts of cryoprecipitated AHF. This plasma is primarily used as a volume expander and is infused over a 4-hour period. Adverse side effects of FFP include chills and fever, allergic reactions, circulatory overload, viral hepatitis, possibly cytomegalovirus (CMV), and citrate toxicity.

The usual FFP unit includes 225 to 275 ml of anticoagulated plasma, which contains about 400 mg of fibrinogen, 200 units of factor VIII, 200 units of factor IX, and other coagulation factors in concentrations of 0.7 to 10 units/ml.

To provide small volumes of FFP needed for the pediatric patient, several methods may be used. A whole unit of FFP can be thawed and aliquoted for use in treatment of several children. However this method may not be cost-effective, since once thawed, the plasma should be used within a 6-hour period.

ABO-compatible FFP is transfused into recipients within 6 hours after thawing using a clot filter at a rate of about 10 ml/min.

Protein fractions (albumin and plasma protein fraction)

Plasma volume expanders of choice are albumin concentrate and its plasma protein fraction (PPF) because they can be heated to 60° C for 10 hours, thereby inactivating the hepatitis virus.

Two main functions of albumin and PPF are to maintain effective oncotic pressure by retaining water in the blood; and secondly, the transportation of nutrients, drugs, pigments, enzymes, hormones, and trace elements throughout the body, since albumin serves as a carrier protein.

The physiochemical quality of stored albumin solutions is influenced by several factors:

1. Albumin prepared from FFP is more stable.

2. Albumin solutions are more stable at 5° C ± 3° C than at room temperature even if stored for up to 5 years.

3. Albumin solution is more stable than lyophilized albumin.

Albumin is used to restore or maintain blood volume in a hypovolemic patient while crossmatching is being completed for transfusion of other blood products. It is also indicated in disorders with excessive loss of albumin and/or depressed synthesis of albumin such as extensive burns.

Administration of a unit of plasma is equivalent to 50 ml of 25% salt-poor albumin or 200 ml of either PPF or 5% albumin in restoring blood volume.[9] The usual rate of infusion of albumin is 5 to 10 ml/min. Filtering is not necessary.

One of the significant side effects of plasma protein administration may be sudden development of hypotension. Rate of transfusion should be slowed until blood pressure gradually returns to normal. Other possible side effects of albumin administration are circulatory overload, microbial contamination of the product, nausea and vomiting, chills, fever, and urticaria.

Antibody concentrates (immunoglobulins)

Immunoglobulins are antibody concentrates prepared from the fractionation of plasma. They contain mostly IgG with little IgA or IgM. Immunoglobulin prepared from plasma is harvested from persons with high titers of specific antibodies following recovery from certain illnesses or deliberate immunization by certain agents (see Fig. 23-1).

Intravenous human immunoglobulins are classified into three categories by preparation: enzymatically modified IgG preparation, chemically modified IgG preparation, and further purified IgG preparations. The enzymatically modified IgG preparation contains approximately 50% intact IgG, which has a half-life as long as several days. Chemically modified IgG preparations are treated with chemical agents possessing a low relative molecular mass. Chemically modified IgG preparation reacts with the globulins and possesses a longer half-life than enzymatically modified IgG preparation. Further purified IgG preparations contain a quantity of intact IgG molecules, including intact Fc-fragments, which are impaired or absent in both chemically and enzymatically modified preparations.

Fc-pieces in the IgG molecule are responsible for phagocytosis of antibody-coated micro-organisms, intracellular killing, and binding of antigen-antibody complexes to Fc-receptors of cells. These preparations have a normal biologic half-life for globulins of between 23 and 28 days.[8]

Immunoglobulins are harvested from plasma of donors who have artificially acquired immunity or donors who have naturally acquired immunity. Preparation of normal immunoglobulins from plasma of the donor retains at least 80% of the protein as assessed by ultracentrifugation, electrophoresis, or gel-filtration chromatography. The liquid immunoglobulin preparation should be stored at $5°$ C $\pm$ $3°$ C and below $25°$ C as a freeze-dried preparation.[8] The liquid preparation can be stored for as long as 3 years.

Immunoglobulin preparations are used as follows: (1) prophylaxis against measles and hepatitis A; (2) hepatitis B prophylaxis; (3) tetanus immunoglobulin for prophylaxis in a nonimmunized wounded patient; (4) rabies immunoglobulin for postexposure prophylaxis; (5) varicella-zoster immunoglobulin for prophylaxis in an immune-suppressed patient exposed to chickenpox; (6) post bone marrow transplant patients to increase immune defenses; (7) Rh (D) immunoglobulin to suppress development of anti-antibodies; and (8) poliomyelitis immunoglobulin for prophylaxis in unvaccinated subjects.[8]

Side effects of immunoglobulins include anaphylactoid responses, which tend to dissipate with slowing of transfusion rate. Some less common side effects are flushing, headache, chills, nausea, and rarely infection with hepatitis B if the immunoglobulin preparation is contaminated with the hepatitis virus.

AUTOLOGOUS TRANSFUSIONS

The concept of autologous transfusion has been considered since the nineteenth century but is rarely used. Autologous transfusion is the infusion of blood or fractions of blood derived from the recipient's own blood.

There are a number of advantages to autologous transfusions. Primarily, the use of autologous blood assures a supply, although somewhat limited, of compatible blood for the recipient and is particularly useful for the rare blood type recipient. Because the patient is receiving his own blood, risks of disease transmission are negligible. Grouping and compatibility errors are minimized and reactions to soluble allergens and exposure to foreign antigens are avoided. Some patients having religious beliefs (e.g., Jehovah's Witnesses) prohibiting acceptance of homologous blood may accept autologous transfusion. Another possible advantage of autologous transfusion systems is that other stored blood supplies are conserved.

Three basic strategies for autologous transfusion have been developed[4]:

1. Predeposit or predonation for future need
2. Salvage of intraoperative blood losses
3. Hemodilution by withdrawing blood immediately following induction of anesthesia and replacement with plasma expanders

Predeposit autologous transfusions are obtained to provide blood for future elective surgery. The donor's suitability for this type of transfusion is determined by the requesting physician who must decide which is safer for the patient—to donate his own blood or to receive it from another donor. Autologous transfusions have no age limits. Units are subjected to typing and other serologic testing, primarily as a check for identity of the unit. The donor may be asked to mark or sign the unit for positive identification at the time of transfusion. This, however, is not useful with surgical procedures.

A potential disadvantage of predeposit autologous transfusions is the red cell deficits may be poorly tolerated during periods of more intensive donations if multiple units are drawn. Some physicians prescribe supplemental iron therapy to optimize red cell production. Another disadvantage of autologous transfusion is the inconvenience to the blood bank personnel for additional processing, storage, and labeling requirements needed for autologous transfusions. Although all these requirements pertain to all blood units, the detail in tracking and safely storing a specific unit for a specific recipient can be extensive.

Salvaged autologous blood is recovered from an operative site, which is processed in some manner and later reinfused. Advantage to this type of infusion is elimination of waiting for grouping and compatibility testing. It has been used successfully in a wide variety of surgical procedures, including open heart procedures, ruptured ectopic pregnancy, hip replacements, and chest trauma. Blood that has been obtained by using continuous flow centrifugation may have grossly hemolysed plasma, which should be removed before reinfusion.

Autologous blood can be obtained after induction of anesthesia by hemodilution of the patient when using heart-lung machines and reinfused at the completion or even during the procedure. Hemodilution has been used in cardiopulmonary bypass for heart surgery and hip replacement and in patients with occlusive cerebral or coronary artery disease. Autoinfusions are contraindicated when salvaged blood may contain viable tumor cells that could be reinfused into the patient. Finally, if the bowel is entered or if the patient has peritonitis, such blood would not be suitable for reinfusion. The blood can be stored up to 24 hours at 2° to 6° C if necessary.

EXCHANGE TRANSFUSIONS

Exchange transfusion is an attempt to replace most or all of the recipient's red blood cells and/or plasma with compatible red blood cells and/or plasma from one or more donors.[5] Exchange transfusion has been used to treat hemolytic disease of the newborn (HDN) caused by Rh, ABO, and other blood group incompatibilities. The exchange transfusion performed to remove damaged red cells and circulating bilirubin from newborn infants with HDN or erythroblastosis fetalis has been drastically reduced with the almost universal use of Rh (anti-D) immune globulin (Rh-Ig). Consequently,

the most common reason to perform exchange transfusion today is for hyperbilirubinemia or other chemical problems in the premature infant.[5] Physiologic hyperbilirubinemia occurs both in the term and premature infant. Increased rate of destruction of red cells coupled with limited capacity of the liver to conjugate bilirubin during the first weeks of the newborn's life can lead to hyperbilirubinemia. This transient delay in liver enzyme adaptation is more prolonged in the premature infant.

Hyperbilirubinemia in the term newborn is commonly associated with ABO hemolytic disease. Hyperbilirubinemia caused by Kell, C, E, and other immune antibodies is much less common. Hyperbilirubinemia may also be associated with breast feeding, hereditary disorders of red cells, certain drugs administered to mother or infant, and intrauterine or other perinatal infections.

In an infant with HDN, the decision to perform an exchange transfusion is made when the cord blood hemoglobin is greater than 11 to 13 g/dl or when the serum unconjugated bilirubin is expected to or does exceed 20 mg/dl.

Early exchange transfusion is usually needed in infants with ABO hemolytic disease even when the cord hemoglobin concentration is greater than 12 g/dl. Transfusions are delivered via the cord to the peritoneal cavity from where they are absorbed into the circulation.

In general, a single unit of blood will allow a two volume exchange of the infant with a removal of 75% to 85% of infant red cells. The following formula can be used for calculating the efficiency of the exchange[5]:

$$\%R = \left[\frac{(V\text{-}S)}{V} \right] N$$

R: The percent of infant cells remaining in circulation after exchange
V: The estimated blood volume of the infant
S: The syringe size or aliquot volume sequentially removed and infused during exchange
N: The number of removal/infusion cycles performed

In removal of bilirubin, exchange transfusion

with a single unit of blood on two separate occasions is better because it allows an interval between exchanges during which additional bilirubin may diffuse from the tissues into the bloodstream.

Effectiveness of phototherapy has greatly decreased the number of exchange transfusions needed. Phototherapy decreases the rate of serum unconjugated bilirubin production by photooxidation of bilirubin into other water-soluble, excretable, nontoxic compounds. Phenobarbital administered to the mother just before delivery or to the newborn reduces hyperbilirubinemia by inducing bilirubin conjugating enzyme activity. Whether exchange transfusion, phototherapy, or phenobarbital is the critical therapy, all are aimed at reducing free unconjugated bilirubin, which can cause permanent brain damage known as kernicterus. Following is a list of reported complications and incidence of mortality in exchange transfusions. Many of these are directly related to the experience and skill of the individual performing the procedure:*

Acid-base and electrolyte complications
  Hyperkalemia
  Hypocalcemia
  Citrate toxicity
  Acidosis
  Hypernatremia
Metabolic
  Hypoglycemia
  Hypothermia
Mechanical
  Umbilical vein perforation
  Hydrothorax
Infection
  Cytomegalovirus
  Endocarditis
Thromboembolic
  Air embolism
  Thromboembolism
  Portal vein thrombosis

Gastrointestinal
  Necrotizing enterocolitis
  Bowel perforation
  Portal hypertension
Cardiac
  Volume overload
  Arrhythmias
  Cardiac arrest
Hematologic
  Thrombocytopenia
  Overheparinization (if heparinized blood is used)
  Graft versus host disease
  Sickling of donor blood
Miscellaneous
  Retrolental fibroplasia
  Intracranial hemorrhage

TRANSFUSION REACTIONS

Over 12 million homologous blood components are transfused annually to approximately 3 million patients in the United States alone. Benefits of these products do not occur without risks. Up to 5%, or 150,000 patients, incur immediate adverse reactions and another 7%, or 210,000, delayed reactions.[10] Although most reactions are not life-threatening, the potential for harm exists with each transfusion, and so the use of blood should not be taken lightly. The physician responsible for the transfusion must assess the risks versus the benefits and transfuse only when the benefits of the transfusion outweigh the risks. The physician also must be capable of recognizing transfusion reactions and be prepared to promptly manage these complications should they occur in the recipient. Table 23-2 summarizes the most frequently developed adverse reactions and their clinical and laboratory features.

TRANSFUSION TECHNIQUES

Transfusion procedures must include selection of needle gauge (refer to each blood product discussed), filter, infusion monitoring devices, and blood warmers.

Filters

Microaggregates of platelets, fibrin, and cell debris begin to accumulate in blood after only a few

---

*Luban, N.L.C., and Keating, L.J.: Hemotherapy of the infant and premature, Arlington, Va., 1983, American Association of Blood Banks.

Table 23-2. Common adverse reactions to transfusion therapy

Reaction	Component/product	Clinical features	Laboratory features
Hemolysis (acute hemolytic transfusion reaction [AHTR])	Whole blood packed red cells	Tachycardia, apprehension/agitation; pain at infusion site, fever, chills, flushing; pain in back, flank, and abdomen; dyspnea and chest pain; generalized bleeding, hypotension/shock, nausea/vomiting; hemoglobinuria	Positive direct antiglobulin (Coombs' test); decreased haptoglobin; elevated bilirubin, hemoglobinuria, hemoglobinemia, hemosiderinuria, methemalbumin, spherocytosis, elevated lactic dehydrogenase, intravascular coagulopathy: hypofibrinogenemia, thrombocytopenia, and decreased factors V and VIII
Hemolysis (delayed hemolytic transfusion reaction [DHTR])	Same components listed for AHTR	Primary alloimmunizations: Subtle 10-14 days after transfusion. Secondary alloimmunizations: See clinical features for AHTR Jaundice Purpura 1-5 days after transfusion	Primary alloimmunizations: Decreased hemoglobin Mild hyperbilirubinemia Red blood cell antibodies. Secondary alloimmunizations: Positive direct antiglobulin Decreased haptoglobin Decreased hemoglobin red blood cell antibodies
Febrile (nonhemolytic) *most common reaction*	Whole blood packed red blood cells; plasma	Fever within 1-2 hours after transfusion. Cold sensation, headache/flushing, tachycardia, palpitations, malaise	No reliable test
Allergic (mild) *second most common reaction*	Plasma constituents	Limited to skin: itching, hives, urticaria, erythema, rash. Anxiety/discomfort	No blood test
Allergic (anaphylaxis)	Plasma in any product	Rapid onset (within minutes of starting transfusion) flushing/dyspnea, wheezing, hypotension/shock. Explosive gastrointestinal symptoms: vomiting, cramping, diarrhea. Anxiety. Tightening chest. Itching. Arrest/death	No blood test
Pulmonary noncardiogenic edema	Whole blood packed red cells, granulocytes, platelets	Anxiety, fever, chills, cough, cyanosis, shock. X-ray: bilateral pulmonary infiltrates. Hypoxia. Respiratory distress. Potentially fatal with rapid onset	

Table 23-2. Common adverse reactions to transfusion therapy—cont'd

Reaction	Component/product	Clinical features	Laboratory features
Circulatory overload	More common with whole blood or excessive volume of any component	Dry cough, hoarseness, rales at base of lungs, cyanosis, dyspnea, feelings of chest tightness X-ray: pulmonary edema Bounding pulse	
Hypothermia	Massive transfusion	Chills, irregular pulse	Decrease blood pH
Hemosiderosis (iron overload)	Red blood cells or whole blood	Hyperplasia, anemia Cardiomyopathy Jaundice Hepatomegaly Fatigue, pallor, dyspnea, tachycardia	Decrease ferritin levels Increase iron concentrations and iron-binding capacity
Graft versus host disease (GVHD)	Lymphocytes Granulocytes Red blood cells	Fever, rash, hepatitis, severe diarrhea Bone marrow suppression Lymphadenopathy Hepatosplenomegaly Hemolytic anemia Pancytopenia	Pancytopenia Abnormal liver function studies
Infection transmission Hepatitis B Hepatitis non A	All blood products except albumin, plasma, protein fraction, and immune serum globulin (hepatitis B and non A, non B)	Fatigue, anorexia, upper quadrant pain, nausea, myalgia, coryza, photophobia, rash, petechiae, pruritis, arthralgia, dark urine, clay-colored stools, cervical adenopathy (hepatitis B and non A, non B)	Elevated liver enzymes: ALT, AST, and ALP Increase serum and urine bilirubin with jaundice HB Ag 2-6 weeks before onset HB Ag 3-6 weeks to 10 weeks Antibodies to B surface antigen, B core antigen, and Be[a] antigen
Cytomegalovirus (CMV)	Fresh whole blood or packed cells	Fever, splenomegaly (40%) Neutropenia Posttransfusion syndrome	CMV antibodies Viremia Atypical lymphocytes of infectious mononucleosis 3-6 weeks after transfusion
Chemical Toxicity Hypercalcemia	Massive transfusion of whole blood (rare) Stored blood cells release K	Gastrointestinal hyperactivity (nausea, vomiting, colic, diarrhea) Vague muscle weakness, paresthesias, flaccid paralysis, apprehension, irregular pulse, cardiac arrest	Hyperkalemia
Dilutional coagulopathy	Massive transfusion	Excessive wound or needle site bleeding Hypotension Disseminated intravascular coagulation Shock Renal ischemia Renal failure	Thrombocytopenia

hours of storage. The number of aggregates progressively increases during storage. They vary in size from 15 to 200 μ and can be filtered out of the blood if appropriate pore size filter is used. One manufacturer produces a burette and pediatric size micropore filter in the same set. Because of lack of pediatric filters, a small nylon mesh containing 170 to 200 micron filters has been used for neonatal transfusions. Micropore filters can be used for platelet transfusions, but regular filters are used for granulocyte transfusions.

Disadvantages encountered with some filters include the following:

(1) There may be relatively small surface area, which may be clotted with debris. When blocked, the increased pressure required to push blood through the filter may cause hemolysis.

(2) Red cell destruction can occur with woven stainless steel mesh micropore filters.

(3) Only one of the filters is designed for the pediatric patient because of the lack of market for these filters.

Infusion monitoring devices

Infusion pumps and syringe pumps are used to control volume and rate at approximately 10 ml/hr. Controlled volume decreases the chance of hemolysis occurring.

Blood warmers

Stored blood may be administered without prior warming, provided it is infused slowly. When blood is given in large quantities over a short period of time or when small volumes must be rapidly given, the blood should be warmed to prevent hypothermia and cardiac arrhythmias. In addition, warmed blood should be administered to patients who have potent cold-reacting antibodies.

Blood may be warmed by passing it through a disposal (plastic) coiled tubing that is immersed in a water bath with a controlled temperature. The warming device monitors bath temperature and alerts the user to above-limit bath temperature, which could cause red cell hemolysis. In the dry heat, blood is passed through a disposable bag that

is exposed to a heated metal surface. This unit also has a temperature display and alarms for overheated conditions.

Blood should never be heated under running hot water or in a microwave oven, because of the difficulty in controlling the temperature and the potential for hemolysis.

Disadvantages associated with the use of some blood warmers may include (1) lost blood volume associated with extra tubing of the system, (2) overheating and subsequent hemolysis of red cells caused by improper temperature control, (3) increased osmotic fragility or rupture of cells resulting from mechanical trauma, and (4) inadequate warming at higher flow rates because of poor heat transfer capacity.

NURSING CONSIDERATIONS

As the transfusionist, the nurse is the last means the patient has to be protected from a transfusion reaction. Consequently, it is imperative for the nurse to double check the following:

1. Patient's name with the name on the transfusion form
2. Patient's ABO and Rh groups
3. Compatibility label
4. Physician's order for designated blood product
5. Patient's identity with blood product's label with another nurse
6. Outdated or abnormal-appearing (cloudy, bubbles) blood.

Before the administration of any blood product, the nurse will focus on reducing the patient's anxiety by explaining why the transfusion was ordered and how the actual procedure will be performed. Nursing assessment of the patient includes recording baseline vital signs and noting any present symptoms exhibited that are similar to a transfusion reaction.

To avoid complications, the nurse must know how to handle the blood product. Blood should be returned to the blood bank if it is not started within 30 minutes after issuance. It is often necessary to hang a primary line of normal saline and piggyback the blood into the line. Each blood product volume should be noted and infused according to age and cardiovascular and renal status of the patient. In patients with cardiovascular disease, the flow rate of blood should be maintained below 2 ml/kg/hr. Medications are never added to blood because the drug may react with the blood or preservative.

Vital signs should be monitored every 15 minutes during the first hour of infusion and every 30 to 60 minutes thereafter. Whole blood and packed and frozen thawed red blood cells are ordinarily administered over 2 to 3 hours. During the infusion and for at least an hour after the infusion, the patient must be assessed for signs and symptoms of a transfusion reaction listed in Table 23-2.

Guidelines used with the patient exhibiting signs of transfusion reaction are as follows:

1. Discontinue blood and resume intravenous saline solution
2. Take patient's vital signs immediately
3. Remain with the patient
4. Notify physician and laboratory
5. Return blood bag and all attached tubing to the blood bank
6. Send to the laboratory the patient's next urine sample labeled "first urine after transfusion reaction"

If no complications occur during or after infusing blood or blood products, the nurse completes the usual routine recording of posttransfusion vital signs, time infusion started and ended, exact volume and blood units, and identification number.

SUMMARY

All blood components, including fresh frozen plasma, carry risks of transmissible disease. Blood components are classified in the same category with prescription drugs and deserve the same considerations. All blood components can stimulate transfusion reactions of varying severity. Red blood cells given to the wrong patient can be fatal. Before a patient receives any blood components, there must be a type and screen for red cells, platelets, fresh frozen plasma, or cryoprecipitate. All blood components are labeled with the identity of the product, expiration date and time, volume, and

blood type. Blood samples for any transfusion service protocols require the patient's full name, history number, date drawn, and the initials of the phlebotomist. Of all transfusion reactions, 95% are caused by clerical error, and court awards in these cases start at $1,000,000.

REFERENCES

1. Basavanthappa, B.T.: Tips for blood transfusion, Nurs. J. India **74**(3):64, 1983.
2. Koepke, J.A.: Blood groups and transfusion therapy, Durham, N.C., 1983, Duke University Medical Center.
3. Alexander, L., and Levine, L.S.: Acute care transfusion manual, Durham, N.C., 1984, Duke University Medical Center.
4. Greenwalt, T.J., and others: General principles of blood transfusion, Chicago, 1977, American Medical Association.
5. Luban, N.L.C., and Keating, L.J.: Hemotherapy of the infant and premature, Arlington, Va., 1983, American Association of Blood Banks.
6. Circular of information for the use of human blood and blood components, Arlington, Va., 1981, American Association of Blood Banks and American Red Cross.
7. Blood component therapy: a physician's handbook, Washington, D.C., 1975, American Association of Blood Banks.
8. The collection, fractionation, quality control and uses of blood and blood products, Geneva, 1981, World Health Organization.
9. Transfusions: What to give, why, how to avoid complications, Patient Care, August 1971.
10. Smith, L.: Reactions to blood transfusions, Am. J. Nurs. **84**(9):1096, 1984.

ADDITIONAL READINGS

Buchholz, D.H.: Blood transfusion: merits of component therapy, J. Pediatr. **84**:1, 1974.
Evaluation of blood warmers, Health Devices, **13**(9):191, 1984.
Laucock: Your blood or mine?, Nurs. Mirror **156**:1, 1983.
Litwin, M.S., and Hurley, M.J.: The filtration of blood, Surg. Annu. **10**:105, 1978.
Oyama: The use of microaggregate filters in blood transfusions, Laboratory Medicine **10**(9):528, 1979.
Sadler, C.: Banking on blood, Nurs. Mirror **156**:15, 1983.
Silvay, G., and Miller, R.: Blood microfilters and the anesthesiologist: a review, Anesthesiology Review December, 1976.
Simpson, M.B.: Transfusion therapy for hematologic diseases and adverse reactions to transfusion therapy. In Koepke, J.A., editor: Laboratory hematology, New York, 1984, Churchill Livingston.
Walker, A.K.: Blood microfiltration: a review, Anesthesia **33**:35, 1978.

CHAPTER 24

Management of infections

MARILYN J. HOCKENBERRY, SUZANNE B. HERMAN, and SAMUEL L. KATZ

Infection in the child with cancer is a major concern and a common occurrence. Increased infection in the compromised patient occurs as a result of four basic defects: a reduction in the number of functional phagocytes, diminished cell-mediated immunity, faulty antibody production, and damage to mechanical barriers that protect against infection.[1]

The type of tumor, state of disease, and intensity of treatment all contribute to the frequency and type of infection. The lowest incidence of infection has been reported in children with solid tumors.[2] Children with acute myeloid leukemia in relapse have an average of one episode of septicemia every 80 hospital days as compared to children with lymphoma who have one episode of septicemia every 1200 hospital days.[3] This difference in frequency of infections is directly related to the intensity of therapy and its related neutropenia.

ETIOLOGY

The single most important factor predisposing a child with cancer to infection is granulocytopenia.[2] Granulocytopenia may be related to the primary disease or may result from treatment. Incidence of infection has been shown to decrease in the presence of an increasing neutrophil count. More than one half of the episodes of infection in children with cancer occur when the absolute neutrophil count is less than 500/mm³.[1,2,4] In some instances, neutrophil function may be impaired in the presence of a normal neutrophil count,[2] particularly in children with leukemia. Decreased chemotaxis and

neutrophil function have been associated with Hodgkin's disease and myelocytic leukemia.[2,5]

Defects in cellular or humoral immunity account for infections associated with specific types of cancer. Impaired immune response to varicella-zoster in patients with malignancies has been well established.[6-9] Abnormal T cell function in conjunction with inadequate specific cell-mediated response to the varicella-zoster virus results in unusually severe infections in these impaired patients. Lymphopenia and a deficiency in T lymphocyte function contribute to the development of viral or fungal infections in children with cancer. The incidence of *Pneumocystis carinii* infection, a protozoan, is also higher in patients with compromised immunity.[10] Patients with lymphoma are particularly susceptible to these infections.[2]

Iatrogenic factors frequently predispose the child with cancer to infections. Organisms are aquired by various sources in the hospital, including food, water, humidifiers, staff to patient transmission, and clothing.[3] Devices that interrupt the skin's natural defense barrier such as intravenous needles, shunts, catheters, respiratory-assist devices, intravascular monitoring lines, transfusions, and hyperalimentation predispose the child to infection. These iatrogenic factors have all been associated with the onset of opportunistic infections in children with cancer.

The malignancy itself may predispose the child to infection. Bronchial obstruction in patients with T cell lymphoma may increase the risk of pneumonia. Urinary obstruction caused by a large mass in the abdomen in children with Wilms' tumor may cause a urinary tract infection.

Treatment for the malignancy may lead to new sources for infection. Stomatitis from chemotherapy may cause septicemia resulting from mouth flora.[3] Rectal fissures and abscesses may serve as sources for overwhelming infections. Children with Hodgkin's disease having a splenectomy are at increased risk throughout their lifetime for overwhelming pneumococcal infections.[3] Specific chemotherapeutic agents such as alkylating agents, antimetabolites, and folic acid antagonists suppress primary and secondary antibody responses and cause delayed hypersensitivity in certain individuals.[2,11] Immunosuppressive agents, especially corticosteroids may interfere with leukocyte mobilization, depress cell-mediated immunity, and impair phagocytosis.[1] These increase the patient's susceptibility to infection while receiving steroids.

CLASSIFICATION OF INFECTIONS

The most common causes of infections in the child with cancer are classified into four major categories: bacterial, viral, fungal, and protozoan. Specific organisms are identified as follows, and this chapter will address each of these infections separately:

Bacterial
  Gram-negative
    Escherichia coli
    Klebsiella
    Pseudomonas
    Serratia
    Proteus
    Hemophilus influenza
  Gram-positive
    Staphylococcus aureus
    Streptococcus pyogenes
    Streptococcus pneumoniae
    Staphylococcus epidermidis
Fungal
  Candidiasis
  Aspergillosis
  Mucormycosis
  Cryptococcus
  Histoplasmosis

Viral
  Varicella-zoster
  Herpes zoster
  Herpes simplex
  Cytomegalovirus
  Hepatitis B
  Epstein-Barr virus
  Measles
Protozoan
  Pneumocystis carinii
  Toxoplasma gondii

Signs and symptoms

Fever is the most common sign of infection in the child with cancer. Fever has also been attributed to malignancies themselves such as leukemia, lymphoma, Ewing's sarcoma, and Hodgkin's disease.[12] However, the following factors suggest microbial infections as a cause of fever versus the malignancy itself:

Presence of skin lesions
Alteration in mental status
Evidence for a consumption coagulopathy
Hemolysis
Hyperventilation
Increased fluid volume requirements
Pain
Oliguria

The detection of an infection in a child with fever in the presence of granulocytopenia is often difficult, since granulocytopenia alters the inflammatory response.[12] An undetected, untreated infection can be rapidly fatal in the child with granulocytopenia. For this reason, it is imperative to evaluate the child with fever and granulocytopenia and to initiate broad-spectrum antibiotics immediately.

Diagnostic evaluation

A detailed history and thorough physical examination are aimed at eliciting even the most subtle signs and symptoms of inflammation. Physical examinations must be repeated frequently, especially when no discernible cause of infection is determined. Routine laboratory tools involved in the evaluation of fever in the child with granulocytopenia are listed in Table 24-1. Surveillance

Table 24-1. Diagnostic tools in the child with granulocytopenia and fever

Blood cultures	Obtain at least two cultures from different sites. If an indwelling catheter is in place, obtain one from it.
Urine culture	Examine urine sediment. A Gram stain may be performed initially if symptoms are present. White cells may be absent secondary to granulocytopenia. Always send urine for culture even in the asymptomatic child.
Throat culture	Obtain a throat culture routinely. Also culture any oral lesion for viral, fungal, and bacterial etiologic findings.
Sputum culture	Obtain sputum cultures when cough, dyspnea, or tachypnea is present. Transtracheal aspirate is sometimes necessary. A Gram stain may be done initially.
Stool culture	Examine Gram stain and guaiac stool when diarrhea is present.
Cultures of skin lesions	Obtain aspirate, culture, and Gram stain of any suspected skin lesion. Use Tzank preparation if there is a question of herpes.
Chest x-ray examination	Obtain routinely in initial evaluation.
Lumbar puncture	In the presence of headache and stiff neck or change in cerebral function, obtain cerebrospinal fluid (CSF) for culture, cell count, glucose, protein, and Gram stain.

cultures from the throat, urine, stool, and nose and at least two blood cultures should be obtained.[13] These blood cultures should be from different venipuncture sites. In the presence of an indwelling catheter, one culture should be obtained through the line. Skin or other mucous membrane lesions should be aspirated for Gram stain and culture. A chest x-ray examination should be performed in the initial diagnostic period regardless of clinical findings.

Even with a comprehensive diagnostic evaluation, a cause for the fever is demonstrated in only approximately one half of the children with granulocytopenia and fever.[12] Numerous infectious processes may take days to weeks to diagnose. Following initial evaluation, broad-spectrum antibiotics should be administered until the underlying cause is identified.

Head and neck infections

Oral mucositis is commonly caused by numerous chemotherapeutic agents. Colonization of drug-induced lesions by bacteria, fungi, and viruses, especially herpes simplex, may result in local infection in the child with granulocytopenia and may result in subsequent septicemia.[13]

Otitis media may be caused by common middle ear pathogens such as *Streptococcus pyogenes, Streptococcus pneumoniae, Haemophilus influenzae,* and less common Gram-negative organisms such as *Klebsiella* and *Pseudomonas*. Therefore, the child with granulocytopenia and fever in the presence of otitis media must be placed on broad-spectrum antibiotic therapy.

Periorbital cellulitis may be seen as a site of infection in the child with granulocytopenia and fever. Herpes zoster and cytomegalovirus have also been identified as infections occurring in the eye. Some patients with disseminated candidiasis may also have eye involvement.[13]

Sinusitis is usually caused by bacteria or fungus. Children with cancer of the nasopharynx are at highest risk for development of sinusitis. Granulocytopenic patients are at risk for aspergillosis or mucormycosis fungal infections.[13]

Lung infections

The lung is the most common site of serious infection in the child with cancer. Specific causes for the infection are related to the child's age, underlying malignancy, disease status, prior or current chemotherapy or radiation, granulocyte count, and microbial colonization.[13] Types of pneumonia vary according to the type of infiltrate and degree of granulocytopenia. The lung infiltrate may appear as a patchy or localized infiltrate or may be interstitial. The specific type of infiltrate may be difficult to detect in the granulocytopenic patient. Patchy or localized infiltrates in the nongranulocytopenic patient are commonly a result of viruses. Patchy infiltrates in the presence of granulocytopenia may be caused by opportunistic Gram-negative bacteria such as *Klebsiella* and *Pseudomonas*.[13] Staphylococcal pneumonia may also occur. Interstitial pneumonia in the child with lymphocytopenia is most commonly caused by *Pneumocystis carinii*. These children may be hypoxemic and tachypneic. Children who have undergone bone marrow transplantation are at risk for developing interstitial pneumonia caused by cytomegalovirus (CMV). In the child with granulocytopenia, Gram-positive and Gram-negative organisms and fungi frequently present as interstitial infiltrates.[13] These children must be followed closely.

Gastrointestinal infections

Esophagitis is most commonly caused by *Candida albicans* or herpes simplex and is characterized by dysphagia and burning retrosternal pain. Fever and granulocytopenia usually accompany *Candida* esophagitis. Barium swallow and/or endoscopy is usually performed to establish the diagnosis. Intra-abdominal infections occur from common intestinal flora and pathogens such as *Salmonella*. Typhlitis, a necrotizing cellulitis of the cecum, occurs most frequently from Gram-negative organisms and has a high mortality in the presence of granulocytopenia. Peritonitis may occur, usually caused by *Clostridium*. Minor fissures and ulcerations of the anorectal mucosa can result in cellulitis. This is most commonly caused by Gram-negative bacteria.[13]

Urinary tract infections

Urinary tract infections occur infrequently in the child with granulocytopenia and fever. Patients at risk for infection are those with tumor obstruction, bladder atony, or catheterization.[13] In addition to bacterial infections, the urinary tract may become infected with fungus, especially *Candida albicans*. Catheterized patients are particularly susceptible to the onset of fungus in the urinary tract.

Skin infections

Local skin infections with bacteria and fungi are seen frequently in the child with cancer and may result in disseminated infection when granulocytopenia occurs. Herpes zoster also disseminates very quickly in the immunocompromised child. Skin lesions may assist in the early diagnosis of generalized infections.

Musculoskeletal infections

Infections of the musculoskeletal system are an uncommon primary site in children with cancer. Atypical infections may occur. Osteomyelitis may be attributed to Gram-negative organisms, fungi, or more common Gram-positive pathogens.

Central nervous system infections

Children who have undergone a splenectomy are at added risk for meningitis and disseminated infection with *Streptococcus pneumoniae, Haemophilus influenzae,* and *Neisseria meningitidis*.[13] Children with granulocytopenia are at risk, although it is uncommon, for meningitis and may demonstrate minimum symptomatology. Fungal meningitis (especially *Candida* or *Cryptococcus*) is usually seen. Focal central nervous system findings in the presence of granulocytopenia may suggest a brain abscess. Encephalitis in the child with cancer is most frequently caused by herpes, varicella, or measles viruses.[13] Ventriculoperitoneal shunts also provide a potential source for infections, often with *Staphylococcus epidermidis*.

Fever of unknown origin

The child with granulocytopenia and fever of unknown origin remains a diagnostic dilemma. Continued antibiotic therapy may mask signs and symptoms of infection. Prolonged use of empiric antibiotic therapy may increase hypersensitivity reactions and toxicities to the drugs. The risk of development of a resistant microbial flora or superinfection is present. At the same time, premature discontinuation may result in significant infectious morbidity and mortality. This dilemma has not yet been completely resolved, and the selection of drugs and the duration of antibiotic therapy in a child with fever of unknown origin remain matters of controversy.

BACTERIAL INFECTIONS

Bacteria are responsible for the most serious acute infections occurring in children with cancer.[11] A significant improvement in survival rates has been seen, since the introduction of antipseudomonal penicillins and aminoglycosides. As many as 80% of patients with leukemias, lymphomas, and previous bone marrow transplants now survive Gram-negative infections.[14] However, mortality continues to remain higher in bacteremic infections caused by pseudomonas.[15] Gram-negative enteric bacteria are the most frequent cause of bacterial infection. Gram-positive bacteria are now seen more frequently at some institutions, the most common organisms being staphylococci and streptococci.[13,14] Gram-negative infections often cause more serious illness than those caused by Gram-positive bacteria.[2] These more severe infections are and in the persistent presence of granulocytopenia (Absolute granulocyte count [AGC] < 200 mm³).[2,13]

Gram-negative infections

Clinical manifestations of Gram-negative bacteria most commonly include septicemia, pneumonia, perianal abscess, urinary tract infection, cellulitis, and osteomyelitis.[13-15] The upper respiratory tract is the most common site of Gram-negative colonization, and the lung is the most frequent site of infection. The organisms are frequently hospital acquired.[16,17]

Escherichia coli, Pseudomonas, and *Klebsiella* are the Gram-negative organisms most commonly causing sepsis in the presence of granulocytopenia.[14,15] Antibiotic therapy for a specific pathogen can be identified in the treatment for Gram-negative

bacteria. Carbenicillin in combination with gentamicin is the treatment of choice for *Pseudomonas.* The combination of cephalothin with gentamicin is synergistic for *Klebsiella* infections and those caused by *Enterobacter, Escherichia coli,* and *Serratia.* Amikacin may replace gentamicin for resistant Gram-negative infections. For further detail of the specific antibiotics see Table 24-2.[18]

Gram-positive infections

Staphylococcus aureus is the most common Gram-positive bacteria causing serious infections in children with cancer.[18,19] Most common clinical findings include pyoderma, cellulitis, osteomyelitis, and pneumonia.[13,20] Septicemia caused by *Staphylococcus aureus* is highly treatable with semisynthetic penicillins even in the presence of persistent granulocytopenia.[12,21,22] In the presence of penicillinase-resistant staphylococci, vancomycin is used. Localized staphylococcal infections should be drained to enhance resolution.[23]

Bacteremia may be caused by other Gram-positive organisms. *Streptococcus pneumoniae* has been identified most frequently in children with leukemia and lymphoma.[23,24]

Empiric treatment of bacterial infections

Antibiotic therapy in the presence of granulocytopenia and fever is implemented before the cause of the fever is known. Specific choices of broad-spectrum antibiotics are dependent on the sensitivities of bacterial organisms found at each institution.[12] A broad-spectrum antibiotic regimen consists of a cephalosporin or semisynthetic penicillin along with an aminoglycoside (See Table 24-2).[12] Dosages and schedules must be carefully assessed to assure effective serum antibiotic levels. Drug dosages should be calculated according to the patient's body weight or surface area. Necessary modifications must be considered for children with organ dysfunction such as hepatic or renal failure (see Table 24-2). This should be monitored by serum peak and trough levels.

Antibiotic therapy in the presence of documented bacterial infection should continue for 7 to 10 days

Table 24-2. Common antibiotics used for fever and granulocytopenia

Drug	Dosage and Administration	Toxicity
Aminoglycosides—For Gram-negative infections—Escherichia coli, Klebsiella, Proteus, Enterobacter, Pseudo- *monas*		
Gentamicin	3-7.5 mg/kg/day every 8 hours over 30 min; peak 4-10 μg, trough 1-2 μg	Renal and ototoxic; observe BUN, creatinine, and urine creatinine clearance; may need to perform hearing testing
Tobramycin	3-5 mg/kg/day every 8 hours over 30 min; peak 4-10 μg trough 1-2 μg	
Amikacin	15-22 mg/kg/day every 8 hours over 30 min; peak 20-30 μg trough 1-2 μg	
Cephalosporins—For Gram-positive infections—penicillinase-producing staphylococci, pneumococci, streptococci. Cefamandole and cefuroxine are effective against *Haemophilus influenzae*. Second generation cephalosporins are effective against Gram-negative infections—E. coli, *Klebsiella* (many new cephalosporins).		
Cefazolin	50-100 mg/kg/day every 8 hours over 30 min	May potentiate renal toxicity when used with aminoglycoside
Cefamandole	50-150 mg/kg/day every 6 hours over 30 min	(Cefamandole—does not penetrate the CSF)
Cephalothin	75-125 mg/kg/day every 6 hours over 30 min	
Cefuroxine	75-150 mg/kg/day every 8 hours over 30 min	(Cefuroxine—highly sensitive to *H. influenzae* and penetrates the CSF)
Antipseudomonal penicillins—For gram-negative infections—Pseudomonas, E. coli, Proteus, Enterobacter. They should not be used alone in suspected Gram-negative infections without bacteria identification.		
Carbenicillin	400-600 mg/kg/day every 6 hours over 30 min	High sodium content—carbenicillin May cause hypernatremia and hypocalemia Allergic reactions in patients sensitive to penicillin Carbenicillin can cause platelet dysfunction
Ticarcillin	200-300 mg/kg/day every 4 hours over 30 min	
Antistaphylococcal agents—For staphylococcal infections		
Methicillin	100-200 mg/kg/day every 6 hours over 30 min	Nephrotoxicity except with nafcillin; nafcillin is preferred over the other antistaphylococcal agents
Oxacillin	100-200 mg/kg/day every 6 hours over 30 min	
Nafcillin	50-100 mg/kg/day every 6 hours over 30 min	

Continued.

Table 24-2. Common antibiotics used for fever and granulocytopenia—cont'd

Drug	Dosage and Administration	Toxicity
Others		
For Gram-positive organisms—penicillinase-producing staphylococci, *Staphylococcus pneumoniae,* streptococci; for anaerobes		
Clindamycin	20-40 mg/kg/day every 6 hours over 30 min	Gastrointestinal toxicity—nausea, vomiting, and diarrhea
For fungal infections		
Amphotericin B		
For *Candida* infections	0.3 mg/kg over 2-4 hours	Renal toxicity—renal tubular defects Potassium wasting effect
For more severe infections	1 mg/kg/over 2-4 hours with escalating doses	
For viral infections—chickenpox and herpes zoster treatment; for severe herpes simplex		
Acyclovir	500 mg/m² every 8 hours for 5-7 days (course may be extended as necessary)	
For *Pneumocystis Carinii* infections		
Trimethoprim sulfamethoxazole (Bactrim, Septra)	Therapeutic dose Trimethoprim 10 mg/kg/day PO divided q12 hours Prophylactic dose Trimethoprim 4 mg/kg/day PO divided q12 hours	May cause bone marrow suppression

after clinical and culture resolution if the granulocyte count is adequate.[3] In the presence of granulocytopenia, 2 weeks of antibiotic therapy after resolution of infection is often recommended. Certain infections, for instance osteomyelitis, require a much longer therapeutic course of antibiotics.

Granulocyte transfusions for bacterial infections

White blood cell transfusions in the granulocytopenic patient with documented septicemia unresponsive to appropriate antimicrobial therapy is thought to be of benefit. Herzig, et al. showed that patients with Gram-negative septicemia, most commonly *Escherichia coli,* had increased survival from use of granulocyte transfusions.[25] Prognosis is improved in patients with an absolute granulocyte count greater than 500 mm³. Improved survival is identified in patients with transient drug-induced neutropenia where the bone marrow will recover.

Prophylactic use of white blood cell transfusions is not recommended. Exposure to white blood cell transfusions is thought to increase the patient's risk for allergic reaction to all blood products. Schiffer noted a 70% incidence of blood product reactions in patients who had previously received granulocyte transfusions. It is also thought that these transfusions jeopardize efficacy of platelet transfusions.

FUNGAL INFECTIONS

Candidiasis, aspergillosis, and mucormycosis are the most frequent fungal invaders. Cryptococcosis and histoplasmosis are also seen in the cancer patient but are not increasing in frequency and do not seem to be correlated with use of intense chemotherapy.[3]

Candidiasis

Most fungal infections in children with cancer are caused by candidiasis. *Candida* infections range from local infection such as thrush and urinary tract infections to more invasive infections leading to widespread dissemination. *Candida albicans* is the species most frequently identified. Other species also implicated are *Candida tropicalis, parapsilosis, krusei,* and *pseudotropicalis*.[25]

Local and superficial infections are usually not difficult to diagnose by use of direct visualization, culture, and biopsy. Disseminated candidiasis often presents a diagnostic dilemma. Blood cultures are rarely positive; however, a postive urine culture may be considered proof of systemic infection.[3,26]

Candida infections are most commonly found in the oral mucosa. Esophagitis characterized by dysphagia and burning retrosternal pain is most commonly caused by *Candida albicans*. Urinary tract infections may also be caused by *Candida albicans*. These infections are usually superficial but can result in disseminated candidiasis in neutropenic patients.[12] Dissemination of *Candida* is often present when neutropenic patients are colonized throughout the gastrointestinal tract.

Oral candidiasis is usually cleared with topical nystatin. Ketaconazole given once daily as oral therapy is now being used for treatment of mucocutaneous candidiasis. It is also being used prophylactically to prevent systemic candidiasis from developing. Vaginal candidiasis can be treated with nystatin vaginal suppositories or povidone-iodine douches. Topical nystatin is used to manage skin lesions. Localized infections must be treated aggressively to prevent systemic involvement.[27]

Amphotericin B is the treatment of choice for systemic candidiasis, severe gastrointestinal disease, and *Candida* infections of the urinary tract, meninges, bone, and lung.[27] Amphotericin B is a toxic drug with possible severe side effects. A test dose of 1 mg is given initially to assess for reactions. Side effects include fever, chills, and hypotension during infusion. These symptoms are often decreased with premedication of Tylenol, Benadryl, and Solumedrol. Demerol can be used during the infusion when chills occur. For those patients who have severe chills without relief from Demerol, Dantrolene has been used with some success. Toxicities of amphotericin include bone marrow suppression and nephrotoxicity resulting in a renal tubular defect which causes potassium wasting, and increased blood urea nitrogen (BUN), and creatinine. The laboratory parameters must be followed closely while the child receives amphotericin. Frequently, potassium supplementation is required in these patients.

Amphotericin must be infused with a dextrose solution because it will precipitate in saline. The drug is light sensitive and should be protected from light until it is administered. Administration is usually over 2 to 6 hours. It has been reported that shorter infusions of 2 hours may result in decreased renal toxicities. Length of treatment varies from 4 to 6 weeks and is dependent on two factors: (1) when the therapeutic response is obtained, and (2) when renal toxicity warns that further exposure to the drug is harmful.[26]

Aspergillosis

The second most common fungal infection in children is aspergillosis. *Aspergillus* is found in dirt, dust, and the air. The most common species isolated from humans and their environment is *Aspergillus fumigatus*. Aspergillosis has been found to cause allergic symptoms such as asthmatic attacks, recurrent bronchitis, or self-limited allergic pneumonitis.

Aspergillosis in the child with cancer is more commonly manifested by tissue invasion rather than the saprophytic or allergic forms of the disease.[3] Typically, patients with leukemia or lymphoma are most often affected.[27] The respiratory tract is usually affected by onset of pulmonary lesions.[3] *Aspergillus* may invade blood vessels and produce thromboses and infarction. Other sites of involvement are the gastrointestinal tract and brain. Diagnosis of aspergillosis is difficult, with blood cultures rarely positive. Aggressive diagnostic procedures such as lung biopsy must be used early in the course of the illness. Early treatment with amphotericin B is imperative to attempt to eradicate the invasion; however aspergillosis remains difficult to treat.[27]

Mucormycosis

Mucormycosis is a life-threatening fungal syndrome caused by the *Mucen, Rhizopus, Absidia,* or *Cunninghamella* species. The disease is most often invasive in immunocompromised hosts who are neutropenic.[25] Central nervous system disease can occur from invasion of the *Mucor, Rhizopus,* and *Absidia* species. In patients with leukemia and lymphoma, the mold can invade the lung and disseminate to the brain. The ''rhinocerebral syndrome'' includes a triad of coma, ophthalmoplegia, and proptosis and occurs in about one third of the cases.[25] Diagnosis is difficult to make with cultures usually not being helpful. Amphotericin B is the only antifungal therapy for the syndrome and must be combined with aggressive surgery to debride areas of involvement.[25]

Pneumonia attributed to mucormycosis in the absence of the rhinocerebral syndrome also occurs. The chest x-ray can vary from a single patchy infiltrate to bilateral diffuse infiltrates to an invasive ''fungus ball.'' Sputum cultures are usually negative, with the diagnosis being made by biopsy. Disseminated mucormycosis may also occur by spreading to the bloodstream from the lungs and invading the liver, spleen, kidney, and brain. Amphotericin B is the treatment of choice in combination with the treatment of underlying neoplastic disease.[25]

Cryptococcosis

Cryptococcus neoformans is an encapsulated yeast found predominantly in the soil and transmitted to man through the respiratory system. Patients with lymphoma and Hodgkin's disease are at risk as a result of altered cell-mediated immunity.[13] The respiratory tract is the portal of entry for the infection although pneumonia is unusual. The fungus usually is seeded through the blood to body organs. The central nervous system is the most common site of involvement presenting with meningitis and brain abscesses.

Diagnosis of cryptococcosis is made with India ink stain of the spinal fluid or by the cryptococcal antigen in the blood or spinal fluid. Treatment is amphotericin B with or without 5-fluorocytosine.[19]

Histoplasmosis

Histoplasma capsulatum typically does not occur more frequently in cancer patients than in other individuals. When it does occur in patients with a lymphoreticular malignancy, it is usually disseminated.[13] Site of infection is most commonly the lung, with a miliary distribution. Dissemination to the reticuloendothelial system results in adenopathy, hepatosplenomegaly, and bone marrow involvement. These signs may be confused with the underlying disease. Careful histologic examination must take place, looking for intracellular yeast forms with Giemsa or methenamine-silver staining. The disease can occur in patients in remission and relapse. Amphotericin B is the treatment of choice.[13]

VIRAL INFECTIONS

Most viral illnesses pose no real threat to the child with cancer. However, more serious viral infections in children with cancer cannot be managed in the same manner as children in the general population. Those viruses include the herpes virus group (including varicella-zoster, herpes hominis simplex, types 1 and 2), CMV, measles, infections occurring after the administration of live virus vaccines; poliomyelitis, vaccinia, measles,[27] and viral hepatitis.[3] These viral infections may cause fatalities or generalized disease in children with malignancies.

Varicella-zoster (chickenpox)

Children with cancer will usually display a similar onset and initial presentation of varicella as children without cancer.[27] Most commonly, the infection is manifested by maculopapular eruptions beginning on the trunk and spreading in crops, with papules that progress rapidly to vesicles. The lesions then crust, scab, and heal over a 3- to 5-day period.[13] Children with cancer are more likely to develop fulminant and prolonged varicella, usually with pneumonia, than other children. It has been reported that as many as one third of children with leukemia who contract varicella may develop disseminated disease with a mortality as high as 20%.[3] Diagnosis is based on clinical signs and symptoms, demonstration of herpes virus particles by electron microscopy, observation of intranuclear inclusions on light microscopy, or culture of the lesions.[27]

All attempts to prevent exposure to the virus should be made. When direct exposure of the child to chickenpox occurs, administration of zoster immune globulin (ZIG) should be performed within 96 hours of the exposure. The dose is given intramuscularly at 0.2 ml/kg with a maximum of 5 ml. This may prevent or at least lessen the severity of varicella. The virus is shed 24 to 48 hours before the eruption of the rash and until all lesions are crusted. An epidemic of varicella in the classroom often requires the child with cancer to remain out of the classroom for an extended period of time.

The use of acyclovir has decreased the morbidity and mortality associated with disseminated varicella.[28] The child developing chickenpox is treated with intravenous acyclovir for 5 to 7 days at a dosage of 500 mg/m^2 every 8 hours.[28]

The question of temporarily stopping cancer therapy after known exposure and before onset of lesions is a controversial subject. It is thought by some that the risk of dissemination is decreased when therapy is not ongoing through the active phase of the disease. Others argue the risk of not adequately treating the underlying malignancy is much greater than the chance of developing disseminated varicella, especially with the recent availability of acyclovir. Presently, most institutions resume chemotherapy in children developing chickenpox once a 5- to 7-day course of acyclovir is completed. Most individuals now feel children exposed to chickenpox should be continued on chemotherapy.

Herpes zoster (shingles)

Herpes zoster (shingles) is a reactivation of varicella virus that can occur in the patient who has a history of chickenpox. Presentation consists of localized pain followed by vesicular eruption in a dermatomal distribution. Lesions undergo a course similar to that of varicella progressing to pustulation, crusting, and scabbing. Incidence in the patient with cancer is higher than the general population. Patients with lymphomas, particularly Hodgkin's disease, seem to be at greatest risk for developing shingles.[29] Although mortality associates with zoster is low, morbidity is great because of the potential for dissemination and neurologic complications.[13]

Treatment of zoster includes meticulous local skin care and observation for secondary bacterial infections. The infection can be treated systemically with acyclovir intravenously for 5 to 7 days at a dose of 500 mg/m^2 every 8 hours.[29] Oral acyclovir is now also available. Vidarabine has also been used to accelerate cutaneous healing of lesions and decrease pain associated with the lesion with relatively mild side effects (nausea and vomiting, hematopoietic suppression).[13,29]

Herpes hominis (simplex)

Herpes simplex infections are generally more severe and prolonged in children with cancer. The virus can cause extensive cellulitis or mucocutaneous lesions in these children. Dissemination can occur with esophagitis and/or necrotizing tracheobronchitis; bronchopneumonia and rarely cutaneous involvement of dermatomes simulating herpes zoster can occur in the immunocompromised patient.[6,27] The treatment of localized lesions is conservative, and topical acyclovir may be used although its efficacy is controversial. Disseminated disease has been treated with antiviral agents such as vidarabine or acyclovir.[27]

Cytomegalovirus

CMV can cause a variety of infections in children with cancer. Frequency of asymptomatic viruria in leukemic patients has been studied longitudinally with repeated sampling is 27%.[13] However, other studies have shown that the frequency of asymptomatic viruria is the same in leukemic and normal children. Evidence of clinical infection with CMV occurs only on rare occasions in children with cancer. The virus can cause pneumonitis, hepatitis, mononucleosis, retinitis, and possibly encephalitis.[13] Frequently, the infection presents with fever, tachypnea, and bilateral diffuse pulmonary involvement. A morbilli form rash is seen infrequently. Clinical diagnosis can be difficult. Infection is confirmed by isolation of the virus, seroconversion, a fourfold titer rise, or presence of intranuclear inclusions in involved organs.[27]

Treatment once the diagnosis is established and the patient is clinically worsening includes fluoruridine (20 mg/kg intravenous push daily × 5 days).[27] Vidarabine has been used both therapeutically and prophylactically without demonstrated effectiveness.

Measles

Annual incidence of measles in the general population has dramatically declined with the advent of the live-attenuated vaccine; however, outbreaks continue to occur. When children with cancer contract the infection, significant problems occur. A giant cell pneumonia may develop without a rash at onset of the illness or as late as 6 months following the onset of infection. Central nervous system involvement may also develop, leading to encephalitis.[13]

Any immunosuppressed patient with a seronegative measles antibody titer and a known exposure to measles should receive prophylactic gamma globulin at a dose of 0.5 ml/kg, with a maximum dose 15 ml.[13] When measles develop, supportive care should be instituted. Prophylaxis should involve *only* passive immunization, since live viruses can cause serious complications in a patient who is immunocompromised.[13]

Hepatitis

Hepatitis can cause extreme morbidity in children with cancer. Viral hepatitis includes at least two types, A and B, which are caused by different agents. Other infections, classified as non-A non-B and delta have also been identified. Type A, known as infectious hepatitis, does not appear to occur more frequently in the immunosuppressed patient. It has an incubation period of several

weeks, is contagious, and is characterized by a short period of abnormal transaminase elevation. Serum hepatitis (type B) has a longer incubation, a longer period of transaminase abnormalites, and is usually a more severe process. Usually type A is acquired by oral route and type B through blood or blood products.[3,13]

Prevention is the main thrust of hepatitis management in the cancer patient. Blood transfusion from only volunteers with a negative hepatitis surface B antigen (HBsAg) should be kept to a minimum if possible. Meticulous hygiene precautions should be employed in caring for immunocompromised patients (needle precautions, wear gloves when drawing blood, good hand washing). Hyperimmune globulin is available should exposure occur to type B. Ordinary immune globulin is effective in prevention of type A.[3,13]

PROTOZOAN INFECTIONS
Pneumocystis carinii

Children with cancer are at an increased risk for *Pneumocystis carinii* infections. Although most infectious processes occur when the patient is neutropenic and in relapse, *Pneumocystis* infections can occur when the patient is in remission and can be fatal for those patients. As many as 6% of children with cancer can develop the infection.[27]

Pneumonitis is the most common clinical presentation of *Pneumocystis carinii*. Symptoms include a dry cough, fever, tachypnea, cyanosis, nasal flaring, and intercostal retractions. X-ray findings demonstrate diffuse bilateral alveolar disease. A low P_aO_2, normal P_aCO_2, and alkaline pH are reflected by arterial blood gases. Presentation can be of a sudden (4 to 5 days) or insidious (1 to 2 months) nature.[13] Diagnosis of *Pneumocystis carinii* includes endobronchial brush biopsy, percutaneous needle aspiration, or open lung biopsy. Open lung biopsy is the most useful diagnostic tool, but it may yield false negative results.[27]

When untreated, *Pneumocystis* infections are fatal in children with cancer. Pentamidine isethionate was formerly the only effective therapeutic agent available for the treatment of pneumocystis infections. This drug had many side effects.[27] Trimethoprim sulfamethoxazole now demonstrates effectiveness against the infection with few side effects. High-oxygen support and ventilation are often required. The value of prophylactic trimethoprim sulfamethoxazole against *Pneumocystis* infections has proven highly effective.

Toxoplasma gondii

Toxoplasmosis is an infection by a parasite that usually is acquired by the ingestion of cyst-containing meat or from the oocyte in cat excreta and soil. The infection in noncancer patients is often subclinical. Those who acquire symptoms with the infection have a self-limited, mononucleosis-like syndrome characterized by fever, malaise, and lymphadenopathy.[13] Some may have pneumonia or a typhus-like rash disease. In immunosuppressed patients, particularly those with defective cell-mediated immunity, the infection can be severe, causing hepatitis, pneumonitis, pericarditis, myocarditis, myositis, and meningoencephalitis. Diagnosis can be made by the biopsy of the protozoa in affected tissues, demonstration of a rise in antibody titer using the Sabin-Feldman dye test, complement fixation, or fluorescent IgM antibody tests.[27] Sulfadiazine and pyrimethamine in conjunction with folinic acid for 30 days or more is the treatment for severe toxoplasmosis.[13]

PREVENTION OF INFECTIONS

The major cause of death in children with cancer is infection. For this reason, measures to prevent infection are a major focus in caring for pediatric cancer patients. Such measures to prevent infection need to be considered when the diagnosis is first made, when the child is hospitalized, and when the child returns to his home and/or school environment.

Hospital environment

Oncology patients are often most at risk for developing infections when they are hospitalized. Transmission can occur from staff to patient, patient to patient, food, air, water, hospital equipment, and medical and surgical manipulations and procedures. Meticulous hand washing is the most important infection control measure that can be taken to reduce microbial transmission. Care must be taken to assure that equipment is clean and sterilized when appropriate, particularly vaporizers and respiratory support equipment. Reusable thermometers should have solutions and containers changed frequently. Many institutions now use electronic thermometers with disposable covers to further minimize the threat of infection. Because of the potential for carrying organisms, plants, flowers, and fresh fruits should be discouraged.

Attention must be given to prevent the transmission of an infection from patients, staff, and visitors to immunocompromised patients with appropriate isolation techniques. Many pediatric settings have sibling visitation programs. The siblings should be screened carefully for infectious diseases before coming into the hospital.

Inspection and care of the skin and mucous membranes are important for detecting and preventing infection. Povidone-iodine skin preparations should be performed before any invasive procedure. Good perineal hygiene to prevent perineal abscesses and urinary tract infections and careful daily inspection for such abscesses are important. Rectal manipulation with thermometers, enemas, and indwelling urinary catheters should be avoided to prevent irritation to the urinary and rectal mucosa. Meticulous mouth care is imperative. Measures should be taken to prevent trauma to the oral mucous membranes. Temperature should be monitored carefully, particularly in immunosuppressed patients.

The preventive measures just mentioned are important for all hospitalized oncology patients. However, some patients may need more intensive programs to prevent infection. There is a wide variation of isolation programs among institutions. Protective isolation is often considered when patients have profound neutropenia (less than 500 granulocytes). Criteria for protective isolation varies. Most facilities have hand washing facilities available near the entrance to the patient's room.

Housekeeping procedures are carefully supervised, with special attention given to furniture and equipment in the room and with disinfectant solutions used for cleaning. Wearing of gowns, gloves, and masks is often required. Nursing staff caring for children with possible infection should not care for patients in protective isolation.

The emotional side effects caused by protective isolation are high, emphasizing the need to provide the child with stimulation and to prevent feelings of emotional isolation. Because of this risk, many institutions do not employ strict protective isolation measures. The issue is controversial, and data addressing the benefits of such procedures in preventing infection are inconclusive.[30]

Total protected environments using laminar airflow rooms are employed in some institutions in particularly high-risk patients such as bone marrow transplant recipients. This system attempts to achieve a relatively sterile environment through complete disinfection of all surfaces of the room. All objects entering the room are steam or gas autoclaved. Patients entering the room are fully decontaminated before entering the room usually with oral nonabsorbable antibiotics, cutaneous antiseptics, and a semisterile diet. This environment greatly reduces the patient's microbial burden as documented by various clinical evaluations. Patients, however, still have an increase of 5% to 25% the number of serious infections found in control patients, with most occurring in the first 4 weeks of isolation.[29,30] The costs of the unit and the psychologic impact of placing a patient in isolation are great. These children must have continuous family and professional staff support during such isolation periods.[31,32]

Prophylactic antibiotics

Recently, the benefits of prophylactic antibiotics in pediatric cancer patients have been evaluated. Trials of various combinations of nonabsorbable antibiotics have been conducted to attempt to achieve gastrointestinal decontamination without a consistent reduction in infectious complications. Other studies have evaluated the use of intravenous systemic antibiotics, in comparison with the oral nonabsorbable antibiotics for preventing fever and infections with comparable results.[13]

Currently, with the use of prolonged oral antibiotic prophylaxis in patients receiving chemotherapy, expected periods of granulocytopenia are being investigated. Trimethoprim sulfamethoxazole regimens are often implemented with some promise in preventing fever and infection; but results are limited, and toxicities such as bone marrow suppression and rashes have been seen.[13,33,34]

Home environment

Good hygienic principles applied to hospitalized care of the pediatric oncology patient should also be practiced at home. Patients and families should be educated about practicing such measures while in the hospital and should be instructed about when to expect blood counts to be low. When the child is neutropenic, crowds should be avoided as should contact with persons known to have infection, with specific instructions for known exposure to the varicella virus. The child should not receive any live virus immunizations. School personnel should be given these instructions and encouraged to notify parents of epidemic situations in the classroom.

Prevention of infection cannot be accomplished with any one modality. Multimodal approaches must be taken, and investigation of such preventive measures must continue, with attention to the benefits and risk of each approach.

REFERENCES

1. Young, L.S.: Infection in the compromised host, Hosp. Prac. **9:**73, 1981.
2. Feigin, R.D.: Opportunistic infections in the compromised host. In Feigin, R.D., and Cherry, J.O.: Textbook of pediatric infectious disease, Philadelphia, 1981, W.B. Saunders Co.
3. Levine, A.S., and Pizzo, P.A.: Managing infections in children with cancer, Pediatr. Ann. **8**(1):65, 1979.
4. Miser, J.S., and others: Septicemia in childhood malignancy, Clin. Pediatr. **20**(5):320, 1981.
5. Holland, J.L., Senn, H., and Banerjee, T.: Quantitative studies of localized leukocyte mobilization in acute leukemia, Blood **37:**499, 1971.

6. Donn, S.M., and Dickerman, J.D.: Fatal recurrent varicella in a child with acute lymphocytic leukemia, Am. J. Pediatr. Hematol. Oncol. **3**(2):183, 1981.

7. Feldman, S., Hughes, W.T., and Daniel, C.B.: Varicella in children with cancer: seventy-seven cases, Pediatrics **56**:388, 1975.

8. Schimpff, S., and others: Varicella-zoster infection in patients with cancer, Ann. Intern. Med. **76**:241, 1972.

9. Feldman, S., and Cox, F.: Viral infections and haematological malignancies, Clin. Haematol. **5**:311, 1976.

10. Robert, N.J., and others: Incidence of pneumocystis carinii antigenemia in ambulatory cancer patients, Cancer **53**(9):1878, 1984.

11. Steinberg, A.D., and others: Cytotoxic drugs in treatment of nonmalignant diseases, Ann. Intern. Med. **76**:619, 1972.

12. Pizzo, P.A.: Infectious complications in the child with cancer. I. Pathophysiology of the compromised host and the initial evaluation and management of the febrile cancer patient, J. Pediatr. **98**(3):341, 1981.

13. Pizzo, P.A.: Infectious complications in the young patient with cancer: etiology, pathogenesis, diagnosis, management and prevention. In Levine, A.S.: Cancer in the young, New York, 1982, Masson Publishing USA, Inc.

14. Rubin, R.H., and Greene, R.: Etiology and management of the compromised patient with fever. In Rubin, R.H., and Young, L.S.: Clinical approach to infection in the compromised host, New York, 1981, Plenum Publishing Corp.

15. Schimpff, S., and others: Significance of *Pseudomonas aeruginosa* in the patient with leukemia or lymphoma, J. Infect. Dis. **130**:524, 1974.

16. Nachman, J.B., and Honig, G.R.: Fever and neutropenia in children with neoplastic disease, Cancer **45**(2):407, 1980.

17. Brown, A.E.: Neutropenia, fever and infection, Am J. Med. **76**:421, 1984.

18. Ladisch, S., and Pizzo, P.A.: *Staphylococcus aureus* sepsis in children with cancer, Pediatrics **61**(2):231, 1978.

19. Kirchner, C.W., and Reheis, C.E.: Two serious complications of neoplasia: sepsis and disseminated intravascular coagulation, Nurs. Clin. North Am. **17**(4):595, 1982.

20. Musler, D.M., and McKenzie, S.O.: Infections due to *Staphylococcus aureus*, Medicine **55**:383, 1977.

21. Feigin, R.D., and Shearer, W.T.: Opportunistic infection in children, J. Pediatr. **87**(4):507, 1975.

22. Pizzo, P.A.: Infectious complications in the child with cancer. II. Management of specific infectious organisms, J. Pediatr. **98**(4):513, 1981.

23. Siber, G.R.: Bacteremias due to *Haemophilus influenzae* and *Streptococcus pneumoniae*, Am. J. Dis. Child. **134**: 668, 1980.

24. Allen, J.B., and Weiner, L.B.: Pneumococcal sepsis in childhood leukemia and lymphoma, Pediatrics **67**(2):292, 1981.

25. Armstrong, O.: Fungal infections in the compromised host. In Rubin, R.H., and Young, L.S.: Clinical approach to infection in the compromised host, New York, 1981, Plenum Publishing Corp.

26. Sauer, S.N., Atwood, P., and Sohner, D.: The challenges of physical care. In Fochtman, D., and Foley, G.V.: Nursing care of the child with cancer, Boston, 1982, Little, Brown & Co.

27. Culbert, S.J., and Van Eys, J.: Principles of total care: physiologic support. In Sutow, W.W., Fernbach D., and Vietti, T.J.: Clinical pediatric oncology, St. Louis, 1984, The C.V. Mosby Co.

28. Prober, C.G., Kirk, L.E., and Keeney, R.E.: Acyclovir therapy of chickenpox in immunosuppressed children: a collaborative study, J. Pediatr. **101**(4):622, 1982.

29. Balfour, H.H., and others: Acyclovir halts progression of herpes zoster in immunosuppressed patients, N. Engl. J. Med. **308**(24):1448, 1983.

30. Crane, L.R., Emmer, D.R., and Giguras, A.: Prevention of infection on the oncology unit, Nurs. Clin. North Am. **15**(4):843, 1980.

31. Ribas-Mundo, M., Grenena, A., and Rozman, C.: Evaluation of a protective environment in the management of granulocytopenic patients, Cancer **48**(4):19, 1981.

32. Pizzo, P.A.: Infectious complications in the child with cancer. III. Prevention, J. Pediatr. **98**(4):524, 1981.

33. Pizzo, P.A., and Schimpff, S.C.: Strategies for the prevention of infection in the myelosuppressed or immunosuppressed cancer patient, Cancer Treat. Rep. **67**(3):223, 1983.

34. Pizzo, P.A., and others: Oral antibiotic prophylaxis in patients with cancer: a double blind randomized placebo controlled trial, J. Pediatr. **102**:(1):125, 1983.

CHAPTER 25

Management of pain

JOANN ELAND

Reliable and valid measures for pain assessment in children did not exist before 1975. There are currently at least three tools developed by nurses. The pain assessment tools described in this chapter can be used by any health professional or parent and convey the subjective phenomena of pain as clearly as possible. Some of the intervention strategies are already employed by many nurses, whereas others reflect a highly specialized knowledge base, which is obtainable from related disciplines. This chapter focuses on children's pain and includes a physiologic perspective, causes of cancer pain, problems specific to children, myths that alter assessment and intervention, assessment tools that have been specifically designed for children, nursing and patient/parent pain relief goals, and nursing interventions. It is written from a clinician's perspective, and the content reflects ideas that work in day-to-day clinical practice.

PAIN THEORY

The Gate Control Theory of Pain introduced in 1965 by Melzack and Wall and revised in 1984 provides the best explanation of pain.[1,2] It encompasses earlier theories and both psychologic and physiologic parameters of the pain experience. It is an appropriate theory from which to plan interventions for pain relief, which will be elaborated upon later in this chapter.

The theory proposes that there are small diameter fibers (A delta and C fibers) that are stimulated by chemicals such as bradykinins, prostaglandins, histamine, and enkephlins (all products of cell injury). There are millions of small diameter fibers in the body, and certain body parts have more small fibers supplying them than others. For example, the skin has many small fibers, whereas the deeper organs within the body have less. Because of the large number of small fibers, the skin is very sensitive to pain, and the pain is easily located. In contrast, abdominal pain such as that associated with appendicitis does not localize until the peritoneum, which has many small fibers, becomes inflamed. Small fibers terminate in a specific spinal cord segment of the dorsal horn known as the substantia gelatinosa.

Large diameter fibers (A beta) inhibit pain and are found everywhere that small diameter fibers are found. Almost everyone has experienced the sharp pain associated with hitting an elbow on a hard surface. The initial response to such an injury is abrupt withdrawal from the offending agent followed by rubbing of the elbow close to the point of injury. Rubbing the elbow near the injury stimulates the large fibers to inhibit pain. Rubbing is more effective than holding the part or pressing on the same spot because the large fiber itself is more sensitive to vibrating sensations. The backrub for abdominal pain or labor pain, transelectrical nerve stimulation, and ultrasound therapy all use large fibers as the vehicle for pain relief. Large fibers also terminate in a specific spinal cord segment within the substantia gelatinosa.[1,2]

A special set of large fibers draws the brain's attention to the injury, and the brain can send messages to the substantia gelatinosa to either minimize pain or make it worse. For example, if a finger is slammed in a drawer, the special set of large fibers would draw the brain's attention to the injury. If the finger was only slightly bruised with no bleeding, most people's central control would send a message to the individual spinal cord segment that the injury "isn't so bad." In contrast, if the same finger was cut in half with excessive blood, bone, and tendon visible, the brain's message would most likely be "now you've really done it, this is serious!" and excitatory pain messages would be sent to the substantia gelatinosa at the level of the injury. There are many individual differences in responding to injury, particularly when the person is a child. Most young children interpret any amount of blood as being "bad" and send excitatory messages to the substantia gelatinosa.

Within the substantia gelatinosa, the T cell acts as a calculator to sum the input from the small and large fibers and the input from the special set of large fibers descending from the brain. If the excitatory messages about pain outnumber the inhibitory messages, the spinal gate is opened and messages about pain are then referred to the brain. If the inhibitory messages outnumber the excitatory messages, the gate remains closed and nothing further happens.

The neospinothalamic tracts, like the small fibers, convey the sensory messages about pain from the spinal gate to the thalamus. The paramedial ascending tracts connect the spinal gate to the thalamus and stimulate the reticular and limbic structures in the brain. Reticular and limbic structures are responsible for the emotions felt with pain such as fear and anxiety. The thalamus receives messages from the individual spinal cord sections via the neospinothalamic and paramedial ascending tracts and acts as a "switchboard" to send messages to other parts of the brain.

Central control, consisting of the cerebrum and thalamus, processes the pain experience. It collects information about time, location, intensity, fear, anxiety, past and present pain experiences and determines how to stop the pain. In the earlier example of the severely cut finger, the brain would process many small fiber messages because many have been injured. As bleeding continues and the finger becomes edematous, more pain-producing chemicals would be released. The special set of large fibers that would draw the brain's attention to the injury would send excitatory messages to the spinal cord segment as opposed to inhibitory messages. Although the injured person would most likely grab the base of the finger, stimulating large fibers, the large fiber input would probably not be great. This would likely result in the opening of the spinal gate and information sent to the central control processes via the thalamus. Central control would process information about the current injury in relation to previous injuries and current emotional distress and make a decision as to what to do to stop the pain. The result of this particular pain would most likely cause the individual to stop the bleeding and seek medical attention.

The Gate Control Theory is useful because it provides a framework for the planning of pain relief interventions. An informed clinician may decide among interventions that will influence the system in many ways. Traditionally, analgesics have been thought of on a continuum from powerful to weak. Morphine sulfate was considered as one of the most "powerful" and aspirin as "weak." Recent research categorizes analgesics according to where they work within the nervous system, providing rationale for combining them. It is now known that morphine sulfate alters the perception of pain and chemically makes large fibers work better, whereas aspirin works at the level of the small fiber to reduce prostaglandin synthesis. If one is attempting to relieve severe pain, it is appropriate to combine aspirin with morphine sulfate because they work at three different action sites. Action sites of drugs and other interventions need to be identified when planning pain relief interventions. By doing this, the system is impacted in as many areas as possible, and the chance of attaining pain relief is maximized. Where specific interventions work within the system will be discussed further under the intervention section of this chapter.

PROBLEMS

One of the single greatest problems of cancer pain in children is making health professionals aware of it as a potential problem. Practitioners are involved in technical aspects of care such as maintaining intravenous infusions, monitoring chemotherapy protocols, treating infections, evaluating blood studies, and identifying remissions and exacerbations, which are appropriate priorities. Little time is given to the topic of pain in basic nursing and medical education.

Staff nurses, by virtue of being with patients 24 hours a day, are witnesses to the pain and suffering of their young patients. Part of the problem with children's pain is the nurses' inability to objectively communicate the pain that they see to their colleagues. Pain is a subjective response to a hurt in contrast to vital signs, which are objectively measured. If a nurse reports of blood pressure of 160/140 mm Hg, another nurse can verify the accuracy of the reading. The numbers 160/140 mean that the patient's blood pressure is much too high and action needs to be taken. A nurse may report that a child is in severe pain, but the severity is not as easily verified. Often the person verifying may say something like, "Jody is not in that much pain, he's just upset." With the blood pressure example, the child's emotional state may be part of the high reading, but action is taken because there may be serious physiologic consequences if the pressure is not lowered. Pain can also have physiologic consequences although they are more subtle. Pain can cause physiologic immobility, worsen shock, lead to ineffective cough postoperatively, and increase anxiety.

MYTHS ABOUT DEALING WITH PAIN IN CHILDREN[3,4]

1. *Children do not experience pain with the intensity that adults do because their nervous systems are immature.* It was once felt that nerves were not completely myelinated at birth, but myelinzation is not necessary for pain transmission.[5-8]
2. *Children recover quickly, or, active children cannot be in pain.* Most adults retreat to their beds when they feel bad, but such is not the case with children. If children stay in their hospital rooms, they are vulnerable to those who want to do anything to them. Therefore the credo of experienced hospitalized children is "keep moving and stay out of your room."
3. *It is unsafe to administer a narcotic analgesic to a child because he may become addicted.* It is unsafe to administer an antibiotic to a child because he may develop anaphylaxis . . . but for some reason that does not prevent children from receiving them. Instead of asking the question "What if Billie becomes addicted?", professionals should ask "What happens to Billie if he is in constant pain?" In a study by Porter and Jick,[9] only four out of 11,882 hospitalized patients became addicted to their narcotics, and all four had prior histories of drug abuse.
4. *Narcotics always depress respirations in children.* In a study by Miller and Jick,[10] only 3 of 3,263 patients developed significant respiratory depression from their narcotic analgesics.
5. *Children cannot tell you where they hurt.* A child will never tell you that she is experiencing a shooting, lacerating, searing pain that begins in the right axilla and radiates down the ulnar deviation of the brachial plexus. But when asked appropriately, a child can tell you where and how much she hurts. However, if an injection is the consistent response to a child who admits to having pain, the child will not continue to tell the truth.
6. *The nurse who wields the needle gets the "guff."* Nurses who give injections to their young patients will never win popularity contests. Injections are not perceived by young children as being worthwhile because they have no time concept and do not realize the medicine is responsible for pain relief. The child who admits to pain gets hurt even further by receiving an injection.
7. *The best way to administer analgesics is by injection.* Probably the worst way to administer analgesics to children is by injection. The best route of administration for analgesics is intravenously, rectally, or orally.

8. *Children always tell the truth about the pain they are experiencing.* As long as the response to admitting to pain is an injection, children will never consistently tell the truth about the pain they are experiencing.

9. *Parents know all the answers about their child's pain.* Eland[11] found that parents do not know all the answers about their children's pain because (a) they have never seen their child in similar circumstances ("this ill"), (b) they may be so consumed by the hospital experience themselves that their responses are not usual, and (c) unfortunately they believe that, "The nurse would know if my child was hurting and would take care of him. I've never seen my child after a '(whatever happened to him)' . . . but the nurse has taken care of *many* children with this problem and would know if he is hurting. A nurse would not let my child suffer."

10. *The child is crying because he is restrained and not because he hurts.* Sometimes children cry when restrained because they know that restraint precedes things that hurt. At other times, youngsters who have had to be restrained for long periods of time do hurt because they have been in one position for a long time.

CAUSES OF SEVERE CANCER PAIN

The adult literature provides information about pathologic destruction that creates pain. Matthews, Zarrow, and Osterholm[12] identified the five leading causes of cancer pain as being bone destruction with infarction; obstruction of a viscus or vessel; infiltration or compression of nerves; infiltration or distention of integument or tissues; and inflammation, infection, and necrosis of tissue. These pathologic changes occur in children but have never been given the same attention given to adults with identical pathologic changes. The types of pain that each of these cause will be addressed in the following paragraphs.

Bone destruction with infarction is the leading cause of cancer pain.[12] Destruction of bone causes a release of prostaglandin, which lowers the threshold of the small fiber. The result of the lowering of the threshold can manifest itself in several ways. The tissue over the affected bone can become extremely sensitive to the slightest stimuli such as a draft or even pressure caused by a bed sheet. Some patients have reported pain from loud noises such as the sound from a stereo speaker when directed at the affected area.

Obstruction of a viscus can be like visceral pain, which is dull, poorly localized, diffuse, and boring, or it can be colicky, cramping, sharp, and severe. It may be present one minute and totally absent the next as the obstructed duct spasms. The abrupt onset and equally abrupt disappearance of this type of pain makes the uninformed practitioner skeptical about the credibility of the pain report unless it is understood that a spasming duct is the cause.

Obstruction of an artery results in ischemic pain, whereas obstruction of a vein causes venous engorgement and edema. Ischemic pain is often described as beating or throbbing. Children with low hemoglobin levels often report ischemic headaches as, "I can feel my heart beat in my head." The pain associated with venous engorgement is diffuse, dull, aching, or burning. The edema associated with venous engorgement can compress nerves and result in numbness, itching, and burning sensations normally associated with neurologic pain.

Infiltration or compression of nerves causes adult patients to use the words sharp, burning, searing, lancinating, or boring to describe it. The pain is located along the course of a nerve or may be referred to adjacent structures. Usually the pain is constant and can be of varying intensity.

Infiltration or distention of integument or tissues causes dull, aching, and stretching sensations that become worse with time. This type of pain can also evolve into ischemic pain depending on the structures involved.

Inflammation, infection, or necrosis of tissue frequently leads to pain and tenderness. Often inflammation or necrosis is a desirable outcome of chemotherapy and/or radiation, but associated release by cellular byproducts can be a source of excruciating pain and suffering.

These pathologic conditions are known to cause severe pain but have been given little attention because of the complexities surrounding the assessment of children's pain. When such pathologic conditions are evident, children need to be evaluated and treated appropriately.

PAIN ASSESSMENT

Pain assessment is complex when the patient is a child but not impossible. Data about pain needs to be collected in at least four categories: documentation of pain-producing pathologic findings from the medical records; objective data, specifically stress response if the problem is acute pain; subjective data from the child, using one of the assessment tools; behavioral changes noted by the child, parents, friends, teachers, and the nurses.

Various pathologic conditions known to cause severe pain in cancer have been discussed. Stress response and vital sign changes associated with it are useful indicators of acute pain. However, caution must be exercised in "across the board" application. Acute pain activates the stress response, and a clinician will see the predictable rise in heart rate, blood pressure, and respiration rate. Specifically, if a child has undergone surgery for the removal of a Wilms' tumor 48 hours previously and becomes restless and fussy, and pulse, respiration, and blood pressure rise from their baseline values, the nurse may conclude that the child is in pain. The nurse has based this decision on observed behaviors, objective data from vital signs and knowledge that incisions usually cause pain in a child 48 hours after surgery. The nurse may also ask the child about hurting. If admitting to pain in the past has resulted in an injection, the child will probably not tell the truth about pain. Most nurses will accept the answer "no" from a child and not intervene even though they have objective evidence to the contrary.

In chronic pain states the body is physically unable to maintain the stress response over time, and vital sign changes may or may not be seen. A child may have chronic pain and show no changes in pulse, blood pressure, or respiration. Unfortunately, many nurses and physicians incorrectly believe that these signs will always be an accurate indicator of pain.

Most children when questioned about pain, will deny it because they fear an intramuscular injection. Forty-nine percent of 242 hospitalized children told Eland that receiving an intramuscular injection was the worst thing that could happen to them.[4] If the response to an admission of pain is an injection, the child will learn not to admit to pain again. A 10-year-old child shared her perception of the hospital pain: "Look what happens to me when I keep quiet . . . bone marrows, IVs, LPs and chemo that makes me throw up. If I say I hurt, who knows what 'they' will do!" The child thought things were bad enough with no admission of symptoms and was fearful of worse consequences if she acknowledged a problem. An 11-year-old denied pain because she was fearful that she would not be dismissed from the hospital if she admitted it.

Children have a very limited vocabulary and may not know the name of the body part that hurts. Melzack and Torgerson[13] found that adults use 141 words to describe pain, whereas Eland[4] found that a majority of hospitalized children between the ages of 4 and 10 know only "hurt" or "owie." Pain is also difficult to describe because it can be many different sensations. Pain can be the sharp, stabbing, searing pain of a destroyed nerve, the throbbing of a vascular headache, or the sharp stinging of a skinned knee. In contrast, concepts such as nausea are primarily a single feeling state, have something concrete that they are associated with, and are easier to learn. Children on certain types of chemotherapy know that chemotherapy makes their stomach feel "funny" and that often after feeling "funny" they vomit. Children very quickly learn that the feeling of nausea and the act of vomiting are related. When a child is in pain there is no objective consequence to make the concept easier to learn. For example, nausea and vomiting often follow chemotherapy, and pain is associated with needles. But pain may occur when there is no event precipitating it, which makes it difficult for children and their caretakers to understand. The pain associated with compression of a ureter by a tumor is not associated with an identifiable event, yet it can be incapacitating. The pain comes, is severe, and then disappears entirely. The child cannot understand what is happening or from where the ''attack'' came. The caretaker may see the expression of severe pain one minute and ''normal'' behavior the next.

When pain has a gradual onset, it may be so subtle that the child experiencing it is not aware of pain until it is removed. Michelle, an 8-year-old, was suffering the long-term effects of a malignant brain tumor, which was most recently manifested by an abrupt onset of paralysis. When asked about her pain, she replied that she had none. However, in light of her radiologic findings, which included vertebral destruction and spinal cord herniation, she was placed on around-the-clock codeine and acetaminophen. Two days later she spontaneously reported that she felt better and was her ''old self.'' When questioned about her previous denial of pain, she said that she did not think she had hurt but attributed her feeling better and becoming her old self to ''those white pills.'' Further questioning of her parents conveyed that Michelle had not been ''herself,'' and her parents had attributed the changes to the progression of the disease. Certainly the disease had progressed, but one can only speculate whether or not Michelle would have returned to her ''old self'' earlier if the pain had not been recognized and alleviated.

Situations similar to Michelle's can be a clinician's nightmare because health care professionals may see behavioral changes but be unable to sort out pain from other subjective feeling states associated with their diagnosis. Frequently, children in pain have little energy, change their eating habits, and become sad, listless, depressed, and withdrawn. These behaviors are legitimized sick role behaviors when the child is undergoing therapy, but all too frequently these behaviors have been attributed to the therapy and never specifically to pain. Oncology nurses and physicians need to look at a child's existing pathologic condition in light of Matthews, Zarrow, and Osterholm's[14] identification of the causes of severe cancer pain. When pain-producing pathologic findings are present, the pain should be treated even when the child or parent is denying any symptoms. Failure to treat pain results in personality destruction equal to the cellular destruction of the pathologic condition itself. Attention to the quality of life issue in children's pain is long overdue.

PAIN ASSESSMENT TOOLS

In the past there were no tools to assess children's pain. Therefore there was no adequate way to measure pain or the success of pain intervention. Fortunately, this is no longer the case. Because no pain assessment tool will work for all children, a clinician working with a specific child needs to experiment with various tools to see what does work and then proceed to pain relief intervention. The tools cited in the following paragraphs have been used specifically with children for a number of years.

The Eland Color Tool was developed to assess pain in the 4 to 10-year-old age group but has been used with younger children, children over 10, and some developmentally disabled adults.[15] It is easy to use, inexpensive, and can be incorporated into a busy clinician's schedule with little difficulty. It is used with body outlines (both front and back views) and crayons or markers (Fig. 25-1). Children select from red, orange, yellow, brown, blue, black, purple, and green colors and use the following protocol.[16]

Ask the child, ''What kind of things have hurt you before?'' If the child does not reply, ask the child, ''Has anyone ever stuck your finger for blood? What did that feel like?'' After discussing several things that have hurt the child in the past, ask the child, ''Of all the things that have ever hurt you, what has been the worst?''

1. Present eight crayons to the child in a random order.

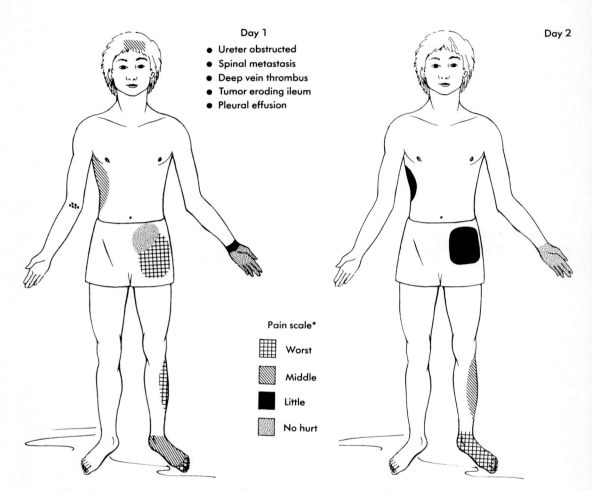

Day 1

- Ureter obstructed
- Spinal metastasis
- Deep vein thrombus
- Tumor eroding ileum
- Pleural effusion

Day 2

Pain scale*

- Worst
- Middle
- Little
- No hurt

Fig. 25-1. Day 1—Tommy, an 11-year-old, was admitted to a hematology unit with the diagnosis of ''rheumatoid arthritis.'' About 20 minutes after he was admitted, he colored this picture. Within the next 24 hours, various scans and biopsy sections revealed he had a ureter obstructed, spinal metastasis, a deep vein thrombus (which had occluded all but one small branch of the saphenous vein). The primary tumor was eroding the ileum, and he had a pleural effusion. Tommy also identified the various venipuncture sites with his ''little'' hurt color. Day 2—The health care team had initiated a morphine drip, and changes in pain were seen with the beginning of what eventually became ''little'' pain as colored by Tommy. *Legend reflects child's choice of color to identify intensity of pain.

2. Ask the child, "Of these colors, which color is like . . . (the event identified by the child as hurting the most)?"
3. Place the crayon away from the other crayons (represents severe pain).
4. Ask the child, "Which color is like a hurt but not quite as much as . . . (event identified by the child as hurting the most)?"
5. Place the crayon with the crayon chosen to represent severe pain.
6. Ask the child, "Which color is like something that hurts just a little?"
7. Place the crayon with the others.
8. Ask the child, "Which color is like no hurt at all?"
9. Show the four crayon choices to the child in order from their worst hurt color to the no hurt color.
10. Ask the child to show on the body outline where they hurt using the crayon for worst, middle, little, or no hurt. Then ask if the hurt is "right now" or "from earlier in the day." Ask why the area hurts.

Children willingly color their hurts and do not color things that are not currently hurting. For example, often a child will not color an intravenous needle that is in place and if questioned will tell you that the IV hurt when it was started but "if you lie very still it doesn't hurt now." Children will also show through their coloring new hurts, indicating advancing pathologic factors that the health care team may not know exist. On multiple occasions coloring of pain has identified bone metastasis, lung metastasis, and neuropathies before existing objective evidence had been obtained. An 8-year-old who had a small cell sarcoma identified an area in her left upper chest as a middle hurt that was sometimes present and sometimes not present. Based on previous experiences with children's coloring, the physicians involved ordered appropriate diagnostic scans and tests and found no pathologic disorder. Two months later lung metastasis was found in the exact area the child had been coloring.

Hester[17] developed the Hester Poker Chip Tool which uses four poker chips as "pieces of hurt."

Four poker chips indicate gradients of pain, from "just a little" to "the most anyone could hurt." This tool is easy to carry around in a nurse's pocket, can be quickly administered, and has the advantage of being something concrete that children readily use to show how much pain they are experiencing.

Visual Analog Scales can be used with children who know numbers. Children can be shown a line with the numbers 1 to 5 (or 1 to 10) under it and asked if "1 represents no hurt and 5 represents the worst possible hurt, where is your hurt now?"

Beyer[16] developed the "Oucher," which combines a visual analog scale with photos of children who are in pain.* The child is asked to show where he hurts along the continuum. The "Oucher" has the advantage of supplying a visual expression of pain with a numerical value. It has the disadvantage in that it is larger than the other tools and not as easily carried around.

Because of the complexities of children's pain, behavioral changes need to be included in the assessment of pain in the child with cancer. Appropriate questions to be asked include the following:

Is the child's sleep interrupted by pain?

Does the child require a daytime nap?

Has the child become a "loner" with few or no friends his own age?

What activities was the child involved with before his illness and can these be continued?

Does the child still attend school and is this something that is realistic and desired by the child?

If he still attends school what does he do after school?

Does he still participate in school social activities?

Does the child participate in other social activities outside of school?

What activities are important to the child that he is not doing but would like to do that might not have been covered in the above questions?

---

*The copyright for the Oucher is held by The University of Virginia Alumni Patents Foundation.

What changing patterns of activity has the school teacher, nurse, or counselor observed?

Can the child focus his attention on the subjects presented?

Has the child's overall classroom performance declined?

When the onset of pain has been gradual, these alterations in activity may be the most useful in tracing the pattern of pain. Previously, these changes have not been viewed as indicative of pain but rather as consequences of progressive disease. Certainly a child's activity level may decline as the result of therapy or uncontrolled disease, but the activity decline may be a symptom of pain. As stated previously, a child may honestly tell a care-taker that he does not hurt when he is in pain because the onset has been so insidious he does not realize it until it has been relieved.

Assessment and intervention are two valuable parts of the nursing process, but a part of the process often forgotten by nurses and their colleagues is the reassessment of pain after the intervention has had time to be effective. A nurse needs to talk with the child and his family to validate the success or failure of the intervention.

GOAL SETTING

A critical step in the nursing process is to establish mutual pain relief goals with the child and family. Rankin[18] found that adult cancer patients and their nurses had different pain relief goals. For nurses it was appropriate to take "the edge off" of pain, but patients were expecting pain relief to the extent that they could be functional in activities of daily living. The same study also found that nurses did not validate success or failure of pain relief interventions with their patients. Nurses also relied on nursing goals, independently evaluated pain relief interventions, and did not communicate with their patients.

Pediatric nurses need to assess a child's pain and discuss with the child and parents what pain relief goals are realistic. The behavioral data collected during the initial assessment phase can be used to help set and evaluate the success of goals. If a child

in pain is sad, quiet, withdrawn, and stays inactive at all times, a measure of pain relief could well be a return to activity and former behaviors. In some cases it is possible to relieve pain entirely and return the child to normal activity. In other cases a goal might be to finish a semester at school or attend a school function such as a holiday party. After setting the goal the health care team can help the child and parent decide what interventions they would like to try in their attempts to reach their goals.

Goals need to be communicated to all members of the health team. A child in pain with limited energies may wish to save all his energies in one day for the hospital school classroom and therefore may not want to take a bath. School is a child's "work" and frequently is the single most important thing to the child. The nurse who is unaware of this child's goal for the day might insist on his participation in a bath and morning care. Nurses must respect a child's goals and acknowledge the child's right of choice in how to use limited energies. Periodically, everyone involved needs to reassess the progress made toward achieving the goals, modify existing goals, and create new goals.

NURSING INTERVENTION

Because it has taken a number of years to develop the assessment tools for children's pain, interventions specific for children have yet to be well documented from a research perspective. Regardless of whether a research base exists, clinicians are faced with the day-to-day reality of children in pain who need interventions immediately. This section will focus on interventions from a nursing perspective and is not all inclusive. As with assessment tools, no intervention(s) will help all children, and the challenge is to find what intervention or combination of interventions will work best for a specific child in pain. Entire texts have been written on many of these interventions and the reader is referred to the bibliography for further reading. There are many pain relief modalities that have been used successfully for adults that have direct application for children, whereas others need modification. The information known about local anesthetics, which is discussed in the next section, is an example of information that has been known for many years but has not been applied to the special problems of children.

"Caines," procedures, and nerve blocks

Anesthesiologists have known for a long time that there are short-, intermediate-, and long-acting local anesthetics. One of the reasons children dislike bone marrow aspirations and lumbar punctures is the infiltration of the intermediate-acting local anesthetic into the tissues, which feels like a million bee stings for a full half minute until the drug takes effect. The stinging is so unpleasant that many children refuse the lidocaine (Xylocaine) or procaine hydrochloride (Novocain). Lidocaine stops stinging 30 to 60 seconds after infiltration and has a duration of about 2 to 3 hours. The stinging associated with chloroprocaine hydrochloride (Nesacaine) lasts about 2 to 3 seconds but the duration of the drug is 15 minutes. If experienced hands are not performing the procedure and it is anticipated that the procedure will last longer than 15 minutes, chloroprocaine hydrochloride (Nesacaine) can be combined in solution with a longer acting local anesthetic such as bupivacaine hydrochloride (Marcaine). Advantages of combining a short- and long-acting local anesthetic for a bone marrow include a 2- to three-second onset of effect (avoiding the sting) and a duration of 8 to 10 hours, eliminating the achiness and soreness that children describe for several hours after the procedure.

Although it may take more time, bone marrow aspirations could be made far less painful by the following methods:

1. Spray the site for 2 to 3 seconds before infiltrating the skin with Frigiderm (ethyl chloride) or put ice on the area.
2. Infiltrate the skin with short-acting anesthetic.
3. Infiltrate the deeper tissue with the short- and long-acting anesthetic combination.
4. Inject a bubble of anesthetic between the periosteum and the bone itself.
5. Perform the procedure.

Most adults' experience with periosteal pain comes from hitting their "crazy bone" in their elbow or striking their shin against an immovable object. Periosteum if the extremely sensitive covering over bone. If periosteum is not injected with anesthetic before a bone marrow aspiration, a sharp stabbing pain continues until the bone marrow needle is withdrawn.

Nerve blocks

Successful nerve blocks can return people to more normal existences without the side effects of more potent systemic analgesics and should be considered for children who might benefit from them. Nerve blocks work by altering small fiber messages. A pain pathway created by the small fiber can be likened to a mud road with deep ruts representing pain. The only way a car (a neurologic message in this case) can go down the road is to drive in the ruts. A nerve block is like a road grader in its attempt to remove the ruts. Success of the road grader is dependent on how many times the road is graded, how dry the road is, and rain in the future. Likewise a nerve block may totally relieve pain after one block or it may take more than one. The long-term duration of the block may vary; some patients may get hours of relief, whereas others may get days or even months.

Nerve blocks are painful. Patients planning to undergo them need to know this from the beginning, but they also need to know that the block may totally relieve their pain. Infiltration of a local anesthetic into intact tissue is painful in itself, but infiltration of a local anesthetic into a painful nerve that has been invaded by malignant cells can be excruciating. Often a physician must locate the affected nerve by placing the needle on a bony landmark, which creates periosteal pain. Patients need to be prepared that a needle may be placed on bone so that they can hold still. Squeezing the nurses hand or yelling is often helpful in these situations, but patients cannot move away from the pain because of damage that can be caused by dislodged needle.

Olness, Spinetta, and Hilgard and LeBaron have

shown that hypnosis is particularly useful in children who have malignancies.[19-23] Hypnosis is thought to work by reducing the number of chemicals that cause fear and anxiety, which are made in reticular and limbic structures. There is also some evidence that hypnosis works in the periventricular and periaqueductal gray areas of central control and produce the body's morphine (see Chapter 29 on coping strategies for children with cancer).

Transelectrical nerve stimulators

I have seen two children suffering severe pain associated with rib destruction from Ewing's sarcoma totally relieved (according to the child) with a transelectrical nerve stimulator (TENS) and an around the clock nonsteroidal anti-inflammatory agent. A 5-year-old child who previously would not leave his bed because of severe pain was found skipping down the hall. When asked if he hurt anymore, his reply was "I'm all better because of the pills and my magic box!"

TENS have primarily been used with adults in chronic pain and represent an area of pain relief that deserves attention for use with children.[22] TENS units deliver tiny amounts of electricity to large fibers (the ones that inhibit pain), and there is some evidence that they cause the body to make its own morphine. The devices consist of small battery packs the size of a bar of soap, which have wires coming from them that are attached to electrodes placed on the skin surface. Currently, there are over eighty companies making TENS units and most have amplitude, rate, and pulse width controls. The settings of these controls vary widely between individuals, but have been used for bone marrow aspiration, lumbar puncture, bone infarction pain, and nerve invasion pain. Visceral types of pain are much more difficult to alleviate with TENS but not impossible.

Distraction

Pediatric nurses have always used distraction with their patients and need to continue doing whatever has worked previously for their patients. Some recent technology can aid nurses in this area. The "walkman-type" portable cassette players are particularly effective for distraction. Children can listen to favorite tapes during painful procedures,[23,24] when trying to relax, and when trying to take their minds off whatever is bothering them. For the young child, a parent's voice reading a favorite story can be a powerful pain reliever. One particularly creative mom recorded her family's bedtime routine for her adolescent who had been hospitalized for 2 months with a lung infection. The normal chaos surrounding five children's bedtime routines was music to a homesick adolescent's ears.

Comfort measures

The most powerful pain interventions have existed for a long time and can be generally classified as comfort measures. Some of these measures contribute directly to pain relief, whereas others aid in pain relief by reducing anxiety and fear. Positioning the patient comfortably relieves pressure on small fibers over bony prominences or may take pressure off of future lines. Arms or legs with intravenous infusions can be supported with pillows or bath blankets. If a patient is lying on his side, pillows should be positioned at the back and between the knees and ankles. Nasogastric tubes should be pinned to gowns or pajamas so that an accidental tug on the tube does not result in discomfort for the patient. Patients who are receiving nothing by mouth, are mouth breathing, or who have nasogastric tubes need frequent mouth care. All patients do not require clean sheets every day. Children particularly need their night-time routines followed, which may include their bath at the end of the day instead of at the beginning. The backrub is another comfort measure that needs to be reintroduced to most nursing units. Backrubs stimulate large fibers (the inhibitory ones) and convey a sense of warmth and caring to central control. Many pediatric patients can be held by those who care about them, but often parents need to be helped to manage all of the tubes and equipment.

Analgesics

Until the mid-1970s, analgesics could not be precisely measured in serum. With the development of radioimmune assay, it is now known that most analgesics have shorter durations than previously believed. Merperidine (Demerol) was once thought to have a duration of 3 to 4 hours but is now known to have a 2 to 3 hour duration.[25] Morphine sulfate's duration is 3 to 4 hours, whereas methadone's (Dolophine) duration is 6 to 7 hours.[26]

Analgesics with the least side effects should be tried initially. If pain is resistant to drugs such as acetaminophen (Tylenol) or aspirin, a trial of a nonsteroidal anti-inflammatory drug (NSAIDs) is probably appropriate. If the nonsteroidal anti-inflammatory drug is not effective, narcotics combined with acetaminophen should be tried. Most nonsteroidal anti-inflammatory drugs compete with acetaminophen or aspirin. Aspirin and acetaminophen work at the level of the small fiber, whereas the nonsteroidal anti-inflammatory agents work at the small fiber and often at the level of the spinal cord. Morphine chemically makes large fibers work better and alters central control's perception of pain, whereas merperidine's only action is to alter central control's perception of pain.

Most patients will have better pain control and will use smaller amounts of analgesics if they are given around the clock (ATC). ATC can be a nursing order when the legal order states "p.r.n." When the idea of ATC is introduced, someone may want to omit the middle-of-the-night dose. If the night dose is omitted, the blood level of the analgesic drops, and the patient is often awakened by pain and cannot return to sleep.

One of the best ways to monitor the success of analgesics is by using an analgesic flow sheet as described by Minehart and McCaffery.[27] The purpose of the flow sheet is to evaluate the safety and effectiveness of the analgesics ordered. The sheet has columns for time of day, pain rating (by the patient), analgesic used, vital signs, level of arousal, plan, and comments. It has the advantage of summarizing all of the data about pain on one specific sheet. A nurse or physician can look at the sheet and follow the success or failure of analgesics. The idea of a flow sheet seems simplistic at first look, but it allows the reader to focus on pain

exclusively. It is also advantageous to use the sheet for outpatients because they can bring the sheet with them to physician appointments or have it at home for the hospice nurse to view. The flow sheet can also be used for monitoring other pain relief interventions and should not be limited exclusively to analgesics.

There are occasions where "normal" doses of analgesics will not relieve pain. If pain has peaked before the administration of analgesics, a usual dose of analgesic will not be effective, and a nurse needs to get an order for a supplemental dose of the drug.

It is sometimes difficult for hospitalized patients to receive analgesics during nursing change of shift activities. Experienced patients and their parents know this and request analgesics early, and inexperienced patients soon become aware of the fact. Unfortunately, early request for analgesics is often misinterpreted by the nursing staff, and such patients and their parents get labeled in a negative sense as "clock watchers." This can be unfortunate because of nurses' unrealistic fears concerning addiction and in some cases the nurse's own need to feel in control of the situation. Such situations also create additional fear and anxiety, which only make pain worse. It is not difficult to understand why patients who control their own analgesics keep their pain under better control with smaller amounts of analgesics.

SUMMARY

The problem of pain control in children with cancer is very complex but far from an impossibility. The pathologic conditions that are known to cause severe pain in adults are present in children. Several assessment tools designed specifically for children are available and must be used to assess pain initially and assess the success or failure of interventions. The area of interventions for children in pain is uncharted territory that needs extensive exploration by those who deal with children and their hurts. Instead of wondering whether or not we should intervene, perhaps it is most appropriate to ask the question, "What is going to happen to the child if we do not?"

REFERENCES

1. Melzack, R., and Wall, P.D.: Pain mechanisms: a new theory, Science **150:**971, 1965.
2. Melzack, R., and Wall, P.D.: The challenge of pain, New York, 1982, Basic Books, Inc., Publishers.
3. Eland, J.: The role of the nurse in children's pain. In Copp, L.A., editor: Recent advances in nursing, Edinburgh, 1985, Churchill-Livingston.
4. Eland, J.M., and Anderson, J.E.: The experience of pain in children. In Jacox, A., editor: Pain: a sourcebook for nurses and other health professionals, Boston, 1977, Little, Brown & Co.
5. Swafford, L.I., and Allen, D.: Pain relief in the pediatric patient, Med. Clin. North Am. **48:**4, 1968.
6. Williamson, P.S., and Williamson, M.L.: Physiologic stress reduction by a local anesthetic during newborn circumcision, Pediatrics **71:**36, 1983.
7. Haslam, D.R.: Age and the perception of pain, Psychonomic Sci. **15:**86, 1969.
8. Kaiko, R.F.: Age and morphine analgesia in cancer patients with postoperative pain, Clin. Pharmacol. Rev. **28:**823, 1980.
9. Porter, J., and Jick, H.: Clinical effects of meperidine in hospitalized medical patients, J. Clin. Pharmacol. **18:**180, 1980.
10. Miller, R.R., and Jick, H.: Clinical effects of meperidine in hospitalized medical patients, J. Clin. Pharmacol. **18:**180, 1978.
11. Eland, J.M.: Children's pain: developmentally appropriate efforts to improve identification of source, intensity, and relevant intervening variables. In Felton, G., and Albert, M., editors: Nursing research: a monograph for non-nurse researchers, 1983.
12. Matthews, G., Zarrow, V., and Osterholm, J.: Cancer pain and its treatment, Semin. Drug Treat. **3**(1):45, 1973.
13. Melzack, R., and Torgerson, W.S.: On the language of pain, Anesthesiology **34:**50, 1971.
14. Matthews, G., Zarrow, V., and Osterholm, J.: Cancer pain and its treatment, Semin. Drug Treat. **3**(1):45, 1973.
15. Eland, J.M.: Minimizing pain associated with prekindergarten intramuscular injections, Issues Compr. Pediatr. Nurs. **5:**361, 1981.
16. Beyer, J.E.: The Oucher: a user's manual and technical report, Evanston, Ill., 1984, Judson Press.
17. Hester, N.K.: The preoperational child's reaction to immunization, Nurs. Res. **28:**250, 1979.
18. Rankin, M.A., and Snider, B.: Nurses' perception of cancer patients' pain, Cancer Nurs. **7**(2):149, 1984.
19. Gardner, G., and Olness, K.: Hypnosis and hypnotherapy with children, New York, Grune & Stratton.
20. Spinetta, J., and Deasy-Spinetta, P.: Living with childhood cancer, St. Louis, 1981, The C.V. Mosby Co.
21. Hilgard, J.R., and LeBaron, S.: Hypnotherapy of pain in children with cancer, Los Altos, Calif., 1984, William Kaufmann, Inc.
22. Mannheimer, J., and Lampe, G.: Clinical transcutaneous electrical nerve stimulation, Philadelphia, 1984, F.A. Davis Co.
23. Clinton, P.K.: Music as a nursing intervention for children during painful procedures, thesis, Iowa City, 1984, The University of Iowa.
24. Eland, J.M.: The use of music as a nursing intervention for children undergoing therapeutic procedures, Unpublished data, 1984.
25. Houde, R.W.: The use and misuse of narcotics in the treatment of chronic pain. In Bonica, J.J. editor: Advances in neurology, New York, 1974, Raven Press.
26. Lipman, A.G.: Drug therapy in terminally ill patients, A. J. Hosp. Pharm. **32:**270, 1975.
27. Meinhart, N.T., and McCaffery, M.: Pain: a nursing approach to assessment and analysis, Norwalk, Conn., 1983, Appleton-Century-Crofts.

CHAPTER 26

Management of nutrition in children with cancer

DEBORAH K. COODY

Malnutrition in children with cancer is a serious yet preventable problem. It is by no means uncommon. Children with Ewing's sarcoma and neuroblastoma appear to be predisposed to malnutrition even at initial diagnosis.[1] In recurrent and metastatic disease, the incidence of malnutrition may approach 40% to 50%.[2] Malnutrition is the consequence of an inadequate intake of nutrients for a body's requirements. It may be secondary to inadequate intake, defects in absorption, or excessive loss of nutrients. In general, the total nutrient demand per body surface area is higher in children than in adults. Therefore nutritional insults manifest themselves more quickly.[1]

This chapter discusses the causes, consequences, assessment, and management of nutritional inadequacy in children with cancer. Such knowledge helps the practitioner to identify children at risk for malnutrition and intervene with appropriate modes of support.

CAUSES OF MALNUTRITION

Causes of malnutrition in children with cancer include mucositis, nausea, vomiting, anorexia, mechanical obstruction, postoperative ileus, malabsorption, and psychogenic food aversion.[3,4] These causes are secondary to disease and/or treatment. Intestinal lymphoma is associated with protein-losing enteropathy, and neuroblastoma can lead to therapy-resistant diarrhea resulting from excessive catecholamine excretion.[5] Burkitt's lymphoma of the jaw or rhabdomyosarcoma of the head and neck can cause functional impairment of the maxilla,

leading to an inability to masticate effectively. Anorexia is associated with disease and treatment, as well as with the psychologic sequelae of both.[5,6] Diagnosis and treatment of cancer can be emotionally depressing for a child and often results in poor appetite.

There is speculation that tumors may place a higher caloric burden on patients than would an equivalent mass of normal tissue. Such a tumor burden would lead to weight loss despite adequate caloric intake. It is speculated that the high incidence of malnutrition seen in children with neuroblastoma may be partially caused by the catabolic effects of catecholamines.[7] Further research is required to substantiate these speculations.

Treatment protocols may include a combined regimen of chemotherapy, radiation therapy, and surgery. Chemotherapeutic agents such as methotrexate, doxorubicin, nitrogen mustard, cis-platinum, cyclophosphamide, and 5-fluorouracil routinely cause severe nausea and/or vomiting. Many of these drugs, particularly methotrexate, cause mucositis and diarrhea because of inhibition of proliferation of the gastrointestinal epithelium.[6,7] The intestinal mucosa of children is especially prone to damage from diarrhea. Radiation therapy to the small and large bowel may cause nausea, vomiting, and diarrhea, resulting in varying degrees of malabsorption of glucose, fats, protein, and electrolytes. In addition, radiation enteritis may cause malabsorptive conditions resulting from intermittent bowel obstruction, ulceration, perforation, and fibrosis.[8,9] Radiation to the head, neck, and upper torso can lead to mucositis, esophagitis, and decreased saliva production. Surgery may contribute to malnutrition through the usual preoperative "nothing by mouth" routine and postoperative ileus. Surgical excision of portions of the small and large bowel can lead to varying degress of malabsorption. Malnutrition itself can lead to malabsorption, which in turn leads to a vicious cycle, intensifying the problem.

Learned food aversion is a cause of anorexia and weight loss in children with cancer. Children develop aversions to familiar and preferred foods in their usual diets when receiving gastrointestinal toxic therapy.[10] Changes in taste acuity in the cancer patient have been observed by many investigators. However, there is controversy regarding the mechanisms by which this occurs.[11]

CONSEQUENCES OF MALNUTRITION

A malnourished child feels ill and often appears to be listless and somber. Severe undernutrition in early life can affect structural and biochemical development of the central nervous system.[12] Malnutrition causes a depression of the immune system, leading to increased susceptibility to infection. The most seriously affected element of immunity is the cell-mediated (T cell) immune response. The incidence of infection is high in malnourished children with cancer as compared with children with cancer who are well nourished. In addition, malnourished children tolerate chemotherapy poorly.[13] Tolerance for chemotherapy is often measured by bone marrow reserve, as evidenced by peripheral blood counts. There is a high correlation between diseases with a 50% or higher incidence of malnutrition and poor bone marrow reserve.[13]

NUTRITIONAL ASSESSMENT
Anthropometric measurements

Malnutrition in adulthood is usually defined on the basis of weight or weight loss. Such a definition cannot be used for children who are actively growing and developing. The most reliable and practical indicator of nutritional status in children is a measurement of weight for height.[14] Body weight is best measured with appropriately sized beam scales. Infant scales should read to the nearest 10 g, and older children scales should read to the nearest 20 g.[15] Children should be weighed unclothed or in a patient gown. During the first 2 years of life, supine length rather than standing height should be measured. Children 24 months of age and older may be measured in the standing position. A stadiometer is the optimum tool to measure height, since platform scales with movable measuring rods do not give accurate readings.[15]

Weight and height are plotted on graphs developed by the National Center for Health Statistics (NCHS).[16] Waterlow and colleagues[17] define overt malnutrition as a weight for height that is 80% of the median. On the widely used NCHS weight for height graphs, this cutoff point is approximately at the 3rd percentile. Therefore, children whose weight for height falls below the 3rd percentile on the NCHS graphs are considered to be overtly malnourished. Children whose weight for height falls below the 10th percentile on the NCHS graphs may be at nutritional risk.

Skinfold thickness measurements are often used to evaluate fat stores in children with cancer. Very precise techniques must be used if the measurements are to be meaningful. The Lange caliper (Cambridge Scientific Industries, Inc., Cambridge, MD 21613) is preferred, since it meets the recommendations of the Committee on Nutritional Anthropometry and the area included within the jaws (30 mm^2) is small enough to be used for infants.[18] Either the Lange or Harpenden caliper can be used for older children and adults. Measurements at a variety of sites are useful, but those most commonly used are the triceps and directly below the scapula.

Biochemical parameters

The most reliable and common indicator of protein inadequacy is the measure of serum albumin. Normal values depend on age, yet a value of 3 g/dl or below is generally indicative of malnutrition.[19] There is no clear relationship between weight for height percent and serum albumin in children with cancer, indicating that the malnutrition in children with cancer is primarily calorie and not protein-calorie malnutrition.

Efforts have recently been made to objectively define "marginal malnutrition" in children with cancer through biochemical parameters. Research has shown that serum albumin is not a sensitive indicator of marginal protein inadequacy, because its half-life is 19 days and levels fall below 3 g/dl only after significant protein depletion occurs.[20,21] Serum transferrin, retinol-binding protein, and plasma thyroxine–binding prealbumin have been investigated as more sensitive indicators of protein-calorie status in children.[22,23] However, none of these parameters is particularly helpful in the routine nutritional assessment of children with cancer.

Dietary history

A common belief is that the dietary history is unreliable and of little benefit in the evaluation of nutritional status. It is indeed unreliable in evaluating the precise intake of specific nutrients. Yet in the general evaluation of dietary intake of calories and major nutrients, the dietary history is a useful tool. There is a high correlation between physical parameters, such as weight for height percentages, and the dietary history.[14] A complete dietary history, a food frequency record, a 4-day food diary, or a 24-hour recall of foods eaten the previous day can be done to determine adequacy of calorie and protein intake. See Fig. 26-1 for an example of a dietary history and Fig. 26-2 for an example of a food frequency record.

Text continued on p. 414.

```
Name _____
Date and time of interview _____
Length of interview _____
Date of recall _____
Day of the week of recall
          1-M    2-T    3-W    4-Th    5-F    6-Sat    7-Sun
     "I would like you to tell me about everything your child ate and
drank from the time he got up in the morning until the time he went to
bed at night and what he ate during the night.  Be sure to mention
everything he ate or drank at home, at school, and away from home.
Include snacks and drinks of all kinds and everything else he put in
his mouth and swallowed.  I also need to know where he ate the food,
but now let us begin."
What time did he get up yesterday? _____
Was it the usual time? _____
What was the first time he ate or had anything to drink yesterday
     morning?  (List on the form that follows)
Where did he eat?  (List on the form that follows)
Now tell me what he had to eat and how much?
(Occasionally the interviewer will need to ask:)
     When did he eat again? or, is there anything else?
     Did he have anything to eat or drink during the night?
Was intake unusual in any way?  Yes_____No_____
     (If answer is yes)  Why? _____
                         In what way? _____
                         _____
```

Continued.

Fig. 26-1. Dietary history. (From Fomon, S.: Nutritional disorders of children, DHEW Publication No. (HSA) 77-5104, Rockville, Md., 1977, U.S. Department of Health, Education and Welfare.)

What time did he go to bed last night?_____
Does he take vitamin and/or mineral supplements?
        Yes_____ No_____
     (If answer is yes) How many per day?_____
                      Per week?_____
    What kind? (Insert brand name if known)
        Multivitamins _____
        Ascorbic acid_____
        Vitamins A and D_____
        Iron _____
        Other _____
Does he eat differently on weekends? Yes_____No_____
    (Describe the differences)_____
_____
_____
Would you describe his appetite as Good?_____Fair?_____Poor?_____
What are his favorite foods?_____
_____
What foods does he dislike?_____
_____
What are his favorite snacks?_____
_____
Who prepares your child's food? (e.g., mother, grandmother, baby
    sitter, brother, sister)_____
Who feeds him?_____
Does he eat alone? Yes_____ No_____
Does he participate in a school lunch, school breakfast, WIC, or other
    feeding program? Yes_____ No_____
Is he on a special diet now? Yes_____No_____
    If yes, why is he on a diet? (check)
    _____for weight reduction (own prescription)
    _____for weight reduction (doctor's prescription)
    _____for gaining weight
    _____for allergy   specify_____
    _____for other reason, specify_____
    If no, has he been on special diet within the past year?
        Yes_____ No_____
    If yes, for what reason?_____
Does he eat anything that is not usually considered food? (e.g., dirt)
    Yes_____ No_____
    What?_____
    How often?_____
Has a doctor or nurse ever told you that he was anemic (had low blood
    count)? Yes_____ No_____
Does he have frequent problems with constipation or diarrhea?
    Yes_____ No_____
Does he complain of sore gums or aching teeth? Yes_____ No_____
Does he have trouble chewing or swallowing? Yes_____ No_____
Is he allergic to any foods? Yes_____ No_____
Does he take any medication regularly?_____
Can he feed himself? Yes_____ No_____
    (With his fingers?_____With a spoon?_____
Can he use a cup or glass by himself? Yes_____ No_____
Does he drink from a bottle with a nipple? Yes_____ No_____

Fig. 26-1, cont'd. For legend, see previous page.

USE OF FOOD FREQUENCY RECORD

Indicate whether or not the child ate the following foods by checking the columns "does not eat" or "does eat" for each item. For each food checked "does eat" write the approximate number of times eaten in a week. If any particular food is eaten less than once a week, do not write anything in the column "times eaten per week."

In some cases more than one food has been listed on a line. If the child does not eat all of these foods, underline the specific food(s). A space has been provided at the end to write in foods not listed that are regularly eaten.

Food	Does not eat	Does eat	Times eaten per week
I. Chicken			
Beef, hamburger, veal			
Liver, kidney, tongue			
Lamb			
Cold cuts, hot dogs			
Pork, ham, sausage			
Bacon			
Fish			
Kidney beans, pinto beans, lentils (all legumes)			
Soybeans			
Eggs			
Nuts or seeds			
Peanut butter			
Tofu			
II. Milk (fluid, dry, evaporated)			
Cottage cheese			
Cheese (all kinds other than cream)			
Condensed milk			
Ice cream			
Yogurt			
Pudding and custard			
Milkshake			
Sherbert			
Ice milk			
III. Whole grain bread			
White bread			
Rolls, biscuits, muffins			
Bagels			
Crackers, pretzels			
Pancakes, waffles			
Cereals (including grits)			

Modified slightly from California Department of Health (1975).

Continued.

Fig. 26-2. Food frequency record. (From Fomon, S.: Nutritional disorders of children, DHEW Publication No. (HSA) 77-5104, Rockville, Md., 1977, U.S. Department of Health, Education and Welfare.)

Food	Does not eat	Does eat	Times eaten per week
White rice			
Brown rice			
Noodles, macaroni, spaghetti			
Tortillas (flour)			
Tortillas (corn)			
IV. Tomato, tomato sauce, or tomato juice			
Orange or orange juice			
Tangerine			
Grapefruit or grapefruit juice			
Papaya, mango			
Lemonade			
White potato			
Turnip			
Peppers (green, red, chili)			
Strawberries, cantaloupe			
V. Lettuce			
Asparagus			
Swiss chard			
Cabbage			
Broccoli			
Brussels sprouts			
Scallions			
Spinach			
Greens (beet, collard, kale, turnip, mustard)			
VI. Carrots			
Artichoke			
Corn			
Sweet potato or yam			
Zucchini			
Summer squash			
Winter squash			
Green peas			
Green and yellow beans			
Hominy			
Beets			
Cucumbers or celery			
Peach			
Apricot			
Apple			
Banana			
Pineapple			
Cherries			

Fig. 26-2, cont'd. Food frequency record.

	Food	Does not eat	Does eat	Times eaten per week
VII.	Cakes, pies, cookies			
	Sweet roll, doughnuts			
	Candy			
	Sugar, honey, jam, jelly			
	Carbonated beverages (sodas)			
	Coffee or tea			
	Cocoa			
	Fruit drink			
VIII.	Other foods not listed that the child regularly eats			

SUGGESTIONS FOR INTERVIEWERS

Information will usually be obtained from the person responsible for feeding the child. Older children may be able to give more reliable information regarding their own intakes than will the responsible adult. The interviewer should judge this in each individual case.

How questions are asked is important. Avoid questions that suggest the correct answers (e.g., Did you have a dark-green or deep-yellow vegetable today?). Avoid expressing approval or disapproval of the foods reported. If you feel there are omissions, ask additional questions: What did he drink with his lunch? What did he have on his toast?

Check carefully for the following information:
    Additions to foods already recorded
        1. Fats: Butter, margarine, honey-butter, peanut butter, mayonnaise, lard, meat drippings, cheese spreads, and others
            Used on toast, bread, rolls, buns, cookies, crackers, sandwiches
            Used on vegetables
            Used on potatoes, rice, noodles
            Used on other foods

Continued.

Fig. 26-2, cont'd. Food frequency record.

2. Sugars: Jam, jelly, honey, syrup, sweetening
   Used on breads, sandwiches, vegetables, fruit, cereal,
   coffee, tea, other foods
3. Other spreads: Catsup, mustard
4. Milk: Cream, half and half, skim milk
   Used on cereal, coffee, tea, desserts, other foods
5. Gravies: Used on bread, biscuits, meat, potatoes, rice,
   noodles, other foods
6. Salad dressings: Used on vegetables, salads, sandwiches,
   other foods
7. Chocolate or other flavored milk (e.g., Quik, Bosco)

Food preparation
1. Preparation of eggs (e.g., fried, scrambled, boiled, poached)
2. Preparation of meat, poultry, fish (e.g., fried, boiled,
   stewed, roasted, baked, broiled)
3. Preparation of mixed dishes—major ingredients used
   (e.g., tuna fish and noodles, macaroni and cheese)
4. Special preparation of food—strained, chopped

Special additional detail about food items
1. Kinds of milk (whole, partially skim, skim, powdered,
   chocolate)
2. Kinds of carbonated beverages (regular, low-calorie)
3. Kinds of fruits (canned, frozen, fresh, dried, cooked with
   sugar added)
4. Kinds of fruit juices, fruit drinks, or juice substitutes

By carrying a few standardized props* it will be possible to obtain
more accurate recording of amounts: a teaspoon and tablespoon; several
sizes of glasses and bowls (including a 4-oz and an 8-oz measure); something to indicate thickness of meat—a ruler or a standard form such as
a model of a slice of bread.

*An assortment of props is available from Nasco, Fort Atkinson, Wis-
consin 53538, or 1534 Princeton Ave., Modesto, California 94352.

Fig. 26-2, cont'd. Food frequency record.

MANAGEMENT

Nutritional support of children with cancer begins at diagnosis. Evaluation of a dietary history and anthropometric measurements at diagnosis allows the professional to have a baseline from which to work. The most important factor in the nutri-tional management of these children is the early detection and aggressive treatment of their nutritional problems. Many children do not meet the criteria for overt malnutrition yet may become malnourished quickly after the onset of cancer treatment. These children fall into the "marginally malnourished category.''[4] Van Eys presents the following predictors of marginal malnutrition in children with cancer: (1) when diseases are present that show a high incidence of malnutrition such as Ewing's sarcoma and neuroblastoma, (2) when there has been inadequate food intake in the face of active disease, and (3) when there has been intensive therapy such as abdominal irradiation or high doses of systemic chemotherapy.[13] Malnutrition can be prevented in these children through monitoring the effects of treatment, emotionally as well as physically, and intervening with appropriate measures.

When nutritional intervention becomes necessary, the gastrointestinal route is used if possible. Techniques to enhance oral nutritional intake include offering frequent smaller feedings, trying chilled and bland foods, providing accessible nutritious snacks, encouraging parents to bring the child's favorite foods from home, and creating a pleasurable and relaxed mealtime experience. A thorough assessment of ethnic food preferences allows the nurse to offer a more tempting variety of foods to the child. One institution has a parent's kitchen and children's dining room, where parents can create meals and share with others and where children can leave their rooms to eat their meals in a more social environment. Special events such as picnics, birthday parties, teen groups, and restaurant outings can be used as vehicles for enhancing nutrition. In the child with persistent anorexia, individualized positive reinforcement techniques may be required. The desire to obtain an identifiable privilege can sometimes override the lack of desire to eat. High-calorie oral supplements can be offered to children with anorexia or to those who have difficulty chewing and swallowing solid foods. Nasogastric feedings of blenderized foods or commercially prepared enteral formulas can be used for children who are unable to swallow, chew, or tolerate food in the mouth. The dietitian can recommend standard formulations, rates of flow for adequate nutrient intake, and special formulations to be used for patients with malabsorption, surgical ileus, and hepatic or renal failure (see Table 26-1). The advantage of enteral feedings is the avoidance of complications of parenteral nutrition. However, enteral feedings are not completely without risk. The patient must have an adequate platelet count for placement of a nasogastric tube. Placing a tube in a patient with thrombocytopenia can lead to a severe bleeding episode. Flexible silastic tubes are tolerated better, since they are softer, of smaller diameter, and less irritating to the nares. Infusion of feedings through a tube placed accidentally into a lung rather than into the stomach can lead to respiratory compromise and infection.

Parenteral hyperalimentation is the most invasive mode of nutritional intervention and therefore requires justification for its use. Failure with other modes of nutritional support in the face of malnutrition or impending malnutrition usually justifies the use of intravenous hyperalimentation (IVH), also called total parenteral nutrition (TPN). IVH is effective in restoring a well-nourished state, since it contains proper amounts of dextrose , amino acids, vitamins, and trace elements (see Fig. 26-3). Since 20% dextrose solutions are destructive to small veins, an indwelling subclavian catheter is usually used to deliver IVH. A dextrose solution of 10% or less may be infused through a peripheral vein. An intravenous fat emulsion of medium-chain triglycerides (Intralipid 10%) is usually delivered in conjunction (IV piggyback) with the dextrose solution two or three times a week so that the patient receives essential fatty acids.

Complications of hyperalimentation include infection, metabolic derangements, and surgical complications such as pneumothorax. Careful surgical insertion techniques and meticulous attention to aseptic management of the catheter help to minimize the risk of sepsis and complications. If thrombocytopenia is present in a child who needs an IVH line, platelet transfusions are delivered through a peripheral IV immediately before insertion of the line. After the line is placed, a chest x-ray examination is done to verify its proper placement.

The IVH line is not used for other fluids, blood products, chemotherapy, or antibiotics. Labeling the tubing ''For IVH Only'' decreases the risk of contamination through entry into the system. The

Table 26-1. Choosing an enteral formula*

	kcal per cc	Protein g/l	Fat g/l	MCT†	mOsm‡ per kg	If age 1 to 3 years need to supplement§:
Routine						
Lactose-containing						
Compleat-B	1	43	43	−	405	Vit. D
Formula 2	1	38	40	−	510	Vit. D
Instant Breakfast	1	58	31	−	615	None (vit. D milk)
Meritene	1	69	34	−	690	None (vit. D milk)
Nutri 1000	1	40	55	−	500	Vit. D, Ca, P, Fe
Lactose-free‖						
Ensure	1.1	37	37	−	450	Vit. D, Ca, P, Fe
Ensure Plus	1.5	55	53	−	600	Vit. D, Ca, P, Fe
Isocal	1	34	44	+	300	Vit. D, P
Isocal HCN	2	75	91	+	740	Vit. D
Magnacal	2	70	80	+	590	None
Nutri 1000 LF	1	40	55	−	380	Vit. D, Ca, P, Fe
Osmolite	1	37	38	+ +	300	Vit. D, Ca, P, Fe
Renu	1	35	40	−	300	Vit. D, Ca, P, Fe
Sustacal	1	61	23	−	625	None
Sustacal HC	1.5	61	58	−	650	None
Travasorb	1	35	35	−	450	Vit. D, Ca, P, Fe
Vitaneed	1	35	40	−	375	Vit. D, Ca, P
Chemically-defined¶						
Criticare HN	1.1	38	3	−	650	Vit. D, Ca, P, Fe
Flexical	1	23	34	+	550	Vit. D, Ca, P, Fe
Portagen	1	34	46	+ +	236	None
Precision Isotonic	1	29	30	−	300	Vit. D
Precision HN	1	44	1	+	557	Vit. D, Ca, P, Fe, Zn
Precision LR	1.1	26	2	+	525	Vit. D, Ca, P, Fe
Travasorb Standard	1	30	13	+	450	Vit. D, Ca, P, Fe
Travasorb HN	1	45	13	+	450	Vit. D, Ca, P, Fe
Travasorb MCT	2	49	33	+ +	475	Vit. D, Ca, P, Fe
Vital HN	1	42	11	+	450	Vit. D
Elemental**						
Vipep	1	25	25	+	520	Vit. D, Ca, Fe
Vivonex	1	21	2	−	550	Vit. D, Ca, P, Fe
Vivonex HN	1	43	1	−	810	Vit. C, D, Ca, P, Zn, Fe
Hepatic failure						
Hepatic-Aid	1.8	48	41	−	900	Vitamins, minerals
Travasorb-Hepatic	1.1	29	14	+	600	Vit. D, Ca, P, Fe, Zn
Renal failure						
Amin-Aid	1.9	18	67	−	900	Vitamins, minerals
Travasorb-Renal	1.4	23	18	+	590	A, D, E, K, folate, minerals, lytes

*From Kevin O'Brien MD.
†Medium-chain triglycerides are easily absorbed fats. "−", less than 20% of fat as MCT; "+", 20 to 49%; "+ +", 50 to 80%.
‡Milliosmoles of solute kg of water; start with no more than isotonic (300 mOsm) and advance as tolerated.
§According to Recommended Dietary Allowances if full caloric intake is met by formula only.
‖Lactose digesting enzymes may be lost from the gut if any diarrhea is present (check stool for "reducing substances").
¶Components selected for easier absorption.
**Protein already broken into amino acids for maximum ease of absorption (for "protein intolerance").

TO PREPARE 1000 CC BOTTLE OF 1A | Date _____

Freamine III 8.5%	_____ g
Dextrose 50%	_____ g
Calcium gluconate 10%	500 mg
Sodium chloride (2.5 mEq/cc)	_____ mEq
Potassium chloride (2.0 mEq/cc)	_____ mEq
Potassium phosphate	(1.0 cc)
Magnesium sulfate 50%	10 mEq

Trace element solution		
Zinc (as sulfate)	1	mg
Copper (as sulfate)	0.5	mg
Fluoride (as sulfate)	25	mcg
Iodide (as sodium salt)	147.5	mcg
Magnese (as sulfate)	0.5	mg	(2.5 cc)
MVI concentrate			(2.0 cc)
Vitamin K (0.2 mg/cc)	1	mg
Folic acid (5.0 mg/cc)	1	mg
Vitamin B12 (10 mcg/cc)	10	mcg
Zinc sulfate	7.5	mg

QS to 1000 cc with sterile water for injection

Bottle 1A to be hung at 0400 every day

TO PREPARE 1000 CC OF 1B

| Freamine III 8.5% | _____ g |
| Dextrose 50% | _____ g |

Sodium chloride (2.5 mEq/cc)	_____ mEq
Potassium chloride (2.0 mEq/cc)	_____ mEq
Potassium phosphate (3 mM/cc)	1.0 cc

Sterile water for injection q.s. 1000 cc

Start Bottle 1A, at 0400 daily and infuse completely, then infuse Bottle 1B for the remainder of the 24 hours, at _____ cc/hr.

Intralipids 10% to be infused IVPB with central IVH (30 cc/kg/day up to 500 cc/day maximal) _____ x/week on (days) _____, _____ cc to be given at _____ cc/hr over _____ hr.

IMED pump to infuse IVH

Bloodwork:
- ☐ SMA 12 on Mondays, Fridays
- ☐ Magnesium every Monday
- ☐ Electrolytes Mondays, Wednesdays, Fridays

Ketodiastix every urine; record on I & O sheet. Weight every AM

Additional orders:
_____
_____
_____

Transcribed by: _____

Unit clerk

_____ Registered nurse

_____ Physician's signature

_____ I.D. No.

Fig. 26-3. Pediatric central IVH. (Used with permission by M.D. Anderson Hospital and Tumor Institute, Houston, Texas.)

1000-cc IVH solution bags are changed at least every 24 hours to reduce the risk of infection, since the 20% dextrose solution is a rich medium for bacteria if contamination should occur. The IV tubing is taped at all terminals to prevent disconnections that could lead to bleeding or bacterial contamination. The IVH is infused through a delivery pump to prevent fluid and dextrose overload or clotting at the catheter tip. Blood chemistries (SMA-12) and electrolytes are checked at least twice a week to monitor for metabolic derangements. The urine is checked for glucose at every void to monitor the body's ability to handle the intravenous glucose load. The patient is weighed daily to assess progress. See Chapter 20 on chemotherapy for care of the long-term access catheter.

SUMMARY

Children with cancer are at risk for malnutrition. Careful monitoring of weight for height percentages from initial diagnosis throughout treatment enables the professional to identify nutritional compromise. Interventions with oral liquid supplements, enteral feedings, and parenteral hyperalimentation enables the child to maintain or regain a well nourished state.

REFERENCES

1. van Eys, J.: Malnutrition in children with cancer: incidence and consequence, Cancer **43**:2030, 1979.
2. van Eys, J., and others: A randomized controlled clinical trial of hyperalimentation in children with metastatic malignancies, Med. Pediatr. Oncol. **8**:63, 1980.
3. De Wys, W.: Nutritional care of the cancer patient, J. Am. Med. Assoc. **244**:374, 1980.
4. van Eys, J.: Nutrition of children with cancer, Front. Radiat. Ther. Oncol. **16**:177, 1982.
5. Waldemann, T., Broder, S., and Strober, W.: Protein-losing enteropathies in malignancy, Ann. N.Y. Acad. Sci. **230**:306, 1974.
6. Ballentine, R.: Common problems and side effects associated with the use of anti-neoplastic agents, Infusion **9**:9, 1977.
7. van Eys, J.: Nutritional therapy in children with cancer, Cancer Res. **37**:2457, 1977.
8. Donaldson, S., and Lenon, R.: Alterations of nutritional status: impact of chemotherapy and radiation therapy, Cancer **43**:2036, 1979.
9. Donaldson, S., and others: Radiation enteritis in children: a retrospective view, clinicopathologic correlation and dietary management, Cancer **35**:1167, 1975.
10. Bernstein, I.: Learned taste aversions in children receiving chemotherapy, Science **200**:1302, 1978.
11. Carson, J. and Gormican, A.: Taste acuity and food attitudes of selected patients with cancer, J. Am. Diet. Assoc. **70**:361, 1977.
12. Winick, M.: Malnutrition and brain development, London, 1976, Oxford University Press.
13. van Eys, J.: Nutritional management as adjuvant in pediatric cancer therapy. In Care of the child with cancer, New York, 1979, American Cancer Society.
14. Carter, P., and others: Nutritional parameters in children with cancer, J. Am. Diet Assoc. **82**:616, 1983.
15. Fomon, S.: Nutritional disorders of children. Rockville, Md., 1977, U.S. Department of Health, Education and Welfare.
16. Hamill, P., and others: Physical growth: National Center for Health Statistics percentiles, Am. J. Clin. Nutr. **32**:607, 1979.
17. Waterlow, J., and others: The presentation and use of height and weight data for comparing the nutritional status of groups of children under the age of 10 years, Bull. WHO **55**(4):489, 1977.
18. Committee on Nutritional Anthropometry of the Food and Nutrition Board of the National Research Council, Keys, A.: Recommendations concerning body measurements for the characterization of nutritional status, Human Biol. **28**:11, 1956.
19. Donaldson, S., and others: A study of the nutritional status of pediatric patients, Am. J. Dis. Child. **135**:1107, 1981.
20. Dudrick, S., and others: A clinical review of nutritional support of the patient, J. Par. Ent. Nutr. **3**:444, 1979.
21. Young, G., Chem, C., and Hill, G.: Assessment of protein-calorie malnutrition in surgical patients from plasma proteins and anthropometric measurements, Am. J. Clin. Nutr. **31**:429, 1978.
22. Ingenbleek, Y., and others: Albumin, transferrin and thyroxine-binding prealbumin/retinol-binding protein complex in assessment of malnutrition, Clin. Chem. Acta **63**:61, 1975.
23. Coody, D., and others: Use of thyroxine-binding prealbumin in the nutritional assessment of children with cancer, J. Par. Ent. Nutr.**7**:151, 1983.

PART IV

PSYCHOSOCIAL ASPECTS OF CARE

CHAPTER 27

Impact of cancer

MARILYN J. HOCKENBERRY

The approach to caring for children with cancer has changed greatly over the past several decades. Twenty-five years ago childhood cancer was perceived as invariably fatal, and coping with the death of a child was the major issue identified in the management of care. As therapeutic modalities progressed, so did length of survival time. Complete continuous remissions became more and more prevalent during the 1970s, and therapy began to be discontinued without evidence of further disease. Recently, the focus of care has evolved from the hope of continued remission to the reality of cure. Cure has historically implied a physical eradication of disease. However, a total cure cannot occur without also addressing the child's mental, emotional, and spiritual well-being. Quality of life for a child with cancer is no longer measured only by how well the disease is eradicated but also by how little treatment affects opportunity for continued growth and development. Fostering a child's efforts to grow and develop within a treatment environment is a complex and major task for the professional. The task requires a knowledge of the child's growth and development needs and an understanding of his perceptions of cancer. Cancer is perceived differently according to age, race, economic status, education, and cultural background. The impact of cancer, in conjunction with the child's and family's developmental status, create a unique situation for each child. This chapter uses a developmental approach to evaluate the child's, family's, and siblings' perceptions of cancer and will assist the health care professional in meeting the multifaceted needs of children with cancer of all ages.

IMPACT OF CANCER: THE INFANT

The infant has no perception of cancer. He is very busy developing an awareness of himself as separate from a significant other.[1] Cancer occurring in the first year of life can alter this development process of self-awareness. Normal processes for differentiation of self from mother may become distorted by physiologic alterations in the infant and by psychologic and emotional trauma affecting the entire family system.[2]

Normal mechanisms designed by nature to meet physiologic and psychologic needs are altered. Cancer must be addressed. The infant's continued growth and development may not initially appear as immediate as the eradication of disease (Fig. 27-1). Developmental processes are altered to fight disease. The infant, however, continues to be unaware of the tragedy being faced and has no real understanding of what is occurring. Separation from mother, pain caused by intrusive procedures, and denial of basic needs such as food and warmth may be experienced by the infant because of treatment. The parents will be unable to explain these intrusions, since the infant has no cognitive understanding of these experiences.

Realization of the infant's lack of perception of cancer can be used to promote the child's continued growth and development. Emphasizing human needs such as warmth, touch, food, and shelter maximizes the infant's ability to adjust to the disease and the intensity of its treatment as shown in Table 27-1.[3] Encouraging the family to foster and provide these basic requirements is of primary concern for professionals caring for the infant with cancer.

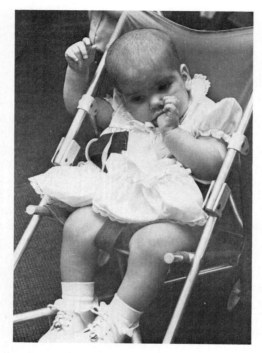

Fig. 27-1. The young infant has no perception of illness.

IMPACT OF CANCER: THE TODDLER

Cancer jeopardizes the toddler's ability to accomplish the task of autonomy.[4] Fears and terrors related to cancer lead to regression, thrusting him back into the safer and more dependent world of infancy. The toddler who regresses to infancy sacrifices autonomy in efforts to decrease stress caused by disease and treatment.[5] Physiologic regression is commonly portrayed by the refusal to carry on with bowel or bladder training. Emotional regression may be evidenced by the refusal to talk, lack of willingness to participate in any interactive games, or inability to display appropriate emotions of anger and frustration. He may even resort to extreme passivity and unresponsiveness. This passivity may continue to alter the child's relationship with his mother or father.

The toddler has no mechanism for perceiving what it means to have cancer.[5] He has no understanding that traumatic procedures such as bone marrow aspirations or lumbar punctures are essential components of adequate treatment. The child only feels the result of treatment, which is pain. This pain is often poorly dealt with, and regression is the easiest most effective coping method used by the toddler. Each intrusive procedure or examination will cause setbacks as the toddler strives to maintain a balance between dependence and independence.[4,6]

Table 27-1. Cancer in the infant: meeting basic needs and supporting developmental tasks

Nurturance	Allow for mother to hold infant as much as possible. Encourage touch. Provide time alone.
Physical comfort	Keep as warm as possible. The infant derives much comfort from mouth, skin, and sense modalities.
Security	Allow parents to remain with infant. Perform procedures and examinations as quickly as possible to decrease time of trauma.
Stimulation	Provide appropriate mechanisms for stimulation. Visual and auditory arousal is essential, even for the critically ill child.
Food	Promote intake as much as possible. Allow for sucking. Strive to minimize events altering the infant's ability to tolerate intake.

Establishment of trust in the toddler is a difficult task. The child has begun to trust others beside mother, yet remains unstable in the ability to separate easily. Onset of cancer involves numerous individuals who must interact with the child. Each individual is threatening to the child, whether it be physician, nurse, social worker, or chaplain (Fig. 27-2). The toddler needs time to be able to explore each individual in his or her own manner.

Parents are often unaware of the importance of setting limits and disciplining the toddler, even when he is ill. The child learns early in the onset of cancer how to manipulate situations to his or her advantage. Temper tantrums are common. Parents forego reasonable methods of control in an attempt to protect the child from further trauma. By doing so, the parents portray inconsistency in their discipline patterns, and the child may overreact emotionally. The toddler, who senses no limitations, is unable to complete developmental tasks essential to promote autonomy.

A mechanism for continuing the development of autonomy is essential to the support of the toddler who has cancer (Table 27-2). The toddler cannot perceive cancer as a threat; however, the treatment clearly causes conflict. Providing him with support systems in the form of discipline and positive reassurance helps him to keep fears and feelings in control.

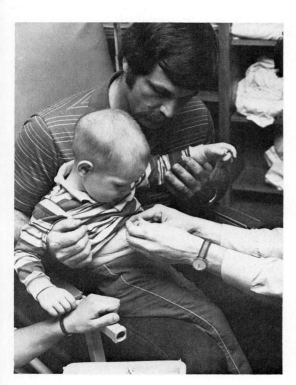

Fig. 27-2. The toddler with cancer struggles between independence and dependency with his parents.

Table 27-2. Cancer in the toddler: meeting basic needs and supporting developmental tasks

Begin physiologic awareness	Promote pursuance of bowel and bladder training. Allow for essential stimulation of motor skills such as walking, talking, fine motor skills.
Autonomy	Encourage independence. Assure parents of toddler's need to participate in activities such as care. Discourage regression by setting limits early in the illness.
Socialization	Continue relationships with other children. Promote activities. Strive to develop the toddler's trust by interacting on a level he or she can comprehend.
Beginning self-awareness	Stress importance of talking to the child and not just with the parents. Include the child in coversations about the illness or treatment. Never talk over the child.
Understanding of limitations	Show consistence with restrictions placed on the child. Clearly define these areas to the child and restate them with each encounter.

IMPACT OF CANCER: THE PRESCHOOLER

By the age of 5 years, the child begins to gather information about who he is.[7,8] He has evolved from a helpless infant to a unique person who begins to think and act independently. Numerous developmental tasks have now been conquered, including walking, talking, and controlling basic body functions. Motor skills are sharpened as physiologic progression and development continues.[9] As these tasks are met, new adventures and experiences are sought.

The onset of cancer in the preschool child disrupts the child's recently organized world and newly developed sense of self. The child has just begun to establish himself as an individual separate from the mother and is now faced with the fear and terror of a disease, which, combined with its treatment, could cause much pain and suffering.[10]

The preschooler may react aggressively to the impact of disease. Drastic changes in the child's environment and daily activities cause frustration and anger displayed in numerous ways. Lack of ability to think concretely or understand what it means to have cancer can cause the child to act out by being angry at everyone, including the parents.[11] It is not uncommon for a preschool child to refuse to acknowledge his parents after a traumatic procedure. Many preschoolers show frustration by throwing toys, biting and hitting significant others and professionals. Other preschoolers may display physiologic regression by refusing to talk, wetting the bed, or lying in a fetal position when hospitalized.[12]

The preschool child continues to develop a sense of what is "good" or "bad." The child continues to be unable to think abstractly and perceives every action as creating either a "good" or "bad" result.[4] Cancer may be perceived as something "bad" that he has caused to occur and that requires punishment.[3] Such a perception of cancer is reinforced by the treatment. Established methods of punishment often consist of pain elicited by spanking or restrictions placed on the child by parents. Treatment is often accompanied by pain and restrictions. The preschool child may perceive pain as punishment for something done wrong and may be too afraid to discuss these thoughts and fears.[5]

Frequently, the young child may become afraid to go to sleep for fear something painful may occur. Dreams may portray needles chasing the child, something eating the child, or even arms or legs being dismembered. Such visions occurring in the child's nightmares are hard to verbally elicit but can often be seen in children's drawings. The young child's feelings and thoughts may also be expressed through stories. Artwork and stories allow the child to work through fears and fantasies brought on by cancer and treatment and can be essential in the development of adequate coping methods[13] (see Chapter 29, Coping Strategies for Children with Cancer).

Perceptions of cancer in the preschooler are not yet fully established.[14] Lack of understanding

Table 27-3. Cancer in the preschool child: meeting basic needs and supporting developmental tasks

Industry	Allow for stimulating activity and independence with play. Provide opportunities for success and accomplishment.
Increased self-awareness	Allow for display of fears and frustrations through drawings, storytelling, play. Allow for verbalization.
Physiologic competency	Promote continuance of increased motor skills, language skills, and control of body functions.
Further socialization	Provide for participation in group games and interaction with children of the same age. Encourage encounters with children in the hospital.
Independence	Allow for independent decisions—only when possible.

brings with it fear and anger as to why painful intrusions must occur. Patience on the part of the professional is essential in establishing trust and maximizing the child's ability to continue to gain independence as a unique individual as shown in Table 27-3.[13]

IMPACT OF CANCER: THE SCHOOL-AGE CHILD

As the child becomes increasingly independent and separate, realization of vulnerability develops.[9] An awareness of the finiteness of the world is evolving at a level that the child is unable to fully comprehend.

The onset of cancer, at a time of increasing independence, autonomy, and vulnerability, may greatly alter the child's self-image.[15] Cancer threatens the process of growth and interferes with the child's concept of body image.[16] It disrupts the establishment of relationships outside the family setting, thereby denying positive socialization patterns that allow for further development of the child as a separate and self-confident individual. The child becomes confused by this disruption yet is not able to fully comprehend its meaning.[10]

Most school-age children have experienced an illness in their lifetime. The child may have had a pet that was sick or a grandparent who was ill. Such exposure increases the child's awareness of what an illness such as cancer means but limits the understanding as to why the disease has occurred. The school-age child now lives under certain established rules and regulations. These rules, established by God, society, and the family allow the child to organize the world methodically. Everything has a cause and a purpose, and the world is more predictable. Cancer occurs at a time when the child's realization of cause and effect becomes even more established.[14] The school-age child, like the preschooler, often sees cancer and its treatment as a punishment for actions or thoughts.[11] Pain caused by treatment adds confusion, especially when individuals tell the child he has done nothing wrong. The child often begins to question why the disease has occurred and may begin to distrust those around. He may withdraw initially, refusing to discuss fears caused by the illness.

Cancer in the school-age child may alter the development of a positive body image.[16] Side effects of the treatment, along with the disease itself, may alter the child's physical appearance. This occurs at a time in the child's life when a positive image of oneself is essential. Alterations in appearance such as hair loss or a change in weight cause the child to become increasingly insecure around others of the same age. Peers who previously knew the child are afraid and uncertain as to what is happening. They withdraw from the child for fear of catching the disease themselves. The child may feel alone and unable to understand why his friends are withdrawing from him. The child may find it easier to express feelings of confusion through play, drawings, or stories, much as the preschool-age child does. This allows the child to become detached from the acuteness of the disease and permits him to test the responses of the individual supervising the play. The child is able to determine the intensity of the situation by observing a professional's reactions to drawings, stories, or play (Fig. 27-3). Fantasies and fears involving monsters and darkness are common and often devour the child. Aggressive behavior is also common when the child is unable to set limits on actions during play. (Therapeutic play is discussed further in Chapter 29, Coping Strategies for Children with Cancer.)

The school-age child is rapidly learning to organize his world.[5] He is becoming more self-confident and independent of others. Because of an increase in rational understanding, the school-age child is able to adjust to situations that previously had caused only frustration and confusion. However, because of his increased autonomy and awareness of the world, the school-age child also experiences increased feelings of confusion and vulnerability. Family and professionals must be aware of this dichotomy and must aim to support a positive self-image and allow for verbalization of the child's confusions and frustrations as seen in Table 27-4.

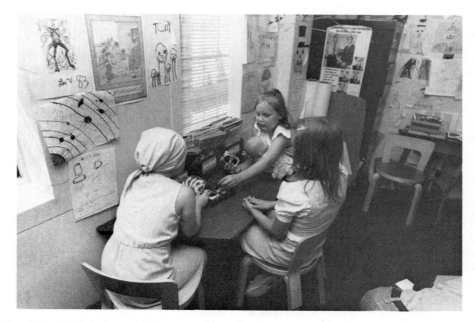

Fig. 27-3. Children frequently interact with each other, expressing thoughts and feelings about chemotherapy.

Table 27-4. Cancer in the school-age child: meeting basic needs and supporting developmental tasks

Positive body image	Create situations for positive reinforcement of child's self-image. Stress side effects as being temporary. Provide ways to decrease effects of treatment.
Increased industry	Allow for continuance of daily activities such as play and school. Support situations for discovery and achievement.
Increased sensory perceptions	Prevent occurrence of sensory loss when possible. Provide opportunities during hospital stay for sensory awareness.
Independence	Support child's self-care and participation in treatment. Provide times in which the child can function without significant others.
Awareness of world	Allow for verbalization of the child's perception of his world. Encourage expression through play and artwork.

IMPACT OF CANCER: THE ADOLESCENT

The adolescent is acutely aware of what development of cancer entails. It alters the adolescent's immediate plans and futuristic goals. Cancer is frightening; it brings with it a realization of finiteness to self and to the universe. It alters time, which is of most importance to the adolescent.[17] Existence is not only for today in the adolescent's mind but encompasses plans for the future. Development of cancer prevents many plans from occurring. The adolescent's entire life-style is altered, no longer

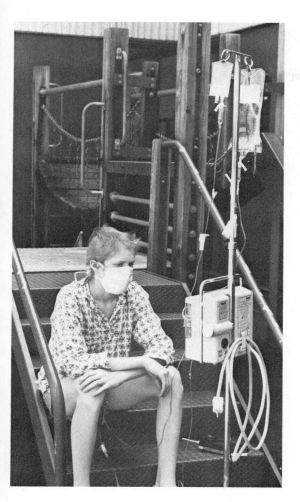

Fig. 27-4. The adolescent with cancer is often lonely and depressed, wishing it had not happened to him.

the young child who strives to continue his role as it was before the disease had occurred.[12]

The adolescent's increased awareness of the severity of cancer may greatly affect the ability to continue previous activities of daily living. The adolescent often becomes depressed and withdraws early in the onset of the disease (Fig. 27-4). It may take months before he is willing to deal realistically with the situation. Silently, the adolescent may become bitter and angry that the cancer has happened to him and not to others. Resignation toward destiny develops and creates a total lack of affect. To cope effectively with the onset of cancer, reorganization of the adolescent's entire life-style must occur.[10]

Adjustment to alterations caused by the disease are often difficult and frustrating. Acknowledgment of the loss of the adolescent's former self may cause confusion as to who he has become. With the acknowledgment, however, comes an understanding of his new world. New roles develop as feelings and fears surface. The adolescent must continue to value himself as a person, irrespective of the disease. Limitations are acknowledged but do not prevent the adolescent's continued self-awareness. Autonomy, a goal that adolescents strive for as they think about the future, is challenged and altered with the onset of cancer.[10] The adolescent becomes dependent on significant others for assistance in meeting even basic needs, and this dependence creates strife and loss of pride.

Emphasis must be placed on integrating the restrictions placed on the adolescent by the disease while maintaining continued autonomy (see Table 27-5). Realization of alterations in life-style must be dealt with while reorganizing his life to endeavor to obtain those goals previously identified.

IMPACT OF CANCER: THE PARENTS

The impact of cancer occurring in a child affects the total family.[18] Parental attitudes and emotions alter perceptions of the disease. Family stability plays a major role in furthering acceptance of cancer in a child. Cancer brings with it feelings of anxiety, fear, depression, and helplessness. Crate

providing time for activities once deemed so essential. Energy must be turned inward to fighting the disease. There is often little energy remaining to allow participation in previous activities. The capacity to tolerate cancer encompasses the adolescent's entire existence.[11] This is different from

Table 27-5. Cancer in the adolescent: meeting basic needs and supporting developmental tasks

Autonomy	Support independence and provide means for autonomy in decision making. Stress importance of this to parents.
Maintaining beliefs and values	Recognize beliefs and values and honor these. Provide positive reinforcement in the development of the adolescent's beliefs. Allow the adolescent to express beliefs and respect them.
Enforcement of self-esteem	Provide situations to reinforce self-esteem. Always treat the adolescent with respect as a unique individual separate from the parents. Strive to know the adolescent personally.
Development of future goals	Encourage development of future goals while assisting the adolescent in dealing realistically with the situation.
Achievement	Stress importance of continued participation in education and other areas of continued improvement. Assist in planning programs to meet the adolescent's needs, realizing the limitations placed on him by the disease.

defines specific stages in one's adaptation to a disease.[10] Initially, disbelief evolves, with family members expressing shock and denial. Inappropriate responses in affect and behavior are common.[10] Effective coping mechanisms help the child and family to adapt to the disease.[18] These mechanisms include: tolerating or relieving anxiety related to the illness; maintaining self-esteem; continuing positive personal relationships; and using available resources to deal with stressful encounters.[19]

Cancer in a child imposes an acute threat to the psychologic and physical well-being of parents.[20] Types of cancer vary in their nature and degree of debilitation, causing different reactions. All families, however, react to the diagnosis of cancer in a similar fashion. Acute anxiety, confusion, and hopelessness are initial reactions. Frequently, there is an inability to recognize the facts and accept the diagnosis as true.[21] Parents may react to the stress through withdrawal or flight. As shock and disbelief subside, an awareness of the intensity of the child's disease develops. Depression, anger, and apathy are frequently manifested, and a sense of loss of control over the future may be expressed.[22]

Factors affecting the parents' ability to adjust vary according to the nature of the disease; prognosis of the child; parental attitudes and emotional balance; adjustment of the child at onset; and threats the disease may have on the child's basic needs.[23] The degree to which cancer restricts a child's activities greatly affects the parents' ability to cope.[24] Excessive guilt is felt if the parents blame themselves for the disease's occurrence. Early support for the parent in working through guilt is essential. Parents must be assisted in making provisions in the home environment for those restrictions placed on the child by the illness. They must seek out ways to carry out the family life-style in the framework of changes brought on by the child's illness.[13]

The age of the child at the onset of cancer may affect the parent's coping methods. The younger child may be totally unaware of the severity of the disease, whereas the teenager has an acute awareness of what it means. This makes it more difficult for parents to hide their fears and concerns. Attitudes of the parents developed over years of experience affect adjustment to cancer. Previous life experiences with similar conflicts cause them to use adequate or inadequate coping skills.[20] Early identification of previous experiences that may hinder the parents' ability to adjust to their child's disease is essential. Open discussion helps to alleviate fears or misconceptions that the parents have developed.

The behavior of the child who has cancer affects the parents. A child who is secure, independent, and has a positive sense of self will adjust more easily to the onset of cancer than one who has not adjusted well to his world.[23] Parents often experience turmoil when their child is having difficulty adapting. It is essential to explore the child's personality to provide support to the parents in dealing with the child. Adaptation to cancer must occur as a family, allowing for emotional adjustment of both parent and child.[24]

Parents may perceive onset of cancer in their child as a personal loss. They no longer have complete control and authority over the child. Realization that the child's existence is being placed in the hands of others may lead to guilt and anguish. Parents often see themselves as failures, as having let the child down. This guilt must be dealt with early. The parents must adjust to changes brought on by the disease. Acceptance by parents is an initial factor in providing the child with an environment in which to adjust favorably.[23] Positive parental attitudes convey acceptance to the child and support self-esteem. Health care personnel can facilitate this adjustment by providing a safe environment in which the parents can gain trust in those involved with their child. The parents must feel that the child is safe within the health care system.

Stress, brought on by the onslaught of cancer, creates unique problems for the parent. Every area of family life is altered. Parents frequently have difficulty in fulfilling their responsibilities at work and in the home.[18] The added stress of cancer may be more than they can handle. Identification of difficulties in fulfilling parental roles is essential to the development of adequate coping mechanisms.[18] Sensitive professionals can assist parents in identifying problems and can guide them in their own adjustment process, thereby enabling them to perform their roles within the family once again.

Outcome of parental stress brought on by the onset of cancer is dependent on several factors.[18] Parents must first comprehend the nature of the disease and must be able to communicate its seriousness to the immediate family members. This is often difficult for the parents who want to protect the siblings and extended family members from grief. This protection often causes difficulty with other family members, especially siblings who may feel neglected and unloved. Without knowing it, the parent may ignore the other children and appear to no longer care about them. Parents who share appropriate feelings of grief and sadness with all family members are able to deal with the stress of cancer more effectively.[20] Sharing feelings allows for participation by all family members in the adjustment period. Constructive exploration of feelings and fears allows for each family member to increase their awareness of the situation. Professionals can help parents identify and build on their strengths, allowing for the development of positive methods for coping (see Table 27-6).[23] With the identification of these strengths, the parent is able to accept the cancer in their child and develop ways in which to carry out their previous lifestyle. This may not occur without drastic change caused by the disease, but the parent who uses strengths and coping skills developed through previous life experiences will be able to create a lifestyle for all family members comparable to that before the onset of cancer in the child.

IMPACT OF CANCER: THE SIBLING

Siblings who lack the ability to understand the intensity of the situation may portray disbelief initially. They often express jealousy toward the affected child, unable to realize the severity of the disease.[13] Siblings may only perceive the increased attention given to the affected child by the parents. Subsequent rivalry is expressed through changes in behavior, school performance, and attitudes toward the affected child.

There are times when the sibling reacts inwardly by mimicking the symptoms of the affected child. He may literally feel the pain the disease is inflicting on his loved one. The sibling may become depressed and may regress, often unable to express fears of losing a loved one. This situation is magnified when the child who has cancer is near the age of the sibling.[13] They may share the same room, same toys, same clothes, same friends, and even the same classroom. The sibling may sense an unbearable loss when the child who has cancer must return to the hospital. Prolonged hospitalization exacerbates the problem for the sibling by bringing about the realization of a possible permanent loss of his loved one.

Table 27-6. Cancer and parents: meeting basic needs and supporting development tasks

Understanding of child's illness	Provide education at parent's level regarding the child's diagnosis, prognosis, treatment plan, long-term goals, alterations in lifestyle. Review these concepts frequently early on to provide the parents with a knowledge base from which to cope with and alter their lifestyle as possible.
Maintenance of family system	Ensure maintenance of intact family system by exploring strengths and identifying weaknesses in the family. Provide support in alleviating those areas that cause added stress to the family (i.e., transportation, work). Stress importance of continued interaction with all family members, especially siblings.
Reorganization of life-style	Assist in providing options to alter those areas in which the family can no longer continue to function because of the disease (i.e., mother can no longer work—seek help with budget, babysitter needed—help explore options in the community).
Recognition of strengths and weaknesses	Identify those strengths in the parents that can be used to support the entire family system. Reassure the parents that they have needs also and must take time to meet these needs. Stress importance of parent having time alone, separate from the child who has cancer.
Continued identity development	As an adult, the parent must remain separate from the child. Stress the importance of the parents' continued involvement with others. Emphasize importance of parents sharing with each other and continuing their relationships as husband and wife.

Table 27-7. Cancer and the sibling: meeting basic needs and supporting development tasks

Participation in the family system	Enforce with the parents the need to continue in the family environment. Stress importance of including the sibling in all family matters.
Discussion of the illness in the family members	Provide time when the sibling visits the hospital for discussion of the ill child's progress. Allow the sibling to ask questions he may be afraid to ask of the parents.
Continued interaction with parents	Stress importance of continued closeness of the ill child and the sibling. Allow sibling to visit hospitalized child.
Understanding of illness affecting family member	Talk with sibling alone, giving concise information on the child's illness. Allow for questions. Reinforce that the disease is not contagious and that the sibling did not give it to the child.

Communication by the parents to the child's siblings provides understanding toward their loved one's disease. It is imperative to discuss cancer and its meaning with even the youngest child.[24] Siblings often think they have caused the child to become ill. Most children at one time or another have wished their sibling would go away, become ill, or even die. The development of cancer may be perceived as something the sibling has caused. It is essential for the family to talk about the disease by stressing that no one caused the child to become ill as shown in Table 27-7. The sibling may fear

acquiring the disease but may be unable to express this concern. His fears can be alleviated through open discussion with the family. Many professionals use books that address issues pertaining to the effects of cancer on the sibling.

It is vital to stress the importance of the parents in continuing their relationship with the siblings.[13] Parents often feel that they must devote all their time to the ill child. This creates an even more difficult situation for the sibling. The sibling must not feel neglected but continually feel a part of the family regardless of the circumstances.

REFERENCES

1. Mahler, M.: Symbiosis and individuation: the psychological birth of the human infant, Psychoanal. Study Child **29**:39, 1974.
2. Illingworth, R.S.: The development of the infant and young child, normal and abnormal, New York, 1975, Churchill Livingstone, Inc.
3. Skerret, K., Hardin, S., and Puskar, K.: Infant anxiety, Matern. Child Nurs. J. **12**(1):51, 1983.
4. Pontious, S.: Practical Piaget: helping children understand, Am. J. Nurs. **82**:114, 1982.
5. Piaget, J., and Inhelder, B.: The psychology of the child, New York, 1969, Basic Books.
6. Sherwen, L.: Separation: the forgotten phenomenon of child development, Top. Clin. Nurs. **5**(1):1, 1983.
7. Erikson, E.H.: Childhood and society, New York, 1950, W.W. Norton & Co., Inc.
8. Gratz, R.R., Zembe, R.: Piaget, preschoolers and pediatric practice, Phys. Occup. Ther. Pediatr. **1**(1):3, 1980.
9. Illingworth, R.S.: The normal child, New York, 1975, Churchill Livingstone, Inc.
10. Bernardo, M.L.: A conceptual mode of children's cognitive adaptation to physical disability, J. Adv. Nurs. **7**:595, 1982.
11. Geist, R.A.: Onset of chronic illness in children and adolescents, Am. J. Orthopsychiatry **49**(1):4, 1979.
12. Mattsson, A.: Long-term physical illness in childhood: a challenge to psychosocial adaptation, Pediatrics **50**(5):801, 1972.
13. Spinetta, J.J.: Living with childhood cancer, St. Louis, 1981, The C.V. Mosby Co.
14. Bibace, R., and Walsh, M.E.: Development of children's concept of illness, Pediatrics **66**(6):912, 1980.
15. Stanwyck, D.J.: Self-esteem through the lifespan, Fam. Community Health **6**(2):11, 1983.
16. Selekam, J.: The development of body image in the child: a learned response, Top. Clin. Nurs. **5**(1):12, 1983.
17. Erikson, E.H.: Identity, youth and crisis, New York, 1968, W.W. Norton & Co., Inc.
18. Kaplan, D.M.: Family mediation of stress, Soc. Work. **18**:60, 1973.
19. Johnson, M.P.: Support groups for parents of chronically ill children, Pediatr. Nurs. **8**:160, 1982.
20. Krouse, H.J., and Krouse, J.H.: Cancer as crises: the critical elements of adjustment, Nurs. Res. **31**(2):96, 1982.
21. Lawrence, S.A., and Lawrence, R.M.: A model of adaptation to stress of chronic illness, Nurs. Forum **18**(1):34, 1979.
22. Townes, B.D., Wold, D.A., and Holmes, T.H.: Parental adjustment to childhood leukemia, J. Psychosom. Res. **18**:9, 1974.
23. Hughes, J.G.: The emotional impact of chronic disease, Am. J. Dis. Child. **130**:1199, 1976.
24. Kellerman, J.: Psychological aspects of childhood cancer, Springfield, Ill., 1980, Charles C Thomas, Publisher.

ADDITIONAL READINGS

Campbell, J.D.: Illness is a point of view: the development of children's concepts of illness, Child Develop. **46**:12, 1975.

Counte, M.A., and others: Stress and personal attitudes in chronic illness, Arch. Phys. Med. Rehabil. **64**(6):272, 1983.

Craig, H.M., and others: Adaptation in chronic illness: an eclectic model for nurses, J. Adv. Nurs. **8**(5):397, 1983.

Crocker, E.: A review of the literature concerning the effects of hospitalization on children, Assoc. Care Child. Hosp. **3**:3, 1974.

King, E.H.: Child-rearing practices: child with chronic illness and well sibling, Issues Compr. Pediatr. Nurs. **5**:185, 1981.

Lewis, K.: Grief in chronic illness and disability, J. Rehabil. **49**(3):8, 1983.

Maier, H.W.: Three theories of child development: the contributions of Erik H. Erikson, Jean Piaget and Robert R. Sears and their applications, New York, 1978, Harper & Row Publishers, Inc.

Pierce, P.M.: Reach: self-care for the chronically ill child, Pediatr. Nurs. **9**(1):37, 1983.

Pless, I., and Pinkerton, P.: Chronic childhood disorders, Chicago, 1975, Year Book Medical Publisher, Inc.

Thomas, D.: The social psychology of childhood disability, New York, 1980, Schocken Books, Inc.

CHAPTER 28

Crisis points in cancer

MARILYN J. HOCKENBERRY

Crisis is defined as an insolvable problem brought on by stressful events, causing loss of equilibrium in an individual.[1] A crisis differs from problems encountered in everyday life, which are dealt with by previously established problem-solving strategies. The onset of a crisis brings forth unresolved feelings, tension, and conflicts that are directly influenced by the present situation.[1] The crisis situation, which is different from anything the individual has previously encountered, prevents the use of any of the coping strategies previously established. The individual finds himself in a state of helplessness.[2]

Adaptation to a crisis situation is contingent on a number of factors. First, a crisis is time limited. Most therapists estimate the initial period to last 4 to 6 weeks.[1] Second, certain amounts of stress are essential to motivate prompt solution of a crisis situation. Third, new methods of coping developed during a previous crisis add to a family's experience and help in developing effective ways of solving problems in the future. Finally, resolution of the immediate crisis is possible only when the individual is able to establish adequate coping skills.[1] Many families have difficulty working toward a positive resolution of stress brought on by a crisis. Family members who communicate effectively with each other are more successful in developing ways of coping with an immediate crises situation.

Diagnosis, treatment, discontinuation of therapy, relapse, and end stage disease are crisis points in the development and management of childhood cancer. Successful coping with each crisis point is related to coping skills and to phases of the illness.[2]

Coping tasks must be resolved in proper sequence within the time frame set by the phases of illness. This chapter addresses each major crisis point in childhood cancer and discusses how the professional can facilitate a family's adaptation and coping.

DIAGNOSIS

The diagnosis of cancer in a child causes psychologic disarray. The initial phase of distress cannot be resolved by ordinary coping strategies.[1] At the time of diagnosis, feelings of anxiety, fear, depression, and helplessness emerge. Disbelief as to how this disease could occur in a child is frequently observed, with parents questioning the diagnosis.

Families frequently experience a prediagnostic phase, a time of questioning the presence of illness in the child. It is a time of grave concern in which parents realize the child is not well yet refuse to accept the reality of the situation.[3] Fears and concerns are unanswerable; no one has yet established what is wrong with the child. The child is usually referred immediately on suspicion of cancer to a major medical center. This facility is often hundreds of miles away from home, which increases the stress placed on the family. They find themselves in unfamiliar surroundings with no one close to provide support.

Some families have unfortunate experiences during this phase. Their child's problem may go undiagnosed for weeks to even months. Numerous diagnostic tests may have been performed without finding a diagnosis. This period of question causes even greater anxiety. Families may become bitter and angry at health professionals who cannot diagnose the problem. This is a time when development of trust in physicians, nurses, and other professionals involved in the child's care is essential.[4] Families must feel that professionals caring for their child truly care.

The official diagnosis is usually heard first by the parents and not the child.[5] Although most parents suspect the diagnosis, most are not prepared to hear the word *cancer*. Parents often react strongly, expressing disbelief, anger, guilt, and grief.[5] They may be unable to hear or understand what the physician is saying and may be physically distressed to the point of losing control of their emotions. The conversation may need to be delayed until the parents regain control of themselves. It is essential for health care professionals to remain patient and supportive to the family during this time. Most information given at the time of initial diagnosis is not retained.[6] Parents and family members may hear the word cancer and nothing else.

Initial discussions with the family gives them a sense of what support systems are available from the health care team. It is the first time in which family members are given a definite plan to solve their problem. Professionals meeting with the family at this time have the ability to establish the beginning of a trusting relationship (Fig. 28-1).

Once the word cancer is heard and families begin to realize what has been said, the most important message families receive is hope for their child. Even the family whose child has a poor prognosis needs to know that individuals caring for their child have hope for the situation. There may be situations in which there is little to no hope for survival, yet professionals must maintain a sense of hope. This may be expressed by comforting the child and stressing that everything possible will be done.

Previous methods of coping will influence the

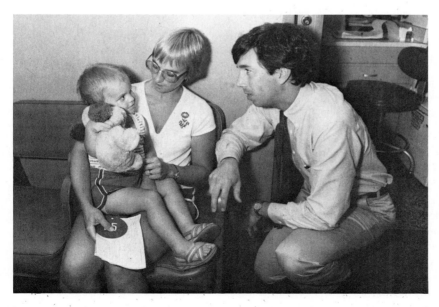

Fig. 28-1. The family with a child newly diagnosed with cancer needs time to establish a trusting relationship with the professional caring for the child.

family's initial reaction to the diagnosis.[7] Experience with illness in other family members and friends may influence their level of perception. Stresses that the family has undergone in the past will influence adaptation to the present illness. Families having previous experiences with cancer in a loved one will have more knowledge regarding the situation yet may have biased ideas and feelings about cancer. Those who have experienced the loss of a loved one to cancer may see no hope in the situation and be more difficult to convince otherwise. Individuals tend to rely on their past experiences to give them guidance in reacting to the present crisis.

It is imperative for the oncology team to give no false reassurances yet at the same time to provide positive support to the situation. Anticipation for the future, no matter how dismal, must be addressed at the initial presentation of the diagnosis.

CASE PRESENTATION

J.G. was a 6-year-old female diagnosed with stage IV neuroblastoma. At the time of presentation, she had an abdominal mass, involvement of the bone marrow and liver, and skeletal metastases. The oncology team met with the family to establish the diagnosis. The physician expressed honestly to the family that J.G. had a type of cancer that was incurable. He went on to express that there were types of therapy that J.G. would ideally respond to and the team would try everything possible to help J.G. Initially, the family responded with shock and disbelief. The father stated he knew that there had been something terribly wrong and that it wasn't just an infection as he had been told previously. They responded with anger at the previous physician who had not been able to diagnose the illness. Their next question was how long did J.G. have to live. The physician appropriately discussed the possibility that J.G. could improve on chemotherapy and that it would help her pain. The question of how long she had to live remained unanswerable.

As seen in the case presentation, once the family has had time to regain control of their emotions, further discussion is necessary to provide information regarding the illness and its effect on the child.[6] It is important for professionals to realize that parents will not be able to retain information

at this encounter. The diagnosis, its prognosis, and type of treatment may be all the information they can process at this time. Future discussion will provide a more detailed explanation of the disease, its treatment and side effects, and concerns for the future. The professional team must make it clear in the first discussion that there will be numerous encounters to further explain the child's illness. Parents should be told that they are not expected to retain everything that is said.

The child must receive an adequate explanation of his disease.[8] Parents frequently hesitate in telling their child of cancer. They worry that the word will produce fear and anxiety in the child. This concern is often their own and not the child's. Most children by school age know the word cancer but are not clear on its meaning. When hearing the word, they may remember a grandmother or another loved one who has died of cancer. Parents may fear the child will think the same thing is going to happen to him. For this reason, parents may wish for the oncology team to tell the child about cancer. Discussing cancer with a child should be done in simple terms that the child can understand. Telling a 6-year-old with leukemia that he has something wrong with the blood for which he must take medicine may be sufficient; whereas, a 17-year-old with osteogenic sarcoma may need a much more complete explanation of the disease, its prognosis, treatment, and side effects. As seen in the following case presentation, the word cancer should be used to prevent the child from hearing it from someone other than those he or she trusts. Parents may be resistant to telling the child of cancer. Honest discussion of cancer, taking into consideration the child's developmental stage, can provide additional support to the family members. Many find it makes the family more relaxed with the diagnosis.[3]

CASE PRESENTATION

P.L. was a 6-year-old girl diagnosed with acute lymphocytic leukemia. She had been well all her life until 2 days before admission when she developed high fever and was taken to the pediatrician. The pediatrician, after finding blasts on her peripheral blood smear, transferred her to a medical center 200 miles away. The diagnosis of leukemia was established the next day. The family reacted appropriately with disbelief as to how she had been well a week ago and now had a possibly fatal disease. The parents were at a loss as to how to break the news to P.L. and asked the oncology team to tell her. When the team entered her room, she was watching TV. The doctor told her they needed to talk about why she had come to the hospital. In simple terms, she was told she had leukemia, a type of cancer that affects the white blood cell. The team went on to explain to her that she would need to take chemotherapy. The chemotherapy would make the leukemia cells go away. P.L. looked concerned and asked, "Will these sticks in the vein hurt me?" The doctor explained that "these sticks" were just like the one she had in her arm when she arrived yesterday. "Oh, that didn't hurt very much," she commented, "but I don't like them." Without pausing, P.L. asked, "Am I going to die?" The doctor calmly assured her that she was not going to die now and that the chemotherapy was used to make the leukemia go away and never come back.

The crisis of the diagnostic period is further intensified by the treatment regimen. The family not only hears the word cancer but now faces chemotherapy, surgery, and radiation therapy. These modes of treatment are frightening within themselves.[9] Unlike other chronic diseases the family is faced with the necessity to treat immediately. There is no time for indecision, and this intensifies the crisis. The family is faced with almost no choice, since their child will die if treatment is not initiated.[4] Family members have no chance to adjust to the diagnosis before making a decision about treatment. The extent of physical and functional impairment is clearly important in influencing the situation.[4] The child with neuroblastoma who is in severe pain may cause the family to make a decision more quickly than the child with Hodgkin's disease who has a painless, enlarged lymph node. The greater the extent of infirmity, the greater the immediacy of the situation.

Reactions to the diagnosis remain complex and varied. Many families state that their immediate response to the word cancer was knowing that their child was going to die. Parent's belief in the fatality

of the disease may lead to a willingness to begin therapy immediately to save the child's life. An essential task in the establishment of adequate methods of coping is the realization that the disease may be fatal.[2] From the moment the family is told of the diagnosis, they must cope with the threat of death. This perception changes the family's previous coping strategies.[4]

Certain families deny the diagnosis of cancer and react with disorganization and apathy. Disbelief in the diagnosis causes conflict between the professional team and family. In these situations, outside advice and second opinions are encouraged and can often provide the family with more support.[3] For families to deal with the diagnosis, they must believe in and begin to develop trust in the professionals caring for their child. The stress of cancer may cause conflict for even the most stable family. Marriages are strained because of the intensity of the situation. The family is separated, both by miles and emotion. The child and mother are often alone because the father and other family members must remain at home to continue work and school. The mother frequently feels abandoned and bitter that she must assume responsibility for the child's care. The father is torn between being with the child and mother and returning home to continue work to support the family.

Several factors influence a family's ability to cope with the crisis of a diagnosis of cancer as seen in Table 28-1.[10] Acute anxiety, brought on by the diagnosis, must be alleviated. As previously discussed, the family must be allowed to regain control of their emotions once they have heard the diagnosis. Assistance in identifying previously established coping skills can provide immediate support to the family.[4] Key individuals who are clearly designated as support figures should be available to provide comfort to family members who are unable to deal with the diagnosis. It is imperative to restore the family system as quickly as possible, since its disruption creates added stress to the situation.[11] All family members must be considered, not only the child with newly diagnosed cancer. This restoration of family function provides a stable

Table 28-1. Diagnosis

Essential coping tasks	Interventions
Gaining control of emotions	Allow time for parents to be alone to grieve
Alleviating acute anxiety	Maintain hope for the child no matter how serious the situation
	Allow the family to express their feelings and fears
Understanding of the diagnosis	Spend time discussing the diagnosis and its meaning before presenting a plan for treatment
Explaining cancer to the child	Using terms the child can understand, tell the child about cancer and its need for treatment
Establishing the treatment regimen	Begin discussions with parents and the child about the treatment regimen and side effects
Preventing anxiety regarding discharge and home care	Begin early to discuss care for the child at home
	Identify key support individuals who will assist the family at home
Allowing for participation of other family members	Discuss with siblings and other family members the child's diagnosis and treatment
	Encourage siblings to visit the child

support to a system that has been greatly disrupted by the onset of illness.

Belief systems are crucial and must be maintained.[11] They are frequently disrupted when families begin to question their belief in a supreme being who should protect children from cancer. It is wise to allow the family to express their feelings regarding their beliefs and values. These are personal aspects of the family system that should be dealt with by each individual. The professional team should not place their own beliefs and values on the family but instead should allow the family to verbalize their thoughts to a nonbiased listener.

Coping with the crisis of cancer requires the development of new attitudes, behaviors, and coping techniques.[12] Family members must work together in establishing a life-style that not only allows for optimum treatment and management of the child with cancer but also provides a way of life comparable to that before the diagnosis.

TREATMENT

Therapy for childhood cancer has evolved from providing comfort to delivering aggressive regimens in hope of cure.[13] Treatment varies in intensity and frequency and is specific to the type of

cancer. Certain regimens may require a family to return to a medical center as frequently as every 3 weeks. The more complex a treatment regimen, the more interference there is with the family's rehabilitation and reintegration.[4]

Cost of care for the child with cancer becomes a major stress factor, second only to the illness. Financial constraints are not only caused by medical expenditures but include such things as transportation to and from the medical center, parking, food, care for other children at home, and clothing for the child. The family income is frequently altered, especially when single parent families are involved when the sole wage earner must miss work and also bring the child for treatment. Financial stresses must be addressed early on by investigating all available programs that may provide support for the family.

Families vary in their resilience and ability to adapt to treatment.[4] The initiation of treatment often accentuates the diagnosis of cancer and forces the family to think about the reality of the situation. There may be much distress with the onset of treatment, which may be short-lived or may continue throughout the whole treatment regimen.

Most treatment for childhood cancer is initiated

in the hospital. This is a time of stress, since many families have just learned of the diagnosis and now must face the treatment. How they cope with the initiation of treatment often gives the oncology team an idea about how they will cope with crisis in the future.[14] Unstable families are identified by their inability to hear anything but the diagnosis. Identifying these families early enables the professional to provide emotional support and to explore appropriate ways for the family to gain adequate coping methods. Other resources in the family and community should be identified early to begin working with the family even before discharge.[4]

It is common for families to become anxious about going home from the hospital after the child has received the first treatment. Their anxiety may be related to feelings of inadequacy in caring for their child and lack of knowledge of the disease, its treatment, and side effects. There should be no rush for discharge. Parents should be encouraged to take the time necessary to establish a basic understanding of their child's disease process, the rationale behind treatment, and the resulting side effects. Families learn at different rates, since learning is affected by educational background, culture, and level of anxiety. Allowing adequate time for family members to grasp basic concepts enables them to feel more comfortable in the care of their child at home.

There will be families who are unable, for reasons such as emotional instability, denial, level of intelligence, or inability to listen during the initial hospitalization, to retain vital information.[5] The professional may find that each encounter produces more stress in family members. These families clearly need time to adjust to the impact of all that has occurred. There may be concern that they will be unable to adequately care for the child with the level of knowledge obtained at initial hospitalization. For these families, identification of a responsible family member or friend is essential. This individual can support the family until they are able to acquire more information and skills regarding the care of the child. Close communication with

the family is essential between treatments to evaluate the child's status at home. Thorough instruction by the oncology team enables the majority of families to leave the hospital with basic skills to care for their child. Most parents feel inadequate initially and require much support from the team. Periodic phone calls to the family give reassurance that they are functioning well at home. Involvement of support personnel in the community setting also gives the family a sense of security, knowing that there is someone close by. The child's local pediatrician and nurse should be included in the child's care from the time of initial diagnosis. Their participation allows for more continuity and lends additional support to the family.

On discharge from the hospital, the family reestablishes a routine that coordinates activities of family members with visits to the treatment center. Work schedules often become altered, and transportation to all scheduled activities sometimes become a problem. The oncology team and local support personnel can help the family establish a workable routine for all members. Understandably, each family member must play a part in developing such a routine.

Siblings often expect that when the child and parents return from the hospital, life will go on as before.[4] When they realize that life is indeed different, resentment and rivalry may occur. It is essential for the sibling to be told about the child's illness. When possible, the siblings should visit the child at the hospital to obtain a better understanding of what being ill entails.[14] Siblings often see their parents with presents and food for the child who is ill and do not understand where the child is or what has happened. Visitation provides the sibling with a more accurate sense of what has really happened. On discharge, the child's siblings should be told that he is still sick, even though he is coming home. They should be told what the child has, and the word cancer should be used.[5] Parents often find it helpful for someone on the oncology team to talk with the siblings. It is encouraged to do this separate from the parents and child to give the sibling an opportunity to ask questions more openly.

CASE PRESENTATION

R.K. is an 11-year-old white male diagnosed with osteosarcoma of the left femur. He underwent an above-the-knee amputation 2 weeks ago and has begun his first course of high-dose methotrexate chemotherapy. R.K. has two younger brothers, ages 6 and 8, who visited him in the hospital. Their parents told them that R.K. has cancer and that was why his leg had to be removed. The parents, concerned with the siblings' level of understanding, asked the oncology team to meet with them. One member of the oncology team who was experienced in talking with siblings met alone with the boys. She explained simply that R.K. had a type of cancer that occurred in his bone. Cancer was described as an abnormal cell that grew and divided into many cells and R.K.'s amputation was necessary to prevent the rapidly dividing cancer cells from spreading. The discussion was stopped momentarily to allow for questions. The 6-year-old timidly asked, "What did they do with my brother's leg after they cut it off?" "What did they use to cut it with?" he continued without waiting for a reply to the first question. The professional simply discussed how their brother was put to sleep and a special type of equipment used only in the operating room was used to remove the leg. She went on to tell the boys how it was important to look at the cells in R.K.'s bone under the microscope and that special slides were prepared from the tissue of his leg. The 8-year-old then asked, "Is R.K. going to die?" The member of the oncology team told the boys that this is an important question because many siblings are worried about death when their brother is diagnosed with cancer. She acknowledged that some children do die of cancer but that the doctors and nurses were going to do everything possible to prevent that from happening to R.K. She then explained that the medicine R.K. had to take when he came to the hospital was to get rid of the cancer so that R.K. would not die.

As seen by the case presentation, siblings must be allowed to verbalize their fears.[4] They may often hesitate to ask questions to their parents and for this reason must have a knowledgeable confidante whom they can depend on to give them simple, honest answers to their questions. Siblings should be encouraged to return to the hospital when their sister or brother receives chemotherapy.

The child recently diagnosed with cancer will need time to readjust to the changed life-style.[16] He may perceive a change in his body image, dependent on its alteration by disease or treatment. It is essential to allow the child to ask questions about his illness and treatment. The child may worry about seeing friends and returning to school. There may be a period of time when the child must miss school, and resentment toward those who are healthy and active may develop. The child needs time for adjustment, and parents must allow the child to regain independence. Parents must balance their own concerns and fears with the child's need to regain integrity and independence.[3]

Onset of treatment is a time when parents further explore their own feelings. It is a phase in which they begin to adjust to the diagnosis and establish an alternate life-style.[3] Treatment places strains on any marriage.[14] Parents often have little time together because of the rigor of treatment schedules and day-to-day family life. It is imperative for parents to communicate with each other. They must learn to depend on one another for strength and support. The professional should emphasize the need for parents to spend time alone with each other. This time should be used for re-establishment of communication and well-needed relaxation. Single parent families have a different kind of stress placed on them. In these families, only one parent is present to carry the burden of the entire family. These families need assistance in identifying individuals to assist with day-to-day tasks.

There are times when families may refuse treatment. This may be a result of religious or moral beliefs or unknown reasons. This places the professional team in an ethical dilemma, since the parents are responsible for decisions regarding the child's treatment. Much time is needed for discussion between the family and the oncology team to assist parents in understanding the implications no treatment entails. There are times when the parents will be overruled by higher authorities when standard treatment is known to be of benefit and yet the parents still choose to refuse treatment. Noncompliance is becoming more of an issue as survival rates continue to improve and each child's course of treatment is examined more closely. Early education does not always prevent noncompliance and may remain an issue for these families throughout treatment.

During the treatment phase, parents learn to cope with many situations. They may develop a rather sophisticated knowledge of their child's disease and treatment, and they become more comfortable in dealing with complications related to treatment. However, at times the responsibility for dealing with these situations becomes overwhelming. Parents may even act inappropriately in the best interest of their child as demonstrated by the following case presentation. There may be a tendency to overprotect and isolate the child in efforts to prevent infection or bleeding.[11] They may need to be reminded of the child's developmental needs and may welcome guidance in how to allow him more freedom. Professionals must continue to offer such

educational reinforcement and emotional support throughout the treatment period (Fig. 28-2).

CASE PRESENTATION

T.J. was 5 years old when he was diagnosed with acute lymphocytic leukemia. His parents were never able to accept the diagnosis and lived in a state of constant fear of relapse. In spite of initiation of psychologic support through weekly conferences with a psychologist, the parents were unable to allow T.J. to begin kindergarten, stating they feared he would become sick at school. They obtained a tutor for T.J. and kept him home for the first year of treatment. By the time T.J. was 6 years old, they had dealt with many of their fears and concerns and were able to allow him to begin first grade. T.J. had a great deal of difficulty interacting with the other children and was unable to participate in many of the group activities. The teacher had to work closely with T.J. to encourage development of social skills. T.J.

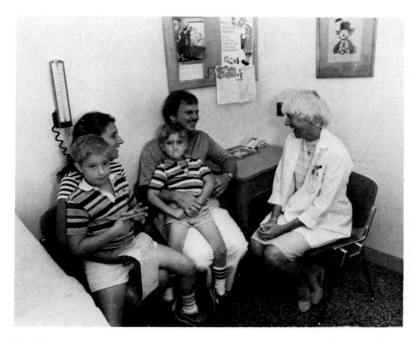

Fig. 28-2. Families have concerns and questions throughout treatment and need continued emotional support from those involved with the child's care.

showed appropriate motor skills for age; he knew his numbers, colors, and how to write his name; but his interactions with the other children showed him to be delayed in social development. He interacted as a pre-schooler. It took 6 months for him to obtain confidence in his interactions with other classmates.

Several principles ensure the development of appropriate coping methods during the treatment phase.[17] All involved must be aware of possible changes in the child's appearance, function, and routines.[18] The child with cancer should participate in decision making and management of care. The child must be given as much control as possible over his environment to promote continued growth and development. Management should be shared by the whole family when feasible as shown in Table 28-2.[18] This prevents jealousy among the siblings and decreases stress in the family. When possible, the child's illness and treatment should be shared with others in his environment to prevent misunderstanding and unwarranted fears. Parents should take control of every situation that allows for decision making to prevent the evolution of uncertainty, passivity, and helplessness.[18]

DISCONTINUATION OF THERAPY

The onset of a chronic illness permanently changes a family. Over time, the family learns to adjust to these changes as the reality of the child's illness is faced. The family and the child have experienced the shock of diagnosis, emotional trauma of treatment, fear of periodic illnesses, and uncertainty of the future. The family has learned to become an effective decision maker regarding numerous aspects of the child's disease.[19] Treatment becomes a way of life. Routine clinic visits, weekly blood counts, and periodic chemotherapy cycles become a part of day-to-day function. The family has adapted to an intense schedule and has established it as a part of their lifestyle. Each fam-

Table 28-2. Treatment

Essential coping tasks	Interventions
Accepting the diagnosis	Allow for continued discussion of the diagnosis with parents and family members
	Reinforce with parents that it is normal to have continued fears and doubts
Understanding treatment and its side effects	Throughout the treatment, continue discussions of treatment and its side effects to increase the family's understanding
Identifying support individuals for the family	Assist the family to identify individuals who will support the family during times of crisis and need
Establishing alternate routines, lifestyle	Provide opportunities for the family to begin re-establishing their lifestyle to meet each family member's needs
	Encourage activities the family participated in before diagnosis
	Stress importance of child's returning to school
Providing support for the child	Allow the child to express his own thoughts and feelings, separate from the parents
	Provide opportunities for age-appropriate play therapy, especially for intrusive procedures
	Provide the child with explanations for any body changes occurring from the disease or treatment
	Allow the child to actively participate in care
Continuing sibling's participation as a family member	Stress importance of including siblings in conversations and care
	Allow siblings to accompany the child to hospital when feasible
	Stress that the parents need to provide time alone with other siblings when at home

ily member becomes accustomed to disruptions and changes in plans. These changes become routine and adaptation becomes an ordinary occurrence.

Most families adapt to treatment and adjust to their change in lifestyle. They become comfortable with their system of managing a family and continuing therapy for the child with cancer. They become knowledgeable in all aspects of care and react to the needs of their child confidently.[4] Importance of treatment is understood in terms of preventing disease recurrence.

The treatment itself becomes a means of security for the child and family. Years of therapy, without evidence of further disease, establishes its success. This security provides the family with the realization that their child can be cured of cancer.[12] As months to years pass, their confidence increases, and they put faith in the treatment the child is receiving. Parents often become compulsive in their attitude toward chemotherapy. They follow regimens without error and become anxious when therapy is altered or delayed. In their eyes, the child's chance for success must not be toyed with.

Cessation of therapy can bring with it new fears for the child and family. Their security is gone. The family can no longer rely on treatment to prevent return of disease. Parents often fear discontinuing therapy more than initiating it. They are no longer overtly fighting disease, and their concern for its return is evident. Preparation for discontinuation of therapy is as essential as initial teaching at diagnosis.[14] It takes months for parents to prepare for this change in attitude. They must begin to perceive their child as having the potential to be cured and must begin to sort out their fears and concerns about discontinuing therapy. When possible, preparation should begin 2 to 3 months before therapy is actually discontinued. During routine chemotherapy visits, discussion should begin regarding the issues of discontinuing chemotherapy. The professional can initiate this conversation by stating therapy would not be stopped unless the oncology team felt it appropriate. Families working with a group of professionals over the course of treatment, trust and rely on these individuals for

guidance. Their trust in the oncology team will make it easier to discontinue therapy. Time must be taken to discuss the family's concerns. Understandably, fear of disease recurrence is great, and questions of when and how the disease may recur are common. It is important to address these issues and allow parents to verbalize their fears.

Parents often feel uncomfortable with how to treat the child after therapy is discontinued.[9] They have developed a way of life that has centered around therapy. Families are hesitant to let go of the security found in previous routine activities such as weekly blood counts, monitoring illness of playmates, preventing exposure to chickenpox, and close observation for fever. For example, frequently parents of children with leukemia who are off therapy experience the trauma of the child being exposed to chickenpox. Previously, they have been told this can be a life-threatening experience, and now the oncology team tells them not to be concerned. Parents continue to be worried and concerned and often cannot comprehend why it is no longer a problem. Parental concerns about changes in their routine and rituals should be taken seriously. Stress can be reduced if time is taken to discuss why certain precautionary measures are no longer necessary. Parents will need time to adapt to these changes. Allowing the family to adapt to these changes enables them to maintain a more stable support system at home.[9] If the family or child feels uneasy about discontinuing blood counts immediately, allow them to continue them for as long as they feel necessary. This is much like a weaning process.

A child learns to adapt to an illness and accepts the treatment as an established way of life.[20] The child grows dependent on therapy but adjusts to alterations the illness makes on his life. This adaptation allows the child to continue to grow and develop within the limitations established by the disease. Discontinuation of therapy changes the child's world once again. The child may not remember his way of life before the illness and must now deal with the changes he will encounter with cessation of therapy.[12]

CASE PRESENTATION

D.B. is a 9-year-old white male diagnosed with non-Hodgkin's lymphoma. He completed 3 years of treatment with no further evidence of disease. Shortly before therapy was discontinued, D.B.'s mother noticed his moods were changing and he would often become irritable for no apparent reason. D.B.'s schoolwork also deteriorated. One week after D.B.'s therapy was discontinued, he had his first nightmare. He awakened in the night, hysterical and unable to recognize his parents. On awakening the next day, D.B. was not able to remember anything about the night before. These nightmares continued on for weeks. A complete workup proved negative for physiologic causes for the changes in behavior or the nightmares. Psychologic intervention was pursued. D.B. began attending a group therapy session for children with cancer. In these sessions, D.B. began to draw pictures and talk about his fears of disease recurrence.

The case presentation demonstrates that the child frequently fears discontinuation of therapy as much as the parents.[9] For years, discussion of therapy has emphasized that it prevents the child from becoming ill. Parents often tell the child that the medications prevent him from becoming sick like he was before beginning therapy. When the child has refused or rebelled against treatment, the rationale is re-emphasized. The child is now faced with no more medication to keep him well. He may be scared that the disease will return yet may be unable to express his fears. Fears and concerns are very real for the child and sensitivity must be used when talking with him. The professional can provide both support and reassurance by assisting the child in identifying fears regarding discontinuing therapy (Fig. 28-3).[12]

Siblings may also question the reason for discontinuing therapy. They too have been told that the child with cancer is receiving therapy to keep him well. They are now told that therapy is no longer necessary. Siblings may become confused and need reassurance that discontinuing therapy does not mean the child will again become ill.[11] Professionals who have developed a trusting relationship with the family may need to talk with the siblings to reassure them that it is safe for therapy to be discontinued.

Cessation of therapy requires adjustment to a new way of life, different from that previously coped with so effectively.[9] The family must begin to balance their feelings of being overjoyed with the child's successful treatment with their fears of disease recurrence.

Adaptation to the situation prevents the child and family from living in constant fear of disease return. As they adjusted to the disease and its treatment regimen, they must adapt to emotional strains brought on by removing their security. Some psychologists have used the term "a roller coaster effect" to define individuals experiencing an illness

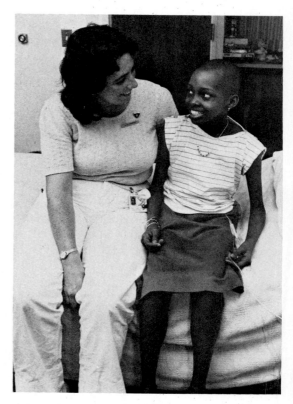

Fig. 28-3. Opportunities to discuss fears and concerns about discontinuing chemotherapy should be initiated by a professional the child trusts.

such as cancer.[21] At times the situation seems so curable, and the life they once knew is attainable again. At other times the situation appears overwhelming, and the future becomes bleak. The family and the child often experience this "high and low" emotional affect after cessation of treatment. Joy and fear are two emotions that are experienced almost simultaneously. Anxiety following discontinuation of therapy will linger for months. Families need constant reassurance that the child is doing well. Even with this reassurance, fear of disease recurrence remains. These fears often are exacerbated on return to the hospital, even for families with a child who has been off therapy for years.

CASE PRESENTATION

F.E. was 14 years of age and had not received therapy for acute lymphocytic leukemia for 4 years. He was returning to the clinic every 6 months and was growing and developing normally. However, the history revealed that for 1 to 2 weeks before each clinic visit during the past year, F.E. would become weak and unable to eat. He would complain of severe headaches, nausea, and at times vomiting. Physical examinations remained completely normal and all diagnostic tests were negative at each clinic visit. Further discussion with the mother gave some insight into the family dynamics. The mother stated

that she worried greatly about F.E.'s disease. They both had come to dread returning to the clinic, even though visits were now every 6 months. She felt that his disease would eventually return, stating she would not be able to cope with it again.

The case presentation reveals that parents play a vital role in relating the seriousness of the illness to the child. Parental reactions to the disease are assumed by the child to be evidence of how well he is doing. Parents are the child's authority. When parents are uncertain or have continued doubts even after years of continued remission, the child senses that fear.[6] Children often become afraid of the disease as a response to the parents' concerns. It is vital for the professional to emphasize the parents' influence on the child's perception. A positive outlook from the parents leads to a positive outlook in the child. Parents who perceive discontinuation of therapy as a positive occurrence and who react with happiness and joy give the child support and courage (Table 28-3). The child and parents need continued support for years after therapy is discontinued. A positive approach facilitates a balance for the family that minimizes the stress caused by cessation of therapy, allowing for continued growth and development without the constant threat of the disease's return.

Table 28-3. Discontinuation of therapy

Essential coping tasks	Interventions
Adapting to discontinuing treatment	Begin discussions several months before therapy is discontinued
	Allow time for parents and child to ask questions and verbalize concerns
Recognizing fear of relapse	Discuss openly the possibility of relapse
	Review concerns for parents and child regarding what to expect if relapse would occur
Realizing parents' impact on the child	Discuss importance of parents' positive attitude and how it affects the child
	Stress importance of verbalizing fears while recognizing the positive situation of discontinuing therapy
Supporting the child's needs and preventing fears	Reassure the child that therapy would not be discontinued unless he was doing well
	Allow the child to express fears separately from parents (provide support and stress need for courage and trust)

RELAPSE

For families with a child diagnosed with cancer, relapse is a word feared beyond all others. Patients never become completely confident that the disease will not return, regardless of length of time since diagnosis. Return of disease brings with it crisis for the entire family regardless of its stability.[3] The initial reaction to relapse may be denial that the cancer has returned. Behavior can be acute, with expressions of grief, rage, and anxiety being overtly displayed. Parents are simply unable to believe or understand why the cancer has returned.[5] Parents should be told the news of relapse separate from the child. This allows for them to express their emotions in privacy, regain control, and prepare themselves for telling the child.

Parents face the dilemma of how to break the news of relapse to the child. The child, regardless of age, has come to understand when parents and professionals are concerned. He must be told of the relapse. Commonly, members of the oncology team tell the child of the relapse. Children often sense that something is wrong by observing the parents' expressions and seeing their tears before a word is said. Honesty is essential, in spite of the pain in telling a child cancer has returned.

Frequently, the relapse comes without warning. Disease recurrence may be found during a routine clinic visit and is a shock to the professionals and to the parents.

Families with a child no longer receiving therapy find it more of a shock than the families with a child presently receiving therapy.[11] They felt that they had succeeded, that the child had completed treatment and responded, that the disease should never return. When relapse occurs, parents feel cheated. They must begin again the long vigil that they had come to know so well.

CASE PRESENTATION

K.B. was an 8-year-old female diagnosed with Burkitt's lymphoma. Six months after diagnosis, she continued to receive chemotherapy without evidence of disease recurrence. At a routine clinic visit, follow-up CT scans indicated return of the primary tumor. Further diagnostic workup revealed extension of the disease into the central nervous system. K.B.'s parents had no idea that a relapse had occurred because she had been doing well at home. The oncology team called the parents into the conference room and told them that they had bad news. The mother looked up in horror disbelief and said, "You can't mean the disease has come back. She's feeling well, she's not sick at all." She broke down and was unable to regain control of her emotions for several minutes. The team waited silently while the father held the mother in his arms. As she regained control, the team told the parents that K.B. had relapsed and that she would need to be told. The parents discussed briefly their plans to admit K.B. to the hospital for further evaluation and a change in chemotherapy. After time alone together, the parents and team sat with K.B. and told her that the cancer had returned. She noticed the shock and grief on her parents' faces when she asked the doctor if she was going to die. Calmly the team discussed with K.B. the fact that everyone was sad that the cancer had returned, but that her therapy was going to be changed to get rid of the cancer again. K.B. was told that she was not going to die now.

As shown by the case presentation, children experiencing relapse are aware of the seriousness of the situation.[5] They have learned that disease recurrence is a bad sign. Parents, as well as the oncology team, repeatedly emphasize with each hospital visit that the disease has not returned. Now the child is told that the disease had indeed returned. Relapse may produce fears in the child that are different from those of the parents. They may fear the side effects of the chemotherapy, or they may wonder if relapse means they will die.[4] The child with cancer may know another child who has relapsed and died and may perceive this as happening to him. The child who has relapsed may ask if what happened to another child will happen to him.

At time of relapse, it is essential to be honest with the child and the family. Hope in the situation must be maintained.[19] The child must be assured that he will remain safe. In most relapse situations, the child can be reassured that he is not going to die now.

The news of the relapse causes a feeling of hopelessness among all family members. Emphasis has been placed on the prevention of disease recurrence, and now they are faced with its presence again. The family and child need professional support to deal with feelings of anger and disbelief. The patient and family must re-establish a sense of control over the situation so that they can begin to adjust to a new set of circumstances. They must again begin the struggle to regain control over the disease. A change in disease status necessitates a shift in priorities.[21] The presence of the disease lends an urgency to the situation not experienced during its remission. The goal now is to eradicate the disease, not to prevent recurrence. The family and child have experienced the presence of the disease at the time of initial diagnosis. Memories of the initial treatment period and the stress brought on by it can cause fatigue, even before therapy is reinstituted. The return of the disease indicates failure, and the family may take this failure as a personal affront to them. Parents frequently feel guilty, as if they should have prevented the disease from returning. Anger returns, causing the parents to question why the disease has recurred in spite of all they had done to prevent its return.

CASE PRESENTATION

J.C. was diagnosed with acute lymphocytic leukemia at 14 years of age. He did well for 2 years of therapy, at which time he presented with a bone marrow relapse. J.C. understood what relapse meant but showed little emotion. He disliked the procedures but always remained passive and quiet. J.C.'s mother was emotional yet very basic in her understanding. Other family members were mentioned by J.C. and the mother but were not involved. J.C. went into remission, and after much discussion with the family and professional team, a bone marrow transplantation was performed. Before the procedures, several conferences were held with the family explaining in detail how involved the transplantation would be. J.C. had no questions and remained passive through the time preceding the transplantation. The mother became increasingly worried and began to express fears of J.C.'s chances for survival. Other family members began to get peripherally involved. The father began to visit but did not show a real understanding of the intensity of the procedure.

The bone marrow transplant took place with remarkable ease. J.C. was hospitalized for approximately 6 weeks and had no serious complications. His bone mar-

row engrafted, and he was in remission.

Over the next year, J.C. continued to come frequently to the clinic. His entire family began to come and often expressed fear and concern regarding his health. J.C. was often depressed but unable to verbalize his thoughts. He was seen routinely by a psychologist who continued to work with him. One year from transplant, J.C. presented with 85% leukemic cells in his bone marrow. J.C. sat quietly in the room and cried. This was the first real emotion he had openly displayed. He said he could not believe it. He had gone through all that (bone marrow transplant) for nothing. J.C.'s family were now very involved, as if, for the first time, they understood the implications of the relapse. Their responses were of shock and disbelief. It was difficult for them to believe that J.C. had relapsed after having a bone marrow transplant. J.C.'s parents felt guilty, questioning why so much had to happen to him. They expressed disbelief in how the transplant could have failed. His father asked if he could have done something to have prevented the relapse.

As seen in the case presentation, parents must be reassured that they have done nothing to cause the disease's return. Family members who have not been involved in the child's treatment may feel increasingly guilty. Their lack of previous involvement creates greater strife. Other family members may feel bitter toward those who have previously not been involved. Frequently, divorced families experience stress when one parent is more involved than the other.[17] The involved parent may blame the other for not being available when the child needed someone. Such accusations lead to increased guilt in the other parent. Divorced parents should be dealt with individually to allow both to feel as if they are essential for the child's support.

Relapse frequently causes more emotional pain than the initial diagnosis.[5] Families have gained an understanding of the illness and its implications. They have come to realize the impact of relapse on the child's chances for cure. A major concern that develops for the family and the child is, "When and how will it all end?" The difficulty in dealing with this concern is that no one knows when or how it will end; nevertheless, hope must be maintained (Table 28-4).

Not all children who relapse will die. Many go on to obtain remission and have no further evidence

Table 28-4. Relapse

Essential coping tasks	Interventions
Alleviating initial shock of relapse	Allow parents to express shock and disbelief
	Provide time for grief before initiating discussion of treatment plan
Understanding impact of relapse	Discuss the seriousness of relapse yet provide hope in the situation
	Offer facts regarding disease's possible outcome
Discussing return of disease with the child	Express importance of being truthful with the child
	Discuss the disease's return with the child and need to begin therapy again (realize the child will perceive the seriousness of the situation by observing parents and staff)
Expressing appropriate feelings of grief	Encourage expression of feelings and need for family to maintain realistic outlook toward the situation
	Identify key support individuals to maintain close follow-up with all family members

of disease. Families whose child has not done well on therapy and continues to have disease spread must eventually face the decision when or if to discontinue therapy. Most families by now have come to trust those professionals involved in the child's care and are able to openly discuss their fears and concerns. Time must be spent in counseling and providing support. Some families refuse to give up and will pursue therapy to the end. These families must be made aware of the treatment as being highly experimental, since phase I therapy is used when other modalities have not been effective. Rational decisions are sometimes difficult when nothing effective remains in treating the child's disease. When the primary goal is to promote the child's well-being and comfort, decisions regarding whether or not to continue therapy are easier to make.

END STAGE DISEASE

Families with a child who has cancer are confronted with the possibility of death at the time of initial diagnosis. Guarantees cannot be made from the health care team, which conveys the uncertainty of prognosis.

The return of the child's disease brings with it the realization of the diagnosis and prognosis.[22] This usually marks the initiation of the family's mourning over the loss of the child. The family has dealt with anger and shock, and their concern changes from "how can we treat the disease" to "how can we make it easy for the child." Although their loss is great, they console themselves with the fact that the child will cease to suffer.[23]

CASE PRESENTATION

L.A. was a 9-year-old with acute lymphocytic leukemia who had two bone marrow and central nervous system relapses over the past year. There were no compatible bone marrow donors. With each relapse, the professional team met with the parents to discuss L.A.'s chances for survival. The parents understood the implications of the relapse and began to deal with the inevitable loss of their child. They began to plan trips together and took L.A. to Disney World. L.A. began to have difficulty tolerating the procedures. His moods changed, and at times he withdrew from those around. At other times he was very open and verbal. During a clinic visit, L.A. met another child who was having difficulty undergoing bone marrows. Two weeks before his death, L.A. stayed with her for one of her procedures and talked her through it. He never openly discussed his death with anyone, but his drawings revealed his thoughts. Shortly before his death he began to draw scenes of the nativity with angels surrounding a stable. L.A.'s parents wanted to keep L.A. at home, and much time was spent with them regarding what would actually take place when he died. The local physician and nurse were involved in supporting the family at home. L.A. died at home without difficulty. The parents returned to the hospital to visit the staff 2 weeks after L.A.'s death. They expressed how peacefully L.A. had died and talked about the future for their family.

Parents facing the inevitable loss of a child from cancer have been through numerous crises since diagnosis but none so difficult as this. As demonstrated in the case presentation, the realization that death will occur alters even the most stable family. The thought of death has occurred frequently since diagnosis, with each setback of the disease lending further credence to the reality that death will occur[24] (see Chapter 32 on terminal care). As the reality of the child's terminal illness becomes inevitable, parents begin to adapt to the anticipated loss.[25] When anticipatory grieving has not taken place, family members experience acute emotional pain, similar to that of parents whose child has died suddenly. Refusal to deal with the child's terminal state causes strife and instability by preventing all family members from accepting the inevitable death of the child. Anticipatory grief can allow the family to begin to establish their lives as separate from the child. When this is begun in a positive manner, the family can identify strengths that will assist in supporting them through the crisis.

There are times when parents or other family members grieve prematurely, causing the child to feel isolated and alone. Professionals must assist the family in accepting the outcome without detaching themselves from the child. No matter how prepared the family may seem before the child's actual death, their grief is exacerbated when it actually occurs.[25]

Intense involvement for weeks to months before the death can result in physical fatigue or collapse of family members. This creates further inability to cope effectively with the crisis. Emotional and physical breakdown prevents the family to continue drawing strength from their support systems. They may no longer feel capable of going on with life. The professional must provide support and assist the family in identifying significant others who can provide stability to the family during these times.

The crisis of end stage disease may last from weeks to months. No one knows when it will end. The state of questioning what each day will bring causes added stress for the family. No definite plans can be made. The family can only await each new day with fear and anxiety. This adaptation period, a phase of waiting for the inevitable, can sometimes assist the family in accepting the loss. Family members commonly portray reactions of disbelief, denial, bargaining, anger, and depression.[24] It is a time when loved ones have no control over the situation.

Knowledge of family attitudes toward religion and death are necessary to lend appropriate support, since beliefs become essential when the disease reaches this stage. Families commonly view their beliefs and religion in one of two ways.[25] Religious background and beliefs may provide further support and give the family added strength in knowing a supreme being is in control of their child. Others may become bitter toward God and blame this supreme being for taking their child from them. Regardless of the attitude taken by the family, all members question the reason for the inevitable death of a child, asking, "What meaning does this have in the deeper order of the universe?"[25]

Children display varied reactions during end stage disease. Their thoughts and perceptions are dependent on age and development. Culture and religious background contribute to their perceptions. Pain is a common fear of death with the child. He may frequently ask how death will feel. Children who are terminally ill often perceive their illness and treatment as worse than their death. They have become tired of prolonged treatment and hospital visits without the hope of getting better.

CASE PRESENTATION

E.B., a 13-year-old, was in the terminal stage of leukemia. His parents were refusing to give up and were asking for E.B. to receive more chemotherapy. E.B. was unable to tolerate procedures without breaking down and crying uncontrollably. He would cry out loudly, "Please no more sticks, I can't take any more sticks." In talking with E.B. after one of these outbursts, he was asked if he knew what would happen if he stopped getting the sticks. He stated calmly that he knew he would die, but he couldn't take anymore procedures. He would rather die than have to live through more procedures. The oncology team was unsure how to react to E.B.'s declaration. He was intelligent, and it was felt that he knew

Table 28-5. End stage disease

Essential coping tasks	Interventions
Accepting the child's impending death	Allow the parents to verbalize their fears of the child's death
	Discuss any questions they may have to decrease their worries and concerns
	When possible, listen to the parents' wishes and demands
Participating in the child's care	Encourage the family to remain involved with the child's care (This involvement will allow the parents to comfort the child while giving the parents a sense of belonging and need. It will also assist in preparing them for the inevitable loss.)
Expressing appropriate emotions	Stress the importance of expressing emotions of grief
	Identify key individuals who will provide comfort and reassurance
	Encourage relatives and significant others to be involved to give parents an opportunity to rest and maintain physical strength
Resolving guilt feelings and sense of helplessness	Reassure parents that they could have done nothing to prevent the child's death
	Assure them that they are doing everything possible by providing comfort and support
	Stress that the most important role is their presence with the child
Planning for future	Stress the need for the family to look toward the future

the meaning of death; but the team was not at ease with E.B.'s statement that he would rather die than have another procedure. E.B. was given time to think about his decision and was asked to discuss it with someone he trusted. E.B. talked with his family and returned to the clinic the next day. He had decided to take no more chemotherapy. He was able to remain as an outpatient for 2 months before developing an infection that eventually led to his death.

E.B. expresses many children's concerns and fears with the numerous painful procedures they must endure. Years of therapy, with seemingly endless procedures, create an ongoing crisis for the child. Their endurance fails. The child in the final stage of disease realizes he is no longer healthy, the disease has returned in spite of treatment. It is at this point that the health care team must discuss with the child decisions regarding further treatment and necessary procedures. The child must be granted some control over life, even in its final stage. As previously discussed, parents may not wish to stop therapy. Their refusal to accept the child's impending death may prevent them from considering the child's wishes. Many children grow tired

of the vigils of chemotherapy and its side effects. They frequently are ready to discontinue therapy before the parents and may plead with the parents to allow them to stop. There is no right or wrong when discussing whether or not to discontinue therapy. The family must all live with their decision and believe they have done everything possible for the child.

Control over the crisis of end stage disease is important for all family members, as well as the child. Involvement allows for acceptance of the impending death and prevents the development of guilt once death has occurred (Table 28-5). End stage disease is the most difficult crisis anyone can encounter. Psychologic, emotional, physical, and spiritual support must be offered for the child and also for all family members (see Chapter 32 on terminal care).

SUMMARY

The crises of childhood cancer—diagnosis, treatment, dicontinuation of therapy, relapse, and end stage disease—alter the family's entire way of life. Previous coping strategies used by the family seem inadequate in dealing with the crises of cancer.

The professional working with the family, must assist in identifying coping strategies that will allow the family to adapt to the illness and its effects on the child.

The professional who is familiar with certain concepts of crisis is better able to help families through them. Some amount of stress is essential to motivate resolution of the crisis. New methods of coping developed during a previous crisis will assist in solving problems in the future. Resolution of the immediate crisis is possible only when families are able to establish adequate coping skills and communicate with each other. Working effectively with families undergoing crises of cancer enables them to remain intact and to function well after the crisis has been resolved.

REFERENCES

1. Lewis, M.S., Gottesman, D., and Gutstein, S.: The cause and duration of crisis, J. Consult. Clin. Psychol. **47**(1):128, 1979.
2. Halpern, H.A.; Crisis theory: a definitional study, Community Ment. Health J. **9**(4):342, 1973.
3. Hughes, J.C.: The emotional impact of chronic disease, Am. J. Dis. Child. **130**:1199, 1976.
4. Spinetta, J.J., and Deasy-Spinetta, P.: Living with childhood cancer, St. Louis, 1981, The C.V. Mosby Co.
5. Ahmed, P.: Living and dying with cancer, New York, 1981, Elsevier Science Publishing Co., Inc.
6. Adams, M.A.: Helping the parents of children with malignancy, J. Pediatr. **93**(5):734, 1978.
7. Cohen, J., Cullen, J.W., and Martin, L.R.: Psychosocial aspects of cancer, New York, 1982, Raven Press.
8. Spinetta, J.J., and Maloney, L.J.: The child with cancer: patterns of communication and denial, J. Consult. Clin. Psychol. **48**:1540, 1978.
9. Koocher, G.P., and O'Malley, J.E.: The domoceles syndrome: psychosocial consequences of surviving childhood cancer, New York, 1980, McGraw-Hill, Inc.
10. Kagen-Goodhart, L.: Reentry: living with childhood cancer, Am. J. Orthopsychiatry **47**(4):651, 1977.
11. Kellerman, J.: Psychological aspects of childhood cancer, Springfield, Ill., 1980, Charles C Thomas, Publisher.
12. van Eys, J.: The truly cured child, Baltimore, 1977, University Park Press.
13. Sutow, W.W., Vietti, T.J., and Fernbach, D.J.: Clinical pediatric oncology, St. Louis, 1983, The C.V. Mosby Co.
14. Ross, J.M.: Coping with childhood cancer: group intervention as an aid to parents in crisis, Soc. Work. Health Care **4**(4):381, 1979.
15. Anderson, J.M.: The social construction of illness experience: families with a chronically ill child, J. Adv. Nurs. **6**:427, 1981.
16. Mattsson, A.: Long-term physical illness in childhood: a challenge to psychosocial adaptation, Pediatrics **50**(5):801, 1972.
17. Kaplan, D.M.: Family mediation of stress, Soc. Work. **18**:60, 1973.
18. Krulik, T.: Successful normalizing tactics of parents of chronically ill children, J. Adv. Nurs. **5**:573, 1980.
19. Krouse, H., and Krouse, J.: Cancer as a crisis: the critical elements of adjustment, Nurs. Res. **31**(2):96, 1982.
20. Geist, R.: Onset of chronic illness in children and adolescents, Am. J. Orthopsychiatry **49**(1):4, 1970.
21. Maddisin, D., and Raphael, B.: Social and psychological consequences of chronic disease in childhood, Am. J. Australia **2**:1265, 1971.
22. Townes, B.D., Wold, D.A., and Holmes, T.H.: Parental adjustment to childhood leukemia, J. Psychosom. Res. **18**:9, 1974.
23. Simetta, J.: Effective parental coping following the death of a child from cancer, J. Pediatr. Psychol. **6**:251, 1981.
24. Martinson, I.M.: Home care for the dying child, New York, 1976, Appleton-Century-Crofts.
25. Sahler, O.J.: The child and death, St. Louis, 1978, The C.V. Mosby Co.

ADDITIONAL READINGS

Adams, D.W.: Childhood malignancy: the psychosocial care of the child and his family, Springfield, Ill., 1980, Charles C Thomas, Publisher.
Bigner, C.M., and others: Childhood leukemia: emotional impact on patient and family, N. Engl. J. Med. **280**:414, 1969.
Clapp, M.J.: Psychosocial reactions of children with cancer, Nurs. Clin. North Am. **11**:73, 1976.
Drotar, D.: Family oriented intervention with the dying adolescent, J. Pediatr. Psychol. **2**:68, 1977.
Kalnins, I.V., Churchill, M.P., and Terry, G.E.: Concurrent stresses in families with a leukemic child, J. Pediatr. Psychol. **5**:81, 1980.
Koocher, G.P., and Sallan, S.E.: Pediatric oncology. In Magrab, P.R., editor: Psychological management of pediatric problems, vol. 1, Early life conditions and chronic diseases, Baltimore, 1978, University Park Press.
Lazarus, R.S.: Patterns of adjustment, New York, 1976, McGraw-Hill, Inc.
Spinetta, J.J.: Adjustment in children with cancer, J. Pediatr. Psychol. **2**(2):49, 1977.
Spinetta, J.J., Rigler, D., and Karon, M.: Anxiety in the dying child, Pediatrics **52**:841, 1973.
Zeltzer, L.: The adolescent with cancer. In Kellerman, J., editor: Psychological aspects of childhood cancer, Springfield, Ill., 1980, Charles C Thomas, Publisher.

CHAPTER 29

Coping strategies for children with cancer

ALEXANDER M. GORDON and PATRICIA H. COTANCH

Most infants, children, and adolescents diagnosed with cancer are previously healthy and normally developing individuals. The diagnosis brings with it certainty of an incredible challenge of maintaining normal development. Although increasing survival rates can be documented and rightfully applauded, what can be said for the quality of patients' lives from an emotional and developmental standpoint? This issue has only just begun to be addressed.[1] As part of this new awareness, experts in pediatric oncology have begun to look more intensely at specific ways to lessen emotional trauma that accompanies various treatment modalities.

Primary treatment modalities that include chemotherapy, surgery, and radiation therapy must be considered traumatic procedures for the child with cancer.[2,3] Various diagnostic and supportive procedures that accompany the treatment modalities include finger sticks, intravenous punctures, bone marrow aspirations, and lumbar punctures.

It has almost become a truism to note that the perceived effects of the disease often pale in the face of the pain that treatment causes. This notion is reflected in the following account by a parent of a child undergoing treatment for leukemia:

During his latest stay in the hospital, Graham asked Maggie, "Why do I get shots all the time that make me sick?" She explained that he had leukemia and that the shots were necessary to make him better.

"I don't want my leukemia to go away," he said sadly.

"Why?" Maggie asked softly.

"Because I will get lots of shots and will get sick."
What he meant was that the cure for the disease made him feel a lot worse than the disease ever had.

It must be emphasized that supporting a child through certain procedures cannot be done without considering numerous factors affecting the child's coping mechanisms. There are a variety of concerns that must be considered for each child[4]:

1. Stage of development
2. Previous adaptive capacity
3. Nature of the parent-child relationship
4. Meaning of the illness to the child and family
5. Current family equilibrium

This chapter can only begin to suggest ways to help the child deal with preparing for and experiencing treatment for cancer. Preparation of the child for traumatic procedures, along with the most recent trends in decreasing side-effects caused by treatment are approached in this chapter.

PREPARATION TECHNIQUES FOR INTRUSIVE PROCEDURES AND TREATMENT
Infant

Obviously, there is no direct way to prepare an infant for treatment.[5] The entire focus for preparation must be with educating the parents.[6] It has been shown that infants can perceive anxiety present in the parent.[7] Providing information, allowing time for information to be processed, and dealing with feelings generated opens the door for parents to set up healthy coping mechanisms.

The diagnostic workup and initiation of treatment usually begin in the inpatient setting. This is a crucial period in the establishment of positive, therapeutic relationships between the family and staff. Parents should be allowed to be present during procedures. Each procedure should be discussed with the parents before they accompany the child to the treatment room. Decisions on who is present during these events should be made in collaboration with the parents.

Toddler

The toddler can benefit from preparation for intrusive procedures.[8] This preparation must include the parents. Although there might be more intricate explanation and opportunity for questions given to parents without the child present, it is imperative that parents be present during the child's preparation. This parental involvement should be allowed to extend through the treatment and into the post-treatment time (i.e., into the treatment room for an IV placement, lead-aproned and in the room for a CT scan, or gowned and present through anesthesia induction for surgery).

Some parents do not want to be with the child for painful procedures or may, at times, be somewhat disruptive. In the former instance they should not be made to feel guilty, and in the latter they should not be placed in the position of being chastised. For those parents who wish to be with their child at these events, the following issues should be discussed:

1. Parents should think in terms of comforting and supporting the child; the staff should perform the restraining role.
2. Parents should try to maintain a neutral emotional state. It is more helpful to the child if parents display their emotional stress outside the procedural setting.
3. Parents should plan ahead what they will say to the child, whether they will explain what is happening or provide for distraction.

The decision of when to tell the child about an upcoming invasive procedure is dependent on a number of factors. Preparation for a procedure generally begins no earlier than the day before the event. The less verbal child might be worked with only just before the procedure. Preparation for a surgical experience, which has many steps to it, should begin at least the day before.

Preparation should include telling the child that something is going to be happening to him.[9] One must keep in mind that it is normal and expected for the child this age to feel the procedure is a form of punishment.[10] The child typically feels he is the cause of the painful procedure despite reassurance to the contrary. It becomes important to say something like, "You did just what I asked you to do," rather than, "You were a good boy."

The preparation experience should include opportunity for the child to play with various equipment that will be used during the procedure. The child may want to practice the event with the materials and a doll. Practice should include identifying phases of the event that hurt or are uncomfortable. The use of a doll serves to depersonalize the event and decreases the stress for the young child. The child may not remember names or functions of the equipment but familiarity is usually helpful. The child's level of development makes it understandable that the distinction between fantasy and reality is somewhat blurred. One must realize that a variety of responses may come from the child. The child may ignore the procedural teaching, intently watch with no desire to touch anything, or may be actively willing to participate by doing such things as using a stethoscope to check a heartbeat.

Remember that the child may choose to use the medical gear in inaccurate ways. To the child who insists on wrapping a tourniquet around a doll's head, one might respond, "You know, the doctor would never wrap it around your neck. He uses the big rubber band or what we call a 'tourniquet' only to make it easier to find one of the veins in your arm, so that he can more easily get the needle in."

During the event itself, support for the child is given through whatever contact is possible—tactile, auditory, and/or visual. A child may find comfort and support in being allowed to have some transitional object with him. This object may be receiving some type of procedure or performing some role under the child's direction. It should be kept in mind that each child will have his own coping style for specific events.

The child with cancer will undergo traumatic procedures in subsequent clinic visits and hospitalizations. Preparation for these repeated events will take on more emotionally charged quality, since the child will have specific experiences on which to reflect. Allowing the child some supervised time to recreate the event allows both for the child to work through feelings and for the adult to reflect on whatever confusion the child may be experiencing. The purpose in all of this activity is the movement toward some sort of mastery of the experience.

Preschooler

If possible, as with the younger age group, parental preparation is crucial. Parents should be told about the procedure or event before the child's being told. This allows parents to begin to work through whatever anxiety and hostility they may feel toward the traumatic procedures. Parents must be used as a resource both before and during the preparation. Ideally, the parents have had experience in the "explaining role" before and can provide the staff with ideas as to what has been effective with the child previously.

One of the most important aspects of preparing parents is to remind them of two behaviors that are quite common and often disturbing in this age group; regression and aggression. Common responses of the preschooler to traumatic procedures, no matter what initial intervention is pursued, may include refusal to talk, withdrawal, problems with elimination, or other behaviors that would be expected at a younger age. Another expected response is anger from the child directed toward those involved in treatment. This anger may be directed most acutely toward parents. Parents must be helped to see that regression and aggression, whether seen in the clinic, hospital, and/or at home, are ways for the child to communicate confusion and frustration with what is occurring as seen in the following case study.

CASE STUDY

R.K. was a 3-year-old female diagnosed with aplastic anemia. Her family included parents and an older and younger male sibling. She was viewed by all who knew her as a delightful, engaging child. Throughout treatment, she needed to spend regular extended periods in the hospital. She very quickly became known as an overly reserved, nonverbal, combative, and generally regressed child. She would typically ignore medical staff who talked to her. She began sucking her thumb fairly regularly during the day. She would go into stormy tantrums in response to anything from an attempt to take her temperature to encouragement to eat her meals. Staff found her to be an increasingly frustrating and unpleasant child with whom to work. They were also concerned with what they saw as a conflict-centered relationship developing between her and her mother. Through discussions and care conferences, the staff working with her was able to take steps to address these concerns. It was agreed that her behavior, although problematic from an interactional standpoint, was indicative of her strength in openly relating her sad and angry feelings about the disruptions occurring in her life. It was up to the staff (and family) to facilitate her ability to keep these feelings from predominating in her life. This concept was interpreted to her parents, and seeking their input and support, the following was included in her care:

1. The staff more consistently/regularly clarified their reasons for coming into her room.
2. Primary nursing was maintained.
3. It was expected that she talk when spoken to, however, no punitive comments were made if she did not.
4. When temper tantrums started, her angry feelings were affirmed by whoever was present. She was reminded that she still must follow through on what might be asked of her.
5. The family was given "permission" not to always be in the enforcing role.
6. The staff involved made an extra effort to spend time with her outside of "procedural" time.
7. R.K. was provided with more supervised time in medical play.

Importantly, these steps took some pressure off both R.K. and her parents. She responded gradually to the consistency in care. Over time she was able to talk more comfortably with selected staff. Thumb sucking eventually stopped. Although her interest in medical play was minimal, she exhibited more drive for other forms of play (recreational, dramatic, fantasy). Temper tantrums still occurred but were less frequent and shorter in duration. Parents relaxed and seemed less embarrassed by their child's occasional combative/resistant behavior.

Expanded experiential knowledge and vocabulary of this aged child justifies the decision to begin preparation before the procedure. Ideally, the extra time simply allows the child more time to tolerate and absorb the information.[11] Nevertheless, it is evident that many parents do not want such extended thought and preparation time. They may with justification feel that the tearful weekends, overabundance of tantrums, and nightmares are simply not worth it. This issue can only be addressed and resolved by listening to the parents, observing the child, and making use of the team approach. Another reality is that treatment decisions may be made that simply do not allow time for preparation. One must then rely primarily on postprocedural work with the child.

When specific preparation of the child is to begin, it must revolve around helping the child develop coping mechanisms for the event.[12] For first-time procedures, it is best to offer simple explanations that might include opportunities to manipulate the equipment; look at drawings, photographs, or videotapes; visit the location of the event; enact the event with a doll; and talk to other children who have experienced the procedure. Primary verbal preparation needs to include statements of what the child will see, hear, feel, taste, and smell. The professional working with the child must be sensitive to the child's being totally overwhelmed. Cues to this overload may include verbal withdrawal, a fearful expression, ignoring the person, or even walking away.

The initial preparation session for a child beginning treatment is the first step in establishing adequate coping methods for the child. Experiencing the event for the first time furthers this process.[13] It is the beginning for establishment of productive relationships among the child, family, and staff (Fig. 29-1). Helping the child through the procedure requires a variety of techniques:

1. Reminding the child, through each step, of the pictures viewed or items previously played with: "Remember how the little girl in the book lay down on the table and held her mother's hand?". . . . . "This felt cool when you rubbed it on your arm earlier today."

2. Allowing the child to hold some transitional object: "I'm glad you brought your stuffed animal with you. . . . It's nice to have a special friend with you."

3. Offering the child a role in the procedure: "Would you like to hold this package? You may cut the tape if you'd like to."

4. Simple distraction, not deception: "Sometimes it helps to count when I'm pushing the needle in. . . ."

5. Responding with empathy to resistant behavior: "I know this hurts because other children have told me so . . . It's okay to be angry about this. I know it's hard to keep still, so we'll give you some help with that."

Other than the specific successful completion of the procedure it may be difficult to determine what makes for a good experience.[14] The hope is for the child not to get too upset and be able to cooperate through completion of the procedure. However, particularly for a first experience, it might be reasonable to expect some children to be overwhelmed and react hysterically. This behavior may clearly indicate the child's fright and wish to let that fear be known.

Working with the child after the procedure provides further opportunities to help the child examine fears and fantasies and work toward gaining better understanding of the event. It is at this phase that play therapy begins clearly to be helpful. Play therapy is based on the concept that children choose to reenact painful, confusing experiences in an effort to gain mastery of the event. These opportunities can be provided in the clinic, hospital, or home setting. For some children, a doctor's box with adhesive bandages, gauze, tape, syringes, or other material can become a valued possession. Some children's zeal for medical play is quite remarkable (Fig. 29-2). Others show very little interest and present an interesting challenge in terms of how much or whether to push medical play.

There are means other than specific play with medical equipment for the child to work through to master specific procedures. The child may want to dictate a story about the experience.[15] Drawing a picture is another way for the child to recreate the experience in such a way that he is in control.[16]

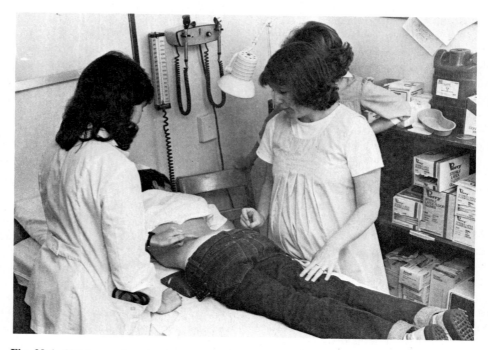

Fig. 29-1. Children undergoing intrusive procedures frequently develop close, trusting relationships with the professional performing the procedures.

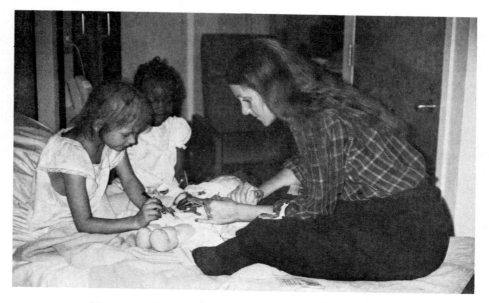

Fig. 29-2. Children with cancer giving chemotherapy to a doll.

These techniques allow for the child not only to express feelings but also to demonstrate whatever misconceptions he may have regarding the procedure. Consider the following thoughts from a hospitalized 5-year-old, as she talked about her first experience with a lumbar puncture:

> The prick hurt a little more. Knowing it had to happen and thinking about it made it hurt a little more. The prick made me get out of the position. It *really* worried me that I got out of the position. I worried about that and it got me through the scary part. The being out of position might make it hurt more. The doctors knew best. The bottom leg got tired. My dad should lift up my top leg.

School-age child

Parents must be a resource for helping the staff determine the pace and style of preparation for the school-age child. Parents usually seem to feel more comfortable in taking an active role in the process. They may feel more confident that their child can be helped to understand the why's and how's of treatment. Ideally, parental presence at various diagnostic or treatment procedures will be preceded by discussion among staff, parents, and the child. There may be times when children in the older range of this group would prefer that parents not be present.

Characteristics of this age group typically offer the opportunity for longer preparation sessions and justify an earlier beginning for preparation time.[6] Ideally, the additional time enhances the quality of the teaching. The child has more time to process information and discuss concerns. At the same time, staff must be sensitive to instances where "more time to think about it," equates to unbearable anxiety. This can be evidenced in the classic stalling attempts by some children before procedures. Usually the longer the delay, the more the child's anxiety is increased.

For this age group the depth of detailed information given may vary greatly depending on the child. What should be common for all children is communicating what the child will experience. This includes what the child may see, hear, feel, taste, or smell. Handling whatever medical equipment is available, reading books, and looking at photographs are helpful for the child's concrete thinking processes. Using a doll and perhaps even labeling it a model for older children (who may reject the idea of "playing with dolls") can be an effective way of communicating to the child what is expected. It can also help determine what support the child may need from those present during the event. For example, the children may offer a variety of ways for the doll/model to get through a procedure, ranging from being quiet and still to holding a parent's hand and crying to recounting a recent plot of a favorite television show.

Given the increased verbal and reasoning skills of this age, important aspects of the treatment time include maintaining both verbal and tactile contact. The message, "Here's what we are doing just as you've been told about," is so crucial to enhancing the development of trust. Both for first time and following procedural experiences, staff and parents must be prepared for angry outbursts. As much as possible, the response to these outbursts should be a calm affirmation of that feeling, "I know this is hard for you, other children feel the same way."

Following the initial procedures, children may choose to work through their feelings and confusion in a variety of ways. Some health professionals note that children may have a need to discuss their experiences from the standpoint of having successfully completed a difficult task. They may want to express this pride through a drawing or story, which they display for all to see. Artwork or story writing may additionally provide a means for expressing and exploring feelings and thoughts (Fig. 29-3 and Fig. 29-4). The anxiety that surrounded the event and may surround future events can be presented with the child in control. The adult's response to these statements can be helpful in complementing the therapy, which the child, in a sense, is providing for himself. These supportive responses should include statements of empathy, reminders that the child is not to blame for the disease, and attempts to clarify the reasons for and techniques of the specific procedures.

This same sort of adult intervention is essential for the child who chooses to recreate the treatment or procedure through play with a doll and appro-

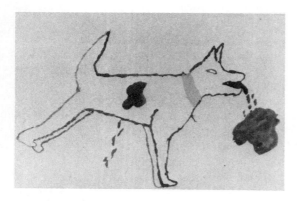

Fig. 29-3. Drawing by a 14-year-old boy diagnosed with nasopharyngeal carcinoma.

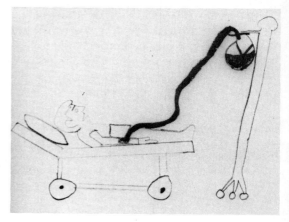

Fig. 29-4. Drawing by a 6-year-old boy with sickle cell anemia receiving red blood cell transfusions following a cerebrovascular accident.

priate medical equipment. Often a staff person taking the voice of the doll/patient can reflect typical concern of children undergoing the particular procedure, both to allow the child to see some legitimacy in his own concerns and to voice some understanding of the why of treatment. There also are benefits to children acting out a treatment scenario simply with a staff person observing and determining areas of confusion, understanding, and general coping abilities in each child. As in any play therapy type of experience, the goal is control for the child, through the chances both to express feelings and to test learning.

Adolescent

For the professional, the adolescent presents a special challenge. The adolescent is a person who continues toward development of a unique personality in the midst of a variety of conflicts. The professional must carefully consider the status of puberty, stage of adolescent development, and related critical issues deriving from both inner instinctive drives and external cultural expectations. Primary concerns of the adolescent revolve around establishing an intact body image and sense of self-esteem; defining his intellectual, sexual, and functional identity; and achieving autonomy.[17]

Cancer and its treatment has the potential to undermine the adolescent's attempts in dealing with these concerns. The adolescent is frequently forced back into a dependent, even passive, state. Social interactions and school life are altered. Thoughts about the future become confused. Given the adolescent's relatively mature thought processes, preparation for treatment and intrusive procedures takes on a new dimension. The question of when to discuss the diagnosis of cancer normally is answered with the reply, as soon as possible. The adolescent has the capacity and needs the time to organize, evaluate, and respond to information about the event. The older adolescent may be more interested in knowing how the treatment fits into his schedule and what it entails. As with younger age groups, the adolescent will continue to look to the parents for support. That relationship may include more serious mutual discussions about treatment and mutual decision making, particularly with older adolescents. The adolescent may demand to know everything the parents have been told. The adolescent might want the parents present at procedures or may request some other trusted adult to be present. There will be times when the adolescent may not want a parent present for either the preparatory teaching or the follow-up.

Once again, preparation should center around what sensory experiences (see, hear, touch) will be encountered and what will be required of him behaviorally. Unlike the younger child, adolescents may be able to understand and visualize their experience of the event before it happens or at least be able to talk more fully about the possibilities. One can often discuss, in more detail, the reasons for and possible outcomes of the treatments and procedures. Although less emphasis is placed on the use of photographs and opportunity for manipulating various medical equipment, these resources should not be overlooked.

One expected result of more intense and detailed teaching is heightened anxiety as exemplified in the following case study.

CASE STUDY

J.H. was a 16-year-old young female with Burkitt's lymphoma. After a year of therapy, she was considered to be disease free. In her initial subsequent visits to the clinic, she was generally ''upbeat'' and pleasantly interactive with staff. She then began to have unexplained bouts with diarrhea and nausea. When admitted to the hospital for further workup, she moved into the depressed and moody state that characterized many of her previous admissions. Those who had known her since the initial diagnosis saw her as much more impatient and less willing to open up to the staff. Her behavior and occasionally her verbalizations gave the message of ''leave me alone . . . why are you continuing to do this?'' She finally was able to confide in certain staff and relate some of her concerns. Foremost in her mind were the clear and honest discussions about Burkitt's lymphoma in which she had previously engaged. These discussions included the message that her cancer was one of the most difficult ones to treat. Indeed, she had not expected to live as long as she had already. The return to the hospital had also interfered with her difficult attempts of re-establishing friendships at home. She was guilty about the continued burden she felt she was to her family and was further deeply bothered by the open-endedness of her condition. Once these concerns were expressed, the staff could affirm them as real and legitimate. From there, they then worked toward helping her develop ways of effectively managing these concerns.

During the procedure or treatment, staff should be prepared to provide empathy and reassurance.

For virtually any problem behavior, part of the response to the adolescent must be, ''Yes, other people your age have felt and acted this way; we know this is difficult for you.'' Except in extreme cases, staff should not arbitrarily take away the individual coping styles of the adolescent.

As a follow-up in the continuation of various treatment modalities, staff can offer the adolescent many resources. As with younger children, the opportunity to recreate the event with models and medical equipment may be helpful. Allowing for expression through the visual or written arts can also provide a means for reviewing information and feelings as seen in the following letter written to Dear Abby (from a children's hospital newsletter):

Dear Abby:
I have cancer and am in the hospital for treatment. The chemotherapy has caused my mouth to be sore. My girlfriend is coming to visit me and I don't know what to do. She kisses very hard, and I'm afraid my mouth will bleed!

Signed, Concerned

Dear Concerned:
No need to worry, simply tell your girlfriend to kiss your ear instead!

Another effective means of information gathering and anxiety sharing is through group therapy.[18] These groups can capitalize on the adolescent's concern for peer acceptance and need to learn of approaches for coping.

Perhaps the most important approach for staff to take when working with adolescents is to let them know someone will always be available to them. Assuming that the formation of identity is a primary task for the adolescent, a trusting relationship can establish a true therapeutic alliance.[19]

It is imperative for one to consider the developmental age of the child when preparing for a procedure that will produce fear and pain. Each child is unique in his ability to perceive the event. Specific fears and concerns must be addressed for each child. Appropriate preparation for treatment paves the way for establishment of effective coping skills that will assist the child in adjusting to the disease and its treatment.

SPECIFIC COPING STRATEGIES FOR INTRUSIVE PROCEDURES AND TREATMENT

Preparation for intrusive procedures and treatment modalities includes development of effective coping strategies. Recent trends have turned to the use of specific modalities that allow the child to regain some control over the situation. These new coping strategies, recently implemented in children with cancer, are most commonly known as relaxation techniques. This section of the chapter presents a detailed explanation of the principles underlying relaxation techniques in children. Examples that have been successfully used with pediatric oncology patients will be explained. Finally, a review of the literature regarding the use of these techniques with children will be presented.

Relaxation techniques

The use of relaxation techniques in children with cancer appears to have three main effects: (1) ameliorates symptoms of disease; (2) decreases treatment-related side effects and discomfort from medical procedures; and (3) allows the children to actively participate in their treatment, thereby offering them some control of a frightening situation. In the pediatric population the most commonly used relaxation intervention is hypnosis and distraction techniques. Hypnosis is defined as a condition in which the individual's conscious state is altered allowing for decreased sensory input. Medical hypnosis remains a drastically under-used intervention with children.[20] Barber[21] states no other psychologic tool known is so efficacious in creating comfort out of discomfort, with none of the adverse side effects associated with the traditional medical treatments of comparable efficacy.

When approaching the pediatric patient with a hypnosis or relaxation intervention, it is important to offer the child an age appropriate explanation. The term *hypnosis* is often frightening, with common misconceptions comparing this relaxation state with "stage hypnosis," a type of magic show. One child related his perception of hypnosis as a mad scientist cartoon character who controlled people and made animal sounds. The child expressed disappointment when he realized he was not going to be made to bark as a dog. He was assured he could bark if he wanted to in his fantasy, but the therapist had no ability to cause him to do so. Interestingly, some children will be intrigued by the novelty of the intervention and others will be frightened.

It is important that the health professional be sensitive to the messages the child is sending. There should always be careful instruction and explanation to prevent anxiety unfounded toward the meaning of hypnosis. Time should be spent assuring the child and family that hypnosis is a self-relaxation technique to assist in gaining control over a situation. It should be stressed that hypnosis does not relinquish control to another individual but promotes self-control.

Hypnosis with children should be done only by a trained therapist capable of dealing with the child's fears and frightening recollections that sometimes occur during trance. On one occasion, we were working with a child who had been instructed to recall a pleasant joyful event. He responded and was quite animated during the trance in describing a prank he had pulled on a playmate. He then began to look sad and started crying while he continued to describe the event in great detail. The prank resulted in him being severely punished and his recall of it allowed him to re-experience the sadness and pain, as well as the initial happy prankish, feeling. The therapist supported the child during the recollection, offering reassurance and emphasizing the child's ability to control and work through an uncomfortable recollection.

Children undergoing hypnosis differ drastically from adults using hypnosis. Unlike adults, children require little or no relaxation induction. Most children become involved in fantasy readily, whereas adults require a prolonged relaxation period where they attempt to set aside inhibitions and concentrate on a pleasant thought. Fantasy is a daily activity for the child and occurs easily without hesitation. We have observed children and adolescents becoming bored with structured progressive muscle relaxation used frequently with adults. A shortened attention span may create this boredom, or children simply may not require this 10- to 20-minute period of relaxation to achieve an altered state of consciousness. Authorities in hypnosis agree that work must be done quickly for the child to achieve a hypnotic state.[22,23]

Adults undergoing hypnosis may select a sedentary relaxing imagery scene such as sitting on the beach, lying in a meadow, or soaking in a hot tub. In comparison, children focus on an action imagery scene such as riding a bicycle, roller skating, running, or swimming. Children prefer imagery themes based on life experiences, requiring unique individualized induction sessions. Attempts at hypnosis induction using a standardized tape recording were unsuccessful with two adolescents who expressed a need to use their own life experiences to create an atmosphere for relaxation.

Age-appropriate vocabulary is essential to provide understanding of the imagery scenes being described by the therapist. Children and adolescents frequently regress and use an imagery scene that is several years behind their stage of development. One 10-year-old recalled a funny experience from his past. As he began to describe this experience, he opened his eyes and spoke in a noticeably less mature manner. After the hypnosis session was finished, the child stated he was 5 years old when the event occurred. It is probably that he experienced spontaneous age regression during hypnosis and was actually communicating as a 5-year-old.

Children seem to be more trusting than adults and have a natural ability to fantasize and imagine. They more easily obtain a somnolent state, occurring frequently even during the initial hypnotic session. Children the ages of 10 to 14 commonly appear to be in deep sleep, yet immediately respond to suggestions such as wiggling their toes or raising their hand. Although children appear to achieve deep trance quickly, they are noticeably slower in awakening. Adults awaken within 5 to 15 seconds in contrast to most of our patients who require as long as 2 to 4 minutes to become fully awake.

During hypnosis, most adolescents and adults keep their eyes closed as compared with younger children who obtain relaxation and even deep trance with their eyes open.[23,24]

Relaxation techniques for reducing pain and anxiety

There are several excellent reviews on the use of hypnosis for pain control in children.[20,23] A systematic investigation was reported by Hilgard and LeBaron[25] where they identified a significant relation between hypnotic susceptibility and pain relief in children receiving bone marrow aspiration. Another study reported a significant reduction in pain and anxiety in adolescents who were receiving lumbar puncture and bone marrow aspiration.[26] Zeltzer and LeBaron[27] compared the use of hypnotic techniques to supportive counseling and distraction in 33 patients undergoing medical procedures. The reports showed that hypnotic techniques were consistently more effective than supportive counseling in decreasing discomfort in the children.

The few studies, many case reports, and personal experiences consistently supported the effectiveness of hypnosis in reducing pain and anxiety during medical procedures. However, Zeltzer and LeBaron[23] present some interesting questions: Are other behavioral interventions more effective? What are potential effective interventions for children less than 6 years of age? Can reduction in pain only be accompanied with active therapist-directed intervention? Can the use of hypnosis and other behavioral intervention be translated into a cost-effective, ongoing program to routinely help children to cope with medical procedures that accompany cancer treatment?

Hypnosis for reducing nausea and vomiting

Behavioral interventions using relaxation, guided imagery, and hypnosis is a new frontier in treatment of chemotherapy-related nausea and vomiting. Previous studies involving adult populations have demonstrated significant reduction of drug-related nausea and vomiting.[28-32]

Fortunately, the diagnosis of cancer in a child has changed from one of a fatal disease to a highly curable illness. The increased survival is largely a result of aggressive drug dose and drug combination chemotherapy, resulting in the devastating side effect of direct and anticipatory nausea and vomiting, which may become progressively worse as the child continues to receive treatment. Children view the chemotherapy and resultant discomforts as being worse than the disease and frequently terminate potentially curative treatment. One study reported that because of side effects of treatment, 33% of the children and 59% of the adolescents prematurely terminated chemotherapy.[33] Severe nausea and vomiting not only cause psychologic stress for the children but also subject them to nutritional deficits, electrolyte imbalance, weakness, increased susceptibility to infections, and disruption of normal childhood activities.[34]

Chemotherapy related nausea and vomiting has repeatedly been reported as a major source of emotional distress in patients of all ages. The following clinical situation is given as an example of how one patient dreaded chemotherapy.

CASE STUDY

S.M. was an 18-year-old male receiving chemotherapy for testicular seminoma. He had surgery to remove the tumor and staging of the disease and then began chemotherapy (which caused severe nausea and vomiting). After his third course of chemotherapy, he underwent a second abdominal/thoracotomy surgical procedure. On the second postoperative day, S.M. was experiencing considerable postoperative pain and had chest tubes, nasogastric tube, peripheral intravenous line, and a central venous line, two abdominal Jackson/Pratt pumps, and a urinary catheter. He was physically and psychologically distressed, which is understandable considering the extensive surgery he had endured. We were discussing the amount of comfort he could look forward to achieving in the following days as his surgical wound healed and the various tubes would be removed and specific behaviors he could choose to use to facilitate this healing process. As we were talking, he turned away and began to cry. S.M. said he felt miserable and believed he could not take any further insults; yet he would

rather face another operation than another course of chemotherapy . . . so great was his dread of chemotherapy.

Five controlled behavioral antiemetic intervention studies have been reported, each producing data that strongly and consistently support the usefulness of behavioral techniques in reducing chemotherapy nausea and vomiting.[28-32] To date, there are no empiric investigations regarding the efficacy of behavioral intervention such as hypnosis in helping children with the adverseness of chemotherapy. There are several encouraging case reports involving children, describing the application of behavioral techniques of hypnosis and imagery exercises.[35-39] Conclusions regarding the effectiveness of interventions in decreasing chemotherapy side effects based on case reports can only be suggestive.[23] There are several systematic investigations describing positive results with the use of hypnosis in children to alleviate chemotherapy nausea and vomiting.[40-43] All are well-done pilot studies carried out by the same group of investigators.

The hypnotic intervention used with children undergoing chemotherapy provides suggestions given in an age-appropriate manner: feelings of safety and comfort, thoughts of restful sleep from the antiemetics, impressions of chemotherapy working effectively, and thoughts of a short hospital stay with the child soon returning home. It is suggested that the child will awaken following completion of chemotherapy feeling thirsty without nausea. Children are encouraged to picture a safe place or a favorite activity where they can escape, becoming relaxed and unaware of the hospital surroundings. Emphasis is placed on each child's own ability to command their own behavior and attain control of chemotherapy side effects.

Relaxation techniques to reduce anxiety and drug-related nausea and vomiting present in children is a new treatment modality that will prove to be of major benefit. Its effectiveness in adults with cancer has paved the way for establishing itself as a therapeutic modality in decreasing untoward side effects of chemotherapy in children.

REFERENCES

1. Spinetta, J.J.; Behavioral and psychological research in childhood cancer, Cancer **50**(Suppl. 9):1939, 1982.
2. Nir, Y.: Psychologic support for children with soft tissue and bone sarcomas, NCI Monograph, No. 56, 145, 1981.
3. van Eys, J., editor: The normally sick child, Baltimore, 1979, University Park Press.
4. Prugh, D.G.: The psychosocial aspects of pediatrics, Philadelphia, 1983, Lea & Febiger.
5. Thompson, R.H., and Stanford, G.: Child life in hospitals: theory and practice, Springfield, Ill., 1982, Charles C Thomas, Publisher.
6. Druske, S.C., and Francis, S.A.: Pediatric diagnostic procedures, New York, 1981, John Wiley & Sons.
7. Mussen, P.H., editor: Handbook of child psychology, ed. 4, vol. 2, New York, 1983, John Wiley & Sons.
8. Mussen, P.H., Conger, J.J., and Kagan, J.: Child development and personality, ed. 3, New York, 1969, Harper & Row, Publishers, Inc.
9. Visintainer, M.A., and Wolfer, J.A. Psychological preparation for surgery patients: the effects on children's and parents' stress responses and adjustment, Pediatrics **56**(2):187, 1975.
10. Brewster, A.B.: Chronically ill children's concepts of their illness, Pediatrics **69**(3):355, 1982.
11. Ritchie, J.A.: Preparation of toddlers and preschool children for hospital procedures. Can. Nurse **75**(11):30, 1979.
12. Menke, E.M.: School-aged children's perception of stress in the hospital, J. Assoc. Care Child. Hosp. **9**(7):80, 1981.
13. Schowalter, J.E.: Be prepared! Pediatrics **68**(3):427, 1981.
14. Oremland, E.K., and Oremland, J.D.: The effects of hospitalization on children, Springfield, Ill., 1973, Charles C Thomas, Publisher.
15. Wallace, N.E.: Special books for special children, Children's Health Care **12**(1)34, 1983.
16. Plank, E.N.: Working with children in hospitals, ed. 2, Cleveland, 1971, The Press of Case Western Reserve University.
17. Hofman, A., Becker, R.D., and Gabriel, H.P.: The hospitalized adolescent: a guide to managing the ill and injured youth, New York, 1976, The Free Press.
18. Schowalter, J.E., and Lord, R.D.: Utilization of patient meetings on an adolescent ward, Psychol. Med. **1**(3):197, 1970.
19. Schowalter, J.E., and Anyan, W.R., Jr.: The family handbook of adolescence, New York, 1981, Alfred A. Knopf, Inc.
20. Gardner, G., and Oleness, K.: Hypnosis and hypnotherapy with children, New York, 1981, Grune & Stratton.
21. Barber, J., and Adrian, C.: Psychosocial approaches to the management of pain, New York, 1982, Brunner/Mazel, Inc.
22. Bandler, R., and Grinder, B.: Frogs into prince, Salt Lake City, Utah, 1978, Loab M. Publishing Co.
23. Zeltzer, L., LeBaron, S.: Behavioral intervention for children and adolescents with cancer, Behav. Med. Update **5**:17, 1983.
24. Morgan, A., and Hilgard, J.: Stanford hypnotic clinical scale for children, Am. J. Clin. Hypn. **21**:155, 1979.
25. Hilgard, J., and LeBaron, S.: Relief of anxiety and pain in children and adolescents with cancer: quantitative measures of clinical observation, Int. J. Clin. Exp. Hypn. **30**(4):417, 1982.
26. Kellerman, J., and others: Adolescents with cancer: hypnosis for the reduction of the acute pain and anxiety associated with medical procedures, J. Adolesc. Health Care **30**(4):85, 1983.
27. Zeltzer, L., and LeBaron, S.: Hypnosis and nonhypnotic technique for reduction of pain and anxiety during painful procedures in children with cancer, J. Pediatr. **101**(6):1032, 1982.
28. Burish, T., and Lyles, J.: Effectiveness of relaxation training in reducing adverse reactions to cancer chemotherapy, J. Behav. Med. **4**:65, 1981.
29. Lyles, J.N., and others: Efficacy of relaxation training and guided imagery in reducing the aversiveness of cancer chemotherapy, J. Consult. Clin. Psychol. **50**:509, 1982.
30. Cotanch, P.: Relaxation training as an antiemetic intervention, Cancer Nurs. **6**:277, 1983.
31. Morrow, G., and Morrell, C.: Behavioral treatment for the anticipatory nausea and vomiting induced by cancer chemotherapy, N. Engl. J. Med. **307**:1476, 1982.
32. Redd, W., and Andrykowski, M.: Behavioral intervention in cancer treatment: controlling aversion reactions to chemotherapy, J. Consult. Clin. Psychol. **50**:1018, 1982.
33. Smith, S.D., and others: A reliable method for evaluating drug compliance in children with cancer, Cancer **43**:169, 1979.
34. Laszlo, J., editor: Antiemetics and cancer chemotherapy, Baltimore, 1983, Williams & Wilkins.
35. Zeltzer, L.: The adolescent with cancer. In Kellerman, J., editor: Psychological aspects of childhood cancer, Springfield, Ill., 1980, Charles C Thomas, Publisher.
36. Hilgard, J.R., and LeBaron, S.: Hypnosis in the treatment of pain and anxiety in children with cancer: a clinical and quantitative investigation, Los Altos, Calif., 1983, William Kaufmann, Inc., (in press).
37. Cotanch, P.: Hypnosis in childhood cancer: a broader therapeutic value, J. Psychol. Oncol. (in review).
38. Hockenberry, M., and Cotanch, P.,: Hypnosis as antiemetic therapy: applications unique to children, Nurs. Clin. North Am. **20**(1):105, 1985.
39. LeBaw, W., and others: The use of self-hypnosis in children with cancer, Am. J. Clin. Hypn. **174**:233, 1975.

40. Zeltzer, L.K., and others: Hypnosis for reduction of vomiting associated with chemotherapy and disease in adolescents with cancer, J. Adolesc. Health Care **4:**77, 1983.
41. Zeltzer, L., LeBaron, S., and Zeltzer, P.: Children on chemotherapy: reduction of nausea and vomiting with behavioral intervention, Clin. Res. **30**(1):138A, 1982.
42. LeBaron, S., and Zeltzer, L.: Reduction of nausea and vomiting associated with chemotherapy in children with cancer: combined hypnotic and non-hypnotic intervention, Int. J. Clin. Exp. Hypn. **30**(3):329, 1982.
43. LeBaron, S., and Zeltzer, L.: Behavioral treatment for control of chemotherapy-related nausea and vomiting in children and adolescents with cancer, Pediatr. Res. **16**(4):208A, 1982.

CHAPTER 30

School re-entry following a diagnosis of cancer

SUZANNE B. HERMAN

School is the child's occupation. It is an essential component of the child's world for both academic and social achievement. Ongoing education is essential for retaining normalcy for the child. The child with cancer, as every child, needs to have a sense of the future. The child needs the stimulation and peer association of school to feel a sense of accomplishment and social acceptance.[1-3] Successful school re-entry must be the goal of all team members involved with the care of the child. This team must include the hospital-based providers, school personnel, community health care providers, and family. Such an extended team is essential for successful school rehabilitation of the child with cancer.

Children with cancer, like all children, must be guided toward the achievement of age-appropriate developmental tasks. These include intellectual growth, development of social skills and peer relationships, and preparation for career and family.[4] Because school is the work place for children, every attempt must be made to assure that the child with cancer has this opportunity despite his affliction. The child must be viewed as a student and not as a patient. For example, elementary school children need the school experience to be totally divorced from medical care and concerns.[5] The return to school for these children is often a reassurance that they are better and can continue with their normal activities. This can decrease anxiety and depression associated with the diagnosis of cancer. Maintenance of pre-illness academic achievement is important for even very young chil-

dren. Children as early as first grade who fall behind academically often feel inferior and will grow to dislike school.[6] Those children who have lasting physical impairments associated with their disease must seek a vocation in which they can function as productive adults.[3]

The peer interactions that occur in school help children develop social maturity. This socialization is important for all children with cancer and is especially important for the adolescent preparing for adulthood. Academically, the high school student with cancer must also look toward graduation from high school and preparation for a career. The adolescent with cancer will also be concerned with issues of mortality and the future, including his potential for becoming a parent.

THE CHILD WITH CANCER IN THE CLASSROOM
The child

Many factors interfere with the child's successful reentry into school. The child undoubtedly misses many days of school during the initial period when the diagnosis of cancer is made. Although much of the maintenance therapy can be administered as an outpatient, school days are missed because of clinic visits and therapy side effects.

The child may fear initial return to the school environment. Often the child has undergone a change in body image and is now "different from his peers." Weight loss or gain and hair loss because of chemotherapy or radiation therapy cause the child to feel self-conscious. Social and physical adjustments must be made. Because the child may fear the responses of the teacher and other students, he may refuse to attend school to avoid potential uncomfortable situations. McCollum states that acceptance or rejection by peers is influenced by "the child's self-confidence, sense of self-worth, and previous status in the group."[7] Children can often be cruel to a child who seems "different or weak," making that child less like themselves. A child who is given excessive attention by the teacher is often disliked by other pupils as well.[8]

School phobia is common for children with cancer and is associated with regressive behavior. Lansky and colleagues[9] found the incidence of school phobia in children with cancer to be 10% of their patient population in contrast to the reported incidence of 1.7% for healthy students. School phobic children with cancer generally had the same complaints of other children exhibiting school phobia, including headache, abdominal pain, and vague aches and pains. The child with cancer who exhibits school phobia symptoms offers a perplexing situation for parents. These physical symptoms may be similar to those first seen at diagnosis, making it difficult for parents to judge if the child's symptoms are related to the disease. Parents often fear relapse of the malignancy, even if the child has been doing well.

When the child has a continuing or recurrent desire to avoid school and is not acutely ill, emotional distress is usually the underlying problem. The younger child, up to about the third-grade level may have separation anxiety. Often the child will sense the reluctance on the part of the parent to let go. The child who is approaching preadolescence may experience school avoidance because of social anxiety, fear of rejection by peers, or fear of academic failure.[7]

School attendance patterns among pediatric cancer patients were studied by Lansky and colleagues at the University of Kansas. Examination of school records of these patients revealed that a significant amount of school was missed by children being treated for cancer. Factors that seemed to influence school attendance included the progression of the child's disease, the population of the town or city in which the child lived, the ordinal placement of the child in his family, the presence of central nervous system chemotherapy, and the sex of the child. From the study results, the researchers speculated that the child most likely to have school attendance problems would be a girl with at least one older sibling living in a large city and experiencing physical limitations because of her disease.[3]

The therapy itself not only affects school attendance but also affects the child's performance and activity while in school. Prolonged nausea, vomiting, and decreased appetite can continue days after chemotherapy has been administered. Decreased activity and fatigue can occur in the child with low blood counts or in one who has had physical limitations associated with the disease. Children receiving central nervous system treatment can have side effects that include nausea and vomiting, lethargy, somnolence, and other neurologic symptoms. Thus the school must have a knowledge of treatment side effects and be flexible to accommodate the child with cancer in the classroom and to encourage his school attendance.

The parents

Parents of the child with cancer may be hesitant to allow him to return to school for fear of the child becoming ill or being injured. This may result in the request for a homebound teacher. Much of this overprotectiveness may stem from separation anxiety occurring between the mother and the child. Parents must be given the support to "let go" to permit the child freedom to experience the school environment, which is essential to his well-being.[9]

Parents of children experiencing school phobia symptoms may have a difficult time maintaining control and discipline over the child. Often the parents feel an underlying sense of guilt for the disease and fear being a "bad parent." This leads to much frustration on the part of the parents, since they are torn between granting the child his desires and pushing the child toward a more normal life-style.[9] Parents often find it difficult to talk with school personnel about the disease, treatment, and prognosis because they feel a need to deny the illness or they do not want to show their emotions to others.[10]

Parents faced with school avoidance problems[8] should be advised to first review the child's health status with a member of the health care team. This will ease the parent's fear and anxiety concerning a possible exacerbation of the child's disease. The next step is to review the child's school experience with his teacher and then to promptly reintegrate the child back into school while offering reassurance and support related to the child's anxieties. When school avoidance continues, the child will become even more apprehensive and may become so frustrated that it becomes a psychologic emergency. In such a case, the child's parents, health care team, and educational and mental health professional must promptly collaborate and intervene with psychologic counseling for the child and family to resolve the problem.

The school

The school personnel and community may be resistant to the child with cancer returning to school. Teachers, untrained in medical areas, often feel frustrated and angry about the added responsibility of a child who is chronically ill. They may feel uncomfortable talking with the child's parents, fearing they might uncover painful feelings. The teacher may react to re-entry into the classroom by isolating the child because of fear about what to expect and how to react if a problem should arise. The teacher may also single out the child and treat the child as a ''favorite'' because of pity or sorrow.[5,10] They may fear the child will have a medical problem while in the classroom that they will not know how to cope with. Some teachers fear such things as uncontrollable bleeding, reactions from medications, or the child passing out in the classroom. Other teachers demonstrate reactions similar to those experienced by the parent. Kaplan[10] found teachers to experience grieving, disbelief, and hope that a miracle will bring cure.

Peers

The peers of the child with cancer are a vital group in assisting with re-entry to school. They can re-establish the child's perception of himself as ''normal'' or ''well.'' The school-age child who is accepted and included by his peers will have more success in normal growth and development toward adulthood.[11] However, peers can adversely affect the rehabilitation of the child. Healthy classmates who do not know or understand the child's diagnosis of cancer often fear or resent the child. Common fears include concern that the disease is contagious or that physical changes occurring in the child with cancer could happen to them. They may fear the child might die and believe their classmate is not the same now that he is ill. Resentment may occur, especially if the child is singled out as a ''favorite'' by the teacher.[8] These concerns of classmates may result in teasing and ridiculing the afflicted child.[11] This consequence results in further isolation.

Peers of adolescents with cancer commonly manifest their anxieties by severing interpersonal relationships, which are so necessary for the teenager. Healthy adolescents may avoid a peer who looks different in an attempt to protect their own sense of physical adequacy.[12]

These problems encountered with peers in both the school-age and adolescent patient can be lessened or prevented with adequate intervention. Interventions that are frequently absent in the child's return to school will be discussed in the following section.

SCHOOL INTERVENTION

Preparing the child for re-entry into the school must begin in the hospital. The hospital-based health care team should initiate this process and elicit early participation of the school personnel and early commitment by the parents and the child. With the support of the health care team, family, and school, they can strive to continue a productive school experience.

On discharge from the hospital, the child should be encouraged to enter school as soon as he is physically able. Occasionally, the child may require a homebound teacher until returning to school is appropriate from a medical perspective. Examples of children who may need a temporary homebound educational program might include the child who is recovering from surgery or the child who is undergoing such intensive chemotherapy, radiation therapy, or physical rehabilitation that it is almost impossible to attend school with any regularity. However, it must be stressed that such programs should be viewed as temporary, and efforts should be made for the child to maintain contact with the school and his peers during this time period.

A strong tie must be established between the parents, the health care team, and school personnel. Responsiveness of the school personnel to the child with cancer will be strengthened if there is communication and cooperation among all involved in the child's care. The teacher must be provided with information about the disease and its treatment. Discussion of how to recognize physical symptoms and problems such as fever, bleeding, and infection must be addressed. Fears by classmates must be addressed by the teacher or by a representative of the health care team. Notions about the communicability of cancer must be allayed. Finally, the teacher must be supported to maintain similar academic, physical, and social expectations for the cancer patient as are held for the other children in the classroom. The parents, with the help of the health care team should meet with the staff to plan how best to meet the child's physical needs. For example, if the child has difficulty climbing stairs because of fatigue, all of his classes might be placed on one level. Should the child have frequent need to use the bathroom, he might be given permission by the teacher to leave the classroom quietly.

The child's academic needs must also be addressed. The parents must try to ensure that the school staff has realistic expectations for the child. It is common for teachers to assume that any learning problem the child has is associated with the malignancy. Rarely is brain damage or mental retardation associated with cancer in children. Learning problems can result from many different sources. They can be related to anxieties associated with school or family life, depression, or as a disturbance in function of the central nervous system.[7]

Children with cancer may have insult to their central nervous system, resulting in a learning problem. This is most commonly caused by cranial irradiation or surgery as treatment for brain tumors or cranial irradiation as central nervous system prophylaxis for acute lymphocytic leukemia. There is a paucity of prospective controlled studies regarding the effect of cranial irradiation and/or intrathecal methotrexate on the intellectual functioning of children with acute lymphocytic leukemia (see Chapter 31 on late effects). Most studies have been retrospective, with few subjects and widely varying results. Meadows and colleagues[13] at the Children's Hospital of Philadelphia evaluated thirty-one children diagnosed with acute lymphocytic leukemia prospectively using standardized intelligence tests during the first month of treatment and periodically thereafter. They found children who received a combination of central nervous system irradiation and intrathecal medications had a significant decrease in overall IQ score, with younger patients being most affected. These deficits were not seen in children who received intrathecal medications without cranial irradiation.[13] Other studies confirm young patients receiving cranial irradiation show a greater decrease in intellectual abilities than patients who are older when treated.[14,15] Eiser[16] found in 28 children studied with acute lymphocytic leukemia with varying combinations of treatment that those who received cranial irradiation were generally of lower intellectual ability. These subjects were not further examined by age.[16] In contrast, studies performed by Obetz and colleagues[17] showed no significant differences in neuropsychologic function related to various central nervous system prophylaxis regimens. Inati and colleagues[15] found school-age children who received cranial irradiation had an 18% rate of learning disabilities, an incidence rate similar to those of school-age children in the community. Copeland

and associates[18] found in a study of 74 patients that central nervous system irradiation of children affects visual-motor and motor skills and partial processing tasks related to arithmetic regardless of the age at diagnosis. Intrathecal chemotherapy alone has not been shown to affect cognitive functioning.[18]

Any child who is suspected of having a learning-related disability should have a comprehensive workup of the disorder. Developmental evaluation clinics and centers are helpful in the diagnosis and treatment of such problems. These tests help to identify specific needs of the child and allow for implementation of specialized programs to assist the child's learning deficits.

THE RE-ENTRY PROCESS

Since the child may miss days of school because of ongoing chemotherapy, radiation therapy, or increased susceptibility to infection, extra help for the student, including home instruction, may be needed. Most school systems are willing to provide homebound teaching for short, frequent absences. This allows the child who may be out of school frequently to attend school when feeling well yet to be able to keep up academically. A telephone conversation between the teacher and a member of the health care team at the time of diagnosis, written material about the disease and its treatment, and availability to the teacher by telephone for problems as they arise serve to increase the teacher's confidence and assist in the child's return to the classroom.

With the support of the child's teacher, other children in the classroom can be prepared for the child's return. When a child must have a homebound program before the return to school, continued communications should be encouraged between the child and his classmates.

The child should be supported in preparing himself to return to school. Because of his diagnosis and changes in body image he may be reluctant to return to the school environment. Positive results have occurred with ''back to school programs'' presented by members of the health care team and the teacher. One such program is the At-Home Rehabilitation Demonstration Project sponsored by the National Cancer Institute, Division of Cancer Control and Rehabilitation. The goal of this project is to make the re-entry into school easier for the child with cancer. A team approach is used, taking advantage of the various community health care professionals' services. This team prepares age-appropriate classroom programs to be presented to the child's class at the time of the child's re-entry into school. This approach has proved to be very positive, helping the patient, peers, and school personnel accept and understand the illness and dispel fears of the disease. Such programs could also be developed by community health educators and school nurses.[19]

In a study by Henning and Fritz,[4] 37 children with diagnoses ranging from leukemia to osteosarcoma showed how re-entry into school could be aided. They suggest four guidelines that have proved useful in facilitating school re-entry of children with cancer: (1) efforts on behalf of the child must be individualized, (2) availability of an experienced professional is essential, (3) activities of medical, educational, and social service professionals must be coordinated, and (4) each child should be treated as if he will do well in school.[9] Ross and Scarvalone[8] developed a program offering a seminar for educators. They found that as a result of the program, school personnel felt more confident and treated the patient more normally. They were able to answer questions from the patient and classmates and could deal more effectively with parents when they are provided with information about the disease and its treatment. Teachers were given some perspective about related psychosocial issues.[8] Reports from similar programs also showed positive results.[1,10,12,20,21]

Goodell[11] focused her intervention on the peers of children with cancer. The educational program was based on the premise that (1) through educating peers of children with cancer, those peers can act as advocates for the child with cancer and (2) through reducing fear by education, teasing and irritating questions would be reduced. Her findings showed that young children were able to return to school more easily than older children and that the program seemed to be a positive factor in easing the process. Preteens were also helped by the program but continued to have problems with the child with cancer "being different."[11] Ross and Ross[22] took an interesting approach to deal with the "being different" and teasing problems. They developed a training program to teach children with leukemia to handle teasing by peers by using certain nonverbal behaviors and verbal strategies. The program made a strong positive impact on the self-confidence of the children who felt that they could now cope with the problem.[22]

Successful school re-entry can be accomplished in the child with cancer. To work toward this goal, there must be a commitment by all involved to strive toward normalcy in the daily activity of the child. School must be perceived as the greatest area of accomplishment and socialization for the child. To make this experience the most rewarding for the child with cancer, a team approach must be used. This team extends from the hospital health care team to the family, school, and community. Communication must remain open. Such open communication will assure that the child's needs are met and that any problem associated with school will be detected early and treated promptly. With successful school reintegration, children with cancer can prosper and strive toward their future goals and achievements.

REFERENCES

1. Kirten, C., and Liverman, M.: Special educational needs of the child with cancer, J. Sch. Health **47**(3):170, 1977.
2. Cyphert, F.R.: Back to school for the child with cancer, J. Sch. Health **43**(4):215, 1973.
3. Cairns, N.V., and others: School attendance of children with cancer, J. Sch. Health **52**(3):152, 1982.
4. Henning, J., and Fritz, G.K.: School reentry in childhood cancer, Psychosomatics **24**(3):261, 1983.
5. Deasy-Spinetta, P.: The school and the child with cancer, In Spinetta, J.J., and Deasy-Spinetta, P., editors: Living with childhood cancer, St. Louis, 1981, The C.V. Mosby Co.
6. Travis, G.: Chronic illness in children, Stanford, Calif., 1976, Stanford University Press.
7. McCollum, A.T.; The chronically ill child, New Haven, Conn., 1975, Yale University Press.
8. Ross, J.W., and Scarvalone, S.A.: Facilitating the pediatric cancer patient's return to school, Soc. Work. **27**(3):256, 1982.
9. Lansky, S.B., and others: School phobia in children with malignant neoplasms, Am. J. Dis. Child. **129**(1):42, 1975.
10. Kaplan, D.M., Smith, A., and Grobstein, R.: School management of the seriously ill child, J. Sch. Health **44**(5):250, 1974.
11. Goodell, A.S.: Peer education in schools for children with cancer, Issues Compr. Pediatr. Nurs. **7**(2-3):101, 1984.
12. Moore, I.M., and Triplett, J.L.: Students with cancer: a school nursing perspective, Cancer Nurs. **3**(4):265, 1980.
13. Meadows, A.T., and others: Declines in I.Q. scores and cognitive dysfunctions in children with acute lymphocytic leukaemia treated with cranial irradiation, Lancet **2**(8254):1015, 1981.
14. Moss, H.A., Nannis, E.D., and Poplack, D.G.: The effects of prophylactic treatment of the CNS system on the intellectual functioning of children with ALL, Am. J. Med. **71**(1):47, 1981.
15. Inati, A., and others: Efficacy and morbidity of central nervous system "prophylaxis" in childhood acute lymphoblastic leukemia: eight years' experience with cranial irradiation and intrathecal methotrexate, Blood **61**(2):297, 1983.
16. Eiser, C.: Intellectual abilities among survivors of childhood leukaemia as a function of CNS irradiation, Arch. Dis. Child. **53**(5):391, 1978.
17. Obetz, S.W., and others: Neuropsychologic follow-up study of children with acute lymphocytic leukemia, Am. J. Pediatr. Hematol. Oncol. **1**(3):207, 1979.
18. Copeland, D.R., and others: CNS irradiation of children found to impair arithmetic-related abilities, Oncology **29**(1):3, 1984.
19. Sachs, M.B.: Helping the child with cancer go back to school, J. Sch. Health **50**(6):328, 1980.
20. Greene, P.: The child with leukemia in the classroom, Am. J. Nurs. **75**(1):86, 1975.
21. Katz, E., Kellerman, J., and Rigler, D.: School intervention with pediatric cancer patients, J. Pediatr. Psychol. **2**(2):72, 1979.
22. Ross, D.M., and Ross, S.A.: Teaching the child with leukemia to cope with teasing, Issues Compr. Pediatr. Nurs. **7**(2):59, 1984.

CHAPTER 31

Late effects of cancer treatment in children

MARY J. WASKERWITZ and JEAN H. FERGUSSON

When a child is diagnosed with cancer, the pediatric oncology team not only works to cure the child of cancer but also strives to provide that child with a high quality of survival. Today quality of survival is as important as survival itself. Each year, 11 out of every 100,000 children in the United States under the age of 15 years are diagnosed as having cancer, according to National Cancer Institute surveys.[1] Cancer treatments that are being used at this time result in a greater than 50% overall survival rate for these children. Some researchers have calculated that by the year 1990 one out of every 1000 persons in the United States who has reached 20 years of age will be a cured cancer patient.[2] These figures document the large numbers of children and young adults who will continue to live after cancer diagnosis and treatment. Ironically, the children and young adults who survive childhood cancer and its treatment may face health hazards caused by the same therapy that allowed them to live.

The term *late effects* is used to describe the broad range of post-therapeutic disabilities that are seen in survivors of pediatric cancers. This chapter delineates and explicates the late consequences of cancer treatment in children from several different perspectives. It begins with a description of the unique chronic problems that are discovered in children who have been diagnosed and treated for cancer. It then concentrates on the effects of cancer treatments on body systems. The specific late outcomes of treatment for the more common forms of cancer in children are included in the text. Early recognition and prompt management of these sequelae may, in some cases, lessen the severity of the residual problems. In other cases, steps may be taken at the time of diagnosis and treatment to prevent some of the long-term toxicities.

Late effects may be caused by either the cancer itself, by its treatment, or by both. Treatment may include surgery, radiotherapy, chemotherapy, or combinations of the three. The nature, timing, gravity, and frequency of the development of late effects are dependent on (1) the location and extent of the primary disease; (2) the type and intensity of the initial treatment; and (3) the age, physiologic, and developmental status of the child at the time of diagnosis and treatment. The time interval between therapy and the onset of later complications is unpredictable. Some residual abnormalities such as surgical amputations or exenterative procedures are clinically obvious. In other cases, late sequelae may represent subtle findings that appear so long after the time of the cancer diagnosis and treatment that the medical-nursing oncology team may not recognize any relationship.

Late effects can involve any organ system. Findings may range from simple laboratory abnormalities to life-threatening complications. The following outline classifies late effects among long-term survivors of childhood cancer. Each item in this outline encompasses an area of physical findings that are commonly affected by cancer and its treatment[3]:

Damage to central nervous system (CNS)
Psychosocial
Neurologic
Intellectual

Impaired growth and development
Gonadal development and reproduction aberrations
Genetic aberrations
Teratogenesis
Oncogenesis
Disruption of function in other organ systems
  Heart
  Kidney
  Liver
  Lungs
  Bladder
  Gastrointestinal tract
  Skeleton

This chapter describes the major late effects that can occur in survivors of childhood cancer. It also presents an appraisal of the probable causes of these sequelae. It concludes with specifications of nursing responsibilities in the assessment and management of late effects in childhood cancer survivors.

CLASSIFICATIONS OF LATE EFFECTS IN CHILDREN
Psychosocial sequelae

For many children the diagnosis of cancer is an event that affects both them and their families for the rest of their lives. Feelings of depression, rage, anxiety, and despair can strain their coping capacities to the limit. Fortunately, many children with cancer grow up to be as well adjusted psychologically as their physically healthy peers, though such positive outcomes are not easily won. The child's personality and his family's personality play a major role in achieving this positive outcome. However, even the most skillful family needs the support and guidance of a compassionate health care team.[4-6]

To date, there are few studies about the late psychologic effects of cancer in childhood. However, studies carried out on populations of children with other forms of chronic disease may be applied to the case of the child with cancer. These studies identify the following general conclusions: (1) children with chronic illness have rates of maladjustment that are higher than those of their peers; (2) features such as age at onset, course and severity of the disease, and visibility and degree of handicap affect the child's overall adjustment; (3) personality attributes such as maturity, intelligence, charm, and sense of humor play a major role in the child's adjustment to illness; (4) individual family resources such as stability, warmth, commitment, and flexibility have a great impact on a child's adjustment; (5) available support systems, quality of care, extended family, friends, and community resources influence the child's adjustment.[4]

There are no major studies demonstrating that children with cancer have a higher rate of maladjustment than any other children. It is certain, however, that cancer, like other chronic illness, creates a cycle of severe stress with an attendant stressful atmosphere that must be dealt with by the child and his family. The outcome of dealing with this stress is the development of coping mechanisms that may or may not be adaptive.

Some research suggests that approximately half of all children with cancer may face certain long-term adjustment problems.[5] Factors that contribute to these problems include (1) uncertainty regarding the duration of the illness and its ultimate outcome, (2) lack of communication between the family and members of the health care team, and (3) lack of openness and honesty in discussing the illness with the patient. A major element that gives way to maladaptive behavior is lack of communication between the child and his family and between the family and the health care team. Unlike many other serious childhood illnesses, cancer often involves an infinite course, for there is always the possibility of a recurrence. For many children, late consequences such as learning disorders serve as a constant reminder of the disease.

Variables that contribute to late psychologic problems in children with cancer are (1) the developmental stage of the child at the time of diagnosis and treatment, (2) the extent of the child's cancer and the rigor of the treatment protocol, (3) the coping resources of the child and his family, and (4) the availability of a multidisciplinary team of health professionals.[4]

In *The Damocles Syndrome,*[5] Koocher describes

the psychosocial consequences of surviving child-hood cancer. Koocher found that the sex of the child did not affect psychologic outcomes; how-ever, he states that family income significantly and positively correlates with favorable psychologic ad-justment. Koocher's data suggests that age at the time of diagnosis and prolonged continuous re-mission of disease are important factors that con-tribute to a lower incidence of psychologic prob-lems. Koocher also found the highest incidence of adjustment problems were seen among survivors of Hodgkin's disease and acute lymphocytic leu-kemia. This finding was attributed to the prolonged course of treatment and its related side effects. Of all the survivors studied by Koocher, those patients who experienced recurrence of disease were found to suffer more long-term psychologic adjustment problems, even when the recurrence was success-fully treated. Children who retained persistent and unresolved concerns about the outcome of their disease seemed to be at greatest risk for late psy-chologic problems.[5]

In summary, Koocher[5] concluded from his stud-ies that survivors of childhood cancer are at greater risk for the development of long-term psychologic problems than are childhood survivors of other chronic but not life-threatening disorders. He found that a number of variables tend to distinguish well-adjusted survivors from those whose adjustment may be compromised. Optimum long-term adjust-ment is influenced by (1) the type of cancer and the number of permanent side effects, (2) the oc-currence of relapse, and (3) the developmental stage at the time of onset.[5]

In another study of late psychologic effects of cancer in childhood, Fergusson[6] concluded that children who have not been told about their diag-nosis have the most severe adjustment problems. Withholding information about the diagnosis from the child inevitably distorts the parent-child rela-tionship and is another variable that contributes toward late psychologic maladjustment. Honesty rather than fabrication is associated with better psy-chologic outcomes for the child.[6]

Meadows and colleagues[8] studied the late social effects of cancer in children. In a review of 93 long-term survivors of childhood cancer, the ed-ucational achievements and employment status of these children as they entered adulthood were stud-ied. Sixty-one percent of those interviewed con-tinued their education beyond high school. Chil-dren who were age 6 to 10 years at the time of diagnosis and treatment had the highest rate of con-tinuing education after high school (72%). Dura-tion of treatment did not seem to influence edu-cational levels. Fourteen percent were unemployed; however, only one patient was over 25 years of age at the time of study. Meadows concluded that al-though survivors of childhood cancer as a whole do not differ from the general population, there are exceptions as described in certain patient subgroups.[8]

Lansky and Cairns[9] wrote that probably the best indication of social rehabilitation in the child with cancer is his willingness to return to school, for school is the work of a child. Children who miss 20 or more days of school per year are not able to maintain good grades. Lansky and Cairns found in a study of 110 children with cancer that school absences were high, even 2 to 3 years after diag-nosis. This absenteeism was associated with other significant problems such as declining grades and acting out.[9]

Discussions of the psychosocial sequelae of childhood cancer must include a recognition of some of the social problems that cancer survivors may confront as adults. Reports of job discrimi-nation, inability to obtain life and medical insur-ance, and being refused college admission or entry into the military service have been gathered.[10] Studies have been initiated at several cancer centers in the United States in an attempt to define these social barriers and to develop proposals for anti-discriminatory legislation for cancer patients.

Neurologic sequelae

Children with cancer who do not receive treat-ment that is directed to the CNS usually have no cause for experiencing neurologic sequelae. In ad-dition, the risk and severity of neurotoxicity are directly proportional to the number and sequence of treatment modalities employed.[11]

In recent years, the multimodal treatment of acute lymphocytic leukemia has included systemic chemotherapy, cranial radiation, and intrathecal methotrexate. This therapeutic approach has greatly improved survival statistics for children with acute lymphocytic leukemia. However, the addition of cranial radiation and intrathecal chemotherapy can produce damage to the CNS.[11] Dementia and seizures have been reported in patients who have received systemic methotrexate without cranial radiation. The severity of methotrexate toxicity is related to methotrexate levels measured in the cerebral spinal fluid. Damage ranging from minor complications such as foot drop to major incidents such as paresis and paralysis are well-known toxicities of spinal cord radiation. Patients treated for primary CNS lesions with cranial radiation in excess of 5500 rad are at high risk for developing residual neurologic sequelae such as blindness, hearing loss, ataxia, hemiplegia, and decreased intellectual functioning.[12] Fortunately, not all children who receive CNS treatment are subject to these problems. Most children who receive combinations of radiation and intrathecal methotrexate do not experience late neurologic sequelae. Children who are less than 3 years of age at the time of treatment are most vulnerable to late neurologic side effects because of the immaturity of their nervous systems.[13] The myelin sheath that completely develops in most children by age 5 years covers neurons and serves as protection from damage for older children.[14] Systemically administered methotrexate can affect CNS tissue by inhibiting the formation of a lipid that is a major component of myelin. Because radiation changes the integrity of the blood-brain barrier, drugs such as methotrexate diffuse more easily into the brain's white matter. There are reports of long-term mild clinical and severe CNS toxicity associated with high-dose intravenous methotrexate in some patients.[15]

Combinations of chemotherapy and cranial radiation are associated with significant CNS damage characterized by evidence of white matter destruction termed leukoencephalopathy. Clinical signs of progressive multifocal leukoencephalopathy are of varying degrees of severity but can include ataxia, restlessness, dysmetria, myoclonic movements, general clumsiness, disorientation, slurred speech, and swallowing difficulty. A computed tomographic (CT) scan will show enhancing hypodensity of the white matter in the centrum ovale and periventricular areas around the frontal horns. There may be moderate ventricular dilatation.[11] Leukoencephalopathy can develop following cranial radiotherapy, particularly when it is combined with intrathecal or systemically administered methotrexate. Radiotherapy increases the permeability of the blood-brain barrier, allowing the concentration of methotrexate to reach toxic levels. Leukoencephalopathy has also been reported in children receiving combinations of chemotherapy intrathecally and CNS radiation for brain tumors and rhabdomyosarcomas[12] (Fig. 31-1).

The effects of excessive cranial and craniospinal radiation have been established. Radiotherapy can injure both the CNS and peripheral nervous system. When neurotoxic manifestations are noted during or shortly after treatment, they are usually mild and transitory; whereas late neurotoxic manifestations may be severe and irreversible.[13] The delayed radiation reaction, cerebral necrosis, is by far the most serious late neurologic sequela. Cerebral necrosis can begin insidiously several months to years after treatment. It is usually diagnosed 1 to 5 years after treatment and can progress to functional impairment or death. Necrosis occurs in areas of the brain exposed to more than 600 rad regardless of whether white or gray matter is within the treatment field.[11]

Vincristine is a chemotherapeutic agent employed in the treatment of many childhood malignancies. Vincristine can be neurotoxic because it disrupts microtubule assembly and alters neuroexcitability. Vincristine neurotoxicity may manifest as diminished reflexes, foot drop, and weakness. This neurotoxicity is usually reversible and is usually abated with a decrease in the administered

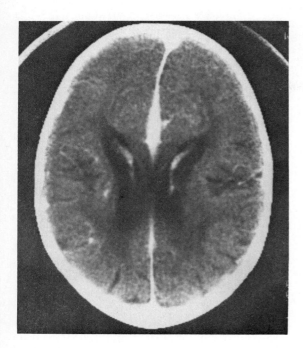

Fig. 31-1. Brain CT scan of child with severe disseminated leukoencephalopathy following radiation therapy and intrathecal chemotherapy. Decreased density of white matter in the centrum semiovale is secondary to leukoencephalopathy.

dosage. Deep tendon reflexes, which are often absent during the course of vincristine treatment, return to normal activity several months after discontinuation of the drug.

Treatment combinations that employ CNS radiation appear to be the most neurotoxic. If CNS radiation must be combined with methotrexate, the least of neurotoxic regimen should be employed. This includes sequential administration of modalities rather than concurrent administration. Methotrexate given during CNS radiation is much more apt to produce severe neurologic sequelae.[11]

Intellectual sequelae

As is true for the development of neurologic sequelae, children with cancer who do not receive treatment that is directed to the CNS usually have no cause for experiencing intellectual sequelae. Studies have documented normal, expected educational achievements without educational delays for children with cancer.[16,17] Neuropsychiatric evaluations of certain patient groups, however, have shown some significant long-term effects of treatment, particularly in the area of cognitive skills.

A study by Eiser[18] describes a group of patients, treated for acute lymphocytic leukemia with cranial radiation and intrathecal chemotherapy, whose intellectual performance was well below matched controls. Significant findings applied particularly to quantitative memory and motor skills but not to language tasks.[18] Other findings have included difficulties in verbal performance and easy distractability. Several other authors report that children who received cranial radiation at an early age appear to be affected more significantly than those who were treated in later years.[19]

Poplack and his associates[20] studied 32 children who received CNS prophylaxis consisting of 2400 cranial rad. These children were tested 19 to 67 months after treatment and scored significantly lower on verbal performance and full scale IQ tests than their peers. The lowest scores were recorded by children who were treated in early childhood.[20]

During the diagnostic period and before CNS treatment was given, Meadows and colleagues[21] administered standardized psychometric tests to a group of 28 children with acute lymphocytic leukemia. The results of these tests were compared with the results of similar tests administered to the children immediately after CNS treatment and again between 2 and 4 years after treatment. There was a normal distribution of scores on both the first and second testings. However, after the third testing, one third of the children were found to be in the subnormal category. Once again, overall testing showed that the greatest changes were in the younger age group. This study suggests effects of cranial radiation and other agents may not become manifest immediately after treatment and in fact may not be appreciated until several years after treatment.[21] Lowered IQ and impairments in neuropsychologic function are attributable to CNS therapy, with cranial radiation probably the most significant agent.[21]

Children with brain tumors receive even more intensive treatment directed to the CNS, often including cranial radiation doses of 2000 to 5000 rad. Late follow-up of these patients reveals that an alarmingly large proportion of them are left with intellectual dysfunction. Etiologic factors that are associated with an increased risk for developing these problems include age less than 2 to 3 years at the time of treatment, radiation dose, primary tumor site, increased intracranial pressure, and extent of radiation field.[22] Significant problems include dementia, learning disabilities, intellectual retardation, and mental retardation.[23,24]

Early recognition of learning disabilities that accompany decreases in IQ will allow teachers to work with both the healthcare team and parents to plan remedial teaching programs for children with cancer. These children will benefit from (1) early assessment of school performance, (2) open patient and family attitudes toward the additional handicap, and (3) honest communication at the time of diagnosis regarding the possibility of these problems.

Impaired growth and development

Growth and development may be impaired to some degree in any child who is afflicted with a chronic illness. For example, many children who have nonmalignant problems such as chronic infection, inflammatory bowel disease, hepatic disease, cardiovascular disease, pulmonary disease, renal disease, and hematologic disease may also present with growth and development disorders.[25] Chemotherapeutic agents that affect the proliferation of all cells in the body and radiotherapy, which has a direct cell-kill effect on radiated structures, seem to be the most common causes of growth and development abnormalities noted in children who have been treated for cancer.

Radiotherapy is implicated in many reported cases of decelerated or decreased growth in children with cancer. Radiation directed at growing bones or at glands responsible for produc-

ing growth-related hormones can delay or stunt growth. Children who are most vulnerable to retarded or arrested bone growth are those who receive radiotherapy during periods of rapid growth. Radiation is especially deleterious when it affects growth centers at the ends of long bones or the spine. Obviously, those persons who receive radiotherapy to bones after they have reached puberty and have completed their adolescent growth spurt will not be as vulnerable to radiation-related growth aberrations.

The pituitary gland is responsible for the production of growth hormone. When cranial radiation strikes the pituitary gland, it can cause pituitary dysfunction. This results in partial or total growth hormone deficiency. The degree of growth hormone deficiency is probably proportional to the total dose of radiotherapy, although some reports indicate that all children may not be equally affected. One study of children with brain tumors treated with 2700 to 5000 cranial rad showed bone age retardation in 9 out of 9 cases and impaired growth hormone response in 6 out of 9 cases.[26] Another study of 21 children with acute lymphocytic leukemia showed that those patients who received prophylactic cranial radiation (1800 to 2400 rad) had lower height velocities during treatment than did patients who had not received radiotherapy or normal controls.[27]

Growth derangements can also be related to hypothyroidism caused by direct beam radiation or scatter to the thyroid gland or by radiation to the pituitary gland, which is responsible for producing thyroid stimulating hormone (TSH).

The precise effect of chemotherapy on skeletal growth is difficult to quantitate. Most studies of growth in children who have received chemotherapy alone indicate temporary growth delays during the period of active treatment. Normal growth rates resume on discontinuation of chemotherapy. The result may be merely that of an ultimate decrease in growth potential.[19]

Some clinical research has been done on the effect of corticosteroids on growth in children. Corticosteroids such as prednisone and dexamethasone are often part of the drug regimen prescribed for children with leukemia, lymphoma, and brain tumors. Because steroids can inhibit the production and release of pituitary growth hormone, they can slow the rate of statural growth and skeletal maturation of children within a few weeks of onset of treatment.[28] There is a tendency for children given growth-suppressing doses of steroids to undergo compensatory growth spurts when doses are reduced or discontinued. The dose of steroids required to produce growth deceleration differs among children; children with some degree of pituitary dysfunction seem to be more affected than children with normal endocrine function.[29] Steroids given on an alternate day basis may allow for hypothalamic and pituitary recovery between doses and hence not result in growth suppression.[30]

Growth charts should be maintained and updated on all pediatric oncology patients. Any child who shows a decreased or abnormal growth velocity warrants further screening. Screening measures include documenting parental heights to consider genetic growth potential, obtaining a wrist x-ray examination for bone age to predict future growth potential, assessing gonadal development, and evaluating pituitary function by obtaining blood studies such as exercise or overnight growth hormone levels and somatomedin C. Somatomedin C is an important peptide growth factor known to be involved in postnatal growth and in the feedback control of growth hormone secretion. A pediatric endocrinologist should be consulted for all children who appear to have growth failure or delay.

Gonadal development and reproduction aberrations

Systemic chemotherapy and radiotherapy to the gonads may affect gonadal development and function of persons treated for cancer. Gonadal dysfunction caused by cancer treatment is related to a number of variables that include age at time of treatment, type of treatment, duration of treatment, and total dose of treatment.

Infertility in childhood cancer survivors has not yet been well documented because until recently,

a large number of children did not survive cancer and grow up to produce their own children. Today, various aspects of radiotherapy and chemotherapy have been implicated in cases of sterility in childhood cancer survivors. Although treatment-induced sterility may be reversible with time, there is no way to predict which patients will recover gonadal function nor how long recovery will take.

Alkylating agents are compounds that interfere with the structure and function of DNA. They are capable of damaging the germ cells and Leydig's cells of the gonads, and are most often cited as the chemotherapeutic agents that can cause gonadal dysfunction and sterility. Cyclophosphamide and chlorambucil are the particular agents that are associated with a high incidence of gonadal failure and sterility. Busulfan, cytosine arabinoside, doxorubicin, and vinblastine have also been associated with sterility in some patients.[31,32]

Factors influencing sensitivity to this drug toxicity include the cumulative dose of the drug received, duration of treatment, and the age, sex, and pubertal status of the patient at the time of treatment. Chemotherapy seems to be less deleterious to gonadal function in prepubertal females than prepubertal males or adults of either sex.[33] For example, women in their forties are more likely to become sterile if they are treated with cyclophosphamide than women in their thirties. In adults, this relationship may be a result of the natural decrease in viable oocytes that occurs with aging.[31] One study cited cumulative cyclophosphamide doses of greater than 365 mg/kg as definitely causing altered spermatogenesis in males.[34] Testicular biopsies on these patients show tubular atrophy.[32] Another study showed that cumulative cyclophosphamide doses as high as 525 mg/kg did not prevent ovulation in females.[34]

In the prepubertal female, chemotherapy may cause primary amenorrhea and absence of secondary sexual development accompanied by elevated serum gonadotropins.[19] Amenorrhea is common among many postpubertal females while they are actually receiving chemotherapy. However, in most of these patients, menses return some time after chemotherapy is stopped.[32] Oligomenorrhea and menopausal symptoms can also occur. The symptoms of this "chemical castration" include emotional upheaval, menstrual aberration, hot flashes, irritability, insomnia, poor self-image, depression, and loss of sexual function.

The effect of chemotherapy on the male testes is to cause germinal aplasia. This manifests itself as oligospermia, loss of libido, and decreased sexual functioning. Drugs such as cyclophosphamide have been implicated in this toxicity. Chemotherapeutic programs that do not include alkylating agents are much less likely to induce testicular dysfunction. The prepubertal testis is relatively insensitive to the cytotoxic effects of cyclophosphamide.[34] Cytotoxic effects of anticancer agents on the postpubertal testis are not necessarily permanent.[19] Gynecomastia has been reported as a complication of treatment with agents such as busulfan, vincristine, and BCNU.

Decreased fertility and even sterility can be caused by radiotherapy to the gonads. Radiation to the abdomen can scatter to the gonads unless they are protected with shielding devices or surgical displacement. One study indicated that fractionated radiation doses were more damaging than single doses.[35] Factors that influence the severity of this toxicity include total radiation dose, radiation regimen, and patient sex, age, and pubertal status at the time of treatment. The severity of the injury and time to recovery are dose dependent. As little as 500 rad to the testes may cause sterility in males.[19] Permanent sterility in females may be induced by as little as 600 rad to the ovaries of an adult female. However, 2000 rad is required to induce sterility in prepubertal girls.[35] Women over 40 years of age appear to be the most sensitive to this dose-related radiotherapy toxicity.[19]

Clinical evaluation of gonadal function can be made during physical assessment of the patient's pubertal status and via specific laboratory tests. The progression of gonadal development is described as stages I through V in the Tanner classification. Gonadal development that does not progress to Tanner stage IV or V is probably indicative of gonadal

dysfunction with decreased spermatogenesis or altered ovarian function. Decreased sperm counts or absence of menses are other clinical indicators of infertility. Increased levels of follicle-stimulating hormone (FSH) and luteinizing hormone (LH) along with decreased levels of testosterone or estradiol are hormonal changes associated with sterility. Young people who have received cytotoxic agents or gonadal radiation need to be counseled about birth control, fertility, and other sexuality issues. The ultimate loss of the ability to parent a child can be fraught with psychologic connotations.[36] The right to select options for or against future parenthood is important for every patient.

Sperm banking should be considered pretreatment for young men as a possible way of circumventing problems such as sterility and mutagenicity. Commercial sperm banks are located throughout the country. Under complete privacy a certain number of sperm ejaculates are collected every other day over a period of 1 to 2 weeks. Initial sperm collection and analysis fees are assessed by sperm banks along with annual storage fees. Some insurance companies will reimburse clients for sperm banking expenses.

Pediatric endocrinologists should be consulted when any of these patients do not show signs of gonadal development by the normally expected ages. Hormonal replacement therapy with oral estrogen or intramuscular testosterone may be warranted to induce secondary sex characteristics development.

Genetic aberrations

There is abundant evidence that underlying genetic predispositions have a profound effect in determining the onset of cancer in childhood.[37] Individuals with certain chromosomal defects are known to have a high incidence of some cancers. For example, children with Down's syndrome are at higher risk for the development of leukemia. Retinoblastoma and neurofibrosarcoma are other forms of cancer that can be inherited and are associated with chromosomal abnormalities. Wilms' tumor and retinoblastoma are two diseases for which actual tumor genes have been identified in some cases.[38] In addition, the offspring of childhood cancer survivors may be at risk for inheriting genetic defects that are brought about by their parents' treatment for cancer.[38]

The offspring of survivors of childhood cancer are at increased risk for having genetic disorders because they may inherit the genes that caused their parents' cancer, and they may acquire new genetic abnormalities that have been induced in the parents' germ cells by therapeutic agents. Only by surveying the incidence of cancer in the offspring of persons treated for cancer can we learn if there is a dominant transmission of disease. Reports of familial cases of childhood cancer raise questions and concerns about genetic aberrations that may be induced in part by cancer treatment.

Therapy for cancer in childhood includes some very potent carcinogens such as ionizing radiation and alkylating agents.[39] Patients who develop second tumors in response to radiation may be those who are genetically predisposed to malignancy. For example, the development of osteogenic sarcoma in a radiated orbit in a child with bilateral retinoblastoma may be attributed to both genetic and environmental factors.[38]

Li[40] reviewed a group of childhood cancer survivors consisting of 84 women and 62 men with a total of 293 pregnancies among them. The survivors were studied in terms of the possible mutagenic effects of their cancer treatments. These patients had histories of diseases that included lymphomas, bone tumors, brain tumors, rhabdomyosarcomas, neuroblastomas, and Wilms' tumors. In some instances, their treatment had included abdominal radiation and chemotherapy. The offspring of these cancer patients who were in remission at the time of conception and during pregnancy had no higher incidence of congenital deformities or other diseases than the general population. Chromosomal studies of some of the offspring did not reveal damage from preconception exposure to chemotherapy and radiotherapy.[40]

The offspring of survivors of childhood cancer constitute a high-risk group for genetic cancer and other genetic abnormalities and should be examined accordingly.[38]

Teratogenesis

Teratogenesis is the production of an abnormal fetus. The teratogenic effects of radiation are well known. When fertilization takes place and either damaged sperm or ovum are involved, spontaneous abortion often occurs.[12] Radiation to the developing embryo produces the most damage during the first trimester, the period of organogenesis and differentiation. During the first 2½ to 3 weeks after conception, the zygote is relatively resistant to harm, and damage to one cell is repaired by replacement from another pluripotential cell. However, during organogenesis and differentiation, each cell plays a major role in the development of organ structure so damage to individual cells contributes to major defects in the developing fetus. During that time the nervous system is particularly sensitive to injury. Fully developed fetal organs and structures are only somewhat sensitive to radiation damage. Toxic effects are less devastating after the eleventh week of gestation.[12]

Animal experiments and other observations clearly show that fetal radiation is teratogenic.[39] Radiation doses in excess of 500 rad commonly result in spontaneous abortion.[40] Studies on the offspring of Japanese women who were pregnant at the time the atomic bomb was dropped at the end of World War II demonstrate a high incidence of microcephaly and mental retardation. Radiation of sperm cells can lead to malformations that could be transmitted through many generations. These mutations in germ cells of mammals can be induced by relatively small doses of radiation. For example, an accumulated dose of radiation to the gonads of 60 to 80 rad may double the incidence of spontaneous mutation in offspring.[39] The genetic consequences of radiation can be greatly reduced if a time interval is allowed between radiation and conception. The exact time allowance needed for humans is not known, though possibly 6 months to 1 year should elapse before a planned concepton follows gonadal radiation.[12]

On the other hand, chemotherapy such as methotrexate administered during the first trimester of pregnancy produces malformations in approximately 80% of aborted fetuses. Alkylating agents such as cyclophosphamide have the potential for terminating early pregnancy, although they are less likely to cause fetal abnormalities.[12]

Oncogenesis

Oncogenesis is the production or causation of tumors. There is some variation in the exact figures stated in current research concerning the incidence of second malignancies in childhood cancer survivors. Many reports indicate that the cumulative probability of one of these persons developing a second malignancy within 20 years from the time of initial diagnosis is as high as 17%.[41] Possibly, this startling figure is related to (1) oncogenicity of the cancer treatment, (2) immune system disturbances induced by the disease or its treatment, or (3) genetic susceptibility of the individual patient. Hence, factors that influence the development of second malignancies include (1) the modality and intensity of the initial cancer treatment, (2) the biology of the primary malignancy, and (3) the state of the patient's immune system and genetic background.

Radiation therapy and chemotherapy have both been implicated as causative factors in the development of second cancers. These treatment modalities used in combination seem to be more oncogenic than either form of therapy used alone.[42] The role of chemotherapy in oncogenesis is less well established than that of radiotherapy. Alkylating agents, which alter DNA, represent the drug classification most often cited as being oncogenic.[42] Because alkylating agents, antimetabolites, antibiotics, and synthetic hormones are all potential mutagens (agents that produce genetic mutations or changes), they are all potential carcinogens (cancer-producing substances). Reports of lymphoma occurring in patients who received immunosuppressive therapy after kidney transplantation imply that these drugs alone can be oncogenic.[41]

The occurrence of benign and malignant second tumors within radiotherapy fields has lessened since megavoltage radiotherapy machines have replaced orthovoltage machines. These newer machines are associated with less absorption of radiation by skin and bone and less radiation scatter. Megavoltage machines also kill more primary tumor cells so fewer malignant cells remain to undergo any future replication or mutation.[43] Bone tumors and soft tissue sarcomas are the most common second malignancies that develop within radiation fields.[31] These radiation-induced second bone tumors seem to occur with somewhat increased frequency in younger patients who have received 1000 rad or more to their primary tumors.[19] The classic story of radiation-induced neoplasms is that of thyroid cancers that developed in a significant number of persons who received approximately 300 rad to an enlarged thymus in infancy.[41]

The suggestion of genetic predisposition to the development of second malignancies relates in part to the large number of children with retinoblastoma who have developed second tumors outside of their radiotherapy fields. The majority of patients who developed these second tumors had bilateral retinoblastoma, which is usually associated with germinal mutations that are inherited and transmitted by the autosomal mode of inheritance.[42]

Listed below are the results of studies that illustrate and describe the incidence of oncogenesis in childhood cancer survivors:

1. Li and colleagues[44] reported: Nineteen second malignant tumors developed in 414 long-term childhood cancer survivors. All but two of these tumors were associated with prior radiotherapy. Another 13 of these patients developed benign tumors.[44]

2. Meadows and colleagues[43] reported: A retrospective analysis of 102 children who developed second malignancies showed that many of the initial tumors were Wilms' tumor and retinoblastoma. Osteogenic sarcoma and chondrosarcoma were the most common second malignancies. Adult cancers or carcinomas, appeared at earlier than expected ages. Radiation was associated with 69 of the

second malignancies. Genetic disease was found in 27 of the 102 patients.[43]

3. The Late Effect's Study Group* registered 200 patients with second malignant neoplasms. One hundred thirty-two of these second malignancies were associated with radiation, and 68 were not associated with radiation. The majority of the 200 primary tumors included retinoblastoma (35), Wilms' tumor (32), brain tumors (24), Hodgkin's disease (22), neuroblastoma (20), and soft tissue sarcomas (20). However, that exact distribution could represent relative survival proportions. The cause of the majority of the 200 second cancers included bone sarcomas (43), soft tissue sarcomas (42), leukemia/lymphoma (33), skin carcinomas (22), brain tumors (21), and thyroid carcinomas (18). Five patients of the 200 developed more than two subsequent malignancies by the time of the study. Only half of the 200 patients survived their second malignancies. Those who developed thyroid and skin cancers usually survived. Patients with bone and soft tissue sarcomas as did less well.[2]

The implications of this high rate of oncogenesis should not totally discourage families of potential childhood cancer survivors who are faced with initial treatment decisions. In the future, modified cancer treatment programs, identification of epidemiologic agents, and proper follow-up to ensure early diagnosis of second malignancies should lessen the incidence and impact of oncogenesis for childhood cancer survivors.

Disruption of function in other organ systems

Administration of chemotherapy and radiotherapy is accompanied by assiduous monitoring for acute toxicity. There is growing awareness that many of these toxicities, which largely affect specific organ systems, may appear insidiously after

cessation of therapy and have the potential to develop into chronic, lifelong problems. Long-term toxicity and disruption of function in the heart, kidneys, liver, lungs, bladder, bone, and gastrointestinal tract can occur in persons who have undergone cancer treatment.

Heart toxicity. Anthracyclines, which include doxorubicin (Adriamycin) and daunorubicin (Daunomycin), have the potential for producing cardiac damage. Anthracycline cardiomyopathy with heart muscle degeneration can be of varying degrees of severity. Primary myocardial dysfunction can progress to congestive heart failure. The signs of this toxicity initially include tachycardia, tachypnea, shortness of breath, dyspnea, edema, hepatomegaly, cardiomegaly, gallop rhythms, palpitations, and pleural effusion. Heart damage can occur after small, single doses of Adriamycin or Daunomycin but is usually associated with high cumulative doses greater than 500 mg/m^2.[19] Prolonged low dose infusions of these drugs may be less damaging than single doses that produce high blood levels of the drugs.[19] The overall incidence of cardiomyopathy after treatment with anthracyclines is less than 10%, with a 1% to 2% incidence at cumulative doses less than 550 mg/m^2 and a 30% incidence at cumulative doses greater than 550 mg/m^2.[33] Patients who receive chest radiation and are elderly or less than 15 years of age are at increased risk for development of this toxicity.[31] Concurrent treatment with other chemotherapeutic agents such as cyclophosphamide and actinomycin D can also influence development of cardiac toxicity.[33] Cardiac toxicity can appear many months after discontinuation of anthracycline therapy.[33] Treatment measures for anthracycline-related congestive heart failure, which may be reversible, include digitalis, diuretics, salt restriction, and activity limitation. Some studies show a 60% to 80% mortality after anthracycline cardiomyopathy has developed[31] (Fig. 31-2).

Radiotherapy to the precordium, with or without adjuvant anthracycline chemotherapy, can induce heart damage with pericardial effusion, constrictive pericarditis, and congestive heart failure. The per-

---

*The Late Effect's Study Group is a 13 institution consortium that systematically recorded the sequelae encountered in 5-year survivors of childhood cancer.

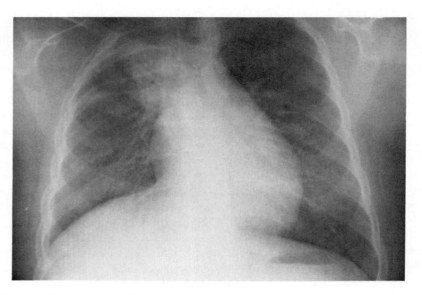

Fig. 31-2. Cardiomegaly in a 13-year-old female with Ewing's sarcoma and lung metastasis at diagnosis. Cardiomegaly occurred 1 year following discontinuation of therapy. She received 1800 rad to the lungs, and a chemotherapeutic regimen that included anthracyclines.

icarditis and pericardial effusions may not produce symptoms and may resolve spontaneously. Constrictive pericardial fibrosis can be fatal. The incidence of postradiotherapy pericarditis is associated with radiotherapy doses greater than 4000 rad.[31] Symptoms of pericarditis include chest pain, dyspnea, fever, venous distention, and friction rub. This toxicity can first appear many years after radiotherapy has been completed.[31]

The diminished cardiac reserve created by anthracycline therapy or radiation to the heart poses a lifelong potential hazard from any physiologic stress that these patients may encounter, even the normal stress of old age. The development of improved cardiac imaging techniques and more effective, less toxic anthracycline analogs should serve to decrease the incidence and severity of cardiac damage in the future.

Kidney toxicity. Chronic nephritis can develop months to years after radiotherapy to the kidneys. It is often associated with proteinuria, azotemia, anemia, and benign hypertension. It may, however, progress to a state of severe renal damage or chronic renal failure with uremia and malignant hypertension. Patients who receive more than 2300 rad to both kidneys are at increased risk for developing radiation nephritis.[33] Concomitant administration of certain chemotherapeutic agents such as actinomycin D can intensify these renal toxicities.

cis-Platinum can cause total renal failure with renal tubular sclerosis, which in turn creates lesions in the distal tubules and collecting ducts. Proper hydration and use of diuretics can minimize this renal toxicity. The administration of high doses of methotrexate must likewise be accompanied by increased fluids and urine alkalinization to limit its potential renal toxicity. Other drugs that can cause long-term kidney damage include BCNU, CCNU, 6-mercaptopurine, Daunomycin, Adriamycin, and cyclophosphamide. In addition, many cancer patients also receive a significant amount of nephrotoxic antibiotics such as aminoglycosides, which can add further insult to the kidneys.

Liver toxicity. Long-term hepatic dysfunction has been associated with radiotherapy to the liver and certain chemotherapeutic agents. The liver is especially sensitive to harm from radiotherapy after any degree of hepatic resection. Liver regeneration will be suppressed if combinations of radiotherapy and chemotherapy (actinomycin D) are given too soon after resection of the liver. Actinomycin D intensifies radiotherapy and can produce hepatic fibrosis.

Methotrexate, chlorambucil, 6-mercaptopurine, Daunomycin, and Adriamycin are other chemotherapeutic agents that are associated with long-term liver toxicity. Toxicities created by these drugs include hepatitis, hepatic fibrosis, and even cirrhosis. Methotrexate hepatic toxicity has been the subject of much research. The incidence of hepatic fibrosis from methotrexate may be as high as 84%.[41] From 2% to 19% of these cases develop into cirrhosis.[31] This liver toxicity can appear gradually, months to years after treatment. It appears that low-dose, daily, oral therapy given over a long period of time results in more hepatic fibrotic changes than do intermittent, higher dose methotrexate regimens.[31] Hepatitic toxicity from 6-mercaptopurine in children with acute lymphocytic leukemia may be as high as 10% to 40%, but is usually reversible with discontinuation of treatment.[19] Other life-style factors such as obesity, alcoholism, and diabetes also influence the severity of liver toxicity. The degree of hepatic fibrosis is best assessed by liver biopsy.

Lung toxicity. Radiotherapy to the lungs at doses higher than 2000 rad can impair their elastic quality.[41] Resultant radiologic abnormalities may be evident in more than half of all patients who receive lung radiation, but only 5% to 15% of these patients become symptomatic.[31] Pneumonitis with dyspnea, nonproductive cough, and fever can develop 2 to 6 months after chest radiation.[31] Pulmonary fibrosis with dyspnea, restrictive ventilation, and decreased exercise tolerance can develop 9 to 12 months after chest radiation.[31] Factors that can influence the occurrence of lung toxicity after radiotherapy include a history of pulmonary resection, concomitant administration of radiosensitizers such as actinomycin D, and concurrent pulmonary infections.

Patients who survive bone marrow transplantation with conditioning regimens that include total body radiation are at high risk for chronic restrictive and obstructive pulmonary disease. One large study reported 21% of patients to have some degree of mild restrictive lung disease that peaked at 1 year after transplant then improved at each subsequent annual testing. Obstructive pulmonary disorders seemed to worsen with time, with symptoms developing as late as 600 days after transplant.[45]

Bleomycin, cyclophosphamide, busulfan, chlorambucil, BCNU, and methotrexate are chemotherapeutic agents that can cause long-term pulmonary toxicity. Bleomycin can create an interstitial pneumonitis and fibrosis with pulmonary function tests that demonstrate ventilation defects, decreased carbon dioxide diffusion capacity, and arterial hypoxemia. Chest x-ray examinations of affected patients show interstitial fibrosis with patchy basilar infiltrates. Cyclophosphamide can produce pulmonary fibrosis, narrowing of the chest, stunted pulmonary growth, and loss of lung volume.

Bladder toxicity. Cyclophosphamide is a drug whose metabolites are excreted primarily through the kidney and can cause cystitis if in contact with the bladder mucosa for a long period of time. Hemorrhagic cystitis of severity ranging from chronic microscopic hematuria to exsanguinating hemorrhage can first appear weeks or years after discontinuation of treatment with cyclophosphamide. The incidence of hemorrhagic cystitis following treatment with cyclophosphamide is between 2% and 40%.[31] Long-term consequences of the hemorrhagic cystitis can include bladder fibrosis that results in decreased bladder capacity and ureteral reflux. Surgical urinary diversion procedures may be required to prevent related renal impairment and exsanguination. Furosemide (Lasix) and fluid intake greater than 3000 ml/m²/day for several hours after the administration of cyclophosphamide will generally prevent the development of subsequent hemorrhagic cystitis.[46]

Bladder or pelvic radiation, most often in doses greater than 4000 rad, can also influence the development of hemorrhagic cystitis.[31] Symptoms of chronic radiation cystitis usually appear a few months to a few years after radiotherapy. These symptoms may make their initial appearance as late as 28 years after treatment.[31]

Gastrointestinal toxicity. Radiation to any segment of the gastrointestinal tract can produce a progressive vasculitis with diffuse collagen deposition and fibrosis. The vasculitis can cause tissue hypoxia, which advances to necrosis, ulceration, and perforation. Collagen deposition and fibrosis can lead to intestinal obstruction. Long-term complications of stricture, malabsorption, and enteritis are other resultant problems. These complications can appear and persist years after completion of the course of radiotherapy.[47] As many as 36% of all children with cancer who receive gastrointestinal radiotherapy will incur some degree of injury to normal tissue within the radiotherapy field.[33] The incidence of these complications increases greatly in patients whose dose of radiotherapy is greater than 5000 rad.[33] Abdominal surgery and use of certain chemotherapeutic agents augment this toxicity. Drugs such as Adriamycin, actinomycin D, methotrexate, hydroxyurea, Daunomycin, and bleomycin have been implicated in the development of these problems.

Any gastrointestinal signs and symptoms that are reported and persist in patients with a history of abdominal radiation bear further investigation. Related signs and symptoms include colic, obstipation, vomiting, abdominal pain, diarrhea, and bleeding. Treatment for this damaged tissue is largely supportive with a low-residue, low-fat, gluten-free diet. Operating on this damaged tissue to relieve symptoms is hazardous because of the limited vascular supply to the tissue and the risk of creating enterocutaneous fistulaes.

Skeletal toxicity. A previous section of this chapter describes the impaired skeletal growth that is caused by radiotherapy. Radiotherapy to growing bones can also result in growth deformities such as spinal kyphoscoliosis, leg length discrepancy, or skull and facial disfigurement. Radiated bones are susceptible to poor healing, fracture, and functional limitation.

Radiation to the face or jaw can cause decreased saliva production with subsequent dental caries and

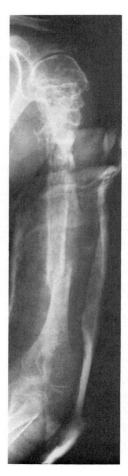

Fig. 31-3. Destruction and fracture of left humerus in a 10-year-old boy with Ewing's sarcoma after receiving 4500 rad. Note the mothy appearance of the bony architecture.

dental abscesses. Cosmetic deformities and dental abnormalities such as incomplete tooth calcification and arrested tooth development can follow maxillofacial radiation, especially if treatment is given in high doses at an early age.[48] In addition, possible chemotherapeutic effects have been recognized in the dental evaluations of cancer patients who did not receive radiation to the mouth area. Findings include poor enamel development, small bicuspid teeth, and a tendency toward thinning of roots with enlarged pulp chambers.[48]

Methotrexate and steroids are drugs that can precipitate skeletal undermineralization and abnormal calcium metabolism, causing osteoporosis and subsequent fracture of bones.

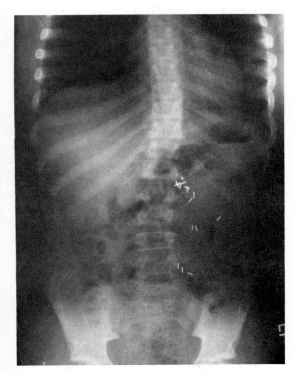

Fig. 31-4. Scoliosis of the dorsolumbar spine of a 9-year-old girl with left Wilm's tumor 7 years following surgery and radiation therapy.

Obviously, orthopedic surgical procedures such as disarticulation, amputation, limb salvage, or any bone removal result in lifelong disfigurement and prosthetic care and management problems (Figs. 31-3 and 31-4).

Other physical toxicities. Many other therapy side effects can create chronic problems that do not resolve. Examples of these are cataract formation from cranial radiation or steroids, hearing loss from *cis*-platinum or ototoxic antibiotics, and prolonged immunosuppression after splenectomy. Other surgical procedures such as enucleation or colectomy are also associated with lifelong management problems.

SIGNIFICANT LATE SEQUELAE OF COMMON PEDIATRIC MALIGNANCIES

It is perhaps somewhat redundant to now describe significant late sequelae found in survivors of the different, common pediatric malignancies in a separate section. The purpose of including this section in the chapter is to allow the reader to develop a point of reference in understanding special problems associated with various diagnoses. The organizational patterns for describing each malignancy's sequelae within this section are likewise unique. This allows the reader to approach each disease in the most logical way, taking disease sites and treatment modalities into account.

Leukemia

Children with leukemia represent the largest population of children with cancer. Children with leukemia now have a greater than 50% chance of survival. Hence, large numbers of children with leukemia are available for late effects research study. This research has focused on the following areas: (1) neuropsychologic disturbances, (2) growth, (3) gonadal function, (4) ophthalmologic aberrations, and (5) second malignant neoplasms.

Neuropsychologic disturbances. One hundred and ten patients diagnosed with leukemia were reviewed in a retrospective study conducted by the

Late Effect's Study Group. The majority of these children had been treated for acute lymphocytic leukemia (ALL). Twenty-one of these children developed significant sequelae. The most frequently occurring sequelae were those related to the nervous system. Eight patients had neurologic deficits. Learning disabilities were reported in five of these patients, encephalopathy in two patients, and a seizure disorder in one patient. All of these children had received combinations of radiotherapy and chemotherapy in an effort to prevent CNS leukemia. Eleven percent of the children who were diagnosed before 5 years of age had developed ongoing deficits in intellectual functioning, which were presumed to be secondary to therapy.[2]

Peylan-Ramu and colleagues[49] evaluated 32 patients with ALL who were treated with 2400 cranial rad and intrathecal chemotherapy. CT scans of the brain obtained 19 to 67 months from the initiation of CNS prophylaxis showed that 17 of these children had abnormalities. Among 11 patients with ALL who had not received CNS therapy, all but one were found to have normal CT scans.[49]

In a study reported by Goff and associates,[50] 43 children with ALL were evaluated for neuropsychologic status 35 to 119 months from the time of diagnosis. Twenty-seven of these children were less than 8 years of age at diagnosis. Twelve members of this group performed poorly in arithmetic skills and immediate memory recall.[50]

A study of intellectual development was described by Eiser and Lansdown.[51] In this study, 15 long-term ALL survivors were compared with matched controls on socioeconomic status, age, and sex. Six older children, ages 6 to 10 years at diagnosis, performed as well as the matched controls in all tasks. However, the younger group of children, ages 2 to 5 years at diagnosis, tended to perform below their matched controls, particularly in tasks that measured memory and motor skills.[51]

Growth. Probert and his associates[52] documented that growth impairment in children with ALL is directly related to the age of the child at the time of treatment. They demonstrated a pronounced reduction in sitting heights of children treated under 6 years of age and those treated during puberty.[52]

Nesbit and others[53] noted a marked decrease in height for children treated with cranial spinal radiation for ALL. Forty-eight percent of 187 children studied were below the 25th percentile for height at 7 years from the time of diagnosis. A statistically significant decrease in height percentiles was observed in both sexes, with females being more affected than males. There was no significant difference observed in the distribution of weight percentiles of these children, either before or after treatment.[53]

Gonadal function. From a study conducted by Nesbit and others[54] of survivors of ALL who had received combinations of chemotherapy and radiation, ovarian failure, as measured by elevated FSH and LH levels, was found to be present in 45% of 58 females studied. The FSH levels were highest in females whose therapy included spinal radiation. In contrast, only 12% of 33 males evaluated had elevated levels of FSH.[54]

Ophthalmologic aberrations. In a recent report, Kline and colleagues[55] estimated the amount of radiation received by the lens of the eye when children with ALL received cranial radiation. It was estimated that children receiving 2400 rad cranial radiation could be receiving more than 500 rad from scatter to the ocular lens.[55] In one study small posterior cataracts were identified on slit lamp examination in 3 of 50 (6%) children with ALL who had received chemotherapy that included steroids and 2400 cranial rad. The examinations were conducted 7 years from the time of diagnosis of ALL.[54]

Second malignant neoplasms. Increased survival in ALL has naturally engendered the reporting of second malignant neoplasms in ALL survivors. The cause of the second cancers is variable, but of note is one alarming report of brain tumors in ALL survivors. Albo and others[56] documented 10 biopsy-proven brain tumors among 468 long-term survivors of ALL who had received systemic chemotherapy, intrathecal methotrexate, and 2400 rad cranial radiation. The cause of this increased incidence of brain tumors is under investigation.[56]

Brain tumors

There are many factors that may contribute to remaining neurologic, physical, and mental defects in children diagnosed with and treated for brain tumors. Many physical abnormalities are present before treatment, including irreparable damage caused by the presence of the tumor itself or the increased intracranial pressure it creates. It is impossible to fully determine whether handicaps that remain after treatment with surgery, radiotherapy, or chemotherapy are caused by malignant disease, its therapy, or inadequate rehabilitation efforts. These handicaps can be severe and multiple, or they can consist of only minor neurologic problems with some degree of intellectual retardation that includes a slowness that delays scholarly achievement and subsequent professional advancement.

The list of possible initial signs and symptoms of brain tumors in children is lengthy. Notably, they include many physical findings that may never improve. These findings include endocrinopathies, seizures, cranial nerve palsies, ataxia, hemiplegia, clumsiness, unsteady gait, strabismus, nystagmus, motor and sensory disorders, blindness, diplopia, difficuclty in phonation, decreased visual acuity, and an inability to walk without aid. Once any of these signs and symptoms occurs, children with brain tumors may experience only minimum relief of symptomatology, if any, at all.

The following studies illustrate some of the profound sequelae found in children who have been treated for brain tumors.

Bamford and others[57] reported on 30 pediatric brain tumor survivors who were 14 months to 15 years of age at diagnosis and 9 to 33 years of age at the time of study.[57] The following sequelae were documented:

1. Cranial nerve palsies: squint (7), facial weakness (4), and dysphagia and palatal weakness (1).
2. Motor abnormalities: ataxia with inability to walk unaided (2), mild ataxia (2), and hemiplegia (4).
3. Visual defects: correctable acuity defects (11), severe visual handicaps (3), and blindness (3).

4. Hearing defects: partial deafness (1) and total deafness (1).
5. Emotional problems found in 13 children: alcoholism (1), suicide attempts (2), depression (4), insecurity (5), emotional lability (6), solitary behavior (7), and aggressive behavior (11).
6. Intelligence: superior (3), average (10), below average (4), educationally subnormal (11), and severely subnormal (2).

The Late Effect's Study Group reported on residual deficits found in 16 of 30 childhood brain tumor survivors.[2] These defects included intellectual dysfunction (8), growth disorders (3), motor dysfunction (3), panhypopituitarism (2), personality disorders (2), seizure disorders (1), visual impairment (1), hearing loss (1), kyphoscoliosis (1), and permanent alopecia (2).

Spunberg and colleagues[58] reported on 14 brain tumor survivors who were less than 2 years of age at diagnosis and 6 to 21 years of age at the time of study. They had received 2400 to 5000 rad of cranial radiation.[58] Sequelae included the following:

1. Neurologic deficits: require seizure medication (5), seizures uncontrolled by medication (2), hearing loss (3), visual acuity loss (3), other cranial nerve deficits (4), hemiplegia or quadriplegia (4), and cerebellar dysfunction (4 gross, 6 fine)
2. Hair regrowth: partial (11) and total (3)
3. Education: attend regular schools (3), dropped out of regular schools (3), attend regular schools with special classes (2), and attend special schools for the handicapped (6)
4. IQ testing scores: 3 above average (90 and above), 3 borderline (70 to 80), 2 mildly retarded (55 to 70), and 5 moderately retarded (40 to 54).

Comments on IQ testing patterns included these: For each patient, verbal score exceeded performance score, reflecting coordination difficulty. Reading skills were generally low. Planning and organization skills were poor. Many survivors exhibited passive, dependent, immature responses. The overall patterns seemed consistent with psychologic stress secondary to illness at an early age, compounded by physical and intellectual handicaps in later years.

Pearson[59] reported the following on a study of sequelae in children with differing brain tumor pathology.

1. CNS late effects in 20 of 31 children with medulloblastoma consisted of blindness (3), partial vision (2), other nerve defects (4), mental retardation (7), and slow performance at school (5).
2. CNS late effects in 4 of 15 children with cerebellar astrocytoma consisted of blindness (1), paresis of right hand (1), and mental retardation (2).
3. CNS late effects in 8 of 12 children with midbrain tumors consisted of cranial nerve defects (3) and intellectual impairment (5).
4. CNS late effects in 12 children with cerebral tumors consisted of residual nerve defects (4), blindness (1), hemiplegia (3), epilepsy (4), hypopituitarism (1), and psychiatric problems (1).

Hodgkin's disease

The late consequences of the treatment for Hodgkin's disease are related to the extent of disease at the time of diagnosis and the treatment protocol. For example, the child with stage I disease, who receives radiation to a single node, will not be exposed to the same hazards as the child with stage IV disease, who is treated with combinations of chemotherapy and radiation.

Children with Hodgkin's disease often undergo laparotomy with splenectomy as part of their initial diagnostic evaluation. Infection and pneumococcal sepsis can follow splenectomy. These children have been reported to have a high incidence of herpes zoster varicella, tuberculosis, and bacterial infections such as Haemophilus influenzae.[12] Karayalcin[12] reports that approximately 8% of these children become septic with a 4% mortality. Daily oral penicillin plays a significant role in preventing disease and is given prophylactically to all splenectomized patients. In addition, the treatment for Hodgkin's disease may impair the ability to respond to immunization for as long as 4 years after the cessation of treatment.[12]

The late effects of treatment for Hodgkin's disease can most easily be categorized by treatment modality. These treatment modalities fall into three categories: (1) radiotherapy, (2) chemotherapy, and (3) treatment that combines chemotherapy and radiotherapy.

Radiotherapy. Because the radiotherapy field for treatment of Hodgkin's disease is often large, many body organs are exposed to radiation. Toxicity to thyroid and lungs is especially significant in these patients. For example, when massive mediastinal adenopathy is treated, little lung tissue can be shielded from the radiation. Sutow[3] reports that incidental radiation of the thyroid in patients with Hodgkin's disease is associated with overt hypothyroidism. The incidence of thyroid dysfunction increases over time. The occurrence of this problem is higher with women and is treated with replacement therapy.[3] Karayalcin[12] describes the incidence of thyroid suppression to be 13% of children with Hodgkin's disease who were treated with radiation.

Chemotherapy. MOPP chemotherapy (nitrogen mustard, vincristine, prednisone, and procarbazine) has long been the standard drug program used to treat Hodgkin's disease. Azoospermia and oncogenesis are recognized side effects of the alkylating agents included in combinations such as MOPP.[3] ABVD (Adriamycin, bleomycin, vinblastine, and DTIC) is a second drug combination that is employed in the treatment of Hodgkin's disease. Increased rates of pulmonary problems have been associated with the administration of bleomycin. Cardiac problems caused by Adriamycin may be increased when mediastinal radiation is included as part of the treatment plan.

Combination radiotherapy and chemotherapy. The use of radiation and chemotherapy in combination for treatment of Hodgkin's disease has resulted in a marked increase in second malignant neoplasms. In a series described by Sutow,[3] there were 177 cases of documented acute myelocytic leukemia (AML) attributable to the treatment of Hodgkin's disease. The incidence of AML in persons with history of Hodgkin's disease is 17: 100,000, which represents a tenfold increase over the general population.[3] AML seen in this group of patients differs from other forms of AML in that it (1) occurs at a younger age, (2) presents with pancytopenia and a megaloblastic bone marrow, (3) does not respond well to treatment, and (4) has a short survival rate.[3]

Rhabdomyosarcoma

In the past decade, the therapeutic management of rhabdomyosarcoma has been greatly modified to avoid many of the mutilating and debilitating procedures or treatments that were needed to cure patients. Chemotherapy and limited radiation therapy now often eliminate the necessity for extensive, disfiguring surgeries.

In a study by Meadows, Krejmas, and Belasco,[2] more than 50% of children with soft tissue sarcoma, diagnosed in 1972, showed substantial residual deficits secondary to therapy for their disease. These sequelae reflect the anatomic sites of disease, the type of surgery required, and the amount of treatment given. For example, a pelvic exenteration may result in problems such as persistent urologic dysfunction, gastrointestinal problems, reproductive dysfunction, sexual problems, and in many instances, psychologic problems. Facial deformities brought on by combinations of treatment may require plastic surgical correction. In this instance, psychologic costs to the child cannot be calculated. Musculoskeletal deficits may occur in both bony structures and soft tissue. Because most of these children have not yet reached their full growth at the time of treatment, the full impact of these disabilities may not become apparent for many years.[2]

If primary treatment has been given to the head and neck area, the child will be subject to long-term dental problems, thyroid problems, hearing loss, cataracts, and possibly learning disabilities. Scarring and fibrosis secondary to surgery and radiation may occur in the orbit, nasopharynx, oropharynx, paranasal sinus, nasal cavity, parotid, cheek, middle ear, larynx, neck, and meningeal lesions.[60] Conductive hearing and visual loss secondary to treatment can be permanent.[2]

A rhabdomyosarcoma that arises in the bladder, prostate, vagina, and uterus may have required exenterative procedures followed by radiation and chemotherapy. The outcome of treatment for these problems may include ureterostomy, colostomy, abdominal adhesions, and abdominal fistulae. Sexual counseling for these children is mandatory, as well as close follow-up for known problems following pelvic or abdominal radiation at high doses coupled with actinomycin D and cyclophosphamide.

As with other childhood malignancies, rhabdomyosarcoma is likewise associated with subsequent oncogenesis. In one report of 200 second neoplasms, 20 of the primary diagnoses were rhabdomyosarcomas, often associated with prior radiotherapy.[2]

Wilms' tumor

Ninety percent of children with Wilms' tumor of favorable histology are now cured of their disease. The National Wilms' Tumor Studies have aimed, in part, to minimize the intensity of treatment of children with Wilms' tumor, thereby eliminating some of the significant late sequelae that had been identified among Wilms' tumor survivors. Fine adjustments in therapy continue to be made to minimize therapy for those children with a good prognosis.

Meadows, Krajmas, and Belasco[2] documented 15 children with significant late effects among 54 survivors of Wilms' tumor diagnosed in 1972. All of the children described as having significant late effects had been treated with surgery, radiation, and combinations of chemotherapy. The most common effects described in this study were splenectomy and gastrointestinal disturbances. Splenectomy had been required for those children whose tumors involved the spleen. Gastrointestinal disturbances were associated with children who had postsurgical adhesions that required treatment. Some children developed small bowel obstruction from adhesions, fibrosis, or intussusception. Other problems described for this group of children also included hepatic damage, renal impairment, cardiac complications, ovarian failure, pulmonary complications, orthopedic sequelae, and second malignant neoplasms.[2]

Severe hepatic damage can occur following radiation to the liver. The degree of damage is related to the volume of liver radiated and the dose delivered. A child with a right-sided Wilms' tumor is more prone to hepatic complications because the right lobe of the liver is included in the radiation field.

Long-term renal impairment with abnormal creatinine clearance has been reported in children with Wilms' tumor.[2] Chronic nephritis is a slowly progressive disorder that may develop in some children, particularly after combinations of actinomycin D and radiation. Abdominal radiation for Wilms' tumor administered to the prepubertal girl may result in ovarian failure, presenting as failure to develop secondary sex characteristics.

Orthopedic deformities in survivors of Wilms' tumor, described by Lanzkowsky, include changes in the vertebral bodies, scoliosis, kyphosis, hypoplasia of the ilium and the rib cage, osteocartilaginous exostoses, and epiphyseal destruction with limb length discrepancy and deformity.[12] In recent years, the radiation dosage employed for Wilms' tumor treatment has been decreased, thereby significantly diminishing the aforementioned effects.[12]

There have been numerous reports of second malignant neoplasms following treatment for Wilms' tumor. Reported second malignancies include soft tissue sarcoma, bone tumors, hepatomas, thyroid carcinoma, and leukemia.[60]

Bone tumors

For children diagnosed with bone tumors, there are obvious sequelae seen in the musculoskeletal system. Amputations, disfiguring surgeries, and growth abnormalities following radiation account for the large number of musculoskeletal sequelae. Issues surrounding long-term orthopedic management after limb-salvage surgeries or amputation and care associated with use of prostheses are discussed in the chapter in this text that is devoted to bone tumors. Obvious physical handicaps such as these are likewise fraught with potential psycho-social sequelae of "always being different from others" and "always getting around a little less well than others." Facial, cosmetic, and neurosensory late effects are seen in this group, and again, are associated with the sites of surgery and radiation therapy.

Other late sequelae in children with a history of bone tumors relate to the specifics of the therapy that has been given. Children with osteogenic sarcoma who have received high-dose methotrexate or *cis*-platinum may demonstrate some degree of renal dysfunction.

Children with Ewing's sarcoma who have received radiotherapy to growing bones can be left with functional limitations, limb length discrepancy, and susceptibility to pathologic fracture. Corrective surgeries, lengthy hospitalizations, and physical therapy are aspects of the expected long-term rehabilitation program for these patients.

Retinoblastoma

For the child with retinoblastoma, late sequelae can include psychologic problems associated with enucleation, sensory deficits, and second malignant neoplasms. While osteogenic sarcoma has been described as developing in the radiated port at the orbit of some patients with retinoblastoma, it also has been reported as the second malignancy in patients with bony disease at sites other than the orbit.[2]

Because retinoblastoma is described as a genetic defect for those individuals with bilateral disease, their progeny have about a 50% chance of developing the disorder.[32] Therefore genetic counseling should become part of the teaching plan at the late effects visit. Long-term care and problems with orbital prostheses are described in Chapter 10 on retinoblastoma.

NURSING RESPONSIBILITIES IN THE MANAGEMENT AND ASSESSMENT OF LATE EFFECTS

The primary goal of late effects follow-up examinations for children and young adults who have been successfully treated for malignancies is to improve their quality of life. Nurses involved in the long-term care of children with cancer must have a broad knowledge and awareness of possible late sequelae to cancer treatment. They must look at the total patient, not just his or her previous primary diagnosis. Of course, oncology nurses cannot possibly be the experts who manage these many newly disclosed patient problems. However, as members of the primary health care team that oversees the patient's overall management, these nurses must develop an awareness of the boundless scope of late sequelae and an organizational plan for thinking about these late effects.

Nursing responsibilities in the management of patients who are long-term survivors of childhood cancer include: (1) developing an awareness of late effects; (2) providing assurance of proper, complete follow-up for all patients successfully treated for malignancies; (3) screening patients for the common known late effects; (4) providing patient education with respect to late effects; and (5) making proper referral to other subspecialists when new problems are identified.

Time must be set aside at each follow-up clinic visit (which likely occurs at only annual intervals) to evaluate the patient's condition and screen the patient for all potential problems. Interval histories must be more thorough than simply asking the patient, "How have you been this year?" A complete review of systems is imperative. Physical assessment must inspect every body part.

For every patient seen in clinic for a late effect's evaluation, the nurse must take into consideration the patient's (1) past diagnosis and sites of disease, (2) type and scope of cancer treatment, (3) age during treatment, and (4) current age and life-style.

For these patients and their families it is, in all likelihood, very alarming to realize that after they have stopped worrying about the diagnosis of cancer and the possibility of death, there may be other, new, long-term problems to complicate their lives. How can these patients be motivated to comply with long-term follow-up requirements now that they feel good and have no actual symptoms of the original cancer?

Education is one way to help patients cope with the possibility of late sequelae. Currently, there is a great or total paucity of patient education materials that define and describe late effects of cancer treatment. It is a nursing responsibility to educate patients and their families about the occurrence and proper follow-up for late sequelae.

The following brief outline can be used as a guide for developing a nursing assessment plan for patients seen in the oncology clinic who have a past history of childhood cancer:

Common finding: damage to the CNS—psychologic
Understand that all patients and their families are at risk for suffering some level of long-term psychologic impairment. All patients and families need long-term support from their pediatric oncology nurses.
Common finding: damage to the CNS—intellectual
Maintain ongoing, formal contact with school personnel from the time of the original diagnosis of cancer.
Document significant school problems as they occur.
Support and foster special education classes for children who are found to be deficient in certain areas.
Recognize patients who are at greatest risk for developing learning problems.
For example, children who received high doses of cranial radiation at an early age are especially vulnerable to this problem.
Common finding: impaired growth and development
Recognize patients at greatest risk for aberrations. For example, children who received craniospinal radiation before reaching their adult height should be closely observed.
Measure and chart patient heights and weights carefully. Accurate growth charts must be kept up on all pediatric patients.
Recognize and follow-up on a significant decrease in velocity on the growth chart of any child.
Common finding: gonadal aberrations
Document the Tanner development stage at each clinic visit.
Develop an understanding of the significant gonadal hormones: FSH, LH, estradiol, and testosterone.
Recognize patients at greatest risk for developing gonadal dysfunction. For example, children who received radiotherapy to pituitary or gonadal sites and patients who have received high cumulative doses of alkylating agents such as cyclophosphamide are at high risk of gonadal dysfunction.

Before treatment begins, initiate sperm banking for teenage boys who wish to participate in such programs.

Encourage frank discussions of future potential for childbirth with all patients who are at an appropriate age for such concerns.

Common finding: disruption of function in heart, kidney, liver, lungs, and other organs

Realize that all chemotherapy side effects that are recognized acutely can become chronic problems. Examples include the following:

Patients who have received Adriamycin or Daunomycin may experience chronic cardiac dysfunction.

Patients who have received *cis*-platinum or high-dose methotrexate may experience chronic renal dysfunction.

Patients who have received methotrexate may experience chronic hepatic dysfunction.

Patients who have received bleomycin may experience chronic pulmonary dysfunction.

Realize that radiotherapy, especially in high doses, can permanently damage the quality of tissue that is included within the radiation port and hence can limit the functional capabilities of that tissue.

Common finding: oncogenesis

Facilitate and maintain communication and contact with all patients after they complete cancer treatment. This allows them to report significant signs and symptoms to their primary pediatric oncology team. Factors related to the initial primary diagnosis and treatment must be available and used in future disease management.

SUMMARY

The first successful cancer treatments seemed to indicate that more treatment produced better results. Unfortunately, those intensive treatments produced serious late consequences. This phenomenon represents a dilemma that continues to plague the medical profession. In the last several years, because of increased numbers of treatment cures, rigorous treatment regimens have been modified for some patients. Today, for some forms of cancer in childhood, we can look forward to a future of curing children with treatments that produce minimum late sequelae.

Health professionals continue to marvel at the adaptability of the human spirit as it attempts to cope with overwhelming odds. Children with cancer and their families do cope. Families do produce young adults who, inspite of the cancer experience, have adapted and are leading fulfilling lives. Problems associated with late effects of treatment do exist for survivors of childhood cancer. Schuler and associates[61] write convincingly about the psychologic burden for children with leukemia and their families. However, an unfortunate event in a child's early life, such as the development of cancer, does not necessarily dictate a blighted adulthood.[62] Given the proper support systems, plus the resiliency of childhood, we need not predict gloomy outcomes for these children. There are opportunities for growth in every lifetime experience. With proper support, children with cancer may be directed toward those opportunities.

Great strides have increased this survivor population. However, the child who has survived cancer and its treatment presents a lifelong challenge to the health profession.[36] As children cured of cancer become adults, health professionals who provide their care must be alert to the unique problems of these, not so rare, young adults coming under their charge, who have survived the rigours of childhood cancer.[31]

REFERENCES

1. Silverberg, E., and Lubera, J.: A review of American Cancer Society estimates of cancer cases and deaths, CA, **33**(1):2, 1983.
2. Meadows, A., Krejmas, N., and Belasco, J.: The medical cost of cure: sequelae in survivors of childhood cancer. In van Eys, J., and Sullivan, M., editors: Status of the curability of childhood cancer, New York, 1980, Raven Press.
3. Sutow, W.: Cost of survival: In Sutow, W., editor: Malignant solid tumors in children, New York, 1981, Raven Press.
4. Sperling, E.: Psychological issues in chronic illness and handicap. In Gellert, E., editor: Psychosocial aspects of pediatric care, New York, 1978, Grune & Stratton.
5. Koocher, G., and O'Mally, J.: The Damocles syndrome: psychosocial consequences of surviving childhood cancer, New York, 1981, McGraw-Hill, Inc.
6. Fergusson, J.: Psychological late effects of a serious illness in childhood, Nurs. Clin. North Am. **11**:1, 1976.

7. Koocher, G.: Psychosocial care of the child cured of cancer, Pediatr. Nurs. **11**:2, 1985.

8. Meadows, A., and others: Childhood cancer survivors: education, employment and reproduction (abstract), Proc. Am. Soc. Clin. Oncol. May 1983, C-294.

9. Lansky, S., and Cairns, N.: Poor school attendance in children with malignancies (abstract), Proc. Am. Soc. of Clin. Oncol. May 1979, C-409.

10. Anderson, J.: Insurability of cancer patients: a rehabilitation barrier, Oncol. Nurs. Forum **11**:2, 1984.

11. Bleyer, W.A.: Neurologic sequelae of methotrexate and ionizing radiation: a new classification, Cancer Treat. Rep. **65**:89, 1981.

12. Karayalcin, G.: Late effects of cancer treatment. In Lanzkowsky, P., editor: Pediatric oncology: a treatise for the clinician, New York, 1983, McGraw-Hill, Inc.

13. Fergusson, J.: Cognitive late effects of treatment for acute lymphocytic leukemia in children, Top. Clin. Nurs. **2**:4, 1981.

14. Jacob, S., Francone, C., and Lossow, W.: Structure and function in man, ed. 5, Philadelphia, 1982, W.B. Saunders Co.

15. Meadows, A., and Evans, A.: Effects of chemotherapy on the central nervous system, Cancer **37**(2):1079, 1976.

16. Li, F., and Stone, R.: Survivors of cancer in childhood, Ann. Intern. Med. **84**(5):551, 1976.

17. Holmes, H., and Holmes, F.: After ten years, what are the handicaps and life styles of children treated for cancer? Clin. Pediatr. **14**(9):819, 1975.

18. Eiser, C.: Intellectual abilities among survivors of childhood leukemia, as a function of CNS irradiation, Arch. Dis. Child. **53**:5, 1978.

19. Jaffe, N.: Late sequelae of cancer therapy. In Sutow, W., Fernbach, D., and Vietti, T., editor: Clinical pediatric oncology, ed. 3, St. Louis, 1984, The C.V. Mosby Co.

20. Poplack, D., and others: Sequelae of central nervous system prophylaxis in patients with acute lymphoblastic leukemia (abstract), Int. Soc. Pediatr. Oncol. September 1978, p. 92.

21. Meadows, A., and others: Decline in I.Q. scores and cognitive dysfunctions in children with acute lymphocytic leukemia treated with cranial irradiation, Lancet **2**:1015, 1981.

22. Kun, L., Mulhern, R., and Crisco, J.: Quality of life in children treated for brain tumors: intellectual, emotional, and academic function, J. Neurosurg. **58**:1, 1983.

23. Duffner, P., Cohen, M., and Thomas, P.: Late effects of treatment on the intelligence of children with posterior fossa tumors, Cancer **51**:233, 1983.

24. Danoff, B., and others: Assessment of the long-term effects of primary radiation therapy for brain tumors in children, Cancer **49**:1580, 1982.

25. Gotlin, R., and Silver, H.: Endocrine disorders. In Kempe, C., Silver, H., and O'Brien, D., editors: Current pediatric diagnosis and treatment, ed. 3, Los Altos, Calif., 1974, Lange Medical Publications.

26. Shalet, S., and others: Growth hormone deficiency in children with brain tumors, Cancer **37**(2):1144, 1976.

27. Wells, R., and others: The impact of cranial irradiation on the growth of children with acute lymphocytic leukemia, Am. J. Dis. Child. **137**:37, 1983.

28. Stempfel, R., and others: Pituitary growth hormone suppression with low dose long-acting corticoid administration, J. Pediatr. **73**(5):767, 1968.

29. Blodgett, F., and others: Effects of prolonged cortisone therapy on the statural growth, skeletal maturation and metabolic status of children, N. Engl. J. Med. **254**:(14):636, 1956.

30. Zutshi, D., Friedman, M., and Ansell, B.: Corticotrophin therapy in juvenile chronic polyarthritis (Still's disease) and effect on growth, Arch. Dis. Child. **46**:584, 1971.

31. Byrd, R.: Late effects of treatment of cancer in children, Pediatr. Ann. **12**(6):450, 1983.

32. Oliff, A., and Levine, A.: Late effects of antineoplastic therapy. In Levine, A., editor: Cancer in the young, New York, 1982, Masson Publishing USA, Inc.

33. Lentz, R., and others: Postpubertal evaluation of gonadal function following cyclophosphamide therapy before and during puberty, J. Pediatr. **91**(3):385, 1977.

34. Schilsky, R., and others: Gonadal dysfunction in patients receiving chemotherapy for cancer, Ann. Intern. Med. **93**:109, 1980.

35. D'Angio, G.: Complications of treatment encountered in lymphoma-leukemia long-term survivors, Cancer **42**:1015, 1978.

36. Kaempfer, S., Hoffman, D., and Wiley, F.: Sperm banking: a reproductive option in cancer therapy, Cancer Nurs. **6**:1, 1983.

37. D'Angio, G.: The child cured of cancer: a problem for the internist, Semin. Oncol. **9**:143, 1982.

38. Knudson, A.: Genetics and the child cured of cancer. In van Eys, J., and Sullivan, M., editors: Status of the curability of childhood cancer, New York, 1979, Raven Press.

39. Schull, W., and Kato, H.: Malignancies and exposure of the young to ionizing radiation, The Cancer Bulletin **34**:85, 1982.

40. Li, F., and Jaffe, N.: Progeny of childhood cancer survivors, Lancet **11**:707, 1974.

41. D'Angio, G.: Late sequelae after cure of childhood cancer, Hosp. Pract. **15**:11, 1980.

42. Ruccione, K., and Fergusson, J.: Late effects of childhood cancer and its treatment, Oncol. Nurs. Forum **11**(5):54, 1984.

43. Meadows, A., and others: Patterns of second malignant neoplasms in children, Cancer **40**:1903, 1977.

44. Li, R., Cassady, R., and Jaffe, N.: Risk of second tumors in survivors of childhood cancer, Cancer **35**:1230, 1975.

45. Sullivan, K., and others: Late complications after marrow transplantation, Semin. Hematol. **21**(1):53, 1984.

46. Vietti, T., and Bergamini, R.: General aspects of chemotherapy. In Sutow, W., Fernbach, D., and Vietti, T., editors: Clinical pediatric oncology, ed. 3, St. Louis, 1984, The C.V. Mosby Co.

47. DeCosse, J.: Radiation injury to the intestine. In Sabaston, D., editor: Textbook of surgery: the biological basis of modern surgical practice, ed. 12, Philadelphia, 1981, W.B. Saunders Co.

48. Jaffe, N., and others: Dental and maxillofacial abnormalities in long-term survivors of childhood cancer: effects of treatment with chemotherapy and radiation to the head and neck, Pediatrics **73**(6):816, 1984.

49. Peylan-Ramu, N., and others: Abnormal CT scans of the brain in asymptomatic children with acute lymphocytic leukemia after prophylactic treatment of CNS with radiation and intrathecal chemotherapy, N. Engl. J. Med. **298**:815, 1978.

50. Goff, J.R., and others: Distractability and memory deficits in long-term survivors of acute lymphoblastic leukemia (abstract), Int. Soc. Pediatr. Oncol., September 1978, p. 151.

51. Eiser, C., and Lansdown, R.: Retrospective study of intellectual development in children treated for acute lymphoblastic leukaemia, Arch. Dis. Child. **52**:525, 1977.

52. Probert, J.C., and others: Growth retardation in children after mega voltage irradiation of the spine, Cancer **32**:634, 1973.

53. Nesbit, M., and others: The effect of successful treatment for acute lymphoblastic leukemia (ALL) on subsequent height of children (abstract), Int. Soc. Pediatr. Oncol., September 1983, p. 76.

54. Nesbit, M., and others: Evaluation of long-term survivors of childhood acute lymphoblastic leukemia (abstract), Proc. Am. Assoc. Cancer Res. May 1982, #419.

55. Kline, R.W., and others: Cranial irradiation in acute leukemia: dose estimate in the lens, Int. J. Radiat. Oncol. Biol. Phys. **5**:117, 1979.

56. Albo, V., and others: Ten brain tumors as a late effect in children cured of acute lymphoblastic leukemia from a single protocol study (abstract), Am. Soc. Clin. Oncol. March 1985, #C-672.

57. Bamford, P., and others: Residual disabilities in children treated for intracranial space-occupying lesions, Cancer **37**:1149, 1976.

58. Spunberg, J., and others: Quality of long-term survival following irradiation for intracranial tumors in children under the age of two, Int. J. Radiat. Oncol. Biol. Phys. **7**:727, 1981.

59. Pearson, D.: Tumours of the central nervous system. In Deeley, T., editor: Malignant diseases in children, South Wales, 1974, Butterworths Co.

60. Maurer, H., and others: Rhabdomyosarcoma. In Sutow, W., Fernbach, D., and Vietti, T., editors: Clinical pediatric oncology, ed. 3, St. Louis, 1984, The C.V. Mosby Co.

61. Schuler, D., and others: Psychological late effects of leukemia in children and their prevention, Med. Pediatr. Oncol. **9**:2, 1981.

62. Kagan, J.: The nature of the child, New York, 1984, Basic Books.

CHAPTER 32

When the dying patient is a child: a challenge for the living

MARTHA BLECHAR GIBBONS

DEATH: A DISTANT PHENOMENON

The present century has witnessed many changes. The age at death has risen dramatically, to a great extent the result of medical and technologic advances. Now there is less likelihood of death in infancy, childhood, and young adulthood, enabling an individual to reach middle age untouched by personal or familial experience with loss.

Family decentralization has decreased the exposure to grandparents in the home. The extended family is no longer a part of every child's growth and development. Many families are separated by long distances, and children are not present as grandparents age and die. Thus the part of the life cycle that culminates in aging and death is vague to the child. The loss of a grandparent may be experienced as a strange and distant phenomenon.

Many children reared in urban settings are not exposed to the life cycle through involvement with pets or wildlife. In school, if a child dies, it is often explained that he "moved away." Exposure through television is misleading, for the "dead" cartoon character all too often comes back to life.

This generally lessened exposure to death has had a dual impact on society. The loss of a loved one in childhood and adolescence is a less frequent tragedy. However, death is no longer perceived as an inevitable fact of life.

Children today are often shielded from discussions of death by parents who have not come to terms with their own feelings about mortality.

Many parents have not been provided with this opportunity, for human death is an experience that is generally denied by the American society.[1]

The consequence of such denial is that people are inexperienced in dealing with the crisis of death and incapable of sustaining grieving friends and family. For the same reasons, health care providers may be no better prepared to cope with death than the distressed families they endeavor to support. It is not unusual for nursing and medical students to encounter death for the first time in the surroundings of the anatomy laboratory!

Parents who are unable to discuss death with each other cannot relate this important concept to their children. In turn, their grandchildren are reared in an environment that attempts to protect them from such "unpleasant" thoughts. The following case illustrates how this cycle continues.

CASE STUDY

A 32-year-old woman was dying of cancer on a unit in the institution where she had been treated for 1 year. Her family requested a conference to discuss concerns they shared, soliciting guidance from staff on what to tell the woman's 3-year-old daughter. In attendance were the maternal grandparents (divorced), paternal grandparents, the dying woman's husband, her best friend, her brother, and his wife.

The initial discussion revealed that all members of the family were experiencing difficulty in sharing their feelings concerning the impending death. The common theme that was verbalized dealt instead with anxiety related to informing the child when her mother died.

493

Each person feared that he or she might have to assume this responsibility. There was concern that the child would suffer from the experience and that "psychologic damage with long-lasting effects" would result.

When asked the reason that the family thought this might occur, there were individual and differing responses. The dying woman's mother recalled how her daughter had reacted as a child when her parents divorced and she could no longer live with her father. "I'm sure she *never* got over it," the mother maintained, intimating that her granddaughter, in turn, would never overcome her own mother's death.

This case illustrates how children can be denied opportunities to experience death as a reality of life. Well-intentioned family members, burdened by their own inability to deal with separation and loss, may project such feelings under the guise of protecting the child.

Given the observations of the pain involved with the acceptance of death, it is not difficult to imagine the complexities encountered when the dying patient is a child.

ASSUMING RESPONSIBILITY FOR THE TERMINALLY ILL CHILD

As a primary care provider, the nurse assuming responsibility for the care of the terminally ill child and his family must be aware of the significance of the last life experiences that they will share together.

The communication process

Communication, so essential from birth throughout life, can decrease in extent and effectiveness as the child and family face death. One of the most important aspects of the responsibility assumed by the person providing care is the facilitation of dynamic communication between the child, family, and inter-relating staff. Such communication ranges from responding to explicit questions posed by the child to lengthy sessions with the entire family and the various consultants involved in the plan of care. Consideration of the following four concepts in communication can significantly enhance the care that is provided during the terminal stages of illness.

An acceptance of personal feelings regarding death. The exploration of personal feelings about death is fundamental to working effectively with the dying patient and his family. It is one of the most important and possibly least tangible qualities required by the care giver.[2] First, one must come to terms with the fact that in grieving for the patient who is dying, the caregiver is also grieving for his own death.[3]

For the child, the natural tendency may be to react spontaneously and to communicate openly and honestly. Those who do not relate reciprocally in this manner may be viewed with caution or even suspicion by the child, who is well aware of deception. The nurse who has not dealt with personal feelings about mortality will have difficulty coping with emotions elicited by the child's approaching death. Such emotions are difficult if not impossible to conceal and may interfere with effective communication. The extent to which the nurse honestly reflects on personal fears, feelings, and thoughts related to death directly influences the ability to assist others in the process. This insight is "tantamount to offering authenticity for pretense in relating to the dying person."[4]

Availability and consistent involvement. Sincerity is another essential quality required by the nurse providing care. It is often assumed that distance should be maintained between the patient and care giver to preserve a professional relationship. In truth, this enables a person who is less willing to become involved to provide care on a continuing basis. Yet, when the dying patient is a child, personal involvement is not only appropriate but necessary.[5] Relating to the child and family in a personal way conveys a willingness to hear what they need to say, when they need to say it.

Availability. Communication is further enhanced by the availability of the key persons providing care. Some children and families will actively solicit the nurse's involvement, identifying needs, and directly requesting guidance and advice. Others will not feel uncomfortable in requesting assistance but will respond when encouraged to share concerns in confidence. Although family communication patterns differ and may alter during the dying process, it is important to remember that it is likely that the family will actually *need* support during this critical time.

The question or topic initially presented by the family in discussions often is not the primary concern. Therefore it may be necessary to devote considerable time in active listening to decipher the significance of the information shared. From the initial contact throughout the duration of the relationship, it is important to identify who will be responsible for the care provided, as well as how, when, and where primary care givers may be contacted. Explanation of alternative resources, as appropriate, should be offered.

Consistency. Once the relationship has been established and there is trust invested in the nurse by the child and family, it is important that the communication patterns be consistent. It is not helpful to facilitate in-depth exploration of feelings and concerns for one session, or to provide vital information needed during one meeting, and fail to initiate follow-up. Although such sessions may not be required frequently, individual needs differ, and it is important to convey readiness when such intervention is warranted. If the nurse initially involved will not be available for a certain period of time, this must be clearly explained and an alternate resource identified. If a significant relationship has developed with the primary care giver and the family expresses a preference to work with this individual, it may be difficult for another staff member to gain the family's confidence. Families during this time are vulnerable and sensitive to differences in performing procedures and care-related tasks. The family may not desire to expend the time and energy required to gain confidence in others; all energies are devoted to supporting the child in terminal illness. However, reassurance that someone is always available conveys a message of concern and justifies the family's feelings that their needs should be prioritized.

Promotion of open communication. The environment that promotes open communication among patients must value such interaction among staff. It is not enough that the nurse assist in facilitating expression among patients and families. Open communication must take place first among the professionals who provide care for those experiencing the crisis of death in the family. Time should be scheduled for staff acknowledgment of (1) the emotional investment required to care for both the terminally ill child and his family and (2) the stresses experienced in providing such care. The sharing of feelings and experiences aroused by caring for chronically ill and dying patients is considered by some health professionals to be necessary to cope effectively with the emotional pressures of working in such a setting.[6]

Whether such sharing takes place between two professionals or within a group setting, the opportunity is provided to gain insight into the management of stressful situations. By clearly defining the feelings resulting from work experience, with the assistance of colleagues, the nurse is better able to identify the cause of the stress and to test alternate methods of coping with it.

Too often, lack of efforts to understand or manage work-related conflict contributes to professional burn-out. Burn-out is "characterized by an emotional exhaustion in which the person no longer has any positive feelings, sympathy, or respect for patients or clients."[7] Burn-out afflicts people within different health and social service professions and plays a primary role in the poor delivery of health care to people in need of such services. Such a phenomenon can be especially damaging when it occurs in a setting where care is provided to the terminally ill child.

Support for the family as a unit. With the crisis of illness and impending death, the roles previously assumed by family members may change. If the child who is dying maintained an active, vital role, someone else in the family may attempt to substitute in the child's absence; however, sometimes no substitute is available. In either case, each family member is affected by the illness. It is important for the nurse to determine how the illness is interpreted by each individual and the family unit as a whole.

For example, a 14-year-old boy with a divorced mother assumed responsibility beyond the societal norm for his age; in the absence of his father, he acquired his father's role. He performed tasks previously completed by his father, and became vital to his mother in assisting in decision making related to family concerns. When the boy was diagnosed with cancer, his mother experienced not only the crisis of his illness, but the loss of a significant personal support. Since there were no other children, no one could substitute in the boy's absence.

It is impossible to treat the child apart from the family. In all aspects of care, the family should be considered a unit, a system in which each member has a certain function. As decisions regarding care are made for the child, the effect of such determinations on the family as a unit must be evaluated.

Methods of communication

As in many situations, when working with a child who is terminally ill, *what* is said to the child and his family may not be as significant as the *manner* in which it is expressed by the care giver.

In many situations it is not necessary for the nurse to lead communication in structured discussions. At times, communication may be more effective if the care giver is alert to messages conveyed by the child and his family. The nurse may employ a nondirectional approach, allowing the child and his family to actively participate in self-expression to the degree that they are physically and emotionally capable. The following methods of communication encourage such interchange.

Life review. The concept of life review was first introduced by a psychiatrist who felt that the mental process of reviewing life experiences when death was imminent was an attempt to resolve lifetime conflicts in preparation for death itself.[8]

The literature examines the use of life review with adults as patients, allowing for reminiscence and the completion of unfinished business in life.[9,10] Expansion of this concept in interventions when the dying patient is a child allows the parents of the dying child to reflect on their life together as a family and the child himself to examine past experiences and present feelings. The tools for life review are most often pictures, which make excellent props for stirring memories.[10]

The parents or the child may indicate the desire to engage in life review. Cues may be statements about what the child "used to look like," "used to be able to do," or "used to enjoy." Frequently the person making such statements will refer to pictures in the room or uncover photographs concealed in a wallet. Consideration of the following points will maximize the potential value of life review as a therapeutic intervention for the child and the family:

1. The use of life review as a supportive intervention does not require that the nurse demonstrate expertise in mental health. Consistent active listening and a concerned focus on the individual(s) will help to promote self-expression, which in essence is the value of life review.

2. Establish objectives to assist in the process of life review.[10] In general, the goal should be to assist the family or patient in acknowledging the significance of the child's life and the time they have shared together. The person assisting should be alert and sensitive to the family's verbal and nonverbal cues and take direction from the information they share. Specific age-appropriate objectives will be discussed.

3. Determine who should be present during the life review session. If the parents initiate the process, assess whether they intend for the child to be involved, and whether he is receptive and ready for such involvement. If the child initiates the session, determine whether he desires other family members to participate. Some children who desire privacy with the nurse will wait for the opportunity to share in confidence.

4. Allow for uninterrupted time in a private area where there are no distractions (a conference room, a section of a playroom). If the dis-

cussion is initiated in a crowded area, suggest moving to a more secluded spot, but do not discontinue the discussion if readiness is apparent.

Life review for the child. The value of life review for the child is inherent in the process of reliving past experiences. The younger child, who views death as separation from loved ones and whose major fears are related to this concept, can be assured that those whom he depends on will not abandon him. This fact can be confirmed by photographs placed near the bed that illustrate family gatherings, pets, and significant objects—concrete examples of how important the child is to the family. Discussions can be focused on particularly memorable events, requiring the child's involvement in describing each photograph to the nurse.

The school-age child, whose developmental tasks include achieving a sense of industry, can be assisted in acknowledging all that has been accomplished in a short life span. Pictures that capture skills the child has mastered, such as swimming or dancing, baseball and soccer, can be introduced as statements of his achievements. The child who is mourning the loss of such meaningful activities because of debilitating disease may be able to take advantage of this opportunity to express feelings that have been repressed. Anger, resentment, sadness, and death-related fears may be conveyed to the care giver who skillfully uses the photographs of past experiences to elicit present concerns.

Terminal illness complicates the developmental stages of adolescence and young adulthood. The individual who is striving to establish identity encounters major difficulties when disease and change in body image interfere with the ability to establish stable traits in self-perception. Life review is a method for exploration of the meaning of an individual's life. By emphasizing the positive aspects of life experiences, the patient can be helped to strengthen and maintain his self-esteem, reduce feelings of loss and isolation, and reaffirm his sense of identity.[9]

Life review for the family. Parents and siblings of a terminally ill child frequently experience the need to share special memories with the nurse who is caring for the child. It is important to understand the significance of such sharing and to respond by assisting them to convey the information when the need arises. In verbalizing memories, the family is initiating important tasks: (1) evaluation of the quality of the life they have shared with the child and the significance of their roles, and (2) anticipatory grief, working toward an acceptance of the child's eventual death and beginning to "let go."

Kubler-Ross[1] advocates that during terminal illness, when there is an opportunity, the family should be encouraged to express their feelings about the person's imminent death, to the extent that this is possible, before the actual occurrence. This serves to mitigate the pain that is experienced after the loved one has died.[1] The following case is an example of life review.

CASE STUDY

The grandfather of a 19-year-old boy diagnosed with rhabdomyosarcoma frequently stood outside the door of the boy's room on the oncology unit. Following the death of the boy's mother from cancer the previous year and subsequent desertion of his father, the boy's grandparents became his surrogate parents.

Several times the man tried to engage staff in a discussion of his family, and occasionally he would show a picture of his grandson "before he lost his hair." Staff politely listened for a brief period, but all were preoccupied with various tasks.

A nurse observed that the man displayed a sense of urgency one morning when he asked her to see his favorite picture of his grandson. The boy had relapsed, and staff were focused on pain management. At first the nurse considered the desire to share a picture representing previous health and vigor strange in contrast to the reality of the boy's poor nutritional status and physical discomfort. However, she consented, and the grandfather produced a wallet filled with pictures of his daughter, who was the boy's mother, and portraits of the family together. The nurse remarked on how much caring and joy was evident in the pictures. The grandfather, spreading the pictures on a stretcher parked in the hall, agreed that the family had experienced wonderful moments together.

He described special memories as he fingered each picture separately.

"You never expect your children to die before you do," he said. The nurse responded by involving him in a discussion of how he and his wife were coping with the boy's terminal illness.

Following the boy's death a week later, the nurse received a letter from the grandfather, describing how much her interest and concern had meant to him on that particular day.

This case illustrates how readiness to engage in life review can go unnoticed by staff, and how valuable the intervention can be once initiated.

Bibliotherapy. Bibliotherapy, in which the reader works out feelings "in concert" with characters in a story, has been recommended by some authorities as an effective way of approaching the subject of death with children and families.[11,12]

Books about illness, death, and other forms of loss can be included in the libraries located in the school, home, and the hospital. There are various theories regarding the introduction of specific books to the child, yet many believe he should be allowed to make his own selection. The adult in attendance may serve as a guide, facilitating self-selection by providing means to attract youngsters to certain books.[12]

Certain books can help children cope with illness, separation, and death. Before using literature with children and their families to introduce these topics, the nurse should read the book and evaluate it for content in relation to the topic, the child's developmental level, and individual needs. After the child has read the book or the book has been shared with him, the nurse can determine the child's understanding of the material by having him relate his impressions. This stimulates questions and allows for correction of misconceptions.[13]

Although the literature offers little documentation that bibliotherapy is effective with the fatally ill child, it appears to be valuable for the following reasons:

1. The child who is seriously ill may gain strength through identification with characters in the book. When the hero in some way conquers or avoids defeat, through identification with the aggressor, the child can achieve mastery of a particularly stressful situation. Through identification with characters and figures who express fears and frustrations, the child may feel less isolated in realizing that others share his feelings. For the child who is able to cope through intellectual mastery of his disease and the treatment plan, reading provides the opportunity to become more informed and to address specific questions. This process aids in decreasing the anxiety he experiences in anticipating the unknown.

2. Books allow the child to discharge repressed emotions. "Through involvement, readers vicariously experience the difficulties and feelings of the characters, leading to catharsis."[12] Books can act as agents that evoke discussions of previously unexpressed feelings in a way that may not be possible with alternate interventions. Such discussions can be particularly valuable with guidance from a sensitive adult who is aware of the significance of the child's feelings.

3. Literature provides the child with suggestions for alternate ways of coping and potential solutions to problems. The child may test out the methods chosen by the characters, or, challenged by the material presented, devise his own way to resolve a particular conflict.

4. Books serve as a useful tool in educating parents about the developmental needs of their children, which become even more significant when the child is fatally ill. Literature provides a foundation for parents to formulate their own explanations about what is happening to the child, to be shared in a manner that meets their individual needs. Parents too may identify with characters in books, in seeking ways to cope with the stresses they are experiencing.

5. Books provide support in that they allow for private exploration of feelings or unite the reader (or person listening to the story) with

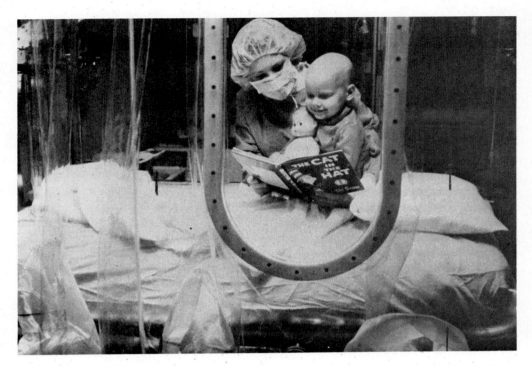

Fig. 32-1. Bibliotherapy. The adult may serve as a guide to the child facilitating effective coping through use of selected literature for the child.

a significant other. The child who prefers not to share his feelings with others may find reading alone a therapeutic experience—in effect, engaging in bibliotherapy himself. For others, the presence of a significant person occupied in storytelling lends a needed sense of security and alleviates anxiety resulting from time endured alone (Fig. 32-1). Such benefits are illustrated in the following case.

CASE STUDY

When his chronic disease became terminal, the 7-year-old boy appeared to have little desire to watch television or to play games. A nurse providing care for several days in succession observed that several books from home lay on a table in the corner of the room. Having failed to interest him with alternate suggestions, she asked if he would like her to read him a book. He nodded without expression but indicated that he preferred the story of a boy and his dog who were separated but later happily reunited.

Although the nurse read the story repeatedly each day, the boy participated in each session with renewed interest. While she read, the nurse observed that his posture became less rigid and his breathing patterns were less labored. Occasionally, he would fall asleep but seemed relieved if when he awoke the nurse was still beside his bed.

However subtle the messages may be, bibliotherapy offers an alternate method for communication. The nurse who is familiar with this tool may find it useful in assessing the child's unique method of coping with his terminal illness.

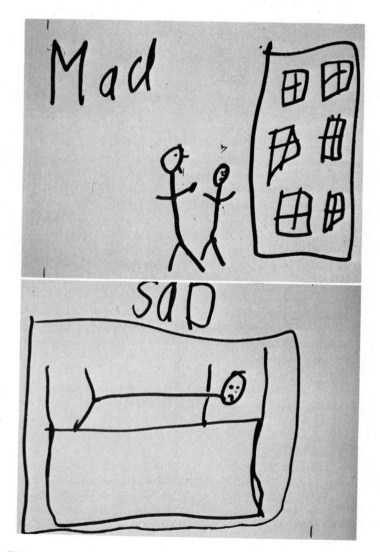

Fig. 32-2. Children may draw pictures to express feelings that they have difficulty verbalizing to others.

Art. Children's drawings have long held a certain fascination for adults. Children illustrate in their drawings how they perceive themselves and the world around them. Professionals have used children's drawings as tools for assessing the developmental maturity of growing children and as vehicles for understanding children's attitudes, feelings, and internal conflicts. Children have difficulty verbalizing these concepts, and art offers a medium for such expression.

In research conducted by Spinetta and colleagues,[14] the Kinetic Family drawings have been used to allow children with cancer and members of their families to document specific attitudinal responses to the cancer experience.

Whether the facility treating the child employs an art therapist or another professional with similar skills, the nurse should encourage expression through the medium of art. It is often helpful to consult a professional knowledgeable in the interpretation of drawings when using art as an intervention with the child. Such consultation can enable the nurse to gain insight into the child's rendition of his disease and treatment. However, lack of such guidance should not prohibit staff from providing opportunities for the child and his family to engage in this form of expression. The process itself, without interpretation, can be a therapeutic intervention.

In all creative play, it is important to encourage children to express their own fantasies rather than to copy the work of others. It is more beneficial for children to draw freely than to follow the lines dictated by a coloring book (Figs. 32-2 and 32-3).

Support groups. Recently a trend in health care has led to the development of groups as a means of meeting patient needs. It has been demonstrated that patients are likely to benefit from such programs and that the group as a supportive intervention has applicability to a variety of settings.[15-17] Support groups for patients and families have been established in institutional settings, community agencies, schools, and neighborhoods—wherever the need arises and the resources are available. Groups have been established on a national scale to offer support to terminally ill patients, their families, and families in bereavement. Many treatment facilities have organized support groups for children with chronic and potentially fatal diseases. In group settings, children are given the opportunity to share concerns with peers who are struggling with many of the same issues.

The nurse caring for the terminally ill child and his family should be aware of the potential value inherent in group participation. Effective support groups facilitate communication and afford a medium for self-expression. Groups acquaint patients and families with vital resources, enhance the development of effective coping strategies, and decrease feelings of hopelessness and isolation by assisting participants to realize that others share similar experiences and are able to function.

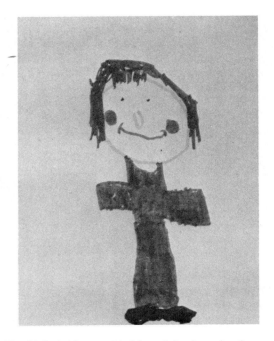

Fig. 32-3. A 10-year-old girl receiving intensive therapy for Ewing's sarcoma drew herself without hands. Her message could be that she was feeling helpless and defenseless, unable to reach out into the environment and interact. Note her "feeble" smile.

Before encouraging patient and family participation, the nurse should evaluate the group to determine its potential value. If possible, the nurse should attend at least one group session. Important aspects to be considered are as follows:

1. What is the purpose of the group, and is it meeting the needs of the participants?
2. Is the group led consistently by one or more qualified facilitators who are familiar with the participants' concerns?
3. Does the group meet at a time that is convenient for its members, and is the meeting place accessible?
4. How long has the group been in operation, and what is the average membership?
5. Who are the participants, and how do they feel about the group?
6. Is the group known locally or nationally, and how is it received in the community?
7. Will the group meet the needs of the patient and family in question?

The nurse should recognize that not every individual will feel comfortable communicating in group settings. Careful patient assessment and group evaluation will help to determine those who will benefit from such participation.

What not to say. In an effort to comfort and console the family in which a child is dying, the nurse at times gropes unsuccessfully for the "right" words to express feelings of concern. It is not unusual for the cliché, "I know how you feel," to be shared unwittingly at the bedside. In return, it is likely that such a statement may be met with a cold, "No, you don't!" with anger and even hostility accompanying this retaliation. In truth, no one other than another parent who has experienced the loss of a child can appreciate the depth of grief and sorrow that is the consequence. It is a result of this fact that a special form of communication often develops among families whose fatally ill children share the same treatment facility.

When words are not necessary

Words are not always necessary to communicate with the dying child and his family. In certain situations nonverbal communication can be an effec-tive method of intervention, as described in the following discussion.

Presence. There is a time when the child and family will not need or desire to discuss the illness and the feelings it elicits. At certain moments the presence of a significant person may be restorative in itself. There are periods when the family will not want to be alone but will be selective of who is included. The actual moment of death may be such a time. A perceptive nurse who is alert to nonverbal clues and direct statements made by the family will be able to determine when such a presence is needed. At such times the presence of a significant person is a therapeutic intervention in itself.

Touch. Touch is a primitive sensation, one of the first to be experienced during birth and continuing throughout life to be an essential component of human development. Touching actions are an effective means of communication. In relating to another person, the setting, cultural background, type of relationship, sex of communicators, ages and expectations of those involved will influence the message conveyed by touch.[18] Touch can be used to express feelings and attitudes by those in helping professions. Caring, concern, and acceptance can be conveyed in the nonverbal mode through the use of touch. For such reasons and more, touch can augment the care provided in terminal illness.

As a therapeutic intervention, massage has been used consistently in the treatment provided for terminally ill patients. Massage, which refers to certain manipulations of the soft tissues of the body, incorporates five basic techniques: stroking (effleurage), kneading (petrissage), percussion (tapotement), vibration, and friction. These actions, performed most effectively with the hands, have potentially beneficial effects on the nervous and muscular systems and the local and general circulation of the blood and lymph.[19]

Research has shown that healing energy can be passed from one person to another, employing the phenomenon of energy transference termed the "laying on of hands."[20]

The therapeutic effects of touch occur so commonly and spontaneously that the potential benefits may be underestimated. For some children, communication through touch can express more than words can convey.

Silence. Care providers who have been patients themselves have related that, when afflicted with a fatal disease, silence can at times be a calming influence. "Silence can say more than all the reassurances."[21] Silence allows for thought and consideration of something previously said. Silence conveys the message that the patient is free to engage in discussion at will—but by his own choice.

The following case illustrates the use of the three methods of nonverbal communication previously discussed. These methods may be initiated by either the patient or the nurse; both can potentially benefit from the experience.

CASE STUDY

In the last hours of her life, the teenage girl was drifting in and out of consciousness. When alert, she would attempt to focus on those around her, but severe mucositis prohibited verbal expression. Her parents requested that the primary nurse be present in the room with them.

Previous experience in caring for the girl led the nurse to suggest a massage, for it tended to alleviate the tension that the girl experienced. The nurse began to massage the girl's neck and back with lotion. The girl sighed, tried to whisper a message, but winced in pain as she tried to form the words with cracked, dry lips. The girl stopped the backrub briefly to reach for the nurse's hand, which she held silently against her face.

Problems encountered in communication

The child's awareness of death. One of the dilemmas most frequently encountered by parents and staff is how to communicate with the child who is dying. Should the child be told his prognosis? Does he sense that he is seriously ill and dying, even when this is not explained?

There are two dichotomous theories concerning the issue of communication with the fatally ill child. The arguments opposing a direct discussion of death with the child are frequently based on theories related to the child's conception of death and the anxiety such a discussion could produce.

Studies indicate that a child's conception of death matures developmentally. Children under 5 years of age appear to view death as reversible—a departure or separation. From approximately 6 to 10 years of age, death is conceptualized as an inevitable, external process often resulting from the actions of others or purposeful forces (God being viewed as such a force). Death is interpreted by these children as punishment for evil thoughts or deeds. Children above the age of 10 begin to conceptualize death as an internal process and universal to all forms of life.[22-24]

There is little debate that the older child with a fatal prognosis, especially an adolescent, can be aware of the seriousness of his illness. Yet some authorities theorize that the fatally ill child under 10 lacks the intellectual capacity to formulate a concept of death and is therefore not aware of his prognosis. It is postulated that if the adult does not discuss the illness and prognosis with the child, the child will experience little or no anxiety related to this subject.[25-28]

Those who contest this approach favor open communication with the dying child and his family. They argue that the normal development of the ability to conceptualize death is accelerated when the child is faced with death at an early age. They state that the awareness of impending death becomes stronger as the child approaches death.[29,30] It has been observed that the fatally ill child reacts to his illness in a different way than the chronically ill child, exhibiting much greater anxiety.[31]

In her study, Waechter[32] found that parents of fatally ill children assumed that their children were unaware of the seriousness of their illness because they had not been informed of their prognosis. When the children were interviewed, however, they responded to projective tests, relating stories concerning loneliness, separation, and death; feelings they had not discussed with the parents. In addition, these children identified the names of specific illnesses. From this study, it is suggested that "knowledge is communicated to the child by the change in affect which he encounters in his total environment after the diagnosis is made and by his perceptiveness of other nonverbal cues."[32]

Whether or not the child is aware of the prognosis, his self-esteem is greatly affected by a chronic illness that becomes terminal. His sense of autonomy is restricted by intrusive procedures and rigorous treatment schedules. His physical integrity is threatened by rapid alterations in body image. Separated from family and friends, he experiences loneliness and isolation. He may attempt to cope by forming relationships with other patients, only to find that other hospitalized children may be transient figures in his life. When death occurs in his environment, on the unit or ward, the staff may attempt to conceal it. As his own illness progresses, staff may unintentionally tend to avoid him at a time when meaningful communication is needed more than ever before. The following case illustrates the consequences of ineffective communication with the terminally ill child.

CASE STUDY

A 14-year-old girl with osteosarcoma failed to respond to the last treatment option available and developed multiple lung metastases. Having previously coped by intellectual mastery of her situation, she became apathetic, lethargic, and disinterested in her appearance. She stated that her body, because of the absence of an amputated right leg, was "ugly."

Her parents were focused on efforts to cope with the symptoms of her father's mental illness, and little energy was spared to attend to her needs. She became increasingly argumentative, and staff tended to spend less time in her room. When she asked direct questions about her prognosis, medical and nursing staff responded in vague generalities.

One evening the social worker and clinical nurse specialist responded to a call from distressed staff who stated that the girl had become "hysterical." She was crying uncontrollably and screaming at all those around her. She lashed out at both visitors as they entered her room.

"Where is everyone when I need them? No one spends time with me anymore; you just come in and change my IV's and leave. Even the play therapists avoid me! None of you will tell me what's going on. I know I'm dying; *I know it, and I'm scared!* You've all abandoned me, and I hate you!"

In this particular case, staff responded to the girl's accusations, acknowledging that they *had* been avoiding her. A plan of care that included multiple disciplines resulted, which supported her in the terminal stages of her illness. Unfortunately, the staff was unaware of their behavior before confronted by her angry outburst.

The theory of communication which has been referred to as the "open approach"[33] provides an environment that is supportive of the child's questions and concerns from the time of diagnosis. During the child's first admission to the treatment facility, open communication may be initiated with the introduction to the hospital and preparation for the procedure and routine to follow. If questions are dealt with from the very beginning, the message will be conveyed that it is acceptable to discuss the illness and all the concerns that are associated with it.

It is important to acknowledge that the illness is serious, and that children can die when afflicted with a serious disease. Denying this truth is a drastic contradiction to the fact that another child may have died on the same ward and does not lend credibility to further statements made by the care giver. Acknowledgment that the illness is serious does not mean eliminating hope. Families often speak of how important it is to maintain hope.[34] For many, hope becomes the lifestream, providing strength to cope with what may follow. Hope assumes many forms as the disease progresses. In the beginning, there is hope that the diagnosis will not be a fatal disease. Once diagnosed, that is replaced by hope that there will be a response to treatment—that treatment will provide a cure. Later, after relapse, there is hope for more time together. And finally, there is hope that death will be peaceful and painless. Hope can be encouraged by sincere statements reflecting the staff's concern for the child and family. Explanations of the rationale for care can be shared in a way that provides evidence to the family that the child's individual needs are of paramount concern.

Reactions of siblings. It is important to include the siblings in the communication process that takes place with the family. All too often the siblings are left at home with friends or relatives, while the child is dying in the hospital.

Several factors have been found to influence the reactions of siblings to the fatal illness of a child. Among these are sibling age and maturity, ability to integrate the meaning of the illness, and the sibling's relationship to the patient.[35] Feelings of anger, guilt, jealousy, competitiveness, despair, isolation, and vulnerability have been observed in children whose brother or sister is dying.[33,36,37] One study found that poor adjustment in siblings of terminally ill children was associated with little communication from the mother about the nature of the disease.[38]

THE TRANSITION FROM CHRONIC TO TERMINAL CARE

Patients with life-threatening illnesses require therapy throughout the course of the disease. At one stage, the goal of therapy is to control and/or cure and to alleviate symptoms associated with the specific disease. When cure and remission are beyond the capacity of the available treatment, intervention focuses on what is termed palliative care. Based on the assumption that the symptoms of terminal disease can be controlled, the goals at this point are to achieve a state in which the patient is as symptom free as possible, alert and comfortable, and free of pain.[39]

In terminal illness, the family, not the patient alone, is considered the unit of care. Kubler-Ross[1] emphasizes that medical and nursing staff cannot truly help the terminally ill patient unless they include his family. The family is defined as those significantly involved: relatives, as well as friends. As discussed earlier, the patient and his family may have had no previous experience with death. Thus it is essential that the dying process be discussed in terms of how it will affect each person involved. The support provided for the patient and family requires the collaboration of many disciplines working as a team, for the problems encountered are many and varied: interpersonal, legal, psychosocial, spiritual, and economic.

Many aspects of terminal care contrast with the care provided earlier. Initially, treatments and procedures, which were focused on control and cure of the disease, were of paramount concern and were therefore given priority. During that period, the patient and the family were expected to adjust to the schedule as determined by the staff. In contrast, the philosophy in terminal care is that the time remaining is precious for the patient and his family. Throughout this period, procedures and treatments deemed necessary for pain relief and comfort are carefully arranged so as not to disrupt the family unit. The care provided during terminal illness should reflect the needs of the patient and family, and communication between those providing care and those receiving it should be open and consistent. The desires of the family unit should be considered in all aspects of planning and in management of the disease. The care provided should be available on a 24-hour basis.[39]

Care for the family unit does not terminate with death. The family in bereavement is at risk emotionally and physically.[40,41] The team that provided care for the deceased is responsible for supporting the survivors.[39] Support for the family is critical when the dying patient is a child. It has been determined that loss of a child produces higher grief intensities in the survivors than either the loss of a spouse or parent.[42]

THE CHOICE: DEATH IN A HOSPITAL, HOSPICE, OR HOME

Recently, a variety of specialty services have been developed dealing mainly with cancer patients. These are called hospices, continuing care units, palliative care units, home care teams, and support teams. The common objectives shared by these services are achieving improved control of symptoms of terminal illness and providing improved emotional, social, and spiritual support for patients and their families. Since 1975 the development of such specialty services for terminal care has expanded rapidly.[43]

Hospice care

The hospice was pioneered throughout England and Europe for centuries as a place of rest for travelers. Today hospice programs have been developed throughout Europe, America, and Canada where the dying patient may receive highly specialized palliative care. These hospices are patterned after St. Christopher's Hospice in Sydenham, England. The common goal is to keep the patient pain free, comfortable, and fully alert during the terminal phases of his illness.

Hospice strives to recognize the individuality in planning for care and death—whether the patient remains at home or enters the facility. The focus is "improving or at least maintaining the quality of life rather than prolonging survival through heroic measures. Care is provided in the setting of a homelike, protective community comprised of family members, staff, volunteers, and members of the broader community."[44] Personnel recognize the patient and family unit as being the center of this service. During bereavement, family members continue to receive this support.

In England, the first hospice for children, Helen House, was opened in November, 1982; it is thought to be the first of its kind in the world. Parents are welcome to stay with their children, and patients requiring terminal care are given priority. The hospice also provides temporary nursing care to children with severe long-term illnesses who are normally cared for at home. This respite is offered by agreement, either at regular intervals for periods not exceeding 4 weeks, or at irregular intervals, to allow families to take a vacation or recover from periods of crisis.[45]

Although 100,000 children die each year in the United States, less than 2% of the 1300 hospices presently in existence accept seriously ill children.[46] The growing concern regarding pediatric hospice has resulted in the establishment of organizations to promote the inclusion of children in existing and developing hospices and home care programs and in the implementation of hospice support through pediatric facilities.[46] Pediatric hospice supports the philosophy that the parents assume the role of primary care giver and have a voice in decisions made regarding the child's care. The

family is supported by an interdisciplinary team throughout the child's illness and during the first year of bereavement.

Home care

The concept of home care for the terminally ill child was the focus of the initiation of the Home Care Project by Ida Martinson in 1972. These efforts were a result of concern regarding the limited availability of home care for the dying and the paucity of resources for the terminally ill child. In this program a home care nurse was available 24 hours a day to arrange visits as dictated by family need, and a personal physician could be contacted at any time.[5]

Similar programs have since been developed.[40,41,47,48] The common observations supporting home care emphasize that family participation in the physical and emotional care of the dying child may reduce feelings of anxiety, helplessness, stress, and guilt. The family may be comforted and aided in resolution of grief following the child's death by the knowledge that they have done everything possible to help their child.[5,40]

Many families choose to allow their child to die at home in response to the child's specific request. Those who prefer hospitalization most often express concern that they will not be able to provide the care required at home and that the experience will be emotionally distressing.[5,40]

Some families attempt to provide care at home and later return to the hospital, citing reasons of inability to cope with the stresses encountered, and lack of confidence in the agency supporting home care. Too often the family may not be introduced to such agencies until late in the stages of the child's terminal disease. Thus the family continues to depend on the staff from the acute care setting to respond to all medical and psychosocial needs. When the transition from hospital to home occurs, the staff who are to provide support while the child is at home are unfamiliar with the family unit. In turn, the family has not been given the opportunity to develop the trust and confidence in the staff, which is so essential to the success of the home care program. Much of this anxiety can be alleviated if community resources are identified for the family at the time of diagnosis. As the disease progresses and the potential need for support at home becomes a reality, staff from the institution providing initial treatment will have established a liaison with the appropriate community agencies. Together, key personnel may work with the family to facilitate the transition from hospital to home.

Hospital care

If the family prefers that the child should die in the hospital or they return after pursuing other resources, it is imperative to support their final decision. The last moments together will become lifelong memories for the survivors. The significance of the roles played by the health care team should never be underestimated. The family may seek guidance from primary care providers in making final decisions regarding their child's death and the bereavement period following.

Much can be done to create a "homelike" atmosphere in a hospital setting. Familiar objects from home which reflect the child's personality may add warmth to the commonly sterile-appearing environment of the treatment facility. Colorful pictures can transform blank walls, and favorite records or tapes can provide sensory stimulation and help to reduce tension. Staff who know the child best and can respond to even the most subtle nonverbal cues should coordinate and participate in the care during the final moments of the child's life.

SUMMARY

The denial of death as an inevitable fact of life has rendered our society unprepared to cope effectively with terminal illness. When the dying patient is a child, the situation is demanding and complex. A knowledge of important concepts and principles regarding terminal care will assist the nurse in meeting the challenge of providing support for the family unit in the last moments of the child's life.

REFERENCES

1. Kubler-Ross, E.: On death and dying, New York, 1969, Macmillan Publishing Co.
2. Jones, R.B.: Life-threatening illness in families. In Garfield, C.A., editor: Stress and survival: the emotional realities of life-threatening illness, St. Louis, 1979, The C.V. Mosby Co.
3. Charles-Edwards, A.: The nursing care of the dying patient, Bucks, England, 1983, Beaconsfield Publishers, Ltd.
4. Krikorian, D.C., and Moffatt, M.W.: Death-related fears, Issues Ment. Health Nurs. 4:1, 1982.
5. Martinson, I.: Home care for the dying child, professional and family perspectives, New York, 1976, Appleton-Century-Crofts.
6. Beardslee, W.R., and DeMaso, D.R.: Staff groups in a pediatric hospital: content and coping, Am. J. Orthopsychiatry, 52(4):712, 1982.
7. Maslack, C.: The burn-out syndrome and patient care. In Garfield, C.A., editor: Stress and survival: the emotional realities of life-threatening illness, St. Louis, 1979, The C.V. Mosby Co.
8. Butler, R.N.: The life review: an interpretation of reminiscence in the aged, Psychiatry, 26:65, 1963.
9. de Ramon, P.B.: Life review for the dying patient, Nursing 83 13(2):46, 1983.
10. Wysocki, M.R.: Life review for the elderly patient, Nursing 83 13(2):46, 1983.
11. Berger, M.F.: Books about death for children, young adults and parents. In Sahler, O.J., editor: The child and death, St. Louis, 1978, The C.V. Mosby Co.
12. Bernstein, J.E.: Books to help children cope with separation and loss, New York, 1977, R.R. Bowker Co.
13. McBride, M.: Children's literature on death and dying, Pediatr. Nurs. 5(3):31, 1979.
14. Spinetta, J.J., and others: The kinetic family drawings in childhood cancer. In Spinetta, J.J., and Deasy-Spinetta, P., editors: Living with childhood cancer, St. Louis, 1981, The C.V. Mosby Co.
15. Loomis, M.E.: Group process for nurses, St. Louis, 1979, The C.V. Mosby Co.
16. Ross, J.: Group intervention as an aid to parents, Psychiatry 33:56, 1979.
17. Gibbons, M.B., and Boren, H.: Stress reduction: a spectrum of strategies in pediatric oncology nursing, Nurs. Clin. North Am., March 1985.
18. Edwards, B.J., and Brelhart, J.K.: Communication in nursing practice, St. Louis, 1981, The C.V. Mosby Co.
19. Pratt, J.W., and Mason, A.: The caring touch, London, 1981, Heyden & Son, Ltd.
20. Krieger, D.: Therapeutic touch: the imprimatur of nursing, Am. J. Nurs. 75:784, 1975.

21. Shlain, L.: Cancer is not a four letter word. In Garfield, C.A., editor: Stress and survival: the emotional realities of life-threatening illness, St. Louis, 1979, The C.V. Mosby Co.

22. Nagy, M.H.: The child's theories concerning death, J. Genet. Psychol. **73:**3, 1948.

23. Safier, G.A.: A study in relationships between the life and death concepts in children, J. Genet. Psychol. **105:**283, 1964.

24. Gartley, W., and Bernasconi, M.: The concept of death in children, J. Genet. Psychol. **110:**71, 1967.

25. Debuskey, M.: Orchestration of care. In Debuskey, M., editor: The chronically ill child, Springfield, Ill., 1970, Charles C Thomas, Publisher.

26. Evans, A.E., and Edin, S.: If a child must die, N. Engl. J. Med. **278:**138, 1968.

27. Ingalls, A.J., and Salermo, M.C.: Maternal and child health, St. Louis, 1971, The C.V. Mosby Co.

28. Yudkin, S.: Children and death, Lancet **1:**37, 1967.

29. Bluebond-Langner, M.: Meanings of death to children. In Feifel, H., editor: New meaning of death, New York, 1977, McGraw-Hill, Inc.

30. Spinetta, J.J., and Deasy-Spinetta, P.: Talking with children who have a life-threatening illness. In Spinetta, J.J., and Deasy-Spinetta, P., editors: Living with childhood cancer, St. Louis, 1981, The C.V. Mosby Co.

31. Spinetta, J.J.: The dying child's awareness of death, Psychol. Bull. **81:**256, 1974.

32. Waechter, E.H.: Children's awareness of fatal illness, Am. J. Nurs. **71:**1168, 1971.

33. Share, L.: Family communication in the crisis of a child's fatal illness: a literature review and analysis, Omega **3:**187, 1972.

34. Frantz, T.: When your child has a life-threatening illness, Association for the Care of Children's Health Publication, 1983.

35. Weiner, I.: Disturbance in adolescence, New York, 1970, John Wiley & Sons, Inc.

36. Giacquinta, B.: Helping families face the crisis of cancer, Am. J. Nurs. **77:**1585, 1977.

37. Kagen-Goodheart, L: Reentry: living with childhood cancer, Am. J. Orthopsychiatry, **47**(4):651, 1977.

38. Townes, B., and Wold, D.: Childhood leukemia. In Pattison, E., editor: The experience of dying, Englewood Cliffs, N.J., 1977, Prentice-Hall, Inc.

39. The International Work Group on Death, Dying, and Bereavement: Assumptions and principles underlying standards for terminal care, Am. J. Nurs. **7**(2):296, 1979.

40. Lauer, M.E., and others: A comparison study of parental adaptation following a child's death at home or in the hospital, Pediatrics **71**(1):107, 1983.

41. Mulhern, R.K., Lauer, M.E., and Hoffman, R.G.; Death of a child at home or in the hospital: subsequent psychological adjustment of the family, Pediatrics **71**(5):743, 1983.

42. Saunders, C.C.: A comparison of adult bereavement on the death of a spouse, child, and parent, Omega **10:**303, 1979.

43. Hunt, B., and Hillier, R.: Terminal care: present services and future priorities, Br. Med. J. **283:**595, 1981.

44. McIver, V.: A time to be born, a time to die, Can. Nurse **76**(8):38, 1980.

45. Site visit by author: Helen House, Oxford, England, June 22, 1984.

46. Fact sheet, 1984, Alexandria, Va., Children's Hospice International.

47. Martinson, I.: Dying children at home, Nurs. Times **76**(29):129, 1976.

48. Lauer, M.E., and Camitta, B.M.: Home care for the dying child: a nursing model, J. Pediatrics **67:**1032, 1980.

ADDITIONAL READINGS

Adams, F.E.: 6 very good reasons why we react differently to various dying patients, Nursing 84 **14:**41, 1984.

Arnold, J./H., and Gemma, P.B.: A child dies: a portrait of family grief, London, 1983, Aspen Systems Corp.

Doyle, D., editor: Terminal care, Glasgow, 1979, Churchill Livingstone, Inc.

Doyle, N.: The dying person and the family, New York, 1972, Public Affairs Pamphlets.

Grollman, E.A.: Explaining death to children, Boston, 1968, Beacon Press.

Kastenbaum, R.J.: Death, society, and human experience, ed. 2, St. Louis, 1981, The C.V. Mosby Co.

Pringle, D., and Taylor, D.: Palliative care in the home: does it work? Can. Nurse **80**(6):26, 1984.

Saunders, C., and Baines, M.: Living with dying: the management of terminal disease, Oxford, 1983, Oxford University Press.

Sternberg, F., and Sternberg, B.: If I die and when I do, exploring death with young people, Englewood Cliffs, N.J., 1980, Prentice-Hall, Inc.

Stoddard, S.: The hospice movement: a better way of caring for the dying, London, 1979, Jonathan Cape Ltd.

Talking to children about death: National Institutes of Mental Health Pamphlet No. (ADM)79-838, U.S. Department of Health, Education, and Welfare Public Health Service, Alcohol, Drug Abuse, and Mental Health Administration.

Index